Textbook of Rapid Response Systems

Michael A. DeVita • Ken Hillman
Rinaldo Bellomo
Editors

Mandy Odell • Daryl A. Jones
Bradford D. Winters • Geoffrey K. Lighthall
Associate Editors

Textbook of Rapid Response Systems

Concept and Implementation

Second Edition

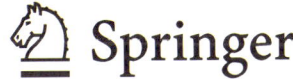

Editors
Michael A. DeVita, MD, FCCM, FRCP
Department of Surgery
Critical Care
Harlem Hospital Center
New York, NY, USA

Department of Internal Medicine
Critical Care
Harlem Hospital Center
New York, NY, USA

Rinaldo Bellomo, MD
Department of Intensive Care
Austin Hospital
Heidelberg, VIC, Australia

Ken Hillman, MBBS, FRCA, FCICM,
    FRCP, MD
The Simpson Centre for Health Services
    Research
South Western Sydney Clinical School
UNSW Sydney, the Ingham Institute
    for Applied Medical Research and
    Intensive Care
Liverpool Hospital
Liverpool BC, NSW, Australia

Associate Editors
Mandy Odell, RN, MA, PGDip, PhD
Royal Berkshire NHS Foundation Trust
Reading, Berkshire, UK

Bradford D. Winters, PhD, MD
Department of Anesthesiology and
    Critical Care Medicine
The Johns Hopkins University School
    of Medicine
Baltimore, MD, USA

Daryl A. Jones
Intensive Care Unit
Austin Hospital
Heidelberg, VIC, Australia

Geoffrey K. Lighthall, PhD, MD
Department of Anesthesia
Stanford University School of Medicine
Palo Alto, CA, USA

ISBN 978-3-319-39389-6   ISBN 978-3-319-39391-9   (eBook)
DOI 10.1007/978-3-319-39391-9

Library of Congress Control Number: 2017933299

This Springer imprint is published by Springer Nature
The registered company is Springer International Publishing AG
The registered company address is: Gewerbestrasse 11, 6330 Cham, Switzerland

Since we have started work in this field, we have met many fantastic clinicians who have worked to improve our knowledge and application of Rapid Response Systems. They are amazing. However, the greatest and most heartfelt impact the editors have encountered is the children, parents, siblings, and spouses who have lost their loved ones due to the failure of a hospital system to respond effectively to deterioration. They have shared their pain with us, and we remember them daily. This textbook is dedicated to the lost loved ones.

Preface

Over 20 years ago, physicians and nurses in separate regions of the globe started work to reduce cardiac arrests by reorganizing healthcare delivery systems. The novel process involved identifying patients who were deteriorating and developed critical illness outside the ICU. Subsequently a response team was notified or "triggered" in later terminology, and these multidisciplinary professionals brought clinical and equipment resources to the bedside very quickly. While they did not supplant the "home" care team, they did augment it by enhancing the resources brought to bear to prevent further deterioration, cardiac arrest, and death. The results were impressive, but because the early studies were before and after trials, the quality of the data was judged by many to be poor and the results inconclusive. Their emphasis on the team response was significant and a controversy of sorts developed over what was the best response team. The first of two consensus conferences allowed these investigators to "compare notes." As a result, they concluded that the team response was only one component of a four-part system, which was named the Rapid Response System (RRS). The second conference reflected the growing appreciation by most investigators that the whole system did not work unless it was reliably "triggered." Without the trigger, there could be no response. Since this report, many investigators have continued to work on this afferent limb of the RRS. Our first two books in this field reflected these two modes of thinking, although we did try to demonstrate how the RRS could be adapted to many other critical and time-sensitive situations in the hospital setting. We devoted many pages in both books related to defining the characteristics of the system, how to create one in hospitals naïve to the process, and how to both improve and expand the process in more experienced settings.

In this third book, the second edition of the Rapid Response Textbook, we have tried to again capture the major trends in RRS implementation and modes of thought. At the 13th annual International Meeting on Rapid Response Systems and Medical Emergency Teams, the new International Society for Rapid Response Systems had its third general meeting. The Society has grown from 15 people in a room in London to well over 100 members from almost 20 countries. The meeting had almost 600 attendees. At this time, some form of RRS (although not named this way in all countries) is required in all or part of about ten countries around the world, and it is becoming more common in many other countries. Indeed, we feel that the

RRS in a sense is becoming an integral part of how acute hospitals function. And the demonstration of its effectiveness is becoming more obvious.

At this 13th meeting, we were struck by an interesting coalescing of data. Initially, in-hospital cardiac arrest rates were between two and eight per thousand admissions. Virtually all organizations implementing RRS effectively, meaning an RRS rate of greater than about 40 per 1000 admissions, showed decreased mortality. However, at this meeting, not one presentation now notes a cardiac arrest rate above 1 per 1000. Thus, in the decade and a half since our first meeting, there has been a one log improvement. This is a stunning achievement and it mirrors the improvements in safety initiatives in the airline industry and automobile industry. The change in scale from 0.6/1000 to 6/10,000 may be confusing at first, but it will serve to reset our frame of vision.

This prompts us to ask, "How low can in-hospital cardiac arrest rates go?" We are not sure of the answer to that, but we do have some thoughts on the matter. First, we would like to distinguish between cardiac arrest responses on the one hand and in-hospital death events on the other. Patients who might live have vital sign abnormalities that are the same as those of patients who are dying. Many patients in hospital are in fact dying naturally and expectedly from their underlying disease. As many as 1/3 of Rapid Response events are triggered for patients who are dying and expected to die. Most of these patients are more in need of palliative care to help promote a safe, painless, and comforting dying process. While some have decried the use of the RRS for patients who are dying, we support it if the patient's death is "out of control" due to pain, distress, or inadequate preparation. We believe that the RRS trigger may be an opportunity to introduce palliation into such patient's care plan. Because of this, we advocate promoting either palliative care skill sets for responders or a close linkage between the RRS and the palliative care team. With this in effect, cardiac arrest rates could drop by perhaps 30 % due to implementation of "not for resuscitation" orders, some of those occurring at or after an RRS event. Second, better triage of hospitalized patients to special care wards may help. More effective triage may be possible through the use of better predictive tools using any one of a variety of severity scoring systems designed to find patients likely to die in the next few hours or days. Patients with elevated risk can have additional resources to bear. Indeed, some investigators have designed systems to not only provide risk estimates but also give decision support to bedside clinicians to promote better care management. Some tools go so far as to alert managers to clusters of high acuity patients. Knowing where (unexpectedly) sick patients are can enable moving resources to up-staff stressed units. These interventions have been shown to help as well, and their use is likely to spread. As they do, expect cardiac arrest rate to fall.

The third intervention which is starting to gain some momentum is continuous physiological monitoring. We are not talking about continuous ECG monitoring which does not signal well early signs of deterioration. We are focusing instead on the continuous monitoring of one or more of the following: heart rate, respiratory rate, level of consciousness, oxygen saturation, and exhaled carbon dioxide. Deterioration of any of these portends trouble. Intermittent monitoring has been used on the general floors of acute hospitals for over a century. However, today's patients are sicker and have more complex interventions which can increase risk of unexpected and sudden deterioration. The unexpected death rate in hospitals among those who are selected high risk and who are monitored is not very different from "healthier" patients selected to not have monitoring. This begs the question of what likelihood of deterioration is sufficiently low to decide to not continuously monitor someone. Because we can never perfectly predict the future, until there is the ability to detect deterioration as it occurs, there will always be unexpected and tragic deaths.

So our answer to the question of "how low can the cardiac arrest rate go?" is "Zero." We feel it is time to target zero cardiac arrest responses in hospital (even though hospital death rates will never fall that low because as we noted, some people are dying from incurable and irremediable illness). We are looking for zero preventable deaths. We are a long way from that goal, but keeping that goal in mind was helpful in other safety initiatives that we would like to emulate.

There are barriers to even aiming for zero. First, the culture change needed to get clinicians to believe that it is a realistic target. Second, the continued change in hospital staffing to enable RRSs to flourish is not easy in some organizations. Additional data and examples from forward thinking hospitals may lead such organizations to progress. A third barrier is cost. Continuous monitoring is expensive, and most hospitals simply cannot see their way to finding the money to invest, let alone consider the return on investment. Fear is another barrier. Some of us have found that some clinicians are more afraid of being blamed for not responding to an alarming monitor than they are of the consequences for the patient of that action. This is a startling observation, but this type of fear of failure exists in all of us to some extent.

There are promoters as well. All clinicians have experienced the situation when they have had to interact with the family of a patient who was not supposed to die. These tragedies impact the clinician in profound ways that may be different and less tragic for the patients themselves and their family, but which are tragic and life altering nonetheless. Some clinicians have left healthcare as a result.

We think the advances in safety that the RRS is promoting will continue to spread and become better. We hope that our textbook is moving beyond the simple introduction of the system and providing resources that can be used to target zero.

The first chapter of the textbook is important. In it, Helen Haskell puts a very personal face on the need for the RRS. These stories moved us so much that we felt they needed to be the first thing the reader of this textbook sees. It will impact in a way that mere numbers cannot. The remainder of the first section is devoted to the patient safety system and the place of RRSs in building the business case and promoting culture change. The second section is geared towards how to create or improve the system. And the final section is focused on assessing the impact and educational interventions to support system improvements.

With the tools in this book, we hope that we will not only help you improve your hospital's safety but also help you to imagine a hospital with a zero cardiac arrest and zero preventable death rate.

New York, NY, USA   Michael A. DeVita
Liverpool BC, NSW, Australia   Ken Hillman
Melbourne, VIC, Australia   Rinaldo Bellomo

Contents

Part II   Creating an RRS

Part III   Monitoring of Efficacy and New Challenges

Contributors

Max Bell, MD, PhD Perioperative Medicine and Intensive Care, Karolinska University Hospital, Stockholm, Sweden

Rinaldo Bellomo Department of Intensive Care, Austin Hospital, Heidelberg, VIC, Australia

Christopher P. Bonafide, MD, MSCE Perelman School of Medicine at the University of Pennsylvania, The Children's Hospital of Philadelphia, Philadelphia, PA, USA

Eliezer Bose, RN, PhD, ACNP-BC Department of Acute and Tertiary Care, School of Nursing, University of Pittsburgh, Pittsburgh, PA, USA

Patrick W. Brady, MD, MSc University of Cincinnati College of Medicine, Cincinnati Children's Hospital Medical Center, Cincinnati, OH, USA

Jeffrey Braithwaite, PhD Faculty of Medicine and Health Sciences, Australian Institute of Health Innovation, Macquarie University, Sydney, NSW, Australia

Richard J. Brilli, MD, FCCM, FAAP Nationwide Children's Hospital, Columbus, OH, USA

Magnolia Cardona-Morrell, MBBS, MPH, PhD The Simpson Centre for Health Services Research, South Western Sydney Clinical School and Ingham Institute for Applied Medical Research, The University of New South Wales, Sydney, NSW, Australia

Jack Chen, MBBS, PhD, MBA (Exec) Simpson Centre for Health Services Research, South Western Sydney Clinical School, University of New South Wales, Sydney, NSW, Australia

Karen Cox, PhD, RN University of Missouri Health, Columbia, MO, USA

Patricia Dalby, MD Associate Professor, Department of Anesthesiology, University of Pittsburgh School of Medicine, Magee-Womens Hospital of UPMC, Pittsburgh, PA, USA

Oluwaseun Davies, MD Critical Care Medicine—Internal Medicine, Adult Critical Care Internal Medicine/Emergency Medicine, University of Pittsburgh Medical Center, Pittsburgh, PA, USA

Edgar Delgado Respiratory Care Department UPMC Presbyterian Shadyside, UPMC Presbyterian Campus, Pittsburgh, PA, USA

Michael A. DeVita, MD, FCCM, FRCP Department of Surgery, Critical Care, Harlem Hospital Center, New York, NY, USA

Department of Internal Medicine, Critical Care, Harlem Hospital Center, New York, NY, USA

Kathy D. Duncan, RN Institute for Healthcare Improvement, Cambridge, MA, USA

Arthas Flabouris, FCICM Intensive Care Unit, Royal Adelaide Hospital and Faculty of Health Sciences, School of Medicine, University of Adelaide, Adelaide, SA, Australia

Donna Goldsmith, RN, PGCert & Dip, MN, PhD Austin Hospital, Heidelberg, VIC, Australia

Gabriella G. Gosman, MD Associate Professor, Department of Obstetrics, Gynecology, and Reproductive Services, University of Pittsburgh School of Medicine, Magee-Womens Hospital of UPMC, Pittsburgh, PA, USA

Kristin Hahn-Cover, MD, FACP University of Missouri Health, Columbia, MO, USA

Leslie W. Hall, MD University of South Carolina, Palmetto Health, Columbia, SC, USA

Melinda Fiedor Hamilton, MD, MSc, FAHA Department of Critical Care Medicine, University of Pittsburgh Medical Center. Director, Pediatric Simulation, Peter M. Winter Institute for Simulation, Education, and Research (WISER), Pittsburgh, PA, USA

Children's Hospital of Pittsburgh Simulation Center, Pittsburgh, PA, USA

Helen Haskell, MA Mothers Against Medical Error, Columbia, SC, USA

Melodie Heland, RN, CritCareCert, GDip. Surgical Clinical Services Unit, Austin Health, Heidelberg, VIC, Australia

Ken Hillman, MBBS, FRCA, FCICM, FRCP, MD The Simpson Centre for Health Services Research, South Western Sydney Clinical School, UNSW Sydney, the Ingham Institute for Applied Medical Research and Intensive Care, Liverpool Hospital, Liverpool, NSW, Australia

Laura E. Hirschinger, RN, MSN, AHN-BC, CPPS Clinic Administration, University of Missouri Health System, Columbia, MO, USA

Marilyn Hravnak, RN, PhD, ACNP-BC, FCCM, FAAN Department of Acute and Tertiary Care, School of Nursing, University of Pittsburgh, Pittsburgh, PA, USA

Elizabeth A. Hunt Department of Anesthesiology and Critical Care Medicine, The Johns Hopkins University School of Medicine, Baltimore, MD, USA

Gabriella Jaderling, MD, PhD Perioperative Medicine and Intensive Care, Karolinska University Hospital, Stockholm, Sweden

Daryl A. Jones Department of Intensive Care, Austin Hospital, Melbourne, VIC, Australia

John Kellett, MD Adjunct Associate Professor in Acute and Emergency Medicine, University of Southern Denmark, Hospital of South West Jutland, Esbjerg, Denmark

David Konrad, MD, PhD Perioperative Medicine and Intensive Care, Karolinska University Hospital, Stockholm, Sweden

Stephen Lam, MBBS(Hons), FRACP, FCICM Department of Critical Care Medicine, Flinders Medical Centre, Bedford Park, SA, Australia

Flinders University, SA, Australia

Bernard Lawless, MD, FRCS (C) Provincial Lead, Critical Care Services Ontario, St. Michaels Hospital, Toronto, ON, Canada

Geoffrey K. Lighthall, PhD, MD Department of Anesthesia, Stanford University School of Medicine, Palo Alto, CA, USA

Patrick Maluso, MD Department of Surgery, George Washington University, Washington, DC, USA

Sonali Mantoo, MD Critical Care Medicine, Harlem Hospital, New York, NY, USA

Andrea Mazzoccoli, MSN, MBA, RN, PhD, FAAN Bon Secours Health System Inc., Marriottsville, MD, USA

Myra McCoig, CPHRM Corp Risk Management, University of Missouri Health Care, Columbia, MO, USA

Marlene Miller Quality and Safety, Children's Center, The Johns Hopkins Hospital, Baltimore, MD, USA

Nicolette Mininni, BSN, RN, MEd, CCRN Nursing Education & Research, UPMC Shadyside, Pittsburgh, PA, USA

Andrew W. Murray, MD Department of Anesthesiology and Perioperative Medicine, Mayo Clinic, Phoenix, AZ, USA

Hadis Nosrati, PhD The Simpson Centre for Health Services Research, Sydney, NSW, Australia

Mandy Odell, RN, MA, PGDip, PhD Royal Berkshire NHS Foundation Trust, Reading, Berkshire, UK

Amy Pearson, RN, BSN Adult Medicine Service Line, Presbyterian Hospital, Albuquerque, NM, USA

John Asger Petersen, EDIC Department of Anesthesia and Intensive Care, Bispebjerg and Frederiksberg University Hospital, Copenhagen, NV, Denmark

Michael R. Pinsky, MD, Dr hc, FCCP, FCCM Department of Critical Care Medicine, University of Pittsburgh, Pittsburgh, PA, USA

Peter J. Pronovost Department of Health Policy and Management, School of Nursing, The Bloomberg School of Public Health, Baltimore, MD, USA

Department of Anesthesiology, Critical Care Medicine and Surgery, The John Hopkins University School of Medicine, Baltimore, MD, USA

David R. Prytherch, PhD, MIEPM, CSci Centre for Healthcare Modelling and Informatics, University of Portsmouth, Portsmouth, Hampshire, UK

Alex J. Psirides Department of Intensive Care Medicine, Wellington Regional Hospital, Wellington, New Zealand

Ajay D. Rao, MD Section of Endocrinology, Diabetes and Metabolism, Temple University School of Medicine, Philadelphia, PA, USA

Stuart F. Reynolds, MD, FRCPE, FCCP Director of Critical Care Services, Spartanburg Regional Healthcare System, Clinical Professor of Critical Care, Medical University of South Carolina, AHEC, Spartanburg, SC, USA

Francesca Rubulotta, MD, PhD, FRCA, FFICM, eMBA Department of Surgery, Intensive Care Unit Charing Cross Hospital, Bariatric Anaesthesia St. Mary's Hospital, Imperial College London, NHS Trust London, London, UK

Babak Sarani, MD, FACS, FCCM Associate Professor of Surgery Director, Center for Trauma and Critical Care Director, George Washington Transfer Center, George Washington University, Washington, DC, USA

John J. Schaefer III, MD Medical University of South Carolina, Charleston, SC, USA

Susan D. Scott, PhD, RN, CPPS, FAAN Office of Clinical Effectiveness, University of Missouri Health System, Columbia, MO, USA

University of Missouri Health, Columbia, MO, USA

Dan Shearn, RN, MSN UPMC Presbyterian Hospital, Pittsburgh, PA, USA

Gary B. Smith, BM, FRCP, FRCA Faculty of Health and Social Sciences, Centre of Postgraduate Medical Research and Education (CoPMRE), University of Bournemouth, Bournemouth, Dorset, UK

Karen Stein, RN, BSN, MSED Department of Nursing Education, University of Pittsburgh School of Nursing, Magee-Womens Hospital, Pittsburgh, PA, USA

David Streitman, MD Assistant Professor, Department of Maternal Fetal Medicine, Saint Luke's Health System Kansas City, Kansas City, MO, USA

Christian Subbe, DM, MRCP Ysbyty Gwynedd, Penrhosgarnedd, Bangor, Wales, UK

Andreas Taenzer The Simpson Centre for Health Services Research, South Western Sydney Clinical School and Ingham Institute for Applied Medical Research, The University of New South Wales, Sydney, NSW, Australia

James Tibballs, MD, MBA, MEd Royal Children's Hospital, Melbourne, VIC, Australia

Shane C. Townsend, MBBS, FANZCA, FCICM, MBA Complex-Wide Adult Intensive Care, Mater Health Services, Brisbane, QLD, Australia

John R. Welch, RN, BSc, MSc Critical Care Unit (T03), University College Hospital, London, UK

Terri Wells, RN, MSN, CCRN Adult Medicine Service Line, Presbyterian Hospital, Albuquerque, NM, USA

Bradford D. Winters, PhD, MD Department of Anesthesiology and Critical Care Medicine, The Johns Hopkins University School of Medicine, Baltimore, MD, USA

Nancy Wise, RNC, BNS Department of Woman Child Birthing Center of Magee-Womens Hospital of UPMC, Labor and Delivery Department, Pittsburgh, PA, USA

Eyal Zimlichman The Simpson Centre for Health Services Research, South Western Sydney Clinical School and Ingham Institute for Applied Medical Research, The University of New South Wales, Sydney, NSW, Australia

Part I

RRSs and Patient Safety

Why Have a Rapid Response System? Cold with Fear: The Patient and Family Experience of Failure to Rescue

Helen Haskell

In this textbook, many authors will present data supporting the impact of rapid response systems and provide guidance for how to create or improve an organization's rapid response system. This chapter is different. It is intended to provide insight into the *human* impact of failing to rescue patients who have serious deterioration while in hospital. The stories in this chapter provide poignant testimony on why rapid response systems must exist. In addition, they will help the reader understand why patients and families should be allowed to activate the system.

As is noted elsewhere in this textbook, the 2014 review by Sir Liam Donaldson and colleagues of the recent National Health Service incident reports finds "mismanagement of deterioration" to be the single most frequent category of preventable death [1]. This well-known but disturbing phenomenon is doubly confounding since not only clinicians but also friends and family are often in attendance as a patient spirals downward. Patients and families are usually well aware when a patient's health status has gone awry, and most feel free to express their concerns to bedside nurses and doctors. Yet families frequently report that their concerns are not heeded [2]. In such situations, few people feel on sure enough ground to try to override the decisions of

medical personnel, and fewer still would know how to do so even if they were confident. What happens to those patients and families who are not rescued? How do these crises play out in the eyes of the family? And what do families see as the solution? Below are four stories from the family member's point of view, beginning with the one I know best, that of my own son, Lewis Blackman.

Lewis's Story

In November, 2000, I was the mother of two high-achieving and to my eyes appealing and well-behaved children, Lewis, 15, and Eliza, 10. Our lives were the usual hubbub of childhood activities and we looked forward for the next number of years to the fixed trajectory of high school and university, the only variables being which universities and where their studies should be focused. Our children were excellent students and the choice was theirs.

Then my husband and I made a fateful decision. Our son Lewis had an indented chest wall, a mild but clearly noticeable case of pectus excavatum. After reading a newspaper article extolling a safe, minimally invasive new surgical repair, we consulted with a pediatric surgeon at a nearby teaching hospital. As it was our understanding that this surgery was best performed before maturity, we determined to proceed before his bones had "hardened." I am ashamed to think how little

H. Haskell, MA (✉)
Mothers Against Medical Error, Columbia, SC, USA
e-mail: haskell.helen@gmail.com

© Springer International Publishing Switzerland 2017
M.A. DeVita et al. (eds.), *Textbook of Rapid Response Systems*, DOI 10.1007/978-3-319-39391-9_1

concern we had about an operation whose seriousness we did not really understand.

Nevertheless, we entered the hospital, as any sensible person does, with trepidation. It is almost unbearable now to think how frightened my son was, though he put on a brave front and his fears were probably only evident to me. His history was taken by a young woman who a few minutes later reappeared wearing a large badge reading, "INTERN," a piece of information that would prove helpful to us later. Other than the intern and a cheerful anesthesiologist in a funny hat, we did not know the roles or identities of anyone in the maelstrom of people who swirled around us.

Though we could not really know, we had no reason to believe that Lewis's surgery did not go well. The problems began afterward. In the recovery unit, Lewis was not urinating. The urinary catheter was suspected and changed, to no effect. Eventually he was discharged, still not urinating, to a room on the hematology-oncology floor. No surgical beds were available.

We had been in hospitals before, but never in a teaching hospital. We were baffled at the lack of attention to our concerns. The intern materialized, now minus her badge. We showed her the empty urine bag and she ordered a bolus of saline solution. Familiar only with the Latin, we puzzled as to why our son was being given "balls" of fluid, eventually concluding, more or less correctly, that it meant simply "a large amount."

We limped through the night and most of the next day on boluses, every one of them initiated by my husband or me. The underlying problem was apparently a reluctance to change the erroneous order that had been written in the postanesthesia unit by the chief resident, though we only discerned that much later. There was no indication that anyone but us ever gave much thought to the lack of urination or to the effect it might have on the many medications our son was taking. The problem was finally solved on the second day after surgery, when an experienced nurse and a pharmacist teamed up to get a junior resident to write a new order. When Lewis finally began urinating at the end of the day, we thought it was a triumph.

For pain relief, Lewis was on epidural hydromorphone and bupivacaine, supplemented by 6-hourly injections of the NSAID ketorolac. At 120 pounds, he was barely within the minimum for the adult dose for ketorolac in the USA, though its use was still off-label due to his age. His pain continued to worsen and the amounts of epidural analgesics, not inconsiderable to begin with, crept continually upward. We still had not learned the identities of the many uniformed people streaming in and out of our room, but we were finding the confusion increasingly disconcerting. We could see that the staff were not communicating about their patients and were giving off-the-cuff opinions that sometimes seemed no more than bluffing.

The weekend arrived, the hubbub subsided, and the hospital fell quiet. The on-call attending rounded on Saturday morning and we did not see him again. Lewis was nauseated, sweating, and itchy, as he had been since day 1. While he didn't get better, he didn't get worse. We lacked the tools to judge, but it was clear he was not going home on Monday as had originally been suggested.

Instead, at 6:30 a.m. on Sunday morning, he was stricken with a sudden new, inexplicable pain in the area of his stomach, quite separate from his surgical pain. This transpired half an hour after a ketorolac injection and in the midst of a shift change. On the children's pain scale, Lewis said in panic, it was 5 out of 5, or more. The night nurse, not yet off duty, answered our call with alarm. A few minutes later she was back with the reassurance that this was "only" an ileus, caused by the narcotics in his epidural.

Thus began the last 30 h of our son's life. The train wreck of his medical care during those hours derived in no small part from that bland assessment, which appeared in retrospect to have had its genesis in nothing more than chatter in the nurses' station. Whatever its origin, the label of "ileus" stuck like a burr, even as Lewis's symptoms made it ever more unlikely to be correct. His pulse and respiration rates gradually rose and his temperature dropped. His blood pressure rose, then fell. Urination again ceased. His eyes became huge black circles, like Franklin

Roosevelt in the weeks before his death. His pain, undiminished, migrated from the epigastric area to his lower abdomen. His belly swelled like a watermelon.

The day nurse stuck to her guns. Today was the day Lewis was supposed to get out of bed and with much assistance he did. From the chair Lewis said, "This was a mistake." Thinking of the whole surgical undertaking, I fervently agreed. But he was focused on the immediate; he was thinking of the logistics involved in getting back in bed and the agonies of vomiting sitting upright with hardware in his chest. Later the nurse said that Lewis should walk to ameliorate his ileus. Since he was too weak to stand, we half-supported, half-dragged him around the ward, stopping every few steps so Lewis could lean on me to rest.

Most of the time, however, Lewis and I were left to our own devices. The nurses were preparing for an inspection the following day and seemed energized by the distraction. When I ventured out of the room I found the silverware rearranged in the kitchen and cheery crayon pictures drawn on the windows. Even our doorplate had been polished. It was a thousand miles away from our universe of pain and fear on the other side.

The nurses seemed unable to see what I was seeing: that my son was going into shock. I had only a vague idea what shock was, but I thought I remembered the symptoms from a junior high First Aid class 35 years earlier. I was very uncertain. I wanted to call Lewis's surgeon, but I did not think anyone would be there to answer the phone in an academic department on a Sunday. I would have liked to go over the head of Lewis's nurse, but I never imagined there might be a supervisor present in the hospital. Our world was the bedside nurse, and I felt helpless to get around her.

Throughout this long day, I had asked repeatedly for a doctor. I did not mean the intern, though I eventually came to suspect that her intermittent visits might have something to do with my requests. I tracked down Lewis's nurse in the break room. She said, "You've just seen the doctor!" Had the intern not been labeled for the OR back on day 1, I would have been thrown into

confusion. Instead I said, "I want a real doctor, not the intern!" I asked for the attending physicians by name. Grudgingly, she agreed to call.

More hours went by. That evening a young man came to Lewis's room. Although I did not know it, he was the same resident who had misprescribed Lewis's IV fluids 3 days earlier. He was wearing a jacket and brought with him a whiff of cold air: although Lewis had entered the hospital wearing shorts and sandals in the warm South Carolina fall, winter had arrived while we were there. The young doctor affirmed the diagnosis of ileus. Lewis's other alarming symptoms, he said, were due to opiate naiveté. Although this explanation left many unanswered questions, I acquiesced. I assumed he was the attending physician I had requested and I thought that if all the nurses and doctors were saying the same thing, they must be right. It never occurred to me that they might all be following each other down a single path.

The story becomes sadder. Around 6 a.m., Lewis's pain vanished, as suddenly as it had come. Lewis and I were disconcerted at this abrupt change, but the team of residents and students who happened by at that moment said, "Oh, good!" 2 h later, the vital signs technician could not detect a blood pressure. Again, no action was taken, because the residents had reported his pain improved, because he showed no signs of cognitive impairment, and because the surgeons were all occupied in the operating room. The lack of BP was attributed to faulty equipment.

By late Monday morning, Lewis's pulse rate peaked at 163. He had lost, we later discovered, 11 pounds. He looked like a small white skeleton in the bed. His father, little sister and I were all in the room, cold with fear as we waited for the doctor to arrive and save the day. Technicians came and went, conducting tests that had been deferred from the night before. While having his blood drawn, Lewis went into cardiac arrest. The code lasted over an hour and the code list included around 20 people. They could not revive him.

The five surgeons who announced his death to us were the first attending physicians we had seen in over 2 days. It was from them that we learned that the doctor we were awaiting had never been called; no one had seen it as an emergency. Though it was nearly more than I could bear, the on-call attending persuaded us to have an autopsy. To their surprise, the autopsy showed a giant duodenal ulcer, presumably associated with the ketorolac, and a blood loss of nearly 3 L. via the underlying eroded gastroduodenal artery. He was 15 years, 2 months, and 2 h old. It was a very casual end for a beloved child, who 5 days earlier held the world in his hands.

These events happened many years ago now. If Lewis were alive he would be a grown man. I have spent nearly every minute of the intervening years working on patient safety, my expiation for failing in the one fundamental duty of a parent. There are few corners of patient safety and quality into which I have not ventured, because there are few errors that were not touched on in his care. But for me the central issues have always remained rapid response and failure to rescue. Our first effort was state-level legislation: the Lewis Blackman Hospital Patient Safety Act, which passed the legislature in our state of South Carolina in 2005 [3]. It was focused squarely on failure to rescue and related issues in Lewis's care. Among its provisions: clinicians were to be identified, with residents labeled as such; patients were to be allowed to speak directly to their doctors and not just through intermediaries; and most important to me, patients were to be given an emergency "mechanism" they could trigger in case of unaddressed medical concerns. This was the most contentious part of the bill, not so much because hospitals objected to the call system as that they were concerned about the implications of telling patients why it might be needed. The law passed unanimously, in part because South Carolina legislators were surprised that these protections did not already exist.

As the years have gone by, we have become more involved with national and international policy. I have seen many reforms and much change in attitude. The question I ask is how much things have really changed for patients. The answer seems to be that much has changed and much remains the same.

Noah's Story

Around the same time Lewis died, 4-year-old Noah Lord had a tonsillectomy for what his surgeon erroneously believed was obstructive sleep apnea. The surgery took place on a Friday morning. For 2 days after he was discharged, Noah was lethargic, was vomiting, and would not eat. Finally, on Sunday morning, Noah's parents took him to the emergency room, where he was treated in the extended emergency department with intravenous fluids for dehydration and IV morphine for his pain. Noah's mother Tanya picks up the story:

His pain improved, but he still was not eating or drinking the entire time he was in the emergency department. The ED staff tried to entice him with slushies and popsicles — anything they could think of, but he wouldn't eat anything. He was extremely lethargic and I was concerned, but they told me that the morphine was making him groggy and it was to be expected.

Noah developed a cough that sounded like he was clearing his throat all the time. I went to the nurses' station to ask if this was normal and was told that this was okay and "not to worry." They were not ED nurses but covering nurses from obstetrics.

While in the ED we saw a variety of different surgeons and nurses but were never really sure who was in charge as they were not identified and often neglected to introduce themselves by name. The surgeon who performed Noah's surgery consulted by phone — and never showed up to examine Noah.

At one time, a woman came in and I grabbed her by the wrist and pulled her over to the bedside and said, "He really is not doing well." I asked the woman to just look at him to help me and she responded, "I am really sorry, but I am just here to take the dirty laundry." At one point an older gentleman poked his head in and said, "How's it going in here?" I responded automatically, "Okay," and then the man disappeared. I found out later that he was the Emergency Department attending physician. I met with him 10 years later and he remembered poking his head in the room and walking away.

A nurse came in and announced that they had talked to Noah's surgeon and that he wanted him sent home with an intravenous line (a peripherally inserted central catheter or PICC line) so he would be able to receive fluids at home. A visiting nurse would come to our home during the evening so Noah would sleep with an IV.

The nurse handed me a paper to sign and I signed it. This was Monday morning following Noah's surgery on Friday. I was so exhausted that I just signed the paper without looking at it. The nurse left the room and I waited for about 3–4 h without anyone coming into the room. So I went to the nursing station again and I told them that I really wanted to talk to a doctor. The nurses' response was, "You can't talk to a doctor; you have been discharged." This was the first time that I realized that the paper I had signed was his discharge paper [4].

Not knowing what else to do, Noah's parents carried their son to the car and took him home, still vomiting. Several hours later, Noah began hemorrhaging from the mouth so profusely that it blocked his airway. His mother, a trained lifeguard, was able to resuscitate him three times, but finally there was a clot she could not clear. By the time the ambulance arrived, Noah was dead.

His mother said, "My world ended the day he died. For years I have looked back on those 3 days and wondered what I could have done differently… Had they listened to me, not just the words I was saying but really taken a moment to see who I was as a person, I think they wouldn't have missed so much" [5].

D.J.'s Story

In 2010, D.J. Sterner, a 47-year-old truck driver undergoing chemotherapy in the hospital, developed acute gastrointestinal distress, with vomiting and extreme pain that could not be controlled with morphine. Here is how his wife, Karen, described it:

The nurse told us that D.J. was just having anxiety, but we thought it was something more serious. His nurse gave him Ativan for anxiety [but] D.J. was in agony all afternoon. His breathing was very shallow, just a pant. We did not realize at the time how serious this was or we would have been out in the hall screaming for help.

Around 3:00 p.m. the nurses began trying to page the doctor to tell him that something was wrong… The nurses made seven calls approximately half an hour to an hour apart up until 7:00 that evening. The doctors never responded. Every time they were called, there was nothing. At one time a doctor who was called assumed that the other doctor had already been to D.J.'s room.

D.J. finally threw his hands up in the air and said, "That's it. I want sedation." I was very surprised because it was totally out of character for him to be complaining of pain. He told us he was scared. He even said to his nurse, "Please make it stop." We knew something was very serious for him to be talking this way.

His nurse checked his respiration around 6:30 p.m. and it was around 20. Then they checked it again around shift change at 7:00 p.m. and it was closer to 30. His blood pressure was really low and his blood oxygen level was 43 percent. At that point his nurse paged another doctor overhead.

By the time the doctor arrived, D.J. had passed out. The nurse called a code and it took only *two minutes* for the resuscitation response team to get to the room. When the respiratory therapist walked through the

> door she said to the assistant next to her, "I knew he was in trouble before I got through the door."
>
> The assistant replied, "Why didn't they call us sooner?" [6].

Karen added, "It has been hard for me because he died in excruciating pain. That is the hardest part for me because I felt like it was unnecessary. I felt as though he was basically being dismissed. I felt as though, because he had leukemia, the hospital really did not feel like they wanted to help him" [7].

Curtis's Story

On a Saturday morning in 2012, 65-year-old Curtis Bentley was admitted to an intensive care unit for bleeding following placement of a cardiac stent and a subsequent change in his anticoagulation regimen. His daughter, Annette, stayed by his side every minute until, awakened by a nurse at 4:00 a.m., she decided to take a much-needed break. Here is her account of the events that followed:

> I stopped at the snack machine, called my husband, and sat for a while in the waiting room. While I was away from my father's room, I heard a Code Blue sound. At first I thought it was for him, but it was for the neighboring patient. I sat a little while longer, but then I had an uneasy feeling. Something told me to go check on him.
>
> I went back and saw that the Code Blue was indeed for the neighboring patient and that many physicians and nurses had responded. However, no one was with my father.
>
> When I walked in, I couldn't see my father's face right away. One leg was hang-ing out of the bed. Embarrassed, I asked him what he was doing, but he did not respond. I asked him a second time as I was covering him up. The TV went to a commercial at that moment and the light hit his face, which was down against the railing. He was positioned like he was trying to get out, perhaps trying to get help. When I looked closer, I saw that my father was taking his last breath. I knew immediately that it was his last breath, as my stepfather had died in my arms. Their last breaths were identical. I ran out calling for help.
>
> A nurse came. During this time I'm yelling, "Where were you…where were you? Why wasn't a code called for him?" She had no answer. I had been in the room with my dad. No nurse had been present. No machine had alerted them to his deteriorating condition.
>
> My father was intubated and placed on life support. I found out by reading his medical records that he had gone into a coma, was brain dead, suffered paralysis and necrosis. No one at the hospital told me that. He was in a coma for seven days and he never came out of it.
>
> A day or so after the code, I talked to the charge/manager nurse about what her staff had done (or rather not done) on that awful morning…I explained to her that there was no one around when my dad coded. No one was at the station monitoring him, nor any of the other patients for that matter—all except for the neighboring patient for whom the Code Blue had been called. The charge/manager nurse told me "Well, when our adrenaline gets going, our focus is on one patient."
>
> I took a deep breath. The tears started rolling. I asked her, "You mean to tell me, if you have 15 patients on ICU, they are going to go uncared for because your focus is on one patient?" She didn't say a word. Then she said, "Somebody is supposed to be at the nurses' station at all times" [8].

The Voice of the Patient

These vignettes reflect a miniseries of circumstances (pediatric hospital, cancer ward, emergency room, intensive care unit) and of patients (healthy children, cancer patients, the anticoagulated elderly). But common to all of them are the reactions of the families: shock, guilt, fear, and an overwhelming sense of helplessness.

A recurring concern among patients is fear of alienating caregivers by not being a "good" patient. Noah Lord's parents carried their lethargic, nauseated son to the car because they felt trapped in the bureaucracy of discharge and, like most patients, were unprepared to violate the social conventions of courtesy in a situation they did not recognize as life-threatening. Noah's mother expressed a common sentiment when she said, "I did not want to go home because I knew it was not the right thing to do, but I also did know how to push back and did not know what to say" [4].

At play is a combination of lack of knowledge and lack of status, with decisions arriving as fiats from a distant authority to whom the family cannot speak directly. The patient and family may feel disconcerted and disempowered, especially if, as is often the case, they lack medical knowledge and do not know how to navigate the hospital system. Family members feel the burden of their lack of knowledge keenly. D.J.'s mother said, "I wish I would have realized at the time how serious this was … I am extremely angry and guilty that I did not realize more myself" [9]. D.J.'s wife Karen adds, "I did not know that we could go to the nurse's superior. If I had known then what I know now I probably would have gone to the charge nurse and said, 'The nurse has called or paged the doctors, but they are not responding. Is there anything else that can be done?'" [7].

Even healthcare professionals are thrown off base and begin to doubt their own judgment when the healthcare providers around them do not appear to be seeing what the professional family member finds obvious and frightening. Jonathan Welch, an emergency physician, recounts his shock upon arriving at the bedside of his mother who had been admitted to the hospital with neu-tropenic sepsis. He says: "My mom's emergency physician and oncologist had taken few, if any, of the essential and obvious interventions needed to save her life. The nurse seemed calm, as if everything was normal. What was their problem? Was I missing something? I felt trapped in an alternate reality where the medical rules were the opposite of everything I'd learned and practiced, where doctors and nurses were oblivious to impending disaster" [10].

Dr. Welch insisted on having his mother transferred to the intensive care unit. But as time went on and she continued not to receive needed interventions, he became more unsure:

> I wish I'd done more at that point—raised hell, insisted on waking both my mom's oncologist and the hospital's intensive care doctor at home, demanded that they come to the hospital. Instead, by that point I felt lost and powerless… I knew there could be a downside to being too demanding in a hospital. I was losing my own confidence as a doctor, becoming instead the helpless son of a sick patient, someone who couldn't get anything at the hospital to work [10].

As with our other stories, the ending is not a happy one. In desperation, Dr. Welch began working to transfer his mother to a different hospital. A new doctor brought on as part of that process finally began treatment but was unable to save his mother.

Patient-Activated Rapid Response

Overwhelmingly, the complaint from families is that their concerns are not heeded and their input not responded to. This is hardly limited to situations of patient deterioration; indeed, a striking feature of some medical stories presented in diary form is the sheer mind-numbing accumulation of minor and not-so-minor insults to the dignity and well-being of the patient, ranging from disregard of hygiene to blind continuation of inappropriate treatments and delayed response to crises [11, 12]. But the consequences of this kind of disregard come most clearly into focus in failure to rescue cases. Especially in cases like those of Lewis Blackman, Noah Lord, or D.J. Sterner, in which patients deteriorate for hours as families ask repeatedly for help, dismissal of the patient voice can undeniably be a contributor to devastating outcomes.

To these families, patient-activated rapid response seems an obvious solution. Historically primarily a North American phenomenon, the idea of a patient-activated emergency system has been largely patient driven and is often presented as a patient "right," even a civil right. Its spread can be credited to a mother, Sorrel King, whose 18-month-old daughter Josie, probably the world's best-known failure to rescue victim, died from an undetected central line infection at Johns Hopkins in 2001. The Kings founded the Josie King Foundation and used part of Josie's settlement to help fund early safety culture work at Johns Hopkins, raising the profile of their work with a widely disseminated video of Sorrel telling Josie's story in a 2002 address at the Institute for Healthcare Improvement (IHI) [13]. In talking about Josie's death, Sorrel emphasized the fact that Josie was not allowed to drink even though she was dehydrated, that Sorrel's concerns about the child's pallor and listlessness were dismissed, and that Josie's cardiac arrest was precipitated by narcotics given in spite of the fact that Sorrel questioned them. Sorrel spoke movingly of the unthinkable experience of removing her child from life support and having Josie die in her arms, while "large snowflakes began falling slowly from the clouds above and the fiery sky turned them a pale pink, like nothing I had ever seen before" [14].

In December, 2004, Sorrel was onstage for a second time at IHI, standing at the end of a line of healthcare leaders from around the USA. The occasion was the introduction of the IHI's groundbreaking Save 100,000 Lives campaign, which would, among other things, make rapid response a byword in American hospitals [15]. Sorrel was there to represent the patient voice, the first time a patient had so publicly been given

consideration as a healthcare stakeholder. When it came Sorrel's turn to speak, she said, "Why can't the patient push the button?" No real answer was given. But one person in the audience did take note: Tami Merryman, Vice President of Patient Care Services at UPMC Shadyside in Pittsburgh. She called Sorrel and asked for her help in establishing a system responsive to patients. Thus was born the patient-activated rapid response system known as Condition H [16].

The concept of patient and family activation was not new—it was implicit in the "emergency mechanism" of the Lewis Blackman Act and also in programs like the universal trigger of UPMC Presbyterian's existing rapid response system, Condition C [17]. But UPMC Shadyside's Condition H (for Help) gave patient-activated rapid response a structure it had previously lacked. Using the story and image of Josie King, Merryman created a complete system with formal triggering criteria (patients were instructed to call if they experienced a medical change not addressed by the health team, a breakdown in care, or confusion over their treatment), a two-tier screening system (a separate Condition H team assessed the patient before calling the rapid response team), a rollout plan, education strategy, and formal assessment tool [18, 19]. These materials were freely available on the Internet and were widely promoted by IHI, the Josie King foundation, and others [20–22]. While individual institutions could and did adapt it in many ways, the Condition H design would provide the basis for most subsequent patient-activated rapid response teams.

Uptake of patient-activated rapid response was buoyed by the Joint Commission's National Patient Safety Goal 16A of 2008, which created the expectation that accredited organizations would "empower staff, patients, and/or families to request additional assistance when they have a concern about the patient's condition" [23]. Promoted by patient advocates, the Joint Commission's language was incorporated into the 2008 omnibus healthcare law of Massachusetts, making it the second state, after South Carolina, to require patient-accessible emergency systems in every hospital [24]. But with the end of IHI's Save 100,000 Lives campaign and its successor, the Save 5 Million Lives campaign, the momentum of broad patient safety initiatives slowed, and the spread of Condition H and similar programs appeared to stall along with it. In Australia, eagerness to comply with the standards of the Australian Commission on Safety and Quality in Health Care appears to have breathed new life into the concept of patient activation, giving rise to programs like REACH in New South Wales, CARE (Call and Respond Early) in the Capital Territory, and the widely publicized Ryan's Rule in Queensland [25–29]. In the United Kingdom, the Call 4 Concern program at the Royal Berkshire NHS Foundation Trust has also shown considerable success [30]. In the USA, however, patient-activated rapid response, while still available in many hospitals, has generally faded into the background.

Beyond Patient Activation

One reason for declining enthusiasm may be the low usage rate that characterizes patient-activated systems, which usually receive only a few calls a month and in some systems almost no calls at all [18, 31]. While this has helped allay some caregivers' apprehensions that patients would overwhelm the team with "frivolous" calls, it presents a distinct challenge to those wishing to maintain awareness of an infrequently exercised option. The reasons for low call volume are debated. Although patients may often be unsure of what constitutes a true medical emergency, the patient population in general predictably demonstrates the same ability inside the hospital as outside it to refrain from calling emergency numbers over unimportant matters. In situations of excessive underuse, poor patient education and fear of retaliation are commonly cited possibilities. When asked, however, patients just as often appear to be concerned about being seen as breaking the bond of trust in a relationship that for them can be both dependent and intimate [32, 33].

In this context, the view of patient activation as a patient right, while a crucial underlying concept, oversimplifies a complex relationship. An illustration of this complexity may be the experi-

ence of North Carolina Children's Hospital, where the first year of a carefully planned program of family activation saw only two calls directly triggered by families, while staff-activated calls increased by 50 percent. Similarly, at Cincinnati Children's Hospital Medical Center, over a period of 6 years, "family concern" was cited as a factor in nearly 6 percent of clinician-initiated rapid response calls, more than three times the total number of family-activated calls. Researchers at the two institutions speculated that an increased awareness and sense of empowerment on the part of bedside caregivers, brought on by the patient-activated rapid response system, may have increased their responsiveness to patient and family concerns [31, 34].

However they are interpreted, accounts like these are indicative of the growing attention being paid to the relationship between the patient and caregiver. The concept of patient and family engagement, and especially the publicly reported HCAHPS (Hospital Consumer Assessment of Healthcare Providers and Systems) patient survey, has done much to change the dynamic between patients and staff in US hospitals [35]. Hospitals now have patient experience officers (sometimes at c-suite level) and send their staff to patient experience conferences [36, 37]. Patient and family engagement, including patient advisory councils and patient involvement in hospital quality efforts, has been a significant component of the US Department of Health and Human Services' successful Partnership for Patients, a national collaborative along the lines of the Save 100,000 Lives campaign [38]. As the concept of patient and family engagement has grown and developed, patient-activated rapid response has come to be seen as part of a web of patient-centered care including such measures as unlimited visiting hours, bedside change of shift, and family-centered rounds. In addition, broader strategies like roving nurses and improvement in situational awareness have been highly successful at driving earlier intervention and reducing adverse outcomes and have been productively paired with patient-activated rapid response [33, 39–41]. Emerging technologies in continuous monitoring, mobile technology, and electronic surveillance promise to further push back detection of patient decline [42]. In this landscape, patient-activated rapid response comes to be seen as an indispensable but far from sufficient component of an integrated quality improvement program, whose possibilities continue to evolve.

The Learning Institution

Researchers have proposed that rapid response data be mined as a sensitive barometer of patient safety, and some organizations now actively analyze rapid response calls as they occur [41, 43–45]. Patient-activated rapid response, whose calling criteria nearly all involve some sort of breakdown in communication, presents an additional possibility. At Cincinnati Children's Hospital Medical Center, where more than 25 percent of patient-activated calls cited "lack of nurse response" or "dismissive interaction from team," Brady et al. suggested that patient-activated calls, especially those not considered to rise to a level of clinical importance, be explored for communication breakdowns and behavioral trends that could represent future safety risks [34].

One problem with these strategies is that, as Hillman et al. point out, the full effect of medical actions may not be evident until after the patient has left the hospital [43]. There is, however, one measure that is sensitive enough to capture all the points along the patient journey. That is patient and family reports—not only in real time as arbiters of their own condition but also of precipitating and succeeding events to rapid response calls, of instances in which the rapid response system should have been triggered and was not, of cases in which the safety net worked, and of cases in which it was not needed—in sum, the patient experience of care.

This is part of a larger picture. As Hillman et al. also note, only the patient can ultimately judge the effectiveness and desirability of procedures, treatments, and the quality of care that accompanied them [43]. There is also an increasing realization that patient accounts can capture serious safety issues that, for various reasons, are not otherwise documented [46]. Even the small sample of patient accounts presented here shows themes that invite follow-up: patients who, like Curtis Bentley, deteriorate while in the ICU; patients whose deterioration is due to inappropriate treatment orders rather than failure to recognize; and the strong correlation of failure to rescue events with night and weekend care. Much light can be shed on these and other issues by listening to families' lived experiences. It bears repeating that the very fragmentation of a system that can lead to adverse events often keeps those who work in it from seeing its larger flaws. It seems apparent that throughout the continuum of care, there are many breakdowns that are clearly visible only to the patient and family.

To patients and families, this is not an academic matter. Not surprisingly, most users want to ensure that their medical systems are safe, and an obvious first step is to share their observations with their healthcare providers. Harmed patients and families, especially, express a nearly universal desire to bring meaning from their experiences by feeling that they are part of change [47]. The structure in which this can occur is now fairly clear, if not easy, and includes both open and honest communication and patient involvement in quality improvement, including event review [48]. But while such changes are occurring, they are not occurring quickly in most organizations. Of the families in this chapter, only two—my own and Josie King's—were able to engage in meaningful and timely discussions with the institutions where harm occurred. The aftermath of most patient stories continues to be a search for answers that in many cases are not forthcoming and a sense of deep despair when this mark of respect is denied to them.

Alyssa's Story

I will leave the final word on this subject to a mother, Carole Hemmelgarn, whose 9-year-old daughter Alyssa died from a hospital-acquired *Clostridium difficile* infection days after being diagnosed with leukemia. Although she now works closely with national safety and quality organizations, Carole suffered through years of distress and uncertainty when the hospital declined to offer explanations, discuss improvement, or engage with her on a personal level over the death of her daughter. Here is Carole's story.

When people think this ends … it never ends. I got a call at 4:18 on a Monday afternoon that she had leukemia, and you know, it rocks your world because it wasn't what you were expecting.

[In the hospital] the people treating her thought she was anxious, she wasn't. She had an infection that was elevated, she was turning septic. Classic case of failure to rescue, her blood pressure was dropping, she needed oxygen, her pulse was increasing, cognitively not there, everyone thought she was sleepy…

After Alyssa died, we were in a state of shock. You took your daughter to the hospital, you came home without her. We walked into the house and had to tell her brother she's no longer alive; what happened?

It was a journey. It took them 3 years, 7 months, 28 days to have an honest conversation with me. All I ever wanted to do was know the truth, so the other people walking into the front doors of the organization would learn from the mistakes and wouldn't have to go through the same thing Alyssa did [49].

It's not something that you want to do, it's something that you have to do … I'd rather she be here than to have to do this, but if I know someone else doesn't have to wake up to an empty bed, or sit at a kitchen table where a chair that used to be filled isn't filled any more, then we're doing a good thing to make the world a better place [50].

References

1. Donaldson LJ, Panesar SS, Darzi A. Patient-safety-related hospital deaths in England: thematic analysis of incidents reported to a national database, 2010–2012. PLoS Med. 2014;11(6):e1001667.
2. Frampton SB, Charmel PA. Transitioning from 'Never Events' to 'Patient-Centered Ever Events.' HealthLeaders Media Oct 16, 2008. http://healthleadersmedia.com/content/QUA-221681/Transitioning-from-Never-Events-to-PatientCentered-Ever-Events. Accessed Nov 2015.
3. Lewis Blackman Hospital Patient Safety Act of 2005. South Carolina Code of Laws § 44-7-3410 et seq. http://www.scstatehouse.gov/sess116_2005-2006/bills/3832.htm
4. Lord T. Not considered a partner: a mother's story of a tonsillectomy gone wrong. In: Johnson J, Haskell H, Barach P, editors. Case studies in patient safety: foundations for core competencies. Burlington, MA: Jones & Bartlett Learning; 2016:143–52.
5. Institute for Healthcare Improvement Open School. Noah's story: are you listening? http://www.ihi.org/education/ihiopenschool/resources/Pages/Activities/NoahsStoryAreYouListening.aspx. Accessed Nov 2015.
6. Sterner K, Ward L. Failure to rescue. In: Johnson J, Haskell H, Barach P, editors. Case studies in patient safety: foundations for core competencies. Burlington, MA: Jones & Bartlett Learning; 2016:277–86.
7. Sterner K. Interview with the author. February 2012.
8. Smith A. Medical error takes a father's life: a daughter's plea for answers. Physician-Patient Alliance for Health & Safety. August 28, 2014. http://thedoctorweighsin.com/medical-error-takes-life-daughters--plea-answers/. Accessed Nov 2015.
9. Ward L. Interview with the author. February 2012.
10. Welch JR. As she lay dying: how I fought to stop medical errors from killing my mom. Health Aff. 2012;31(12):2817–20.
11. Deed M, Niss M. The last collaboration. London: Friends of Spork; 2012.
12. Lindell L. 108 days. Webster TX: March 5 Publishing; 2005.
13. Institute for Healthcare Improvement Open School What happened to Josie? http://www.ihi.org/education/IHIOpenSchool/resources/Pages/Activities/WhatHappenedtoJosieKing.aspx. Accessed Nov 2015.
14. King S. Josie's story. New York: Atlantic Monthly Press; 2009.
15. Berwick D, Calkins DR, McCannon CJ, Hackbarth AD. The 100,000 lives campaign: setting a goal and a deadline for improving health care quality. JAMA. 2006;295(3):324–7.
16. Kenney C. The best practice: how the new quality movement is transforming medicine. New York: Perseus Books; 2008.

17. Haskell H. The case for family activation of the RRS. In: DeVita M, Hillman K, Bellomo R, editors. Textbook of rapid response systems: concept and implementation. New York: Springer; 2011. p. 197–206.

18. Dean BS, Decker MJ, Hupp D, et al. Condition HELP: a pediatric rapid response team triggered by patients and parents. J Healthc Qual. 2008;30:28–31.

19. Greenhouse PK, Kuzminsky B, Martin SC, Merryman T. Calling a condition H(elp). Am J Nurs. 2006; 106(11):63–6.

20. Institute for Healthcare Improvement. Resources. condition H (Help) brochure for patients and families. http://www.ihi.org/resources/Pages/Tools/ConditionHBrochureforPatientsandFamilies.aspx. Accessed Nov 2015.

21. Josie King Foundation. Foundation programs: Condition Help (Condition H). http://www.josieking.org/page.cfm?pageID=18. Accessed Nov 2015.

22. Robert Wood Johnson Foundation. Promising practices on patient satisfaction and engagement: Condition H staff validation tool. http://www.rwjf.org/en/library/research/2008/06/condition-h-staff-validation-tool.html. Accessed Nov 2015.

23. The Joint Commission on Accreditation of Healthcare Organizations. 2008 National Patient Safety Goals, Hospital. 2008.

24. The General Laws of Massachusetts Part I, Title XVI, Chapter 111: Section 53F. Chapter 305 of the Laws of 2008, an act to promote cost containment, transparency, and efficiency in the delivery of healthcare. Requests for additional assistance for deteriorating patients.

25. New South Wales Clinical Health Commission. Programs partnering with patients. REACH–patient and family escalation. http://www.cec.health.nsw.gov.au/programs/partnering-with-patients/pwp-reach#ir. Accessed Dec 2015.

26. Kidspot Health You have the right to demand medical attention. May 2015. http://www.kidspot.com.au/health/family-health/real-life/you-have-the-right-to--demand-medical-attention?ref=category_view%2Creal-life. Accessed Dec 2015.

27. Queensland Health Ryan's rule: consumer/family escalation process. https://www.health.qld.gov.au/cairns_hinterland/html/ryan-home.asp. Accessed Dec 2015.

28. Adams L. Patient, family and carer escalation. Managing the deteriorating patient, Melbourne. 2014 Sept 22. http://www.slideshare.net/informaoz/lynette-adams. Accessed Nov 2015.

29. Harris J. This Queensland mum knew her baby was ill so invoked Ryan's Rule. Kidspot Health, 2015 Apr 29. http://www.kidspot.com.au/health/baby-health/real-life/this-queensland-mum-knew-her-baby-was-ill-so-invoked-ryans-rule. Accessed Dec 2015.

30. Odell M, Gerber K, Gager M. Call 4 Concern: patient and relative activated critical care outreach. Br J Nurs. 2010;19(2):600–2.

31. Ray EM, Smith R, Massie S, et al. Family Alert: implementing direct family activation of a pediatric rapid response team. Jt Comm J Qual Patient Saf. 2009;35:575–80.

32. Hueckel RM, Mericle JM, Frush K, Martin PL, Champagne MT. Implementation of Condition Help: family teaching and evaluation of family understanding. J Nurs Care Qual. 2012;27(2):176–81.

33. Gerdik C, Vallish RO, Miles K, Godwin SA, Wludyka PS, Panni MK. Successful implementation of a family and patient activated rapid response team in an adult level 1 trauma center. Resuscitation. 2010;81:1676–81.

34. Brady PW, Zix J, Brilli R, et al. Developing and evaluating the success of a family activated medical emergency team: a quality improvement report. BMJ Qual Saf. 2015;24:203–11.

35. US Centers for Medicare & Medicaid Services. HCAHPS: patients' perspectives of care survey. https://www.cms.gov/Medicare/Quality-Initiatives-Patient-Assessment-Instruments/HospitalQualityInits/HospitalHCAHPS.html. Accessed Nov 2015.

36. Boehm L. The evolving role of the healthcare chief experience officer. San Jose CA: Vocera Experience Innovation Network; 2015.

37. The Advisory Board Company. Hospitals put patient experience officers in the C-suite. 2014 Mar 25. https://www.advisory.com/daily-briefing/2014/03/25/hospitals-put-patient-experience-officers-in-the-c-suite. Accessed Nov 2015.

38. US Centers for Medicare & Medicaid Services. Partnership for patients: patient and family engagement. https://partnershipforpatients.cms.gov/about-the-partnership/patient-and-family-engagement/the-patient-and-family-engagement.html. Accessed Nov 2015.

39. Hueckel R, Turi J, Kshitij M, Mericle J, Meliones J. Beyond rapid response teams: instituting a "rover team" improves the management of at-risk patients, facilitates proactive interventions, and improves outcomes. Crit Care Med. 2006;34(12):A54.

40. Brady PW, Muething S, Kotagal U, et al. Improving situation awareness to reduce unrecognized clinical deterioration and serious safety events. Pediatrics. 2013;131(1):e298–308.

41. Beckett DJ, Inglis M, Oswald S, et al. Reducing cardiac arrests in the acute admissions unit: a quality improvement journey. BMJ Qual Saf. 2013;22:1025–31.

42. Bates DW, Zimlichman E. Finding patients before they crash: the next major opportunity to improve patient safety. BMJ Qual Saf. 2015;24:1–3.

43. Hillman KM, Lilford R, Braithwaite J. Patient safety and rapid response systems. MJA. 2014;201(11):654–6.

44. Iyengar A, Baxter A, Forster AJ. Using medical emergency teams to detect preventable adverse events. Crit Care. 2009;13:R126.

45. Amaral AC, Shojania KG. The evolving story of medical emergency teams in quality improvement. Crit Care. 2009;13(5):194.

46. Weissman JS, Schneider EC, Weingart SN, et al. Comparing patient-reported hospital adverse events with medical record review: do patients know something that hospitals do not? Ann Intern Med. 2008;149:100–8.

47. Halpern MT, Roussel AE, Treiman K, Nerz PA, Hatlie MJ, Sheridan S. Designing consumer reporting systems for patient safety events. final report (prepared by RTI International and Consumers Advancing Patient Safety under Contract No. 290–06–00001-5). AHRQ Publication No. 11–0060-EF. Agency for Healthcare Research and Quality: Rockville MD; 2011.

48. Carman KL, Dardess P, Maurer ME, Workman T, Ganachari D, Pathak-Sen E. A roadmap for patient and family engagement in healthcare practice and research. (Prepared by the American Institutes for Research under a grant from the Gordon and Betty Moore Foundation, Dominick Frosch, project officer and fellow; Susan Baade, program officer.) Palo Alto CA: Gordon and Betty Moore Foundation. 2014. www.patientfamilyengagement.org. Accessed Dec 2015.

49. Daley J. For Colorado mom, story of daughter's hospital death is key to others' safety. Colorado Public Radio. 2015 Feb 17. http://www.cpr.org/news/story/colorado-mom-story-daughters-hospital-death-key-others-safety. Accessed Nov 2015.

50. MedStar Health. Alyssa's story: including patients and families in delivery of care. https://www.youtube.com/watch?v=3SfrQnwRIjU. Accessed Nov 2015.

Rapid Response Systems: History and Terminology

Bradford D. Winters and Michael A. DeVita

Principles

The Rapid Response System (RRS) concept has matured substantially since its inception in the early 1990s when critical care physicians, primarily in Australia; Pittsburgh, PA; and the UK started asking some crucial questions regarding patients who deteriorated and often arrested on general hospital wards prior to their admission to the ICU. Specifically, they asked exactly what is happening to general hospital ward patients in the minutes and hours prior to their cardiorespiratory arrests and whether we can do something to intervene and halt these deteriorations before the patient arrests or nearly arrests. This was a sea change in thought and perspective since, at that time, resources focused on resuscitation were primarily concerned with how to improve performance of CPR and ACLS rather than preventing the event to start with. Critical care physicians were well aware, in a general sense, that patients admitted or readmitted to the ICU from the general ward uncommonly went from "just fine" to critically ill. This sense was confirmed by early studies that clearly showed that arrests and deteriorations were not sudden but rather commonly heralded by long periods of obvious hemodynamic and respiratory instability that was often unappreciated by general ward providers [1–17]. The development of critical illness on the general ward was rarely "sudden," only suddenly recognized.

Given this result, critical care physicians reasoned that if we could create usable criteria for general ward staff to use in the early recognition of impending deterioration and empower these staff members to bring a team of critical care physicians and/or nurses outside of the ICU to the bedside, we could improve the outcomes of these patients. Data from these studies of the antecedents to arrest provided the basis for developing the physiological criteria that were put into place for general ward staff to use as a guide for making the decision to call for help [13–17]. Intensive care unit staff (physicians, nurses, respiratory therapists) were the first providers chosen to form the team that would come to the patient's bedside to evaluate, stabilize, and help create a new care and triage plan. Through sheer will, and often working

B.D. Winters, PhD, MD (✉)
Department of Anesthesiology and Critical Care Medicine, The Johns Hopkins University School of Medicine, Zayed 9127 1800 Orleans Street, Baltimore, MD 21298, USA

Department of Surgery, The Johns Hopkins University School of Medicine, Zayed 9127 1800 Orleans Street, Baltimore, MD 21298, USA
e-mail: bwinters@jhmi.edu

M.A. DeVita, MD, FCCM, FRCP
Department of Surgery, Critical Care, Harlem Hospital Center, 506 Lenox Avenue, New York, NY 10037, USA

Department of Internal Medicine, Critical Care, Harlem Hospital Center, 506 Lenox Avenue, New York, NY 10037, USA
e-mail: michael.devita@NYCHHC.ORG

M.A. DeVita et al. (eds.), *Textbook of Rapid Response Systems*, DOI 10.1007/978-3-319-39391-9_2

in isolation without the support of the health community, these critical care clinicians created a new patient safety and quality initiative, long before patient safety and quality became a national and international concern and had the attention of the public and policymakers [18–48].

These early programs were often referred to as Medical Emergency Teams (METs), although other terms, such as Condition C Teams, Patient At-Risk Teams, and Critical Care Outreach Teams, were also used. This linking defined activation criteria to a response team and empowered the general ward staff to summon that team and has resulted in the development of a powerful patient safety and quality initiative that has enjoyed wide adoption in the USA, Australia, New Zealand, Canada, and the UK and ever-increasing acceptance around the world. The first International Conference on Medical Emergency Teams was held in Pittsburgh, PA, in May 2005. Subsequent conferences have been held each year again in Pittsburgh and also in Toronto, Canada; Miami, Florida; Copenhagen, Denmark; and Arnhem, the Netherlands. The RRS concept has reached such significance that the Institute for Healthcare Improvement (IHI) included Rapid Response Systems as one of its six "planks" for improving patient in its "100,000 Lives" Campaign [49]. Additionally, the essential principles of the RRS were embraced by the Joint Commission (the accreditation organization for US hospitals) as a mandate for American hospitals in the form of National Patient Safety Goal 16 and 16A [50]. While this goal did not specifically require hospitals to create Rapid Response Systems, the implementation of this specific patient safety and quality initiative was widely embraced as the best and most appropriate response to this mandate making RRSs ubiquitous in American hospitals. RRSs are the logical solution for meeting this requirement and providing patients with the safety net they need to help prevent medical deteriorations from progressing and degenerating into an arrest and death. While other solutions have been proposed to meet these goals, such as increased nurse-to-patient ratios, hospitalist services, and others, none has the practicality and body of evidence in their favor like RRSs.

The most recent development has been the official inauguration of the International Society for Rapid Response Systems (http://rapidresponsesystems.org/) in 2014 whose goal is to support the implementation and further development of Rapid Response Systems around the globe. Evidence continues to accumulate in support of this important patient safety and quality intervention (Chap. XX).

One of the primary goals of RRSs is to prevent cardiorespiratory arrest and therefore the very high mortality known to be associated with such in-hospital events. Since the physiological instability that precedes the arrest is usually evident for substantial periods of time prior to the arrest, there is significant face validity to the notion that RRSs should result in a reduction in the incidence of cardiac arrest and mortality. Additionally, RRSs should be able to, through early recognition and intervention, reduce unanticipated ICU admission. By catching problems early in their course, it is envisioned that patients not only will not arrest but also may not even require ICU care and be able to be managed on the general ward. This helps to keep ICU beds open for other patients and improve throughput. Likewise, with reductions in serious deteriorations and complications, length of stay should also decrease. Even when patients still require transfer to an ICU as a result of their deterioration, in principle, having the early intervention afforded by an RRS should have the patient arriving in the ICU in better condition than without such a system. The expected benefit in this circumstance is reduced ICU and hospital mortality and reduced ICU and length of hospital stay.

The foundation for achieving these goals is an underlying principle and strength of RRSs, namely, that RRSs address the mismatch between the patient's needs and the available resources on the general wards [51]. This imbalance between what the patient needs (human resources, monitoring, specialized equipment, and medications) and what the general ward can provide (staffing, monitoring, and policy limitations) is at the center of these deteriorations. RRSs are commonly activated by nurses who determine that the patient is seriously ill and cannot be managed under the current circumstances. These circumstances may include staff/acuity limitations, inadequate care plans, and/or new events such as sepsis. Through rapid assessment and intervention, new plans can be developed and communicated to the ward staff and primary service and resource/needs imbalances accounted for resulting in an effective triage and care plan for the patient. Often the patient requires triage to a higher level of care to achieve a rebalancing of resources and needs, but if needs are reduced through RRS intervention, that rebalancing can be achieved with the patient remaining on the ward.

Many of these goals and benefits have been realized through the implementation of RRSs, while some have been less successful and yet others not well evaluated [18–48]. While outcome measures such as mortality are important to clinicians, regulators, and patients, other measures of RRS success and positive impact need to also be considered. Some of these include process of care measures (such as meeting sepsis management guidelines and appropriate institution of Not for Resuscitation status and especially addressing end-of-life care since general ward deteriorations often highlight a patient's underlying severity of illness and likelihood of survival to hospital discharge) [52–54], patient and nursing satisfaction [55–57], and especially the value RRSs bring to staff education in the recognition and management of the critically ill patient who presents as such outside the walls of the ICU [58, 59]. In fact, this last goal and benefit of RRSs may be the most underappreciated, although in many ways the most important. RRSs change culture, and culture is a crucial element of the health systems in which we work. RRSs are not just teams; they are systems in themselves that include a component that emphasizes and educates in the early detection of problems and a component that responds to the call for help.

The RRS functions within a greater system that spans from the patient, through the providers, and their environment up to the departmental, hospital, and institutional level. This realization requires that RRSs have two additional components besides the activation process and a responding team. The first is an evaluative

element that continuously assesses the performance of the RRS and helps to inform the hospital quality improvement (QI) process [51]. Institutions such as the University of Pittsburgh have used their RRS to scrutinize all of their arrest and MET calls in an ongoing QI process that has had great impact for their hospital [60]. The second component is a governance and administration structure [51]. This helps to develop, implement, and, most crucially, maintain and improve the RRS program. The work of the evaluation/QI element and the governance/administrative structure has been greatly improved in the last 2 years with the addition of RRS data fields to the American Heart Association's (AHA) National Get with the Guidelines (GWTG) database [61]. From this database, useful reports and comparisons can be generated to support the RRS and provide feedback to general wards and ICUs. For example, reports on RRS activations within 24 h of an ICU discharge can be extremely helpful to the ICU for determining appropriate triage decisions. While these two additional components are not absolutely essential to having an RRS, they enhance its effectiveness, role, and status within the hospital system and are well worth consideration for those programs that do not already have them in place.

RRSs have become a great agent for change, encouraging and empowering ward staff to ask for help for their patients. The archaic concept, often held and promulgated by physicians and occasionally others, that calling for help is "a sign of weakness" is washed away by the RRS as it changes the culture to an understanding that the patient and his/her well-being is the primary concern of all providers and that calling for help is the sign of the wise and caring clinician.

Terminology

It is important to have a clear understanding of the terminology for Rapid Response Systems so as to get the most from this book and any review of RRS literature. Historically, the early RRSs were most commonly called "Medical Emergency

Teams" or METs, although other terms were also used, including Medical Emergency Response Teams (MERT), Patient-At-Risk Teams (PART), Critical Care Outreach Teams (CCOTs), and eventually Rapid Response Teams (RRTs). Some of these terms are used interchangeably in places such as Australia where RRT and MET often mean the same thing. While hospitals and institutions often create specific names for their programs based on local preferences and the desire to use something memorable to encourage utilization (some of which are quite creative), consensus has been developed on specific terminology that should be used when reporting and sharing information and data in the public forum (publications, research articles, etc.) [51, 62]. The term Rapid Response System refers to the entire system for responding to all patients with a critical medical problem. Most broadly, this can include the Cardiac Arrest Team (Code Team) and the MET as well as other specialized teams that may exist within the hospital, such as a Difficult Airway Response Team or Stroke Team, although most commonly and preferably the term RRS is used to refer to systems that seek to prevent deterioration and arrests rather than respond to arrests. This term encompasses both the recognition process (the activation criteria and the activation process) and the responding team. These two subcomponents are referred to as the afferent and efferent limbs of the RRS, respectively. Additional confusion may arise when the Code Team and the MET are one and the same in terms of personnel but take on different roles depending on the patient's situation (arrest versus deterioration) though many institutions have performed this integration well and can lead by example. Often it is local culture and resources that determine these structures.

The historical MET and similar systems are now defined through consensus based on the team structure and functionality [51]. Teams that include physicians along with nurses, but may also include respiratory therapists and others, are properly called Medical Emergency Teams, which have full capability for assessment, treatment, and triage planning, while teams that do not include physicians as responders and rely on nurses and others only are referred to as Rapid Response Teams (RRTs). These nurse-led RRTs often have physician consultation available, but the physician does not respond to the bedside as a member of the initial response. RRTs often provide an intermediate range of capability since nurses cannot write orders for therapy. Exceptions to this are the nurse practitioners and physician assistants in the USA, who can prescribe a range of orders. As such, true RRTs are able to assess and provide some level of stabilization, but if needs and resources are severely out of balance, the patient is likely to require triage to a higher level of care. To date, there is very little data to support having an MET versus an RRT. It is not that the evidence suggests they are equally capable, which they very well be, but that there are essentially no head-to-head comparisons of the two team structures for outcomes or process measures. As such the decision as to which team to create is often determined by local resources and culture. Teams that provide follow-up service and surveillance on patients discharged from the ICU on a regular basis, as well as response to any deteriorating general ward patient that may or may not have been in an ICU previously, are described as Critical Care Outreach Teams (CCOTs). These teams are often staffed by nurses (though some CCOTs do have physicians), and therefore their response to deteriorating patients would be an RRT-type response team. Other terms, such as Patient-At-Risk Team, may be used as the local name for the program, and hospitals may choose to call their system an RRT even though it has physicians as responders; such names should only be for local use and should be avoided in the literature when publishing results for the RRS intervention. So that proper comparisons may be made, the preferred nomenclature should describe the response component of the RRS as an MET, RRT, or CCOT based on these consensus definitions.

As mentioned previously, another important terminology distinction to consider is the difference between the process of recognition that the patient is deteriorating and that of the teams that respond. The process and criteria used for triggering the call for help are called the afferent limb, while the response to that call, the team, is the efferent limb. While both work in concert as a system, their separate nomenclature and consideration are important. Many think of the efferent limb as the RRS, but the afferent limb is perhaps more important, since this is where the recognition is made that the patient needs help. Providing a responding team is of less benefit if the patient has already progressed to the point where arrest is imminent; the earlier the recognition is made, the better. Some have argued that it may not even matter who comes to help the patient (a critical care team, a hospitalist team, or the primary service) as long as it is recognized that help is needed early enough to make a difference. The importance of early recognition was addressed by the first Consensus Conference on Medical Emergency Teams and then further emphasized by the special Afferent Limb Consensus Conference convened ahead of the third International Conference on Medical Emergency Teams and continues to be emphasized in the literature and at the international meetings. In these forums, the question of how RRSs might improve their identification of seriously ill general ward patients is considered and debated. The report of the first Consensus Conference [51] indicates that RRS should use clear methods of detection for identifying "emergent unmet patient needs" and deteriorations. Objective criteria are preferred, and several identification systems exist, including direct vital sign parameters and various scoring systems [51, 63–79]. Early data suggests that technological solutions are going to be essential for better monitoring and detection in the mostly ambulatory general ward patient population but that we still are struggling to determine what best needs to be monitored and how. This is an area of very active research with many exciting possibilities likely to result in the next few years [80–84].

The efferent limb also continues as an area of active research. New education modalities and strategies such as simulation are being used to improve team performance and function and prepare teams for unusual or rare scenarios. The kind of team that makes up the efferent limb probably does matter—not so much by what their title is,

but rather by how well they are prepared and how well they work as team members [85–87].

Summary

RRSs have grown substantially since their inception almost two decades ago to become a robust strategy for improving patient care and healthcare culture. The interventions have become the standard of care in an increasing number of countries around the world including the USA, the UK, Australia, and New Zealand. Europe is moving toward greater adoption as well. Some clinicians who support these initiatives have striven to be evidence based and thorough, resulting in an ever-expanding body of literature and experience that points to RRSs as a successful systems-based solution to the problem of deteriorating general ward patients and the imbalance of resources necessary to care for them. Clear definitions and nomenclature have aided this process. By working to improve the afferent and efferent limbs of RRSs through methods best suited to their uniqueness and melding them into an effective system, RRSs can continue to be a developing and dynamic patient safety and quality of care improvement paradigm.

References

1. Sax FL, Charlson ME. Medical patients at high risk for catastrophic deterioration. Crit Care Med. 1987;15(5):510–5.
2. Schein RM, Hazday N, Pena M, Robin BH, Sprung CL. Clinical antecedents to in-hospital cardiopulmonary arrest. Chest. 1990;98(6):1388–92.
3. Bedell SE, Deitz DC, Leeman D, Delbanco TL. Incidence and characteristics of preventable iatrogenic cardiac arrests. J Am Med Assoc. 1991;265(21):2815–20.
4. Daffurn K, Lee A, Hillman KM, Bishop GF, Bauman A. Do nurses know when to summon emergency assistance? Intensive Crit Care Nurs. 1994;10(2):115–20.
5. Smith AF, Wood J. Can some in-hospital cardiorespiratory arrests be prevented? A prospective survey. Resuscitation. 1998;37(3):133–7.
6. Buist MD, Jarmolowski E, Burton PR, Bernard SA, Waxman BP, Anderson J. Recognising clinical instability in hospital patients before cardiac arrest or unplanned admission to intensive care. A pilot study

in a tertiary-care hospital. Med J Aust. 1999;171(1):22–5.

7. Hillman KM, Bristow PJ, Chey T, Daffurn K, et al. Antecedents to hospital deaths. Intern Med J. 2001;31(6):343–8.

8. Hodgetts TJ, Kenward G, Vlachonikolis IG, et al. Incidence, location and reasons for avoidable in-hospital cardiac arrest in a district general hospital. Resuscitation. 2002;54(2):115–23.

9. Kause J, Smith G, Prytherch D, et al. A comparison of antecedents to cardiac arrests, deaths and emergency intensive care admissions in Australia, New Zealand, and the United Kingdom—The ACADEMIA study. Resuscitation. 2004;62(3):275–82.

10. Hillman K, Bristow PJ, Chey T, et al. Duration of life-threatening antecedents prior to intensive care admission. Intensive Care Med. 2002;28:1629–34.

11. Franklin C, Mathew J. Developing strategies to prevent in-hospital cardiac arrest: analyzing responses of physicians and nurses in the hours before the event. Crit Care Med. 1994;22(2):244–7.

12. McGloin H, Adam SK, Singer M. Unexpected deaths and referrals to intensive care of patients on general wards. Are some cases potentially avoidable? J R Coll Physicians Lond. 1999;33(37):255–9.

13. Goldhill DR, White SA, Sumner A. Physiological values and procedures in the 24 h before ICU admissions from the ward. Anaesthesia. 1999;54(6):529–34.

14. Morgan RJM, Williams F, Wright MM. An early warning scoring system for detecting developing critical illness. Clin Intensive Care. 1997;8:100.

15. Stenhouse C, Coates S, Tivey M, Allsop P, Parker T. Prospective evaluation of a modified early warning score to aid earlier detection of patients developing critical illness on a general surgical ward. Br J Anaesth. 2000;84:663P.

16. Subbe CP, Kruger M, Rutherford P, Gemmel L. Validation of a modified early warning score in medical admissions. Q J Med. 2001;94(10):521–6.

17. Hodgetts TJ, Kenward G, Vlachonikolis IG, Payne S, Castle N. The identification of risk factors for cardiac arrest and formulation of activation criteria to alert a medical emergency team. Resuscitation. 2002;54(2):125–31.

18. Lee A, Bishop G, Hillman K, Daffurn K. The medical emergency team. Anaesth Intensive Care. 1995;23:183–6.

19. Goldhill DR, Worthington L, Mulcahy A, Tarling M, Sumner A. The patient-at-risk team: identifying and managing seriously ill ward patients. Anaesthesia. 1999;54(2):853–60.

20. Bristow PJ, Hillman KM, Chey T, et al. Rates of in-hospital arrests, deaths and intensive care admissions: the effect of a medical emergency team. Med J Aust. 2000;173(5):236–40.

21. Buist MD, Moore GE, Bernard SA, Waxman BP, Anderson JN, Nguyen TV. Effects of a medical emergency team on reduction of incidence of and mortality from unexpected cardiac arrests in hospital: preliminary study. Br Med J. 2002;324(7334):387–90.

22. Ball C, Kirkby M, Williams S. Effect of the critical care outreach team on patient survival to discharge from hospital and readmission to critical care: non-randomised population based study. Br Med J. 2003;327(7422):1014–6.

23. Leary T, Ridley S. Impact of an outreach team on re-admissions to a critical care unit. Anaesthesia. 2003;58(4):328–32.

24. Bellomo R, Goldsmith D, Uchino S, et al. A prospective before-and-after trial of a medical emergency team. Med J Aust. 2003;179(6):283–7.

25. Kenwood G, Castle N, Hodgetts T, Shaikh L. Evaluation of a medical emergency team one year after implementation. Resuscitation. 2004;61(3):257–63.

26. Priestley G, Watson W, Rashidian A, et al. Introducing critical care outreach: a ward- randomised trial of phased introduction in a general hospital. Intensive Care Med. 2004;30(7):1398–404.

27. Bellomo R, Goldsmith D, Uchino S, et al. Prospective controlled trial of effect of medical emergency team on postoperative morbidity and mortality rates. Crit Care Med. 2004;32(4):916–21.

28. DeVita MA, Braithwaite RS, Mahidhara R, Stuart S, Foraida M, Simmons RL. Use of medical emergency team responses to reduce hospital cardiopulmonary arrests. Qual Saf Health Care. 2004;13(4):251–4.

29. Garcea G, Thomasset S, McClelland L, Leslie A, Berry DP. Impact of a critical care outreach team on critical care readmissions and mortality. Acta Anaesthesiol Scand. 2004;48(9):1096–100.

30. MERIT Study Investigators. Introduction of the medical emergency team (MET) system: a cluster-randomised controlled trial. Lancet. 2005;365(9477):2091–7.

31. Jones D, Bellomo R, Bates S, et al. Long term effect of a medical emergency team on cardiac arrests in a teaching hospital. Crit Care. 2005;9(6):R808–15.

32. Jones D, Opdam H, Egi M, et al. Long-term effect of a medical emergency team on mortality in a teaching hospital. Resuscitation. 2007;74(2):235–41.

33. Jolley J, Bendyk H, Holaday B, Lombardozzi KAK, Harmon C. Rapid response teams: do they make a difference? Dimens Crit Care Nurs. 2007;26(6):253–60.

34. Dacey MJ, Mirza ER, Wilcox V, et al. The effect of a rapid response team on major clinical outcome measures in a community hospital. Crit Care Med. 2007;35(9):2076–82.

35. Chan PS, Khalid A, Longmore LS, Berg RA, Kosiborod M, Spertus JA. Hospital-wide code rates and mortality before and after implementation of a rapid response team. J Am Med Assoc. 2008;300(21):2506–13.

36. Tibballs J, Kinney S, Duke T, Oakely E, Hennessy M. Reduction of pediatric in-patient cardiac arrest and death with a medical emergency team: preliminary results. Arch Dis Child. 2005;90(11):1148–52.

37. Tibballs J, Kinney S. Reduction of hospital mortality and of preventable cardiac arrest and death on introduction of a pediatric medical emergency team. Pediatr Crit Care Med. 2009;10(3):306–12.

38. Brilli RJ, Gibson R, Luria JW, et al. Implementation of a medical emergency team in a large pediatric teaching hospital prevents respiratory and cardiopulmonary arrests outside the intensive care unit. Pediatr Crit Care Med. 2007;8(3):236–46.

39. Sharek PJ, Parast M, Leong K, et al. Effect of a rapid response team on hospital-wide mortality and code rates outside the ICU in a children's hospital. J Am Med Assoc. 2007;298(19):2267–74.

40. Zenker P, Schlesinger A, Hauck M, et al. Implementation and impact of a rapid response team in a children's hospital. Joint Comm J Qual Patient Saf. 2007;33(7):418–25.

41. Buist M, Harrison J, Abaloz E, Van Dyke S. Six-year audit of cardiac arrests and medical emergency team calls in an Australian teaching hospital. Br Med J. 2007;335(7631):1210–2.

42. Jones D, Egi M, Bellomo R, Goldsmith D. Effect of the medical emergency team on long-term mortality following major surgery. Crit Care. 2007;11(1):R12.

43. Mailey J, Digiovine B, Baillod D, Gnam G, Jordan J, Rubinfeld I. Reducing hospital standardized mortality rate with early interventions. J Trauma Nurs. 2006;13(4):178–82.

44. Tolchin S, Brush R, Lange P, Bates P, Garbo JJ. Eliminating preventable death at Ascension Health. Joint Comm J Qual Patient Saf. 2007;33(3):145–54.

45. Offner P, Heit J, Roberts R. Implementation of a rapid response team decreases cardiac arrest outside of the intensive care unit. J Trauma. 2007;62(5):1223–8.

46. Story D, Shelton A, Poustie S, Colin-Thome N, McIntrye R, McNicol P. Effect of an anesthesia department-led critical care outreach and acute pain service on postoperative serious adverse events. Anesthesia. 2006;61:24–8.

47. King E, Horvath R, Shulkin D. Establishing a Rapid Response Team (RRT) in an academic hospital: one year's experience. J Hosp Med. 2006;1(5):296–305.

48. Hunt EA, Zimmer KP, Rinke ML, et al. Transition from a traditional code team to a medical emergency team and categorization of cardiopulmonary arrests in a children's center. Arch Pediatr Adolesc Med. 2008;162(2):117–22.

49. 100K Lives Campaign. www.ihi.org/IHI/Programs/Campaign/Campaign. Accessed 10 Jul 2009.

50. Joint Commission National Patient Safety Goals. www.jointcommission.org/patientsafety/nationalpatientsafetygoals/. Accessed 10 Jan 2010.

51. Devita M, Bellomo R, Hillmam K, et al. Findings of the first consensus conference on medical emergency teams. Crit Care Med. 2006;34(9):2463–78.

52. Sebat F, Musthafa AA, Johnson D, et al. Effect of a rapid response system for patients in shock on time to treatment and mortality during 5 years. Crit Care Med. 2007;35(11):2568–75.

53. Jones DA, McIntyre T, Baldwin I, Mercer I, Kattula A, Bellomo R. The medical emergency team and end-of-life care: a pilot study. Crit Care Resusc. 2007;9(2):151–6.

54. Chen J, Flabouris A, Bellomo R, Hillman K, Finfer S. MERIT study investigators for the Simpson Center and the ANZICS Clinical Trials Group, the Medical Emergency Team System and not-for-resuscitation orders: results from the MERIT study. Resuscitation. 2008;79(3):391–7.

55. Jones D, Baldwin I, McIntyre T, et al. Nurses' attitudes to a medical emergency team service in a teaching hospital. Qual Saf Health Care. 2006;15(6):427–32.

56. Galhotra S, Scholle CC, Dew MA, Mininni NC, Clermont G, DeVita MA. Medical emergency teams: a strategy for improving patient care and nursing work environments. J Adv Nurs. 2006;55(2):180–7.

57. Salamonson Y, van Heere B, Everett B, Davison P. Voices from the floor: nurses' perceptions of the medical emergency team. Intensive Crit Care Nurs. 2006;22(3):138–43.

58. Buist M, Bellomo R. MET. The emergency medical team or the medical education team? Crit Care Resusc. 2004;6:88–91.

59. Jones D, Bates S, Warrillow S, Goldsmith D, et al. Effect of an education programme on the utilization of a medical emergency team in a teaching hospital. Intern Med J. 2006;36(4):231–6.

60. Braithewaite RS, Devita MA, Mahidhara R, et al. Use of medical emergency teams (MET) responses to detect medical errors. Qual Saf Health Care. 2004;13:255–9.

61. American Heart Association National Registry for CPR. www.nrcpr.org. Accessed 23 Jan 2010.

62. Cretikos M, Parr M, Hillman K, et al. Guidelines for the uniform reporting of data for medical emergency teams. Resuscitation. 2006;68:11–25.

63. Subbe CP, Davies RG, Williams E, Rutherford P, Gemmell L. Effect of introducing the modified early warning score on clinical outcomes, cardiopulmonary arrests and intensive care utilisation in acute medical admissions. Anesthesia. 2003;58(8):797–802.

64. Goldhill DR, McNarry AF. Physiological abnormalities in early warning scores are related to mortality in adult inpatients. Br J Anaesth. 2004;92(6):882–4.

65. Goldhill DR, McNarry AF, Mandersloot G, McGinley A. A physiologically-based early warning score for ward patients: the association between score and outcome. Anaesthesia. 2005;60(6):547–53.

66. Sharpley JT, Holden JC. Introducing an early warning scoring system in a district general hospital. Nurs Crit Care. 2004;9(3):98–103.

67. Gardner-Thorpe J, Love N, Wrightson J, Walsh S, Keeling N. The value of Modified Early Warning Score (MEWS) in surgical in-patients: a prospective observational study. Ann R Coll Surg Engl. 2006;88(6):571–5.

68. Jacques T, Harrison G, McLaws M, Kilborn G. Signs of critical conditions and emergency response (SOCCER): a model for predicting adverse events in the inpatient setting. Resuscitation. 2006;69:175–83.

69. Harrison GA, Jacques T, McLaws ML, Kilborn G. Combinations of early signs of critical illness

predict in-hospital death—the SOCCER study (signs of critical conditions and emergency responses). Resuscitation. 2006;71(3):327–34.

70. Subbe CP, Hibbs R, Williams E, Rutherford P, Gemmel L. ASSIST: a screening tool for critically ill patients on general medical wards. Intensive Care Med. 2002;28(suppl):S21.

71. Haines C, Perrott M, Weir P. Promoting care for acutely ill children. Development and evaluation of a paediatric early warning tool. Intensive Crit Care Nurs. 2006;22(2):73–81.

72. Duncan H, Hutchison J, Parshuram CS. The pediatric early warning system score: a severity of illness score to predict urgent medical need in hospitalised children. J Crit Care. 2006;21(13):271–9.

73. Subbe CP, Gao H, Harrison DA. Reproducibility of physiological track-and-trigger warning systems for identifying at-risk patients on the ward. Intensive Care Med. 2007;33(4):619–24.

74. Bell MB, Konrad D, Granath F, Ekbom A, Martling CR. Prevalence and sensitivity of MET-criteria in a Scandinavian University Hospital. Resuscitation. 2006;70(1):66–73.

75. Green A, Williams A. An evaluation of an early warning clinical marker referral tool. Intensive Crit Care Nurs. 2006;22:274–82.

76. Cretikos M, Chen J, Hillman K, Bellomo R, Finfer S, Flabouris A. MERIT study investigators. The objective medical emergency team activation criteria: a case-control study. Resuscitation. 2007;73(1):62–72.

77. Smith GB, Prytherch DR, Schmidt PE, Featherstone PI, Higgins B. A review, and performance evaluation, of single-parameter "track-and-trigger" systems. Resuscitation. 2008;79(1):11–21.

78. Smith GB, Prytherch DR, Schmidt PE, Featherstone PI. Review and performance evaluation of aggregate weighted "track-and-trigger" systems. Resuscitation. 2008;77(2):170–9.

79. Santiano N, Young L, Hillman K, et al. Analysis of medical emergency team calls comparing subjective to "objective" call criteria. Resuscitation. 2009;80(1):44–9.

80. Smith GB, Prytherch DR, Schmidt P, Featherstone PI, et al. Hospital-wide physiological surveillance. A new approach to the early identification and management of the sick patient. Resuscitation. 2006;71(1):19–28.

81. Watkinson PJ, Barber VS, Price JD, Hann A, et al. A randomised controlled trial of the effect of continuous electronic physiological monitoring on the adverse event rate in high risk medical and surgical patients. Anaesthesia. 2006;61(11):1031–9.

82. Tarassenko L, Hann A, Young D. Integrated monitoring and analysis for early warning of patient deterioration. Br J Anaesth. 2006;97(1):64–8.

83. Pyke J, Taenzer AH, Renaud CE, McGrath SP. Developing a continuous monitoring infrastructure for detection of inpatient deterioration. Joint Comm. J. Safety and Quality. 2012;38(9):328–31.

84. Tanzear AH, Pyke J, Herrick MD, Dodds TM, McGrath SP. A comparison of oxygen saturation data in inpatients with low oxygen saturation using automated continuous monitoring and intermittent manual data charting. Anesthesia and Analgesia. 2014;118(2):326–31.

85. DeVita MA, Schaefer J, Lutz J, Wang H, Dongilli T. Improving medical emergency team (MET) performance using a novel curriculum and a computerized human patient simulator. Qual Saf Health Care. 2005;14(5):326–31.

86. Wallin CJ, Meurling L, Hedman L, Hedegård J, Felländer-Tsai L. Target-focused medical emergency team training using a human patient simulator: effects on behaviour and attitude. Med Educ. 2007;41(2):173–80.

87. Jones D, Duke G, Green J, et al. Medical emergency team syndromes and an approach to their management. Crit Care. 2006;10(1):R30.

Ajay D. Rao and Michael A. DeVita

Introduction

Studies focused on hospital outcomes have proven to be conflicting with regard to the rapid response system irrespective of whether the responders are medical emergency teams (METs) or rapid response teams (RRTs). On the one hand, several studies have shown improved hospital outcomes [1–4], yet on the other hand, there have been some studies that have also shown negative outcomes [5–7]. Several recent meta-analyses have concluded that there is a benefit in both mortality and cardiac arrest rate in hospitalized patients outside the ICU [8]. Although some ambiguity and skepticism remain, many hospitals have implemented METs and RRTs to promote patient safety and to satisfy regulatory requirements to find deterioration and respond in a planned fashion.

A.D. Rao, MD
Section of Endocrinology, Diabetes and Metabolism,
Temple University School of Medicine,
Philadelphia, PA 19140, USA

M.A. DeVita, MD, FCCM, FRCP (✉)
Department of Surgery, Critical Care, Harlem
Hospital Center, 506 Lenox Avenue, New York, NY
10037, USA

Department of Internal Medicine, Critical Care,
Harlem Hospital Center, 506 Lenox Avenue,
New York, NY 10037, USA
e-mail: michael.devita@NYCHHC.ORG

Quantifying the benefits of any form of rapid response system requires not only information about the constituents (what type of professional) of the response team; it also involves analysis of the triggers that set off the response. Specifically, detailed assessment of the afferent limb (i.e., the calling criteria, the reliability of detecting deterioration, and the adequacy of the triggering mechanism) can shed light on why (or why not) the efferent limb of the MET or RRT is effective [9]. Indeed, some have argued that the most important part of the RRS is a robust triggering mechanism to reap most of the benefits of an RRS [10, 11]. In addition, one might expect that a hospital's quality improvement efforts may be abetted by review of events preceding a cardiac arrest or rapid response event [12]. Hospitals may bring different material and personnel resources to bear in either the response or the review of events. The skills of the responders may impact outcome. Because of these considerations, it is obvious that the response—RRT or MET—is a system event and not exclusively a team event [13]. In this chapter, we will describe and provide an overview of the rapid response system.

Overview

In 2004, experts convened to describe and create a common terminology for teams that respond to patient deterioration outside the ICU. At that time, the participants of the consensus conference recog-

© Springer International Publishing Switzerland 2017
M.A. DeVita et al. (eds.), *Textbook of Rapid Response Systems*, DOI 10.1007/978-3-319-39391-9_3

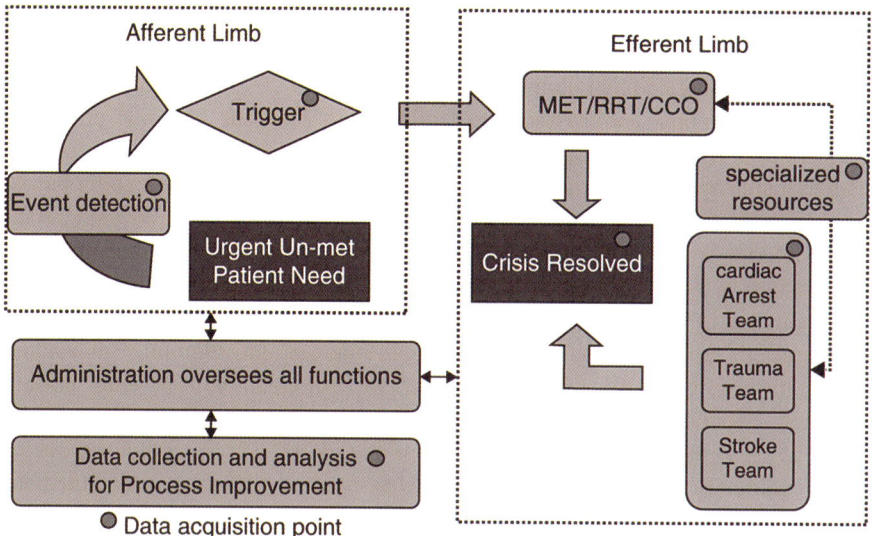

Fig. 3.1 Rapid response system structure. When patients have critical unmet needs and as a result are at risk for imminent danger, the afferent limb detects the event and triggers a systemic response. The response provides resources to stabilize and, if needed, triage the patient to a location where resources meet the patient's needs. Data are collected to determine event rate, resources needed, and outcomes and to enable an analysis of events to prevent or prepare for future events. An administrative mechanism is needed to oversee all components and to provide resources to facilitate the system, for example, educational interventions. *MET* medical emergency team, *RRT* rapid response team, *CCO* critical care outreach

nized a critical observation: All organizations that had successfully created a planned team response had also made a series of interventions in their organizations beyond the mere creation of a team. They therefore recognized and defined the rapid response system [9]. The RRS has four components: the afferent limb, the efferent limb, the quality improvement limb, and the administrative limb (Fig. 3.1).

The Afferent Limb

The afferent (or event detection and response trigger) limb is one of the most important components of the rapid response system (RRS). This is most likely related to the fact that many failures within the health system's ability to manage deteriorating patients originate in the afferent limb. In other words, a patient may deteriorate without rescue if he or she is not assessed, or if assessed, the person doing the assessment does not recognize a critical state, or if recognized, a call for help not made, or if made, the responders not arrive (Fig. 3.2).

Each step in the chain of event recognition and response triggering can be easily broken, leading to an unsafe outcome—failure to respond to a patient in crisis. In the sense that the afferent limb is responsible for identifying a crisis and triggering a response, it may be the most important component because without it there can be no response. These steps are described by Smith in the first four links of the "Chain of Prevention" [10]. The afferent limb may also be the most error-prone component of the rapid response system because of the many steps in the process and the fact that patients are often not continuously observed.

Logistically, the afferent limb can be divided into several components: [1] the selection/diagnostic/triggering criteria, [2] human and/or technologic monitoring (with alarm limits), and [3] a mechanism for triggering response. In addition, the administrative limb (to be discussed later) impacts on the afferent limb through implementation and oversight of educational processes for the totality of hospital workers to understand their role in the afferent limb. Each one of these components poses

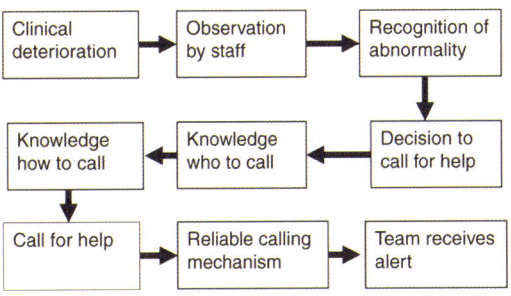

Fig. 3.2 Steps in the afferent limb

unique challenges to any hospital's attempt to create an RRS as they may require a change from traditional hospital culture. These are described more fully in Chaps. 8, 9, and 16, which also deal with the afferent limb.

Virtually all reported rapid response systems rely heavily on an objective set of calling criteria. There is regional and interhospital variability in the types of criteria and the actual limits. In the UK, for example, an early warning score is calculated from a number of physiologic variables. In Australia and the USA, the "MET criteria" are single parameter triggers, for example, a high or low respiratory rate. We will note, however, that a subjective assessment can be a valuable tool for RRS triggering as well. This relies on the staff's feelings of being "worried" about a patient. This criterion is usually used in conjunction with the first two systems, but this system is effective in allowing nurses to call for help based on their clinical instincts. Santiano et al. showed that while "nurse worried" is the most common calling criterion, most patients who have a call based on this criterion also met at least one of the criteria in the single parameter system [14]. Others have shown that the reliability of crisis detection and team triggering is increased if objective signs are used [15, 16]. In actuality, although most published criteria consist of a variety of objective measures, many organizations have also included an option for a provider who is "worried." This essentially represents a fallback position to support a staff member who may be unsure of making a call. In a study from Australia, over one-half of "worried" calls ended up falling into one of the other objective calling criteria categories [10]

Nevertheless, many times the objective criteria are not recognized or not felt to be sufficient to promote a call. Thus, the subjective criteria reinforce the objective and may be sufficient by themselves to elicit a call.

In general, the most common hospital personnel responsible for triggering these criteria have been nurses, although other hospital personnel, families, visitors, and patients themselves have triggered the system. The RRS has enabled nurses to exert their own independent judgment in calling for help through a preset system that goes "around" usual hospital hierarchy [17].

More calls decrease the cardiac arrest risk (Chen). Furthermore, it is important that triggering an RRS response should be the inherent responsibility of all hospital personnel. It has been up to each organization to determine which criteria will be used and, more importantly, to educate the staff accordingly. Finally, it may be important to standardize calling criteria across institutions, and the UK in 2012 moved in that direction in the creation of a National Early Warning Score (NEWS) and requirement that all National Health Service hospitals use it (Royal College of Physicians). Time will tell regarding whether there is additional benefit to this level of standardization. As a final point, standardizing the triggering criteria has the benefit of improving the resourcing of RRS because it enables quantifying more accurately the event rate [18].

The Efferent Limb

The efferent limb consists of the resources that are brought to bear, both personnel and equipment. Thus the efferent limb is more than the response team. The components of the efferent limb, including the types of teams that may be created to deal with a host of different critical situations, are described in Chaps. 18–23. The intention is to restore balance to a situation where the patient's needs exceed the resources available at a time when the patient's status is critical and time is of the essence. For most crises, the efferent limb intends to enable critical care resources to get to the patient's bedside without bureaucratic, sociological, or logistical barriers. Nevertheless, nurses often continue to choose to call the patient's primary physician, regardless of how long an RRS has been in place [19].

The responders, who are members of the efferent limb, and the type of equipment required are described in detail in Chaps. 24 and 25. There are four common models that have been identified: the primary response team (consisting of the patient's physician team along with nursing and respiratory care support) [11], the medical emergency team (consisting of a physician-led group of professionals), the rapid response team (which does not include a physician responder unless called by the team), and the critical care outreach team (a nurse team that proactively seeks to prevent RRS calls or respond to events) [9]. Patient-at-risk teams (PART), when led by nurses, have proven to be effective in reducing ward cardiac arrests [20].

Examples of critically unbalanced resource-to-needs situations include an acute trauma or fall, acute hemorrhage, a lost patient, an obstetric emergency, an unruly patient or family member, or even a staff member who is despondent over committing an error that caused patient harm. The standard MET or RRT will not have the skill set or equipment to manage these situations. Specialized skills are required. To make patients as safe as possible, each of these situations should have a planned triggering mechanism and a planned response team with appropriate training.

At the outset of creating an organization's RRS, it is unlikely that facilities will create all the teams we have identified in this textbook. It is only through continuous quality efforts that development of the resources becomes recognized as a need. We and others have found that events that trigger the RRS are examples of situations in which patients were in danger [12]. To prevent future dangerous situations, a hospital must have a quality apparatus attached to the RRS. This quality limb should both attempt to prevent critical events and improve the response to those events. Both require careful data collection, analysis, and provide feedback to responsible administrative and clinical personnel. These individuals or teams can create needed new processes to attend to both preventive and responsive measures. This limb is addressed in Chaps. 4, 5, 6, 7, 31, 32, and 34.

The Administrative Limb

The third component of the rapid response system is the administrative limb. This limb is responsible for marshalling both personnel and equipment resources. Initial efforts might be focused on improving the cardiac arrest response program, with particular attention to organizing the responders and overcoming equipment barriers. Different types of defibrillators should be avoided because it leads to inefficiencies in equipment use and costly repairs because of the need to maintain spare parts inventories as well as education needs for engineers and clinicians. Hospital administrators working with clinicians can create a business plan to standardize defibrillators and crash cart contents. The result will likely be reduction in costs and educational needs, as well as clinically better use of the equipment. Perhaps the most important function of the administrative limb is education. It is obvious that the response team should have focused education on (1) the clinical syndromes that cause a patient deterioration and (2) the method of working together as a team. What is not as obvious, but is equally important, is the need to educate the entire staff of the hospital regarding the rapid response system. Staff need to understand the rationale for the team, what constitutes a crisis, and how to trigger a response. Coordinated educational plans for staff result in higher call rates [16].

Recent work in this field has stressed the importance of a "Chain of Prevention," to assist hospitals to structure their care processes to prevent and detect patient deterioration and cardiac arrest [10]. The Chain of Prevention starts with education of the whole hospital regarding the importance of vital signs in detecting deterioration and the need to react reliably and efficiently. The chain links education, monitoring, detection of abnormality, recognition of the deterioration, calling for help by triggering the rapid response system, and finally the responders coming to assist. Smith argues convincingly that this chain needs to be taught to all hospital personnel much the same way that basic life support and advanced cardiac life support are.

The Quality Improvement Limb

Without a strong quality improvement limb to collect and report data, action by the administrative limb may not be focused or effective in structuring a response to patient needs. The need to prevent cardiac arrests by responding sooner to patient deteriorations may not be obvious to all practitioners or administrators. Collecting data regarding the antecedents to cardiac arrest and frequency of cardiac arrest events can help provide a foundation for education and other interventions to gain improvement. A clinical decision that a response team of critical care clinicians is needed may not be feasible without the data that administrators and clinical leaders needed to analyze to foster change.

There are many potential examples of the way quality improvement teams and the data they generate can impact both the afferent and efferent limbs function. Quality improvement efforts involving the afferent limb are now demonstrating that capturing vital sign data (as frequently as possible) is needed if every patient deterioration is to be assessed and recognized. As a result of this quality improvement data, some are calling for continuous vital sign monitoring for traditionally unmonitored patients [21, 22]. Intermittent monitoring provides the requirement of a human-technology interaction and is usually of lower cost. Of course, abnormalities may occur in between assessments, allowing the potential for missing an evolving event for minutes to hours, depending upon the monitoring interval and the specific time of the occurrence relative to the monitoring timetable. Continuous monitoring would likely prevent (or reduce) the occurrence of undetected deterioration; however, it does have major drawbacks worth considering. Additional research in the quality improvement realm are needed to sort out the clinical and financial benefits and costs of an intervention of this type. Moving to an "all patients monitored" hospital will require not only a strong administrative limb to deal with cost and cultural obstacles but also the data from the quality improvement limb to support the rationale and measure success (or failure).

Summary

In summary, the rapid response system is indeed an integrated system of care. At its best, it requires development and integration of the four limbs of the system. Each limb has a specific goal and place in the chair of care. Each is important to all other pathways of the rapid response system. Most importantly, the degree of development and integration directly affects the effectiveness of the other limbs.

References

1. Bellomo R, Goldsmith D, Uchino S, Buckmaster J, Hart GK, Opdam H, et al. A prospective before-and-after trial of a medical emergency team. Med J Aust. 2003;179:283.
2. Bellomo R, Goldsmith D, Uchino S. Prospective controlled trial of effect of medical emergency team on postoperative morbidity and mortality rates. Crit Care Med. 2004;32:916.
3. Buist MD, Moore GE, Bernard SA, Waxman BP, Anderson JN, Nguyen TV. Effects of a medical emergency team on reduction of incidence of and mortality from unexpected cardiac arrests in hospital: preliminary study. BMJ. 2002;324:387.
4. DeVita MA, Braithwaite RS, Mahidhara R, Stuart S, Foraida M, Simmons RL. Use of medical emergency team responses to reduce hospital cardiopulmonary arrests. Qual Saf Health Care. 2004;13:251.
5. Hillman K, Chen J, Cretikos M, Bellomo R, Brown D, Doig G, et al. MERIT study investigators: introduction of the medical emergency team (MET) system: a cluster-randomised controlled trial. Lancet. 2005;365:2091.
6. Kenward G, Castle N, Hodgetts T, Shaikh L. Evaluation of a medical emergency team one year after implementation. Resuscitation. 2004;61:257.
7. Chan PS, Khalid A, Longmore LS, Berg RA, Kosiborod M, Spertus JA. Hospital-wide code rates and mortality before and after implementation of a rapid response team. JAMA. 2008;300:2506.
8. Chan PS, Jain R, Nallmothu BK, Berg RA, Sasson C. Rapid response teams: a systematic review and meta-analysis. Arch Intern Med. 2010;170(1):18.
9. DeVita MA, Bellomo R, Hillman K, Kellum J, Rotondi A, Teres D, et al. Findings of the first consensus conference on medical emergency teams. Crit Care Med. 2006;34:2463.
10. Smith GB. In-hospital cardiac arrest: is it time for an in-hospital 'chain of prevention'? Resuscitation. 2010;81(9):1209–11.
11. Howell MD, Ngo L, Folcarelli P, Yang J, Mottley L, Marcantonio ER, et al. Sustained effectiveness of a

primary-team-based rapid response system. Crit Care Med. 2012;40(9):2562–8.

12. Braithwaite RS, DeVita MA, Mahidhara R, Simmons RL, Stuart S, Foraida M, et al. Use of medical emergency team (MET) responses to detect medical errors. Qual Saf Health Care. 2004;13:255.

13. DeVita MA, Bellomo R, Hillman K, Kellum J, Rotondi A, Teres D, et al. Findings of the first consensus conference on medical emergency teams. Crit Care Med. 2006;34(9):2463–78.

14. Santiano N, Young L, Hillman K, Parr M, Jayasinghe S, Baramy L-S, et al. Analysis of medical emergency team calls comparing subjective to "objective" call criteria. Resuscitation. 2009;80(1):44.

15. Sakai T, DeVita M. Rapid response system. J Anesth. 2009;23(3):403.

16. Foraida MI, DeVita MA, Braithwaite RS. Improving the utilization of medical crisis teams (Condition C) at an urban tertiary care hospital. J Crit Care. 2003;18(2):87.

17. Tee A, Calzavacca P, Licari E, Goldsmith D, Bellomo R. Bench-to-bedside review: the MET syndrome–the

18. Jones D, Drennan K, Hart GK, Bellomo R, Web SA. Rapid response team composition, resourcing and calling criteria in Australia. Resuscitation. 2012;83(5):563–7.

19. Jones D, Baldwin I, McIntyre T, Story D, Mercer I, Miglic A, et al. Nurses' attitudes to a medical emergency team service in a teaching hospital. Qual Saf Health Care. 2006;15:427.

20. Pirret AM, Takerei SF, Kazula LM. The effectiveness of a patient at risk team comprised of predominantly ward experienced nurses: a before and after study. Intensive Crit Care Nurs. 2015;31(3):133–40.

21. Taenzer AH, Pyke JB, McGrath SP, Blike GT. Impact of pulse oximetry surveillance on rescue events and intensive care unit transfers: a before-and-after concurrence study. Anesthesiology. 2010;112(2):282–7.

22. DeVita MA, Smith GB, Adam SK, Adams-Pizarro I, Buist M, Bellomo R, et al. "Identifying the hospitalised patient in crisis"—a consensus conference on the afferent limb of Rapid Response Systems. Resuscitation. 2010;81(4):375.

challenges of researching and adopting medical emergency teams. Crit Care. 2008;12(1):205.

Measuring Safety

4

Bradford D. Winters, Peter J. Pronovost,
Marlene Miller, and Elizabeth A. Hunt

Introduction

It has been a decade and a half since the Institute of Medicine brought to the public's attention the significant problems with patient safety in our healthcare system [1]. Since then patient safety and quality has been vigorously pursued by providers, hospitals, the government, and other payers. The healthcare community has worked to

B.D. Winters, PhD, MD (✉)
Department of Anesthesiology and Critical Care Medicine, The Johns Hopkins University School of Medicine, Zayed 9127 1800 Orleans Street, Baltimore, MD 21298, USA
e-mail: bhwinters@jhmi.edu

P.J. Pronovost
Department of Health Policy and Management, School of Nursing, The Bloomberg School of Public Health, 1909 Thames Street, 2nd Floor, Baltimore, MD 21231, USA

Department of Anesthesiology, Critical Care Medicine and Surgery, The John Hopkins University School of Medicine, Meyer 297 600 N Wolfe Street, Baltimore, MD 21298, USA

M. Miller
Quality and Safety, Children's Center, The Johns Hopkins Hospital, 600 N. Wolfe Street, Sheikh Zayed Tower, Baltimore, MD 21287, USA

E.A. Hunt
Department of Anesthesiology and Critical Care Medicine, The Johns Hopkins University School of Medicine, 600 N. Wolfe Street, Sheikh Zayed Tower, Baltimore, MD 21287, USA

educate themselves on methods to improve safety and strived to execute interventions toward the goal of improving patient safety and quality [2, 3]. Despite a decade and a half of effort, it is unclear if we have made progress. We still have much to do, and the science of safety needs to mature more rapidly to meet the needs of patients. We especially need to develop effective methods for evaluating the impact of our interventions so that we know what works and where to best invest our resources. This is especially true as payers (e.g., the US Centers for Medicare and Medicaid) have begun to tie reimbursement to the reduction and elimination of certain adverse events.

Fifteen years on, patients and families are still asking "have we made progress"? They want assurances that the care they are receiving is safe. They want to know if they, or their loved ones, are less likely to be injured or die as a result of medical care. Currently, there are only a handful of areas where we can say this is so. We can tell them they are less likely to develop a catheter-associated bloodstream infection. We can tell them they are less likely to have a cardiac arrest in hospitals that have a rapid response system (RRS). They are less likely to have a medication error. Unfortunately, we cannot tell them we have reduced all harms. We need to continue to strive to develop interventions that work and prove it through rigorous metrics. We need to provide evidence of success to patients, families, and those who pay for healthcare.

© Springer International Publishing Switzerland 2017
M.A. DeVita et al. (eds.), *Textbook of Rapid Response Systems*, DOI 10.1007/978-3-319-39391-9_4

Measuring and improving safety is a difficult task. By their very nature, few safety measures lend themselves to examination by the gold standard of evidence-based medicine, randomized blinded placebo-controlled trial. Blinding is often impossible, randomization difficult, and placebo groups may even be viewed as unethical. Moreover, the context in which an intervention is implemented can influence its effect. Controlling for the Hawthorne effect is very difficult and may obscure otherwise effective interventions. This problem is thought by many to have been at least partly responsible for the failure of the MERIT trial to demonstrate a difference in the case of RRSs. We have come to understand that the foundation for success in improvement in patient safety is the active change from a culture of tolerance for unsafe care to a culture that seeks to eliminate preventable harm. Changing culture is a formidable challenge. Measuring that change and the impact it exerts is almost equally difficult. Rising to the challenge is essential to answering our patients and their families; honestly, "yes, you will be safe from unintended harm" [2, 3].

This chapter provides an overview of the issues in measuring patient safety and presents a framework for measuring and improving safety. It is important to recognize that safety is a component of the broader concept of "quality," which also includes care that is effective, efficient, patient centered, timely, and equitable [4]. The boundaries between these concepts often overlap, and measures can often bridge several categories. For example, is the failure to use an evidence-based therapy a safety measure—a mistake of omission—or an effectiveness measure? Is a complication, such as a catheter-related bloodstream infection, a safety or effectiveness measure? For these examples, the answer may be either or both. In terms of understanding whether we have made an improvement, the distinction is less important than having a valid measure. Thus, in this chapter, we will use the term "safety" to represent both safety and effectiveness.

Approach for the Organizational Evaluation of Patient Safety

Donabedian's approach to measuring quality of care—evaluating how we organize care (the structures), what we do (the processes), and the results we obtain (the outcomes)—also applies to measuring safety [5]. Many institutional efforts to improve safety focus on structural measures, such as policies and procedures [6], and while they are an important component of the overall framework, they by themselves are inadequate to achieve results. Institutions should also measure processes (how often certain aspects of safe and effective care were performed) and outcomes (how often certain complications occurred). Unfortunately these are generally more difficult to develop and collect than structural measures and, as a result, are often not well represented in the framework [7, 8]. Not all institutions are able to measure all three contemporaneously, and while process and outcome measures are generally preferable to structural measures, measuring safety is best served by knowing all three.

Generally, process and outcome measures are rates that include a numerator and denominator, but not all measures of safety can, or should, be presented as rates. For example, a single episode of harm (such as the failure to rescue a single deteriorating patient) may be statistically insignificant in terms of a measure such as in-hospital mortality, but the circumstances that led to that failure may be sufficient to trigger an organizational change of great impact. Analysis of single events as well as overall rates can be illustrative. If organizations do not recognize and learn from such single episodes in addition to developing knowledge of adverse event rates and process adherence rate, they will fail to maximize safety improvement. Analysis of multiple single episodes may lead to recognition of patterns that further provide insights into opportunities for safety interventions. Additionally, measurement of rates is resource intensive and not feasible for every type of medical error. Therefore we strike a balance between rates in some circumstances and other analyses for different ones. Ultimately such "data gathering" and learning need to be feasible within the institutional structure.

Along with the ability to learn, many other aspects of an organization's culture have a significant impact on safety [9, 10]. In aviation, changes in culture, as opposed to technology, have been responsible for much of the advancements in safety over the last several decades [9, 11]. Within healthcare, communication failures are a common cause of sentinel events [12] (www.jointcommission.org), and miscommunication has central cultural underpinnings (hierarchy, command structure, etc.). Indeed, communication patterns within an organization are a strong reflection of the existing culture. Thus, the measure of both organizational learning and culture may provide insight into an organization's measure of safety.

Measuring patient safety requires universally and mutually agreed upon standardized definitions and methods, including how to adjust for risk and confounding factors. W. Edwards Deming once said, "There is no true value of anything that is measured; change the method of measurement and you change the result" [13]. Unless we develop and agree upon metrics for everyone to use, our ability to share our developed knowledge and make it generally applicable will be severely limited.

There are multiple ways to measure each area of patient safety. For medication safety we can have a structural measure, such as computerized physician order entry; a process measure, such as prescribing errors; or an outcome measure, such as adverse drug events. Moreover, each category (structure, process, or outcome) can be measured in multiple ways. For example, the methods of surveillance for evaluating adverse drug events— many of which use self-reported events, with the numerator being how the adverse event is defined and the denominator being either patient, number of patient days, or dose—vary widely (Table 4.1) [14–18] and which method is most "correct" is unclear. The result may vary but they may all be "correct." In the absence of standardized definitions, comparisons within and between institutions are problematic [19, 20]. Even with standard definitions, there is concern that comparing outcomes among hospitals is not scientifically sound, nor fair, with differences influenced by insufficient risk adjustment (hospital characteristics, patient populations, etc.) and random error rather than variations in patient safety [8, 19–21].

In addition, the context in which an intervention is implemented (its staff, resources, leadership, etc., that is, its culture) can influence the impact of an intervention. It is naive to believe that interventions will be equally effective in all healthcare organizations in which they are

Table 4.1 Sample of methods to measure medication

Study	Number studied	Numerator	Denominator	Assessed by	Rate of events
Leape et al. NEJM 1991	30195 records	Disabling adverse events	Per record reviewed/admission	Physician reviewer	3.7 per 100 admissions
Lesar, Briceland JAMA 1990	289411 medication orders/1 year	Prescribing errors	Number of orders written	Physicians	3.13 errors for each 1000 orders
Lesar, Briceland Stein JAMA 1997	1 year of prescribing errors detected and averted by pharmacist	Prescribing errors	Per medication orders written	Pharmacists, retrospectively evaluated by a physician and two pharmacists	3.99 errors per 1000 orders
Cullen, et al. Crit Care Medicine 1997	4031 adult admissions over 6 months	Adverse drug events	Number of patient days	Self-report by nurse and pharmacists, daily review of all charts by nurse investigators	19 events per 1000 ICU patient days

implemented. Context matters. Yet context should not be viewed as static but rather as dynamic and malleable leading to better understanding of mechanisms. In basic science, how genes turn on and off, how proteins fold, and how receptors bind were once context; these are now mechanisms and the target for therapies. Likewise, how culture influences outcomes, how leadership drives improvement, and how teamwork impacts on patients are context and, with robust science, will be mechanism and the target for interventions.

Based on this background, our approach to evaluating patient safety at the organizational level has four components and prompts the institution to answer the following four questions: (1) how often do we harm patients, (2) how often do patients receive the interventions they should, (3) how often do we learn from our mistakes, and (4) how well have we created a culture of patient safety? This framework is presented in Table 4.2.

Measuring Defects

To measure safety, we often estimate reliability in defects per unit, or sigma, with 1 sigma defined as defects per units of 10, 2 sigma as defects per unit of hundreds, 3 sigma defects per thousand, 4 sigma defects per ten thousand, 5 sigma defects per hundred thousand, and 6 sigma defects per million. Measuring safety is difficult, and the methods are evolving [8]. To measure safety and

quality, we need valid and reliable numerators (defects) and denominators (risk pool). Often we are not clear regarding the unit of analysis for either the numerator or the denominator. For example, in RRSs, a common numerator is the number of cardiorespiratory arrests. How this is measured may vary. One hospital may choose to include all "code" calls because it is easy to glean from administrative databases, while another hospital may choose to require that there be clear documentation of pulselessness or cessation of breathing which requires a more labor-intensive review of medical records to quantify. For denominators, is the appropriate measure the total number of admits or the number of admits who are not "Do Not Resuscitate"? The defect rate can be influenced significantly by the chosen numerator/denominator and can sometimes make comparisons across institutions problematic.

In addition, it may be unclear what the unit of analysis should be for the denominator. The choice can change performance. For example, the specialty of anesthesiology changed its denominators from minutes of care to per case. Thus, if an average anesthesia case is 100 min, the defect rate could change 2 sigmas without any change in safety.

Measures are often chosen based on their ease of collection as mentioned above for "code" calls. While this may improve data collection, they may not reflect the true impact of the safety intervention. There may be measures that better define the impact of the intervention but are difficult to obtain. For example, in RRSs, mortality

Table 4.2 Framework for an institutional scorecard for patient safety and effectiveness

Domain	Definition	Example from department of anesthesiology
How often do we harm patients?	Measures of healthcare-acquired infections	Bloodstream infections Surgical site infections
How often do patients receive the interventions they should?	Using either nationally validated process measures or a validated process to develop a measure, what percentage of patients receive evidence-based interventions	Use of perioperative beta blockers Elevation of head of bed in mechanically ventilated patients Rates of postoperative hypothermia
How often do we learn from our mistakes?	What percentage of months does each area learn from mistakes	Monitor percentage of months in which the department creates a shared story
How well have we created a culture of patient safety?	Annual assessment of safety culture at the unit level	Percentage change in culture scores for each care area

data is usually analyzed based on total in-hospital mortality because all hospitals have administrative records for this. However, since many patients with end-stage diseases are likely to not survive their hospitalization (thereby questioning why they are being hospitalized in the first place instead of going to hospice care), a better metric might be unexpected mortality. Unfortunately this is more labor intensive to collect and injects its own biases (subjectivity of "end-stage") into the calculus.

While metrics are crucial, we run the risk of creating measures of safety as though the goal was based on increasing the number of identified defects rather than actually learning from those defects. We become almost too focused on the "metric" to the exclusion of all else. In this haste we have often compromised validity. Many organizations use rates of self-reported adverse drug events as a measure of safety without recognizing that, as for all outcome measures, variations in the method of data collection/definition/data quality, case mix, and quality, as well as chance, influence outcomes [19]. Changes in these rates may, or may not, reflect what we have learned from them. Moreover, variations in data quality and case mix are likely to be far greater than the variation in safety, which limits our ability to make inferences about quality of care from these measures.

Measures of safety and quality must be important, usable, scientifically sound, and feasible. Importance and usability are value judgments that are typically made by the group, institution, or organization that decides to measure a particular area. Importance is relative, and usability refers to its ease of use by those who seek to directly improve safety, especially frontline providers. Scientifically sound refers to validity and reliability. An indicator is deemed valid if the following criteria are met (www.rand.org) [22]:

- Adequate scientific evidence or professional consensus exists supporting the indicator.
- The indicator actually measures what it purports to measure (good sensitivity, specificity, positive predictive value, and negative predictive value).

- There are identifiable health benefits to patients who receive care specified by the indicator.
- Based on experience, health professionals with significantly higher rates of adherence to an indicator would be considered higher-quality providers.
- Most factors that determine adherence to an indicator are under the control of the health professional (or are subject to influence by the health professional, such as smoking cessation).

An indicator is considered to be feasible if [22]:

- The information necessary to determine adherence is likely to be found in a typical medical record.
- Estimates of adherence to the indicator based on medical record data are likely to be reliable and unbiased.
- A reliable measure produces similar results when measurement is repeated.

Unfortunately there are often trade-offs between validity and feasibility of data collection. Often the better the validity of the measure, the greater is the workload required to collect it making it less feasible. The converse is also often true where easily collected measures may be less valid.

It is also important to distinguish whether we are measuring the reliability of a process (what we do) or an outcome (the results we get). While RRSs may be able to reduce the incidence of arrest (outcome), we know that failure to activate the MET is stubbornly common despite criteria clearly existing in the patient (process measure). Intuitively, outcome measures are more appealing than process measures, yet measuring outcomes poses an added risk for bias that often leads to little or no useful information [19, 23]. Outcomes for rare adverse events may require extensive data collection periods (years) making them less useful to frontline providers. Process measures may have a more direct impact on the common experience in healthcare. Also we presume that improved compliance with process measures has a beneficial effect on outcomes. Reliability of an outcome measure can also be influenced by variations in the methods of surveillance, in methods of data collection and definitions, in case mix, in true variation in safety, and in random error [23]. We also need to recognize that the value of some defects lies solely in learning from the numerator; the costs of obtaining an appropriate denominator may be prohibitive.

Among institutions, variation in safety and quality is often significantly smaller than variation of other variables. In healthcare, we need to work toward standardized measures of reliability. One excellent example is the National Nosocomial Infections Surveillance (NNIS) program (now called the NHSN) that provides standardized methods to monitor rates of healthcare-acquired infections [13]. Evidence-based processes of care (defects of omission) lend themselves to monitoring rates. However, we currently only have a limited number of validated process measures. A more diverse group of quality measures is needed in general and in RRSs in particular.

So, how do we select measures? W. E. Deming again provides some guidance. Measures should be selected to optimize learning, that is, ensure the measure has face validity—is it important to the person expected to use the data? To develop measures that are clinically meaningful, we need the combined input of diverse and independent sources and apply methodological rigor. For example, the exposure risk (denominator) for a failed extubation is an attempted extubation. Yet rates of failed extubation are often presented using patients or ventilator days as the denominator [24].

Given this, what are some possible measures of safety for RRSs? Unanticipated intensive care unit (ICU) admission, in-hospital mortality, and the incidence of cardiorespiratory arrest are commonly used measures, and, while they all seem to be relevant, each has potential problems. For example, unanticipated ICU admission lacks validity. While the intuitive expectation and goal would be that early intervention by the RRS would reduce this rate, we know that whether a patient remains on the general ward or moves to the ICU is based on several factors including

culture and especially on the resources-to-needs ratio for that patient as well as all of the other patients on the general ward. This resource (mostly nursing)-to-needs ratio is also fluid over time and may be very different across institutions. Given this, we do not know whether an increase or decrease in this outcome translates to high-quality care.

As mentioned previously, arrest seems to be a valid measure, but the definition of arrests and how arrests are "counted" matters. Preferably, there should be clear documentation that the patient was pulseless or had stopped breathing to qualify as an arrest.

Total hospital mortality, as mentioned earlier, fails to account for the exposure group. A certain portion of hospital mortality is not preventable. Some patients are not likely to survive their hospital stay at the time of admission. Additionally, a patient directly admitted to the ICU who then dies in the ICU and is never on the general ward couldn't possibly be exposed to the RRS intervention. Both of these types of patients are counted in total mortality. Defining what is preventable and non-preventable is much more difficult, and this choice of denominator may lead to very different results.

More relevant and valid metrics may include unexpected mortality, changes in severity scores on the general ward or on admission to the ICU, institution of end-of-life (EoL) care interventions, how often the RRS is activated when patients meet criteria, measures of delay in activating the RRS, etc. Several of these potential metrics are process measures. Recent evidence suggests that RRSs can have a positive impact on process measures such as appropriate institution of "Not for Resuscitation" status [25] and implementing early goal-directed fluid resuscitation for severe sepsis and septic shock [26]. These types of patient safety and quality measures deserve more research especially in the area of RRSs.

In addition to the choice of numerator for RRSs, we need to be careful about choice of denominator. Although admissions (and sometimes discharges) are used commonly as the denominator, patient days may be a more valid denominator. A patient's risk for arrest is influenced by, among other things, the length of time they are in the hospital. The longer a patient is in the hospital, the greater the risk. Hospital mortality and length of stay may be measures of safety for RRSs, but, as with all outcome measures, case mix will significantly influence these outcomes making comparisons among hospitals difficult to interpret [23]. As long as a hospital does not change a product line, case mix within a hospital is relatively constant, making changes in mortality rate within a hospital potentially important and measurable.

We can also measure context and culture. In fact, the RRS intervention is a major paradigm shift in acute care hospital culture away from one of "patient ownership" and rigid hierarchy to one that is focused on getting the necessary resources to a patient in need regardless of which clinical service they may be on. The RRS can be an agent of change in the safety and teamwork culture of the hospital. There are multiple tools to measure culture and scores on culture, which can be linked to process and outcomes to better understand context. Standardized tools to measure leadership and team behaviors can also be linked to process and outcome measures [27]. Finally, qualitative analysis of context (asking staff to reflect on what worked and what did not) can help develop conceptual models and hypothesis that can later be tested.

How Might We Improve Safety?

There are many examples of nearly flawless highly reliable systems from nuclear power to commercial airlines to auto racing pit crews. These systems have in common standardized processes, specified roles, high levels of training and education, and a culture dedicated to high performance. Processes are repeatedly rehearsed until a high degree of fidelity is achieved. Thus, despite the high-risk nature of many of these systems, their safety and performance rates are excellent.

How might these systems inform patient safety? Virtually all organizations are aware of the need to improve patient safety, and most have committed to doing so either through their own initiative or in response to regulators and payers. The drive to improve patient safety is still relatively new in healthcare despite the decade and a half since the Institute of Medicine's (IOMs) call to action, and culture change takes effort and time. We must view healthcare delivery as a science as well as an art if we are to improve safety and quality. Standardization of processes and applying scientific methods can help achieve higher levels of fidelity and reduce the defects that imperil our patients.

A Framework to Improve Reliability

In healthcare, most of our processes are between 1 and 2 sigmas. For a wide variety of processes, patients can rely on receiving the interventions they should half the time or 1 sigma [28]. For some outcomes, defects are 2 to 3 sigmas—for example, catheter-related bloodstream infection rates and rates of ventilator-associated pneumonia are typically between 1 and 20/1000 catheter or ventilator days, respectively [13, 29]. Some notable exceptions include anesthesiology and in transfusion medicine that are estimated to be 4 or 5 sigmas (defects/10,000 or 1,00,000) [30, 31], but there is clearly room for much improvement.

Improving reliability first depends on creating a culture of safety where the entire care team makes the patient their singular focus according to which they create and implement common goals. A culture of safety allows all members of the care team to speak up when they have concerns and listen when others voice concerns. It also creates a "zero-tolerance" attitude toward defects. Next comes standardization, specifying what is done and when it should be done [32–34]. This contrasts with traditional practice in which the "art of medicine" and "eminence-based medicine" trump the science- and "evidence-based medicine"—individual caregiver practice is unstructured and at times appears chaotic (i.e., caregivers do what they want, when they want). In the ICU, the therapies that a patient receives depend more on who is making the rounds, rather than what the evidence suggests resulting in defects in the 1–2 sigma range. Blood banking approaches the reliability of non-healthcare settings such as commercial aviation because they are standardized. Without standardization, reliability will remain at 1–2 sigma imparting a significant toll on patients.

An important aspect of standardization is to simplify or reduce complexity. Every step is a process that has an independent probability of failure. As such, processes that have five steps are more likely to fail than those that have four, three, or two steps. While there are defenses in most systems that may catch mistakes, if we reduce the number of steps in a process, we have a higher probability of improving reliability. Rather than building additional steps as barriers to errors, we need to focus on building more robust defenses into a fewer number of steps.

For example, in the effort to eliminate catheter-related bloodstream infections (CRBSI), it was noted that the operator often had to obtain the equipment for insertion from many different sources. This often led to missing or erroneous items requiring the operator to break sterility in order to get them or worse do without. The "line cart" was instituted as a mobile central location for all supplies necessary for central catheter insertion. This reduces complexity and contributes to the operator's adherence to central line insertion guidelines. For RRSs, the hierarchal nature of who to call for a deteriorating patient may lead nurses to have to "run through" an extensive list of providers prior to finding one who knows the patient and can respond. Simplifying the process to activating the MET/RRT leads to improvement.

A second aspect of standardization is ensuring that evidence is translated into practice. Evidence-based therapies that can reduce harm are often not translated into practice because, while significant efforts are made in developing therapies, little effort is made to determine how to best deliver these therapies. One model [35] designed to address this problem is based on five key components: (1) focus on systems rather than individual patients, (2) engage local multidisciplinary teams to take ownership of the initiative, (3) cre-

ate centralized support for the technical aspects, (4) encourage local adaptation, and (5) create a collaborative culture within the local unit and larger system. Specific steps include summarizing the evidence, identifying local barriers to implementation, and measuring performance to ensure all patients receive the intervention.

Successful use of this model to support standardization depends also on creating and sustaining the culture of safety. This can be achieved using strategies such as the Comprehensive Unit-based Safety Program (CUSP) [36]. While CUSP and other teamwork strategies are a local process at the unit level (e.g., ICU or ward) and RRSs are a hospital-wide intervention, the two can easily complement each other. For example, institutional support of the RRS is necessary to provide the resources it needs, but barriers to RRS activation, resulting in low utilization rates, primarily need to be addressed at the unit level.

We also need to identify and learn from defects. This involves creating independent checks to identify defects. A significant challenge we face in healthcare is developing a shared definition or concept of a defect. This can be a challenge due to different providers viewing an event from different perspectives (physician vs. nursing point of view) as well as differing perspectives in the literature (the evidence) and inherent variability leading to more than one choice. Ultimately, staff needs to come to an agreement for analysis and eventually implementation of interventions designed to reduce or eliminate the defect. A strong culture of safety helps to drive this.

To learn from defects, we need to investigate what went wrong and make recommendations for improvement. The Learning from Defects Tool (Table 4.3) is one such strategy that helps uncover what happened, why it happened, and what must be done to fix the defect. It differs from root cause analysis (RCA), commonly used by institutions for evaluating sentinel and other critical events, in that while it seeks to answer these questions, it also focuses on mitigating factors that may have ameliorated the harm. This has value for application to other defects and processes besides the one at hand. These steps—(1) create a culture of

Table 4.3 How to investigate a defect

Problem statement: Healthcare organizations could increase the extent to which they learn from defects

What is a defect? A defect is any clinical or operational event or situation that you would not want to happen again. These could include incidents that you believe caused a patient harm or put patients at risk for significant harm

Purpose of tool: The purpose of this tool is to provide a structured approach to help caregivers and administrators identify the types of systems that contributed to the defect and follow up to ensure safety improvements are achieved

Who should use this tool?
• Clinical departmental designee at morbidity and mortality rounds
• Patient care areas as part of the Comprehensive Unit-based Safety Program (CUSP)
All staff involved in the delivery of care related to this defect *should be present when this defect is evaluated*. At a minimum, this should include the physician, nurse, and administrator and others as appropriate (e.g., medication defect includes pharmacy, equipment defect includes clinical engineering)

How to use this tool: Complete this tool on *at least one defect per month*. In addition, departments should investigate all of the following defects: liability claims, sentinel events, events for which risk management is notified, case presented to morbidity and mortality rounds, and healthcare-acquired infections

Investigation process
I.   Provide a clear, thorough, and objective explanation of *what happened*
II.   Review the list of factors that contributed to the incident and check off those that negatively contributed and positively contributed to the impact of the incident. *Negative contributing factors* are those that harmed or increased risk of harm for the patient; *positive contributing factors* limited the impact of harm
III. Describe how you will reduce the likelihood of this defect happening again by completing the table. List *what* you will do, *who* will lead the intervention, *when* you will follow up on the intervention's progress, and *how* you will know risk reduction has been achieved

Investigation process
I.   **What happened?** (Reconstruct the timeline and explain what happened. For this investigation, put yourself in the place of those involved in the event as it was unfolding, to understand what they were thinking and the reasoning behind their actions/decisions when the event occurred)

An African American male >65 years old was admitted to a cardiac surgical ICU in the early morning hours. The patient was status-post cardiac surgery and on dialysis at the time of the incident. Within 2 h of admission to the ICU, it was clear that the patient needed a transvenous pacing wire. The wire was threaded using an IJ Cordis sheath, which is a stocked item in the ICU and standard for pulmonary artery catheters, but not the right size for a transvenous pacing wire. The sheath that matched the pacing wire was not stocked in this ICU, because transvenous pacing wires are used infrequently. The wire was threaded and placed in the ventricle, but the staff soon realized that the sheath did not properly seal over the wire, thus introducing risk of an air embolus. Since the wire was pacing the patient at 100 %, there was no possibility for removal at that time. To reduce the patient's risk of embolus, the bedside nurse and resident sealed the sheath using gauze and tape

II.   **Why did it happen? Below is a framework to help you review and evaluate your case.** Please read each contributing factor and evaluate whether it was involved and, if so, whether it contributed negatively (increased harm) or positively (reduced impact of harm) to the incident

Contributing factors (*example*)	Negatively contributed	Positively contributed
Patient factors	–	–
Patient was acutely ill or agitated (*elderly patient in renal failure, secondary to congestive heart failure*)	–	–
There was a language barrier (*patient did not speak English*)	–	–
There were personal or social issues (*patient declined therapy*)	–	–
Task factors	–	–
Was there a protocol available to guide therapy? (*Protocol for mixing medication concentrations is posted above the medication bin*)	XX	–

(continued)

Table 4.3 (continued)

Were test results available to help make care decision? (*Stat blood glucose results were sent in 20 min*)	–	–
Were tests results accurate? (*Four diagnostic tests done; only magnetic resonance imaging [MRI] results needed quickly—results faxed*)	–	–
Caregiver factors	–	–
Was the caregiver fatigued? (*Tired at the end of a double shift, nurse forgot to take a blood pressure reading*)	–	–
Did the caregiver's outlook and perception of own professional role impact on this event? (*Doctor followed up to make sure cardiac consultation was done expeditiously*)	–	–
Was the physical or mental health of the caregiver a factor? (*Caregiver was having personal issues and missed hearing a verbal order*)	–	–
Team factors	–	–
Was verbal or written communication during handoff clear, accurate, clinically relevant, and goal directed? (*Oncoming care team was debriefed by outgoing staff regarding patient's condition*)	–	–
Was verbal or written communication during care clear, accurate, clinically relevant, and goal directed? (*Staff was comfortable expressing concern regarding high medication dose*)	–	–
Was verbal or written communication during crisis clear, accurate, clinically relevant, and goal directed? (*Team leader quickly explained and directed the team regarding the plan of action*)	–	–
Was there a cohesive team structure with an identified and communicative leader? (*Attending physician gave clear instructions to the team*)	–	–
Training and education factors	–	–
Was the caregiver knowledgeable, skilled, and competent? (*Nurse knew dose ordered was not standard for that medication*)	XX	–
Did the caregiver follow the established protocol? (*Provider pulled protocol to ensure steps were followed*)	–	–
Did the caregiver seek supervision or help? (*New nurse asked preceptor to help mix medication concentration*)	–	–
Information technology/computerized physician order entry factors	–	–
Did the computer/software program generate an error? (*Heparin was chosen but digoxin printed on the order sheet*)	–	–
Did the computer/software malfunction? (*Computer shut down in the middle of provider's order entry*)	–	–
Did the user check what was entered to make sure it was correct? (*Caregiver initially chose .25 mg but caught error and changed it to .025 mg*)	–	–
Local environment factors	–	–
Was adequate equipment available and was it working properly? (*There were two extra ventilators stocked and recently serviced by clinical engineering*)	XX	–

(continued)

Table 4.3 (continued)

Was operational (administrative and managerial) support adequate? (*Unit clerk out sick but extra clerk sent to cover from another unit*)	–	–
Was the physical environment conducive to enhancing patient care? (*All beds were visible from the nurse's station*)	–	–
Was enough staff on the unit to care for patient volume? (*Nurse ratio was 1:1*)	–	–
Was there a good mix of skilled and new staff? (*A nurse orientee was shadowing a senior nurse, and an extra nurse was on to cover the senior nurse's responsibilities*)	–	–
Did workload impact the provision of good care? (*Nurse caring for three patients because nurse went home sick*)	–	–
Institutional environment factors	–	–
Were adequate financial resources available? (*Unit requested experienced patient transport team for critically ill patients, and one was made available the next day*)	–	–
Were laboratory technicians adequately in-serviced/educated? (*Lab technician was fully aware of complications related to thallium injection*)	–	–
Was there adequate staffing in the laboratory to run results? (*There were three dedicated laboratory technicians to run stat results*)	–	–
Were pharmacists adequately in-service/educated? (*Pharmacists knew and followed the protocol for stat medication orders*)	–	–
Did pharmacy have a good infrastructure (policy, procedures)? (*It was standard policy to have a second pharmacist do an independent check before dispensing medications*)	–	–
Was there adequate pharmacy staffing? (*There was a pharmacist dedicated to the ICU*)	–	–
Does hospital administration work with the units regarding what and how to support their needs? (*Guidelines established to hold new ICU admissions in the emergency department when beds are not available in the ICU*)	–	–

III. How will you reduce the likelihood of this defect happening again?

Specific things to be done to reduce the risk of the defect	Who will lead this effort?	Follow-up date	How will you determine the risk is reduced? (action items)
Bedside nurse called Central Supply and requested pacing wires and matching sheaths be packaged together	Bedside nurse	1 week	Supplies are packaged together

safety, (2) standardize what and when actions are done, and (3) identify and learn from defects—provide a framework to improve reliability.

Unfortunately standardization runs into many barriers, particularly among physicians. Often outside regulators, such as The Joint Commission in the USA, are relied upon to force this change in culture. This was in fact the case for RRSs as it took The Joint Commission requiring, as one of its patient safety goals (#16) for 2009, that hospitals implement better systems to respond to deteriorating patients on general hospital wards (www.jointcommission.org). While they did not explicitly require RRSs by name, this was the logical choice to meet this requirement, and RRSs, in some fashion, became nearly universal across the USA over the next couple of years. The concept of physician autonomy is deeply ingrained in the practice of medicine and is often at odds with the need to standardize practice. When physicians are asked to relinquish their autonomy in order to standardize practice, we need to be sure that those standards are just and wise and supported by the best evidence possible. Regulations may be an important tool for driving standardization and culture change, but far too many processes rely on this strategy alone, and the process by which these standards are developed needs to be transparent with the full account of risks, benefits, and cost estimates considered [37]. Rapid response systems, as a patient safety intervention, have been perhaps one of the most rigorously evaluated approaches to reducing harm outside of healthcare-acquired infections (CRBSIs, etc.). While they may be a "Band-Aid" solution to the defect of poor response to deteriorating patients on general wards, all of the evidence and wisdom to date suggests they are the best solution currently available.

To date, most efforts to improve standardization of evidence-based therapies in healthcare have focused on practice guidelines: a series of conditional probability or "if yes then 'x'" statements [35]. Given that some of these can be 100 pages or more such as the US Centers for Disease Control and Prevention's guidelines for preventing CRBSI, it is not surprising that the use of guidelines alone has met with little success [38, 39]. Under time pressure, it is difficult for caregivers to think in terms of conditional probabilities [40], and guidelines tend to be designed for physicians, ignoring other crucial team members who can act as a redundant independent check. Checklist tools can aid in this process and have led to significant improvements in aviation, nuclear power, and rail safety. They are routinely used in more and more areas of medicine including in the operating theater and in the ICU [29] and can be used to monitor performance, with each item serving as a process measure of quality and safety [7, 41]. Measurement then becomes a tool to improve performance.

Why RRSs Can Improve Safety

Rapid response systems are well grounded in the science of safety as outlined above. In most adverse events, miscommunication (delays, incorrect information, lack of information, wrong person at the receiving end, etc.) is central to the system failure. With deteriorating patients, anyone of these may occur as well as someone not speaking up (perhaps due to a sense that admitting they needed help was a sign of their inability to handle a situation they thought they should be able to handle), or if they did it was not heeded because of a hierarchical or punitive culture. With RRSs, frontline staffs are empowered—indeed encouraged—to call the MET/RRT when they are concerned. This requires a strong culture of safety that puts the patient above all else. The RRS identifies problems early, when there is still time to recover from them. As such, RRSs are based on sound safety theory and would be expected to improve safety as well as act as agent of culture change.

Conclusion

The science of measuring safety is gradually maturing. Some measures of safety lend themselves to rates, while others do not. We have described an approach for organizations to answer the question, "Are patients safer?" We also have summarized the issues regarding measuring and improving reliability and provided a framework for improving safety. With these measures, we defer to the wisdom of caregivers and administrators to identify and mitigate safety concerns, but also attempt to provide a framework to assist the caregiver with safety efforts. The need to improve quality and safety is significant, and hospitals are continually learning how to accomplish this goal. Rapid response systems are grounded in safety theory and offer the promise to reduce patient harm. While imperfect, the current data would suggest they do.

References

1. Kohn LT, Corrigan JM, Donaldson MS (Eds). To err is human. Building a safer health system. Washington, DC: National Academies Press; 2000.
2. Altman DE, Clancy C, Blendon RJ. Improving patient safety—5 years after the IOM report. N Engl J Med. 2004;351:2041–3.
3. Wachter RM. The end of the beginning: patient safety five years after "To Err Is Human." Health Aff. 2004; 23:1–12.
4. Committee on Quality of Health Care in America, Institute of Medicine. Crossing the quality chasm: a new health system for the 21st century. Washington, DC: National Academies Press; 2001.
5. Donabedian A. Evaluating the quality of medical care. Millbank Mem Fund Q. 1966;44:166–206.
6. Paine LA, Baker DR, Rosenstein B, Pronovost PJ. The Johns Hopkins Hospital: identifying and addressing risks and safety issues. Jt Comm J Qual Saf. 2004;30:543–50.
7. Rubin H, Pronovost PJ, Diette G. The advantages and disadvantages of process-based measures of health care quality. Int J Qual Health Care. 2001;13:469–74.
8. Pronovost PJ, Nolan T, Zeger S, Miller M, Rubin H. How can clinicians measure safety and quality in acute care? Lancet. 2004;363:1061–7.
9. Sexton JB, Helmreich RL, Thomas EJ. Error, stress, and teamwork in medicine and aviation: cross-sectional surveys. BMJ. 2000;320:745–9.
10. Shortell SM, Marsteller JA, Lin M, et al. The role of perceived team effectiveness in improving chronic illness care. Med Care. 2004;42:1040–8.
11. Sexton JB. The link between safety attitudes and observed performance in flight operations. Columbus, OH: Ohio State University; 2001.
12. Pronovost P, Weast B, Bishop K, et al. Senior executive adopt-a-work unit: a model for safety improvement. Jt Comm J Qual Saf. 2004;30:59–68.
13. Division of Healthcare Quality Promotion, National Center for Infectious Disease, Center for Disease Control. National Nosocomial Infections Surveillance (NNIS) System Report, data summary from January 1992 through June 2003, issued August 2003. Am J Infect Control. 2003;31:481–98.
14. Bates D, Leape L, Cullen D, et al. Effect of computerized physician order entry and a team intervention on prevention of serious medication errors. JAMA. 1998;280:1311–6.
15. Flynn E, Barker KN, Pepper GA, Bates DW, Mikeal RL. Comparison of methods for detecting medication errors in 36 hospitals and skilled-nursing facilities. Am J Health Syst Pharm. 2002;59:436–46.
16. Lesar TS, Briceland L, Delcoure K, Parmalee JC, Masta-Gornic V, Pohl H. Medication prescribing errors in a teaching hospital. JAMA. 1990;263:2329–34.
17. Lesar TS, Briceland L, Stein DS. Factors related to errors in medication prescribing. JAMA. 1997;277:312–7.
18. Leape L, Cullen D, Clapp M, et al. Pharmacist participation on physician rounds and adverse drug events in the intensive care unit. JAMA. 1999;282:267–70.
19. Lilford R, Mohammed MA, Braunholtz D, Hofer TP. The measurement of active errors: methodological issues. Qual Saf Health Care. 2004;12(suppl II):ii8–ii12.
20. Hayward R, Hofer TP. Estimating hospital deaths due to medical errors: preventability is in the eye of the reviewer. JAMA. 2004;286:415–20.
21. Cook DJ, Montori VM, McMullin JP, Finfer SR, Rocker GM. Improving patients' safety locally: changing clinician behaviour. Lancet. 2004;363:1224–30.
22. Brook R. The RAND/UCLA appropriateness method. AHCPR Pub. No. 95–0009. Rockville, MD: Public Health Service; 1994.
23. Lilford R, Mohammed MA, Spiegelhalter D, Thomson R. Use and misuse of process and outcome data in managing performance of acute medical care: avoiding institutional stigma. Lancet. 2004;363:1147–54.
24. Pronovost P, Jenckes M, To M, et al. Reducing failed extubations in the intensive care unit. Jt Comm J Qual Improv. 2002;28:595–604.
25. Jones DA, McIntyre T, et al. The medical emergency team and end-of-life care: a pilot study. Crit Care Resusc. 2007;9:151–6.
26. Sebat F, Musthafa AA, et al. Effect of a rapid response system for patients in shock on time to treatment and mortality during 5 years. Crit Care Med. 2007;35:2568–75.
27. Chan KS, Hsu YJ, Lubomski LH, Marsteller JA. Validity and usefulness of members reports of implementation progress in a quality improvement initiative: findings from the Team Check-up Tool (TCT). Implement Sci. 2011;6:115.
28. McGlynn EA, Asch SM, Adams J, et al. The quality of health care delivered to adults in the United States. N Engl J Med. 2003;348:2635–45.
29. Berenholtz S, Pronovost PJ, Lipsett PA, et al. Eliminating catheter-related bloodstream infections in the intensive care unit. Crit Care Med. 2004;32:2014–20.
30. Romano PS, Geppert JJ, Davies S, Miller MR, Elixhauser A, McDonald KM. A national profile of patient safety in U.S. hospitals. Health Aff (Millwood). 2003;22:154–66.
31. Zhan C, Miller MR. Excess length of stay, charges, and mortality attributable to medical injuries during hospitalization. JAMA. 2004;290:1868–74.
32. Reason J. Combating omission errors through task analysis and good reminders. Qual Saf Health Care. 2002;11:40–4.
33. Reason J. Managing the risks of organizational accidents. Burlington, VT: Ashgate Publishing Company; 2000.
34. Weick K, Sutcliffe K. Managing the unexpected: assuring high performance in an age of complexity. San Francisco: Jossey-Bass; 2001.
35. Pronovost P, Berenholtz SM, Needham D. Translating evidence into practice: a model for large scale knowledge translation. BMJ. 2008;377:963–5.

36. Pronovost P, Berenholtz SM, et al. Improving patient safety in intensive care units in Michigan. J Crit Care. 2008;23:207–21.

37. Matthews S, Pronovost P. Physician autonomy and informed decision making. JAMA. 2008;300:2913–5.

38. Grol R. Improving the quality of medical care: building bridges among professional pride, payer profit, and patient satisfaction. JAMA. 2001;286:2578–85.

39. Gross PA, Greenfield S, Cretin S, et al. Optimal methods for guideline implementation: conclusions from Leeds Castle meeting. Med Care. 2001;39(8 suppl 2):II85–92.

40. Klein G. Sources of power: how people make decisions. Cambridge: Massachusetts Institute of Technology; 1999.

41. Rubin H, Pronovost P, Diette G. From a process of care to a measure: the development and testing of a quality indicator. Int J Qual Health Care. 2001;13:489–96.

Medical Trainees and Patient Safety

Stephen Lam and Arthas Flabouris

As the next generation of medical practitioners, medical trainees form an important part of the medical profession. They contribute to patient care, administrative and quality activities, research and teaching. Their progression through training evolves through accumulated expertise which is associated with a gradual reduction in clinical supervision and increased autonomy. Assessment is typically both formative and summative and continues until the trainee is considered safe to practise without further supervision and gains the relevant qualifications.

Patient profiles and illness types (or 'case mix') and available health resources determine the healthcare provision that is required from medical trainees. In turn, the learning environment for trainees is determined by the case mix to which they are exposed along with other factors such as level and quality of supervision, resources and working conditions. Thus, there is a 'shared dependence', where patients depend on trainees to provide safe and competent care, whilst trainees rely on the clinical environment and patient encounters to gain quality training and experience. It is important to note that 'safe' practice within this context refers to the provision of sufficient trainee support and oversight so that their involvement in patient care does not result in patient harm [1].

The risks to patient safety associated with this relationship can be broadly categorised as:

- Those specific to supervision and the involvement of trainees in healthcare delivery.
- Those associated with the roles and responsibilities typically assigned to trainees.
- The clinical environment.

Safety Issues Specific to the Supervision and Involvement of Trainees in Healthcare Delivery

Preparing Undergraduates for Supervised Clinical Training

The quality of a trainee's learning depends on what they already know [2]. When exposed to clinical practice, they attempt to make sense of new experiences by using their existing knowledge. The primary role of medical schools is the education of medical students, preparing them with the necessary knowledge and skills for structured, supervised practice in acute

S. Lam, MBBS(Hons), FRACP, FCICM (✉)
Department of Critical Care Medicine, Flinders Medical Centre, Flinders Drive,
Bedford Park, South Australia 5042, Australia

Flinders University, PO Box 3040, Unley, South Australia 5061, Australia
e-mail: stevelamski@hotmail.com

A. Flabouris, FCICM
Intensive Care Unit, Royal Adelaide Hospital,
Adelaide, South Australia, Australia
e-mail: Arthas.Flabouris@health.sa.gov.au

© Springer International Publishing Switzerland 2017
M.A. DeVita et al. (eds.), *Textbook of Rapid Response Systems*, DOI 10.1007/978-3-319-39391-9_5

care facilities. Increasingly this role has had to compete with research and other non-teaching activities. In the 1990s, the medical curriculum was criticised for being too rigid, with overuse of didactic teaching methods and rote memorisation [3, 4]. Since then, the emphasis of undergraduate training and examination has shifted towards patient-oriented knowledge and problem-based learning [4–7]. The adoption of patient-based learning methods has been undertaken with a view to improving the link between undergraduate training and postgraduate provision of patient care as it engages students with the problems they are likely to encounter in medical practice [5–8]. Similarly, team-based knowledge also has a focus on patient-orientated knowledge, with the main difference being students learn both medical knowledge and its application within a team framework. This is particularly useful as lack of training in team interactions, crisis management and conflict resolution are identifiable deficiencies linked to patient harm [9].

Recognition of the importance of practical skills assessment has led to the use of examination techniques such as the observed structured clinical examination (OSCE). This type of teaching methodology that incorporates structured clinical, objective, multidisciplinary, problem-based instruction with OSCE or computer simulation-based assessments has been shown to be effective [4, 10, 11]. Whilst clinically oriented, these teaching methods employ simulated scenarios with minimal, if any, provision of direct healthcare and hence carry no risk to patient safety.

Undergraduate training should also cover specific topics such as human factors in patient safety and the impact of complexity on patient care. Ideally, aspects related to patient safety should be incorporated into existing patient or team-based learning methods. Within a controlled environment such as simulation, students can be taught to recognise and respond to errors.

The importance of undergraduate education in 'professionalism' has also been recognised [12, 13]. Its importance with respect to patient safety

is emphasised by the fact that clinicians who have been disciplined by state medical-licensing boards are three times as likely to have displayed unprofessional behaviour whilst in medical school [14].

Supervising and Teaching Postgraduate Trainees in Clinical Practice

Trainees learn and provide care via an apprenticeship model in the clinical setting. This supervised practice also forms a vital component of trainee assessment since summative examinations have limited capacity to examine procedural skills or real-world clinical competence [15]. Medical trainees have either (a) not completed the amount of training deemed necessary by the corresponding governing authorities to be recognised as suitable to practise without supervision, (b) not yet demonstrated achievement of the minimum level of competence required for independent practice in a formal assessment process (such as specialist college examination) or (c) been deemed by an authoritative body to require further training or period of supervision (such as remedial training or following extended leave from clinical work).

Trainee supervision is thus crucial for achieving patient safety [16–19]. In order for supervisors to be effective teachers, they must not only be sound in the delivery of clinical care but also knowledgeable in educational theory and competent in their skills of assessment, mentoring and feedback [16].

Significant skill is required by both the trainee and supervisor in order to fulfil certain key elements of patient safety including:

1. Supervisor presence and/or availability
2. Supervisor competency in delivering a safe educational experience during healthcare delivery
3. Situational awareness by both the trainee and supervisor, consisting of familiarity with the trainee's abilities as well as the task in hand

The supervision of postgraduate trainees in their provision of patient care is adjusted according to their level of experience and assessed competency. Predictable illness clinical pathways can be used to oversee clinical performance, but senior clinical oversight remains essential.

The mere presence of a supervisor does not guarantee patient safety during the performance of a procedure. Even under direct supervision, a suboptimally performed manoeuvre can result in an immediate procedural complication before the supervisor is able to intervene. It is important that both the trainee and supervisor are aware of the trainee's degree of competence, as well as the resource, environmental and patient specific circumstances that may challenge the trainee beyond their safe boundaries of competency. Similarly the supervisor can adjust the extent of their supervision (e.g. proximal or remote) based upon an assessment of the risks to the patient and educational opportunities that may be afforded to the trainee [19].

Failure of unsupervised trainees to seek appropriate assistance is considered a major cause of preventable medical errors and is often related to a lack of situational awareness arising from poor judgement of the clinical situation, a trainee's own abilities, or both [9, 20–22]. Thus it is important that trainees develop skills in self-evaluation and an understanding of their own abilities and limitations. This requires considerable accumulated experience and expertise and therefore cannot be expected of trainees until close to completion of their training. Trainees may also lack the expertise required to completely assess the task at hand and therefore underestimate, or be unaware of, immediate issues which may adversely impact upon patient safety. Varying familiarities of supervisors with their trainees and trainees with their own abilities and tasks to which they have been assigned are considered to be prominent reasons contributing to 'seasonal' fluctuations in patient outcomes (the 'July effect') [20, 21, 23].

Safety Issues Associated with the Roles and Responsibilities Assigned to Trainees

Medical issues requiring provision of care can be separated into those associated with an already identified medical condition (e.g. provision of elective surgical procedure or selection of an investigation or drug treatment for a known problem) and those associated with an acute undifferentiated medical condition (e.g. sepsis of unknown aetiology, idiosyncratic drug reactions, undifferentiated shocked states).

Ideally the right trainee should be selected for the right procedure and the right patient. Involving trainees in elective procedures and management of known entities in a controlled environment is relatively straightforward since safety issues are somewhat more predictable. However, the needs of hospital patients extend well beyond this [24]. As outlined above, trainees depend heavily on their supervisors to judge their abilities and limitations and provide appropriate supervision for each particular task. However, the typical hospital hierarchical models of medical care delivery in teaching hospitals often place trainees at the front line of patient care where issues relating to their junior level of skill, environmental challenges and level of supervision combine to create the potential for compromised patient safety.

In a typical teaching hospital routine aspects of general patient care, such as prescription of intravenous fluids and medication, are often assigned to trainees. The relatively simple nature of these tasks and the sheer magnitude of the demand for such tasks also results in them bypassing senior staff for reasons relating to healthcare resources, economics and hierarchy [25]. For the same reasons, trainees frequently manage these issues unsupervised and receive little feedback unless an adverse event is the result [26]. Amongst these tasks are those arising from unanticipated changes in patient condition and, as yet, unidentified or unresolved issues. The seriousness of the clinical situation in these circumstances varies considerably, and their management often requires expertise well beyond that of junior trainees. The mode of presentation of medical emergencies may also be subtle or nonspecific, and their early recognition and timely management is crucial to patient safety and outcome [27–33]. Subtle indicators of a more severe underlying process can be easily overlooked amongst the burden of routine trainee tasks.

Complications in clinical medicine include misdiagnosis, suboptimal or inappropriate treatment plans and errors in execution such as prescription, follow-up or communication. Studies of hospital inpatients who suffered unexpected adverse events have found that many had significant physiological derangements prior to those events, often with documentation of review by medical staff which was not followed by an appropriate escalation of care, thus highlighting the possible preventability of such these adverse events by more timely intervention [31–33].

There is significant diurnal variation associated with in-hospital care, and the high frequency of minor medical issues arising in ward care requires 24-h 'on-call' medical cover. Doctors on-call outside of normal working hours usually manage these issues and incidences with 'skeleton' levels of staffing and resources, during long duty hours that extend into the night [25, 34]. On such shifts, medical trainees are often given a wide range of smaller, less focused tasks. Several tasks for multiple patients may be allocated to the same individual trainee, often simultaneously, and often from different areas of the hospital. The priority of such tasks may vary for reasons ranging from the level of perceived urgency of the patient's clinical condition to the need to meet required time frames and deadlines (e.g. awaiting transfer to the operating room). As such, medical trainees are often faced with the need to triage priorities and handle important tasks with multiple distracting issues under significant time pressure [25]. Additionally, a single trainee is often assigned the role of providing care for patients belonging to different clinical teams, with the goal being to 'troubleshoot' until the primary care team arrives to take over during normal working hours. In instances where they are

not part of the primary care team, they are often unfamiliar with the patient, and when they are part of the primary care team, they are working 'overtime' hours [34, 35].

Difficult working conditions can compromise performance in a manner not restricted to medical trainees, but any profession in general. These characteristics of on-call shifts can hinder task completion, cognitive processing and the ability to correctly separate impending disasters from more minor complaints and issues [24, 25]. In recognition of this, specific taskforce-derived measures to improve trainee education and patient safety have been implemented with mixed and often disappointing results [35–40]. To some extent, this difficulty in achieving clear improvements may reflect the inherent nature of the service required, rather than being purely related to faults within the current paradigms of hierarchy and task allocation.

Trainees, and indeed non-hospitalist and critical care trained specialists in general, may lack the necessary skills set to recognise and optimally manage high-risk patients and medical emergencies. Yet hospital systems often place these practitioners at the front line of patient care in many circumstances and so are the first to encounter such patients, often alone and under difficult circumstances. The need for other means of compensating for these weaknesses in the system have been recognised and developed. Important examples of this include systems which detect medical emergencies as early as possible and with less reliance on higher levels of expertise in the 'first-responder' and organised systems of response when potential issues are identified.

The Clinical Environment

Delivering care in a hospital setting has become increasingly more complex and risky [24]. The population is ageing with increasing co-morbidities, changing disease demographics, increasing complexity and choice of healthcare technology and patients with chronic and often terminal conditions finding themselves 'trapped' in acute care facilities due to the lack of available chronic and aged care facilities [24]. Meanwhile hospitals seek to achieve cost efficiency through reducing acute hospital beds, streamlining inpatient care, staff reductions and greater emphasis on home care. In such an environment, education can become less of a 'core' activity and viewed as more of a 'luxury' despite recognition of its positive contribution to patient safety [25].

Rapid growth in technology and scientific advances resulting from better understanding of complex disease processes has fuelled the growth of medical specialisation [24]. Highly technical proceduralists and specialists are now limiting their practice to specific diseases, organs or parts of the body. Because of the associated technical complexity and cost of such procedures, many of these services are being restricted to academic and acute care medical facilities. As a result, there has been a decline in the number of medical practitioners devoted to comprehensive and holistic care. Medical specialisation has been described as fragmented and confusing to patients and general practitioners alike, with risk to the perception of medicine as an integrated profession [24, 41, 42].

In association with these changes, quality of care and patient safety has gained an increasing emphasis, in particular as medical errors have been identified as a leading cause of patient harm [41]. Trainees are at risk of exposing patients to harm because of lack of experience, knowledge and technical skills whilst working in a complex and dynamic environment with limited resources and supervision [24, 25, 41].

Patient Safety and Medical Trainees in Training Institutions

Training Requirements and Supervision in an Era of Medical Specialisation

Complicated patients need practitioners who are able to manage undifferentiated illnesses, often in conjunction with multiple specialist teams and/or other generalists. Focussing on one area of practice with specialist training invariably leads to a lack of knowledge and experience in other areas. This therefore highlights two important areas of need in an environment of specialist practitioners and trainees: first of all skill sets in all doctors for recognition and participation in team management of medical emergencies and, secondly, availability of general and critical care specialists to supervise trainees from other specialty disciplines.

The various causes of adverse events have been widely recognised as being multifactorial and highlight the importance of technical competency, problem-solving skills, communication, and system design in the delivery of high-quality medical care. These are therefore considered vital components of postgraduate education [27, 41, 43].

The need for postgraduate training to maintain skills required for whole-patient care during undifferentiated illness presentation and acute emergencies is more crucial than ever in an era of increasing specialisation. A framework of competences for all doctors has been suggested in respect to addressing the recognition and response to deteriorating patients [44]. At the very least, medical trainees should be taught to distinguish warning signs that may herald progress towards a serious adverse patient event, recognise their own limitations and be empowered to refer as appropriate, or seek, critical care involvement during times of medical crises. Skill sets considered crucial include the measurement, monitoring and interpretation of vital signs, triage, emergency planning and preparation, team organisation and leadership, record keeping and escalation of response through appropriate referral processes. Preparation for such training should begin in the undergraduate years and progress throughout general medicine training prior to specialisation. Critical care training modules for postgraduates provide a broad exposure to acute critical care. Since opportunities for specialty trainees (and their fully qualified specialist supervisors) to regularly perform or practise these skills are infrequent, the use of simulation technology and provision of reaccreditation sessions is extremely valuable [4].

Support for the concept of 'hospitalist' practitioners has risen from the recognition of the need for supervision of specialist trainees and attendance of hospital inpatients by practitioners with a broad range of knowledge and skills [45–47]. This includes the critical care domains of intensive care and emergency medicine, which promotes coordinated, whole-patient acute care for inpatients [48] and the more recent recognition of the need for acute general medicine and acute general medical units [49, 50].

Medical Trainees and Systems for Identifying and Responding to At-Risk Patients

Whilst important general medical skill sets have been outlined above, the degree of medical expertise required to identify and optimally manage high-risk patients and medical emergencies can extend far beyond that which could be realistically achieved and maintained in non-hospitalist and noncritical care specialist doctors. Therefore, methods for early detection of at-risk patients and medical emergencies acting in concert with systems for organised response remain crucial for patient safety. Systems for early recognition which are simple to use, highly sensitive during the performance of routine nursing or medical observations and with minimal reliance on high levels of critical care expertise in first responders have been developed and widely recommended [51].

Too often the most junior doctors are left to recognise and manage inpatients following acute deterioration. Ideally, the hospital response to acute patient deterioration should be immediate, organised and predetermined and involve a team of appropriately trained and resourced clinical staff. Achieving such a collaborative, coordinated and patient-centered care approach encourages collective responsibility for the care of patients across professions and healthcare teams. However, the required skills and multidisciplinary, coordinated team approach may not be consistent with the reality of a junior doctor acting in isolation within a hospital ward.

A good example of an organised multidisciplinary response is the trauma team, a system which has been shown to reduce preventable deaths [52–54]. As demonstrated in this book, a team that responds to acute medical emergencies other than cardiac arrest for hospital inpatients is a concept that has been specifically developed for acute inpatient deterioration and is becoming increasingly popular [55–58]. Similar to trauma teams, rapid response teams provide an organised response with simple pathways of activation. They complement, as well as compensate for, deficiencies in the skill sets of trainees and non-critical care specialists working in the front line of patient care, who often encounter high-risk hospital patients and medical emergencies alone and without the necessary skills.

Summary

With changing hospital patient demographics and rapidly advancing healthcare technology, it is becoming increasingly important for healthcare systems to evolve to meet their new challenges.

Medical trainees provide not only routine and straightforward care but also emergency and complex medical care within acute healthcare facilities. Postgraduate training and medical team structures often place junior trainees at the forefront of identifying and responding to the acutely deteriorating inpatient. This requires them to deal with issues ranging from the trivial to the more complicated and often subtle presentations of acute medical emergencies. Their ability to recognise acute patient deterioration and subsequently know when to alert, and/or participate in the response to these events as part of, or in conjunction with, hospital rapid response teams is crucial to minimising serious adverse events for such patients.

For medical trainees to safely and efficiently fulfil their roles in emergent and elective patient care, undergraduate and postgraduate training will need to provide them with the appropriate skills, environment, and clinical exposure which is balanced between specialisation and acute general medicine.

Simple to use, highly sensitive methods to identify patients at risk of serious illness, even during routine nursing or medical observation, coupled with rapid response systems involving teams with expertise in undifferentiated clinical scenarios are becoming increasingly important to maximise patient safety in an environment that also fosters the theoretical and practical instruction of trainees.

References

1. Kapp MB. Legal implications of clinical supervision of medical students and residents. J Med Educ. 1983;58:293–9.
2. Dyrbye LN, Harris I, Rohren CH. Early clinical experiences from students' perspectives: a qualitative study. Acad Med. 2007;82:979–98.
3. Christakis NA. The similarity and frequency of proposals to reform US medical education: constant concerns. JAMA. 1995;274:706–11.
4. IOM (Institute of Medicine). Redesigning continuing education in the health professions. Washington, DC: The National Academies Press; 2010.
5. Chantler C. National health service: the role and education of doctors in the delivery of health care. Lancet. 1999;353:1178–81.
6. Howe A, Campion P, Searle J, Smith H. New perspectives—approaches to medical education at four new UK medical schools. BMJ. 2004;329:327–31.
7. Jones R, Higgs R, Angelis C, Prideaux D. Changing face of medical curricula. Lancet. 2001;357:699–704.
8. Dornan T, Bundy C. What can experience add to early medical education? Consensus survey. BMJ. 2004;329:834–40.
9. Singh H, Thomas EJ, Peterson LA, et al. Medical errors involving trainees. A study of closed malpractice claims from 5 insurers. Arch Intern Med. 2007;167:2030–6.
10. Hill D, Stalley P, Pennington D, Besser M, McCarthy W. Competency-based learning in traumatology. Am J Surg. 1997;173:136–40.
11. Rogers PL, Jacob H, Rashwan AS, Pinsky MR. Quantifying learning in medical students during a critical care medicine elective: a comparison of three evaluation instruments. Crit Care Med. 2001;29:1268–73.
12. Learning objectives for medical student education—guidelines for medical schools: report I of the Medical School Objectives Project. Acad Med. 1999;74:13–18.
13. Cruess SR, Cruess RL. Professionalism must be taught. BMJ. 1997;315:1674–7.
14. Papadakis MA, Teherani A, Banach MA, et al. Disciplinary action by medical boards and prior behavior in medical school. N Engl J Med. 2008;353:2673–82.
15. Smee S. Skill based assessment. BMJ. 2003;326(7391):703–6.
16. Farnan JM, Petty LA, Georgitis E, et al. A systematic review: the effect of clinical supervision on patient and residency education outcomes. Acad Med. 2012;87:428–42.
17. Australian Curriculum Framework for Junior Doctors. http://www.cpmec.org.au/curriculum.
18. Iglehart JK. Revisiting duty-hour limits—IOM recommendations for patient safety and resident education. N Engl J Med. 2008;359:2633–5.
19. Kilminster SM, Jolly BC. Effective supervision in clinical practice settings: a literature review. Med Educ. 2000;34:827–40.
20. Grieg PR, Higham H, Nobre AC. Failure to perceive clinical events: an under-recognised source of error. Resuscitation. 2014;85:952–6.
21. Singh H, Petersen LA, Thomas EJ. Understanding diagnostic errors in medicine: a lesson from aviation. Qual Saf Health Care. 2006;15:159–64.
22. Kennedy TJT, Regehr G, Currie R, et al. Preserving professional credibility: grounded theory study of medical trainees' requests for clinical support. BMJ. 2009;338:b128.
23. Young JQ, Ranji SR, Wachter RM, et al. "July Effect": impact of the academic year-end changeover on patient outcomes. A systematic review. Arch Intern Med. 2011;155:309–15.
24. Crossing the quality chasm: a new health system for the 21st century. http://books.nap.edu/catalog/10027.html.
25. IOM (Institute of Medicine). Resident duty hours: enhancing sleep, supervision, and safety. Washington, DC: The National Academies Press; 2009.
26. Lack CS, Cartmill JA. Working with registrars: a qualitative study of interns' perceptions and experiences. Med J Aust. 2005;182:70–2.
27. McQuillan P, Pilkington S, Allan A, et al. Confidential inquiry into quality of care before admission to intensive care. BMJ. 1998;316:1853–8.
28. Hillman K, Bristow PJ, Chey T, et al. Antecedents to hospital deaths. Intern Med J. 2001;31:343–8.
29. Franklin C, Mathew J. Developing strategies to prevent inhospital cardiac arrest analyzing responses of physicians and nurses in the hours before the event. Crit Care Med. 1994;22:244–7.
30. Bedell SE, Deitz DC, Leeman D, Delbanco TL. Incidence and characteristics of preventable iatrogenic cardiac arrest. JAMA. 1991;265:2815–20.
31. Schein RM, Hazday N, Pena M, Ruben BH, Sprung CL. Clinical antecedents to in-hospital cardiopulmonary arrest. Chest. 1990;98:1388–92.
32. Kause J, Smith G, Prytherch D, Parr M, Flabouris A, Hillman K, Intensive Care Society (UK), Australian and New Zealand Intensive Care Society Clinical Trials Group. A comparison of antecedents to cardiac arrests, deaths, and emergency intensive care admissions in Australia and New Zealand, and the United Kingdom—the ACADEMIA study. Resuscitation. 2004;62:275–82.

33. Garrad C, Young D. Suboptimal care of patients before admission to intensive care is caused by a failure to appreciate or apply the ABCs of life support. BMJ. 1998;316:1841–2.

34. Philibert I, Taradejna C. Chapter 2. A brief history of duty hours and resident education. In: Philibert I, Amis S (eds.) The ACGME 2011 duty hour standards: enhancing quality of care, supervision, and resident professional development. Chicago, IL: Accreditation Council for Graduate Medical Education; 2011.

35. Nasca TJ, Day SH, Amis Jr ES. ACGME duty hour task force the new recommendations on duty hours from the ACGME task force. N Engl J Med. 2010;363:e3.

36. Desai SV, Feldman L, Brown L, et al. Effect of the 2011 vs 2003 duty hour regulation-compliant models of sleep duration, trainee education, and continuity of patient care among internal medicine house staff. A randomised trial. JAMA. 2013;173:649–55.

37. Landrigan CP, Rothschild JM, Cronin JW, et al. Effect of reducing interns' work hours on serious medical errors in intensive care units. N Engl J Med. 2004;351:1838–48.

38. Volpp KG, Rosen AK, Rosenbaum PR, et al. Did duty hour reform lead to better outcomes among the highest risk patients? J Gen Intern Med. 2009;24:1149–55.

39. Fargen KM, Rosen CL. Are duty hour regulations promoting a culture of dishonesty among resident physicians? J Grad Med Educ. 2013;5:553–5.

40. Moonesinghe SR, Lowery J, Shahi N, et al. Impact of reduction in working hours for doctors in training on postgraduate medical education and patients' outcomes: systematic review. BMJ. 2011;342:d1580.

41. Kohn LT, Corrigan JM, Donaldson MS, Molla S. To err is human: building a safer health system. Washington: National Academy Press; 2000.

42. Phillips RA, Andrieni JD. Translational patient care. a new model for inpatient care in the 21st century. Arch Intern Med. 2007;167:2025–6.

43. Wilson RM, Runciman WB, Gibberd RW, et al. The quality in Australian health care study. Med J Aust. 1995;163:458–71.

44. National Institute for Health and Clinical Excellence. Acutely ill patients in hospital: recognition of and response to acute illness in adults in hospital, (NICE guideline no 50). London: NICE; 2007.

45. Farnan JM, Burger A, Boonayasai RT, et al. Survey of overnight academic hospitalist supervision of trainees. J Hosp Med. 2012;7:521–3.

46. Wachter RM, Goldman L. The emerging role of hospitalists in the American health care system. N Engl J Med. 1996;335:514–7.

47. Wachter RM. Hospitalists in the United States—mission accomplished or work in progress? N Engl J Med. 2004;350:1935–6.

48. Hauer KE, Wachter RM, McCulloch CE, Woo GA, Auerbach AD. Effects of hospitalist attending physicians on trainee satisfaction with teaching and with internal medicine rotations. Arch Intern Med. 2004;164:1866–71.

49. Recognising and responding to clinical deterioration: use of observation charts to identify clinical deterioration. Australian Commission on safety and quality in health care. http://www.safetyandquality.gov.au/wp-content/uploads/2012/02/UsingObservationCharts-20091.pdf.

50. Kramer MHH, Akalin E, Alvarez de Mono Soto M, et al. Internal medicine in Europe: How to cope with the future? An official EFIM strategy document. Eur J Intern Med. 2010;21:173–5.

51. Byrne D, Silke B. Acute medical units: review of evidence. Eur J Intern Med. 2011;22:344–7.

52. Pagliarello G, Dempster A, Wesson D. The integrated trauma program: a model for cooperative trauma triage. J Trauma. 1992;33:198–204.

53. Shackford SR, Hollingworth-Fridlund P, Cooper GF, et al. The effect of regionalization upon the quality of trauma care as assessed by concurrent audit before and after institution of a trauma system. J Trauma. 1986;26:812–20.

54. Draaisma JM, de Haan AF, Goris RJ. Preventable trauma deaths in the Netherlands—a prospective multicenter study. J Trauma. 1989;29:1552–7.

55. Lee A, Bishop G, Hillman KM, Daffurn K. The medical emergency team. Anaesth Intensive Care. 1995;23:183–6.

56. Stenhouse C, Coates S, Tivey M, Allsop P, Parker T. Prospective evaluation of a modified early warning score to aid detection of patients developing critical illness on a surgical ward. Br J Anaesth. 2000;179(6):663P.

57. Kerridge RK, Saul WP. The medical emergency team, evidence-based medicine and ethics. Med J Aust. 2003;179:313–5.

58. Goldhill OR, Worthing L, Mulcahy A, Tarling M, Sumner A. The patient-at-risk team: identifying and managing seriously ill ward patients. Anaesthesia. 1999;54:853–60.

Ken Hillman, Hadis Nosrati,
and Jeffrey Braithwaite

The concept of organisational culture is one that we all probably consider that we understand. However, it remains challenging to gain a consensus on exactly what it means.

Organisational or 'corporate' culture has been described as the implicit, invisible, intrinsic and informal consciousness of the organisation which guides the behaviour of individuals and which, in turn, is shaped from their behaviours [1]. Organisational culture can affect, and be affected by, healthcare performance, is amenable to manipulation and is based on the assumptions that healthcare organisations have identifiable cultures, that culture is related to performance and that a culture can be altered to change the performance [2]. These concepts are foreign to many practising clinicians and can be difficult for many of them to relate to.

K. Hillman, MBBS, FRCA, FCICM, FRCP, MD (✉)
The Simpson Centre for Health Services Research, South Western Sydney Clinical School, UNSW Sydney, the Ingham Institute for Applied Medical Research and Intensive Care, Liverpool Hospital, Locked Bag 7103, Liverpool BC, NSW 1871, Australia
e-mail: k.hillman@unsw.edu.au

H. Nosrati, PhD
The Simpson Centre for Health Services Research, Sydney, NSW 2052, Australia

J. Braithwaite, PhD
Faculty of Medicine and Health Sciences, Australian Institute of Health Innovation, Macquarie University, Level 6, 75 Talavera Road, Sydney, NSW 2109, Australia

Hospital Culture and the Need for Rapid Response Systems

Rapid response systems (RRSs) operate across the entire organisation. They require the support of all clinicians as well as the hospital administration. It is not surprising therefore that the system may be more successfully accepted in some organisations than others. In fact, in the largest study on RRSs, there was so much variability among the hospitals which were assigned with a RRS to the study group that approximately 100 hospitals would have been necessary to demonstrate any statistical difference between the control and intervention groups [3]. In other words, it appeared that some organisations implemented the system more effectively than others and this may have been related to the way staff within the organisations related to each other as well as other collective properties such as morale, organisational focus as well as difficult to define concepts such as commitment to the organisation's goals and even pride. This is consistent with the result of a recent systematic review to identify how organisational and cultural factors mediate or are mediated by hospital-wide interventions such as RRS. The article suggested that, while associations between organisational factors, intervention success and patient outcomes were difficult to measure [4], effective leadership and clinical champions, adequate financial and educational resources and dedicated promotional

© Springer International Publishing Switzerland 2017
M.A. DeVita et al. (eds.), *Textbook of Rapid Response Systems*, DOI 10.1007/978-3-319-39391-9_6

activities appear to be common factors in successful system-wide change.

The culture of hospitals may also have been a major reason why there was an obvious need to manage serious illness on the general floors of a hospital in a different way. Before the implementation of RRSs, there was a high incidence of potentially preventable deaths [5–8]. Part of the problem was that patients were being suboptimally managed on the general floors of acute hospitals [9, 10]. Many patients who died [11], had a cardiac arrest [12] or were admitted to an ICU [13] had prolonged and documented periods of deterioration before the event.

We need to examine the way hospitals work and the way that the culture of a hospital may have influenced the suboptimal care of patients on the general floors. Another way of defining culture is expressed as the 'way we do things around here'. Historically, the management of patients in hospitals has been designed around the admission of a patient 'under' the care of a specialist physician. That physician is responsible for the care of the patient. However, the physician is almost never in the hospital for 24 h every day. In fact, it is common practice that they visit patients for less than 10 min each day. Not so many years ago, the most junior member of the admitting team in the United Kingdom was called the 'Houseman'. They were assigned this title because they were expected to live in the hospital 24/7 for the first year of their training. They were then promoted to senior house officer (SHO), as they climbed the promotion ladder and continued their apprenticeship. The SHO worked hours that would be unacceptable today but had the occasional days off, unlike the Houseman.

The remnants of this system remain. The admitting specialist usually works with a team of more junior or trainee doctors. Currently it is more common that, while there are always doctors in the hospital, they may not inevitably be members of the admitting team. It is becoming more common for doctors working in hospitals to work in shifts in order to cover the hospital at all times. As such, there may not be a member of the admitting team always caring for the patient but doctors working shifts, reporting to the admitting

specialists as necessary and when there are problems with particular patients.

At the same time, nursing staff are the only clinicians continuously at the patient's bedside. While their role has changed in some ways, they still largely act under the orders of the admitting medical team. This has important implications for patients who are deteriorating on the general floors of an acute hospital.

Nursing staff measure vital signs and either manually or electronically enters them in charts. However, nurses are not empowered or trained to intervene according to the abnormality. Nurses usually have to navigate a rigid hierarchical medical system in order to seek help for their patient. They would call the most junior member of the medical team who would rarely be trained in advanced resuscitation [14]. Further assistance up the medical hierarchy would be sought, as necessary, to doctors who are usually not proficient in all aspects of caring for the seriously ill and deteriorating patient.

Over the last 30 years, there has been an increasing trend to specialise in medicine [15]. This has many advantages. Doctors become increasingly proficient in their areas of expertise. The need to maintain knowledge and skills usually mean that they can barely keep up with their own journals, books and meetings. While admitting teams used to care for all aspects of their patients' care, this became more difficult as the patient's problems moved outside the admitting team's expertise. The more junior members of the medical hierarchy did not have the appropriate training to care for complex, seriously ill patients and, when further advice was sought from more senior members of the admitting team, who had become specialised in their own areas and no longer had the appropriate skills, knowledge and experience to care for the seriously ill. While specialists can, and do, refer patients for opinions outside their own areas of expertise, research has shown that the admitting team has difficulty in even recognising that a patient is deteriorating [9, 16]. As such, many patients suffered potentially avoidable death and serious adverse events and death [11, 12, 17].

The challenge of caring for the deteriorating and at-risk patients on general floors is compounded by the changing population of patients in acute hospitals [18]. Patients are now older with multiple co-morbidities and having complex interventions with an increased rate of complications [19]. There is also pressure to decrease the length of stay, resulting in only the more complex and at-risk patients remaining in hospitals. In fact, patients who are subject to rapid response calls have a higher mortality and are as seriously ill as patients in an ICU [20, 21].

As a result, we have a perfect storm. Acute hospitals now have a population of patients where the level of illness of the patients on the general floors is often as great as those in the ICU. The culture of the hospital or the 'way we do things around here' is built around admitting a patient 'under' a specialist who only sporadically sees the patient and whose skills do not necessarily include recognising and managing serious illness. The specialist is supported by a team of more junior or training doctors who also do not have the appropriate skills to care for seriously ill patients. The bedside nurses' involvement is limited to observing and recording. They are not empowered or trained to intervene in deteriorating patients. Thus, the culture of acute hospitals remains, in essence, much the same as it has for over a century but is no longer appropriate for the needs of patients in acute hospitals.

The Impact of a RRS on Hospital Culture

The implementation of a RRS almost certainly has an impact on the culture of an acute hospital. The system is one of the first organisation-wide patient safety initiatives. Usually the various tribes such as doctors, nurses and administrators in a hospital act independently from each other.

For a RRS to function, these barriers have to be broken down. As a result of implementing a RRS, nurses are empowered to bypass the usual hierarchical medical system; the admitting specialist is bypassed; other specialists, usually from an ICU, operate outside their usual silo in order

to manage patients on the general floors; and hospital managers need to support and fund the system. Thus, the culture of the organisation has to change significantly as a result of the implementation of a RRS. The most important cultural change is that the system is built around patient not professional imperatives.

Junior doctors no longer have to 'lose face' by calling for assistance as a standardised system is in place which makes it compulsory for them to summon help when certain criteria are met. Similarly, nursing staff no longer feel bound to follow historical and rigid ways of operating. They are empowered to be genuine advocates for their patients. Specialists in the hospital are no longer bound to put professional etiquette before patient safety.

Above all, patients are attended to at an early stage of their illness rather than delaying until a cardiac arrest occurs.

A RRS operates within the complexity of an acute hospital. Because it has been constructed around patient needs, staff are 'allowed' to break age-old conventions.

The way we currently measure culture has limited bedside credibility or utility, and, as such, it is difficult to estimate the influence of culture on patient outcomes and clinical practice [22].

The implementation of a RRS allows us to approach the concept of culture from a different direction. Instead of using elusive measures of culture to evaluate the effectiveness of the implementation of a RRS, we propose that the effectiveness of the implementation of a RRS could be indirectly affected by the culture of the organisation.

The effectiveness of a RRS can be evaluated by measuring the outcomes that it is designed to improve. These include deaths and cardiac arrests. However, a RRS is not designed to prevent death when it is inevitable as in terminally ill patients. As such we use the term 'unexpected' deaths which is the sum of all deaths expressed as/1000 admissions but not including patients who are designated as do not attempt resuscitation (DNAR) [23, 24]. We also use the term 'potentially preventable' to further refine the utility of mortality as an outcome [23, 24]. This refers to deaths which are preceded by

RRS calling criteria within 24 h of death which have not been acted on appropriately and, similarly, cardiac arrests where the rate is refined by using 'unexpected' and 'potentially preventable' [23, 24].

One could suggest that the effectiveness of a RRS, one of the few organisation-wide systems in acute hospitals, is related to how effectively the various silos in a hospital operate together.

Similarly, the outcome indicator of the number of rapid response calls/1000 admissions is directly associated with the reduction in cardiac arrest and death rates in a hospital [25]. Thus, the effectiveness of the implementation process is measureable and may be related to the acceptance by staff of the system, as well as the ability to function as a team and communicate well. These are all features of 'how we do things around here'.

The rapidity of how well the RRS is implemented and how effective it is may also be related to organisational culture. We know that it may take several years for a RRS to be effectively implemented [26].

The culture of the organisation may influence the ability to learn together and co-operate effectively.

It is not inconceivable that the implementation of one unique patient-centred and organisation-wide system would facilitate other such initiatives. The presence of a RRS may highlight a serious deficiency in acute hospitals. Almost one-third of all calls are to patients who have end-of-life issues (EoL) [27]. In other words, the diagnosis of dying in acute hospitals is less than ideal. Even when these patients are recognised, their management is often sub-standard [28].

Thus, we have another group of patients who fall between the cracks under the existing 'way of doing things around here'. The model of RRS could facilitate other patient-centred approaches. For example, in the case of patients at the EoL, they may be recognised by certain criteria. Obviously, these would be more complicated than those used to recognise deteriorating patients. The 'response' would vary depending on many factors such as the particular stage of the dying process.

However, a common component of this response would be an honest and transparent discussion with the patient and carers in order to agree to an appropriate management plan.

In summary, while culture is an elusive concept and difficult to measure, it has an effect on the way RRSs are implemented. Organisational culture may also be influenced by the very implementation of the RRS itself.

References

1. ScholzC. Corporate culture and strategy—the problem of strategic fit. Long Range Plann. 1987;20(4):78-87
2. MannionR, DaviesHTO, MarshallMN. Cultures for performance in health care. Maidenhead, UK: Open University Press2005.
3. MERIT Study Investigators. Introduction of the medical emergency team (MET) systems: a cluster randomised controlled trial. Lancet. 2005;365(9477):2091-2097
4. Clay-WilliamsR, NosratiH, CunninghamFC, HillmanK, BraithwaiteJ. Do large-scale hospital- and system-wide interventions improve patient outcomes: a systematic review. BMC Health Serv Res. 2014;14:369
5. BrennanTA, LeapeLL, LairdNM, HerbertL, LocalioAR, LawthersAG, et al. Incidence of adverse events and negligence in hospitalized patients: results from the Harvard Medical Practice Study I. N Engl J Med. 1991;324:370-376
6. WilsonRM, RuncimanWB, GibberdRW, HarrisonBT, NewbyI, HamiltonJD. The quality in Australian Health Care Study. Med J Aust. 1995;163:458-471
7. VincentC, NealeG, WoloshynowychM. Adverse events in British hospitals: preliminary retrospective record review. Br Med J. 2001;322:517-519
8. Kohn LT, Corrigan JM, Donaldson MS, editors. To err is human: building a safer health system. Washington, DC: National Academy Press; 2000.
9. GoldhillDR, SumnerA. Outcome of intensive care patients in a group of British intensive care units. Crit Care Med. 1998;26(8):1337-1345
10. ForaidaMI, DeVitaMA, BraithwaiteRS, StuartSA, BrooksMM, SimmonsRL. Improving the utilization of medical crisis teams (Condition C) at an urban tertiary care hospital. J Crit Care. 2003;18:87-94
11. HillmanKM, BristowPJ, CheyT, DaffurnK, JacquesT, NormanSL, et al. Antecedents to hospital deaths. Intern Med J. 2001;31:343-348
12. ScheinRMH, HazdayN, PenaM, RubenBH, SprungCL. Clinical antecedents to in-hospital cardiopulmonary arrest. Chest. 1990;98:1388-1392
13. HillmanKM, BristowPJ, CheyT, DaffurnK, JacquesT, NormanSL, et al. Duration of life-threatening antecedents prior to intensive care admission. Intensive Care Med. 2002;28:1629-1634

14. PerkinsGD, BarrettH, BullockI, GabbottDA, NolanJP, MitchellS, et al. The acute care undergraduate teaching (ACUTE) initiative: consensus development of core competencies in acute care for undergraduates in the United Kingdom. Intensive Care Med. 2005;31: 1627-1633

15. Donni-LenhoffFG, HedrickHL. Growth of specialization in graduate medical education. J Am Med Assoc. 2000;284:1284-1289

16. McQuillanP, PilkingtonS, AllanA, TaylorB, ShortA, MorganG, et al. Confidential inquiry into quality of care before admission to intensive care. Br Med J. 1998;316(7148):1853-1858

17. ChenJ, HillmanK, BellomoR, FlabourisA, FinferS, CretikosM, The MERIT Study Investigators for the Simpson Centre and the ANZICS Clinical Trials Group. The impact of introducing medical emergency team system on the documentation of vital signs. Resuscitation. 2009;80:35-43

18. HillmanK, JonesD, ChenJ. Rapid response systems. Med J Aust. 2014;201:519-521

19. NguyenY-L, AngusDC, BoumendilA, GuidetB. The challenge of admitting the very elderly to intensive care. Ann Intensive Care. 2011;1:29

20. BuistM, BernardS, NguyenTV, MooreG, AndersonJ, et al. Association between clinically abnormal observations and subsequent in-hospital mortality: a prospective study. Resuscitation. 2004;62:137-141

21. MercerI, BellomoR, KattulaA, BaldwinI, JonesDA, McIntyreT. The medical emergency team and end-of-life care: a pilot study. Crit Care Resusc. 2007;9:151-156

22. MannionR, DaviesH, HarrisonS, KontehF, GreenerI, McDonaldR. Quantitative explorations of culture and performance relationship. Changing organisational cultures and hospital performance in the NHS. Birmingham, UK: National Institute for Health Research, Service Delivery and Organisation Programme2010. p. 42-72.

23. HillmanK, AlexandrouE, FlabourisM, BrownD, MurphyJ, DaffurnK, et al. Clinical outcome indicators in acute hospital medicine. Clin Intensive Care. 2000;11(2):89-94

24. CretikosM, ParrM, HillmanK, BishopG, BrownD, DaffurnK, et al. Guidelines for the uniform reporting of data for medical emergency teams. Resuscitation. 2006;68(1):11-25

25. ChenJ, BellomoR, FlabourisA, HillmanK, FinferS, CretikosM, MERIT Study Investigators for the Simpson Centre and the ANZICS Clinical Trials Group. The relationship between early emergency team calls and serious adverse events. Crit Care Med. 2009;37(1):148-153

26. SantamariaJ, TobinA, HolmesJ. Changing cardiac arrest and hospital mortality rates through a medical emergency team takes time and constant review. Crit Care Med. 2010;38(2):445-450

27. JonesD, BagshawSM, BarrettJ, BellomoR, GaurayB, BucknallTK, et al. The role of the medical emergency team in end-of-life care: a multicentre prospective observational study. Crit Care Med. 2012;40(1): 98-103

28. LorenzKA, LynnJ, DySM, ShugarmanLR, WilkinsonA, MularskiRA, et al. Evidence for improving palliative care at the end of life: a systematic review. Ann Intern Med. 2008;148:147-159

Creating Process and Policy Change in Healthcare

Stuart F. Reynolds and Bernard Lawless

The word "policy" is often bantered about, and it is assumed that everyone has or uses a fundamental definition for policy and, hence, policy development. In broad terms policy can refer simply to a "plan of action" or "statement of aims or goals." However defined, it is then difficult to interpret who is involved in policy planning and what are the key functions of policy development, policy implementation, and subsequent evaluation. To better understand some of these nuances, William Jenkins defines policy as a set of incremental decisions taken by a political figure or group regarding the prioritization of goals and the means to achieve these goals. James Anderson describes public policy as a purposive course of action aimed at dealing with a problem identified by the government [1]. These begin to capture some of the key elements of public policy making and the inherent link to government as a key player in policy development and implementation.

Traditionally, policy to support large-scale implementation has not been rooted in scientific evidence and frequently has not even been well supported by anecdotal evidence [2]. The relative lack of scientific rigor is secondary to the inherent complexity of randomizing policies to the whole populations or communities, achieving agreement of measurement and analysis, maintaining internal integrity, and timing interventions with data collection and the inherent political nature of the evaluation process [2–4]. Even focused healthcare policies seem to rarely be evaluated owing to difficulties in monitoring multiple activities, the challenges of observing for disparate effects, or prolonged timelines that do not allow for observing meaningful change.

Thus, many policies and innovations need to be evaluated from a social science paradigm rather than the archetype of traditional medical science evaluation [5]. A social science paradigm enriches the evaluation by examining why certain innovations are readily adopted and sustained while others are rejected or do not perform. Systematic evaluative approaches must be utilized to provide a realistic form of evaluation.

Further challenges in policy implementation are directed by politicians or decision-makers who are less interested in science or health impact and more interested in financial implications or views of particular groups and communities [4]. The process of "evidence-based policy making" is further complicated by the fact that barriers to communication exist between researchers and decision-makers. Each profession may utilize specialty-specific terminology which is not fully

S.F. Reynolds, MD, FRCPE, FCCP (✉)
Director of Critical Care Services,
Spartanburg Regional Healthcare System,
Clinical Professor of Critical Care, Medical
University of South Carolina, AHEC 101 East Wood
Street, Spartanburg, SC 29303, USA
e-mail: sreynolds@srhs.com

B. Lawless, MD, FRCS (C)
Provincial Lead, Critical Care Services Ontario,
St. Michaels Hospital, Toronto, ON, Canada,
M5B 1W8

© Springer International Publishing Switzerland 2017
M.A. DeVita et al. (eds.), *Textbook of Rapid Response Systems*, DOI 10.1007/978-3-319-39391-9_7

understood by the listener. In addition, differences in priorities and the interpretation of findings further hinder policy development and implementation.

The policy cycle makes up the regular business of government. It strives to be incremental, continuous, and systematic, thereby aligning policy and organizational priorities. Despite what may appear to be a good model for prospective planning, the creation of new public policy often occurs as a response to a tragic situation. A recent example is the US government response, through its agencies, to the hospital-acquired infection by Ebola of two critical care nurses; the response was delayed and initially inappropriate. A distant example but more germane to the topic of rapid response systems is the province of Ontario's response to the severe acute respiratory syndrome (SARs) in 2003.

Cursory review of crisis will result in stopgap measures; however, comprehensive, systematic analyses of these crises often reveal fundamental problems with current policy or processes. In the case of SARs, comprehensive analysis revealed problems with access to critical care, critical care capacity issues, and a paucity of system integration. It became clear these issues would be magnified in the event of pandemic and were guaranteed to worsen because of the aging population. This event set in motion the transformation strategy for critical care in the province of Ontario—specifically, the development of a critical care policy that was resourced and linked to measurement and accountability.

Key to the success of policy development, implementation, and sustainability is appropriate support through funding, provision of personnel, leadership, and a constant check with clinical appropriateness. Greenhalgh et al. have noted a correlation between successful, sustained change and dedicated resource provision resulting in successful implementation and sustainable change [6]. Ovretveit and Staines in their evaluation of a large-scale long-term quality improvement program in Sweden noted that a defined minimum level of investment in infrastructure is necessary for sustainable change and coined the term "investment threshold" [7]. Staines [8] recent follow-up demonstrated clini-

cal outcome improvement in critical care and process improvement throughout the health system; and this was attributed, in part, to ongoing investment.

Implementing the RRS: A Case Study in the Theory of Policy

The theoretical underpinnings of policy and planning are instructive in understanding the implementation and success of a rapid response system. The development of a provincial rapid response system, known as the Critical Care Response Team (CCRT) project, was a cornerstone of the Critical Care Transformation Strategy in Ontario, Canada. It became readily apparent that a properly implemented rapid response system was well positioned to improve access to critical care services and mitigate demand through its integration throughout the hospital system. In principle, the RRS proactively identifies patients before physiologic collapse and potentially differentiates between those whom would and are not likely to benefit from critical care interventions.

Rapid response systems (RRS) are a challenging healthcare innovation. As with other large-scale healthcare innovations, RRS's result in a dynamic sociologic interplay thus presents similar implementation, sustainability, and evaluation challenges as those ascribed to policy implementation.

Rogers [9] in his book, *Diffusion of Innovations*, defined an innovation as an idea, a practice that is perceived as new by an individual or an organization. The diffusion of the innovation is the process whereby the innovation is communicated through members of a social system.

Rogers suggests that in order to obtain widespread acceptance, an innovation needs to demonstrate a *relative advantage*. This requires that the new idea must offer significant improvements over current practice. This is supported by other scientists' attributions that engagement in change is increased when there is a genuine belief that the innovation provides better patient care or reduces workload [10, 11].

Innovations with minimal *complexity* are more apt to be successful because complex interventions become infinitely more complex when brought to scale [9, 12]. Finally, when people see the results of an innovation, the *observability* increases the likelihood that the innovation will be both utilized and accepted.

Current data suggests that patients in acute hospitals are at risk of adverse events, including cardiac arrest and death. Most of these adverse events are predictable and therefore preventable, often through simple interventions [13, 14]. The relative advantage of an RRS is that it provides a systematic mechanism to both identify and respond to patients at risk of clinical deterioration. This is significantly better than traditional medical practice, where the patient is required to significantly deteriorate prior to obtaining expert critical care consultation and interventions, even to the point of having a cardiac arrest [15, 16]. The RRS concept is not a complex notion, but rather a common sense innovation—the quintessence of an ounce of prevention—rather than a pound of cure—or in the case of an ICU often pounding for a cure. Finally, a RRS is not restricted to the four walls of an ICU; instead the impact is readily and consistently observed throughout the hospital.

If an innovation appears to have sufficient merit, on the basis of relative advantage and simplicity, the degree to which it is adopted depends on the characteristics of those within the social system [16]. The diffusion of innovation theory identifies characteristics of those who, within an organization, are apt to support change or innovation. Early support can be expected from those within the organization who themselves are *innovators*. *Early adopters* are usually well integrated within the organization. They are usually opinion leaders, successful and often thought of as role models. *Early majority adopters* are characterized by frequent interactions with peers but are unlikely to be opinion leaders and tend to deliberate before adopting new ideas. *Late majority adopters* are characterized as skeptical and cautious, and their motivations for change arise from pressure from peers and economic sources. The last groups to adopt, or most likely to not adopt,

are unfortunately referred to as *laggards*. Greenhalgh et al. attribute individual adoption to various psychological antecedents—specifically the individual's willingness to try new things and the individual's ability to use innovation [4].

An effective communication strategy will increase the number of people willing to adopt an innovation. Stakeholder input and response to concerns improve adoption [6]. Therefore, these actions by leaders will be helpful with initial design and subsequent acceptance of an innovation. Communication during implementation that clearly defines goals and responsibilities with opinion leaders, team members, end users, and administration is imperative.

From an RRS perspective, it is important to seek out the change agents, clinical champions, opinion leaders, and innovators within the hospital system. Providing these innovators with the time to promote change maximizes benefit [17, 18]. Change agents are those who embody characteristics which promote change through engagement of staff and articulation of the foundation of the innovation or vision [10]. It is particularly important to promote the vision and obtain acceptance by administration. Such approval is a prerequisite to build a foundation of system wide acceptance and ensure that there is alignment of RRS goals with organizational values, thereby improving the chance of RRS success.

Rapid response systems have the opportunity to be a readily accepted innovation on the basis of need alone. Dodgson and Bessant [19] determined the success of an innovation relies on the recipient of the innovation to do something with the resource provided. In other words, it's not good enough to create an RRS; but it needs to be utilized to be successful. This explains the relationship between the uptake of service (adoption) of RRS and reduction in cardiac arrests and other adverse events [20, 21]. The question needs to move from does the innovation work to why does it work and in what context. This "realist evaluation" sets the stage for sustainability, as innovations reset a system equilibrium. Thus, measurement and reevaluation must be performed in order to respond to the changing environment [22, 23].

The first focus during policy implementation should therefore be on diffusion of the innovation, creating an environment that will allow the innovation to thrive. Therefore, program acceptance or utilization is a reasonable first outcome measure for the RRS. Understanding first that medical help and ICU consultation via the RRS are available is an important and essential first step. Subsequent steps can focus on fine-tuning the utilization and practice patterns of the RRS. While patient-centered and economic outcomes are the eventual proof positive of the RRS's efficacy, early valuation of the intervention may not be attainable. An example of the latter point was demonstrated in the 6-month RRT intervention in the MERIT trial [21], wherein the inability of MET hospitals to significantly reduce adverse outcomes was interpreted as ineffectiveness of the intervention, rather than the incomplete diffusion of a simple innovation with an obvious relative advantage. Thus policy and implementation science may not only inform the nature and means of advancing a particular innovation, but may also provide a clearer set of process outcomes to track at different stages of its implementation.

References

1. Anderson JE. Public policymaking: an introduction. Boston: Houghton Mifflin Company; 2003. p. 1–34.
2. Letherman S, Sutherland K. Designing national quality reforms: a framework for action. International J Qual Health Care. 2007;19(6):334–40.
3. Shimkhada R, Peabody JW, Quimbo SA, Solon O. The quality improvement demonstration study: An example of evidence-based policy-making in practice. Health Res Policy Syst. 2008;6:5.
4. Davies P. Policy evaluation in the United Kingdom. Seoul, Korea: KDI International Policy Evaluation Forum; 2004.
5. Berwick D. The science of improvement. JAMA. 2008;299(10):1182–4.
6. Greenhalgh T, Robert G, Macfarlane F, Bate P, Kyriakidou O. Diffusion of innovations in service organizations: systematic review and recommendations. Milbank Q. 2004;82:581–629.
7. Ovretveit J, Staines A. Sustained improvement? Findings from an independent case study of the Jonkoping quality program. Qual Manag Health Care. 2007;16:68–83.
8. Staines A, Thor J, Robert G. Sustaining improvement? The 20-year Jönköping quality improvement program revisited. Qual Manag Health Care. 2015;24(1):21–37.
9. Rogers EM. Diffusion of innovations. 4th ed. New York: The Free press; 1995.
10. Della Penna R, Martel H, Neuwirth EB, Rice J, Filipski MI, Green J, et al. Rapid spread of complex change: a case study in inpatient palliative care. BMC Health Serv Res. 2009;9:245.
11. Bradley E, Webster T, Baker D, LaPane K, Lipson D, Stone R, et al. Translating research into practice: speeding the adoption of innovative health care programs. Issue Brief. 2004. www.commonwealthfund.org/Publications/Issue-Briefs/2004/Jul/Translating-Research-into-Practice.
12. ExpandNet. Practical guidance for scaling up health service innovations. www.expandnet.net/PDFs/ExpandNetWHO%20Nine%20Step%20Guide%20published.pdf.
13. McGloin H, Adam S, Singer M. The quality of pre-ICU care influences outcome of patients admitted from the ward. Clin Intensive Care. 1997;8:104.
14. McQuillan P, Pilkington S, Allan A, et al. Confidential inquiry into quality of care before admission to intensive care. BMJ. 1998;316(7148):1853–8.
15. Schein RM, Hazday N, Pena M, Ruben BH, Sprung CL. Clinical antecedents to in-hospital cardiopulmonary arrest. Chest. 1990;98(6):1388–92.
16. Buist MD, Jarmolowski E, Burton PR, Bernard SA, Waxman BP, Anderson J. Recognizing clinical instability in hospital patients before cardiac arrest or unplanned admission to intensive e care. A pilot study in a tertiary-care hospital. Med J Aust. 1999;171(1):22–5.
17. Perla J, Bradbury E, Gunther-Murphy C. Large-scale improvement initiatives in healthcare: a scan of the literature. J Healthc Qual. 2013;35(1):30–40.
18. Soumerai S, McLaughlin TJ, Gurwitz JH, et al. Effect of local medical opinion leaders on quality of care for acute myocardial infarction. JAMA. 1998;279(17):1358–63.
19. Dodgson M, Bessant J. Effective innovation policy: a new approach. New York: Routledge; 1996.
20. Jones D, Bellomo R, Bates S, et al. Long term effect of a medical emergency team on cardiac arrests in a teaching hospital. Crit Care. 2005;9:R808–15.
21. MERIT Study Investigators. Introduction of the medical emergency team (MET) system: a cluster randomised controlled trial. Lancet. 2005;365(9477):2091–7.
22. Reynolds S. Sustainability of RRS presentation. International rapid response system and medical emergency team symposium. Toronto 2008.
23. Pawson R, Tilley N. Realistic evaluation. London: Sage; 1997.

The Assessment and Interpretation of Vital Signs

John Kellett

Introduction

Vital signs are the simplest and probably the most important information gathered on hospitalized patients. After almost a century of neglect, vital signs are now an area of active research. A vital sign could be defined as any patient feature that predicts outcome, indicates the need for specific treatment, or which can be used to monitor clinical course. Some patient features, such as date of birth and sex, are stable, whereas others, including the four traditional vital signs, are dynamic and can change from moment to moment. Several such features have been proposed as additional vital signs. Pain [1], breathlessness [2], oximetry [3, 4], mental status [5], functional status, and mobility [6] have all been proposed as vital signs. In addition to diabetic patients, blood glucose is an essential measurement in patients with alerted mental status, and it has also been proposed as one of the criteria that identifies sepsis [7]. Other laboratory tests and biomarkers might also be considered as vital signs. This chapter will discuss the assessment and interpretation of these extra vital signs as well as the traditional ones.

The Four Classic Vital Signs

The four classic vital signs are respiratory rate, temperature, pulse rate, and blood pressure. Although their measurement has been standard practice for over a century, over this time there have been surprisingly few attempts to quantify their clinical performance. Until recently the largest study of respiratory rate was performed by Hutchinson in 1846 [8], and the largest studies on fever remain those performed by Wunderlich in the nineteenth century [9]. Amazingly the ominous significance of low temperatures has only recently been appreciated [10, 11], and the mortality risk associated with transient hypotension only reported for the first time in 2006 [12]. It was not until 1966 that the prognostic significance of the relationship between a high heart rate and low blood pressure (i.e., the Shock Index) was recognized [13] and not until 1997 that combining vital signs into early warning scores was proposed [14].

What Is the "Normal Range" of the Four Traditional Vital Signs?

The "normal" range for a medical test has been traditionally defined as being within two standard deviations of the mean of the healthy population.

J. Kellett, MD (✉)
Adjunct Associate Professor in Acute and Emergency Medicine, University of Southern Denmark, Hospital of South West Jutland, Esbjerg, Denmark
e-mail: jgkellett@eircom.net

© Springer International Publishing Switzerland 2017
M.A. DeVita et al. (eds.), *Textbook of Rapid Response Systems*, DOI 10.1007/978-3-319-39391-9_8

This does not mean that all values outside the statistically normal range are necessarily associated with illness or an increased risk of death. Conversely values within the normal range may occasionally be associated with illness and death if the patient is sick, while occasionally healthy individuals can present with a persistent abnormality of one vital sign and remain well. Rather than this statistical approach, Bleyer et al. attempted to define vital sign values in terms of their associated mortality. They reported the ranges of vital signs associated with a 5%, 10%, and 20% in-hospital mortality during multiple observations made on 42,430 consecutive patients admitted to an American tertiary care hospital from January 1, 2008, and June 30, 2009 [16]. They defined a "critical" vital sign as one associated with an in-hospital mortality of 5% or more and found that usually patients had at least two vital signs within the critical range. If no vital signs were in the "critical" range, patients had an in-hospital mortality of only 0.24%, while three or more abnormal vital signs increase the risk 19-fold [16].

Bleyer et al.'s findings do not completely agree with the in-hospital mortality associated with the admission vital signs on 75,419 patients admitted to Thunder Bay Regional Health Sciences Center (TBRHSC), Canada, between 2005 and 2010 [17] (Table 8.1). The overall mortality of Bleyer et al.'s patients was lower than TBRHSC patients (1.8% versus 2.8%). However, the prevalence of different vital sign values is broadly similar in both patient populations (Figs. 8.1–8.5). Although the mortality rates at high and low vital signs were higher in the TBRHSC patients, the ranges of all the vital signs associated with the lowest mortality were similar in both patient populations – even though the mortality rates in these ranges were statistically different, these differences were so small as to be of little clinical importance. An alternative approach would be to accept that the vital sign values assigned a score of zero by the well-validated UK National Early Warning Score (NEWS) could be considered to be "normal," since they have been shown to be associated with no increased risk of death within 24 hours [15].

Table 8.1 Ranges of vital signs associated with different rates of in-hospital mortality as reported by Bleyer et al. and those admitted to Thunder Bay Regional Health Sciences Center (TBRHSC)

			In-hospital mortality		
Vital sign		Study	5–9%	10–19%	>20%
Systolic blood pressure (mmHg)		Bleyer et al.	70–79	60–69	<60
		TBRHSC	90–99	80–89	<80
			≥200		
Heart rate (beats per minute)		Bleyer et al.	120–139	140–169	≥170
		TBRHSC	100–119	120–149	≥150
			20–29		
Breathing rate (breaths per minute)	Low	Bleyer et al.	8–11	<8	
		TBRHSC	≤10		
	High	Bleyer et al.	28–31	32–35	≥36
		TBRHSC	22–25	26–29	≥30
Temperature (degrees C)	Low	Bleyer et al.	34.5–34.9	<34.5	
		TBRHSC	35.0–35.4	34.5–34.9	<34.5
	High	Bleyer et al.	39.0–39.9	≥40	
		TBRHSC	≥40		
Oxygen saturation (%)		Bleyer et al.	≤90		
		TBRHSC	91–93	87–90	<87

Table 8.2 Proportion of patients and mortality rates associated with a NEWS of zero and the ranges of vital signs with the lowest mortality rates in patients reported by Bleyer et al. and Thunder Bay Regional Health Sciences Center (TBRHSC) patients (see Figs. 1–5)

		NEWS = 0			
		Proportion of patients		In-hospital mortality	
		Bleyer et al.	TBRHSC	Bleyer et al.	TBRHSC
Systolic blood pressure	*111–219 mmHg*	92%*	84%	2.1%*	2.2%
Heart rate	*51–90 bpm*	71%	73%	1.6%	1.9%
Respiratory rate	*12–20 bpm*	61%	65%	1.9%	1.9%
Temperature	*36.1–38.0 °C*	63%*	78%	1.8%*	2.3%
Oxygen saturation	*≥96%*	55%	70%	1.9%	2.1%
		Vital sign ranges with the lowest mortality			
		Proportion of patients		In-hospital mortality	
		Bleyer et al.	TBRHSC	Bleyer et al.	TBRHSC
Systolic blood pressure	*100–200 mmHg*	66%	83%	2.1%	2.5%
Heart rate	*50–90 bpm*	71%	73%	1.6%	1.9%
Respiratory rate	*16–20 bpm*	51%	61%	1.8%	1.6%
Temperature	*36–38 °C*	63%*	78%	1.8%[a]	2.3%
Oxygen saturation	*95–99%*	60%	79%	1.9%	2.0%

bpm beats or breaths per minute; [a] extrapolated from incomplete data provided in Ref. [16]

With the possible exception of breathing rate, the in-hospital mortality associated with NEWS ranges assigned a score of zero roughly corresponded to those of both Bleyer et al.'s and TBRHSC data (Table 8.2) and is also consistent with current single-parameter MET "track and trigger" systems [18].

Pulse Rate

Sir William Osler, while neither defining bradycardia nor tachycardia, remarked that a slow pulse was sometimes normal and that Napoleon had a pulse rate of only 40 beats per minute [19]. The accepted limits for heart rate have long been set at between 60 and 100 beats per minute [20]; however, these recommendations are "traditional" and not based on any systematic clinical studies [21]. Although the lower and upper limit of normal for the pulse rate of 60 and 100 beats per minute was "generally agreed" and endorsed by the New York Heart Association in 1953 [20], they were never confirmed by any systematic

clinical investigations. Only relatively recently has Spodick et al. reported that the mean heart rate for men and women was 70–75 beats per minute with two standard deviation limits of 43–93 beats per minute in men and 52–94 beats per minute for women. There was no significant change from ages 50 to 80 [21]. Nevertheless, it is still a common practice for beta-blockers to be held, even in those with a recent myocardial infarction, if the pulse falls below 60 beats per minute. However, sinus bradycardia occurs in normal children [22] and adults [23, 24], particularly during sleep when rates of 30 beats per minute and pauses of up to 2 s are not uncommon [23, 25]. Bradycardia may also be seen in the absence of heart disease in the elderly [26], has no adverse effect on longevity [27], and is of no prognostic significance in otherwise healthy subjects. It is hard to interpret the significance of the increased mortality associated with heart rates below 40 beats per minute observed in TBRHSC and Bleyer et al.'s patients, as heart rates this low only occurred in 0.1% of patients (Fig. 8.1).

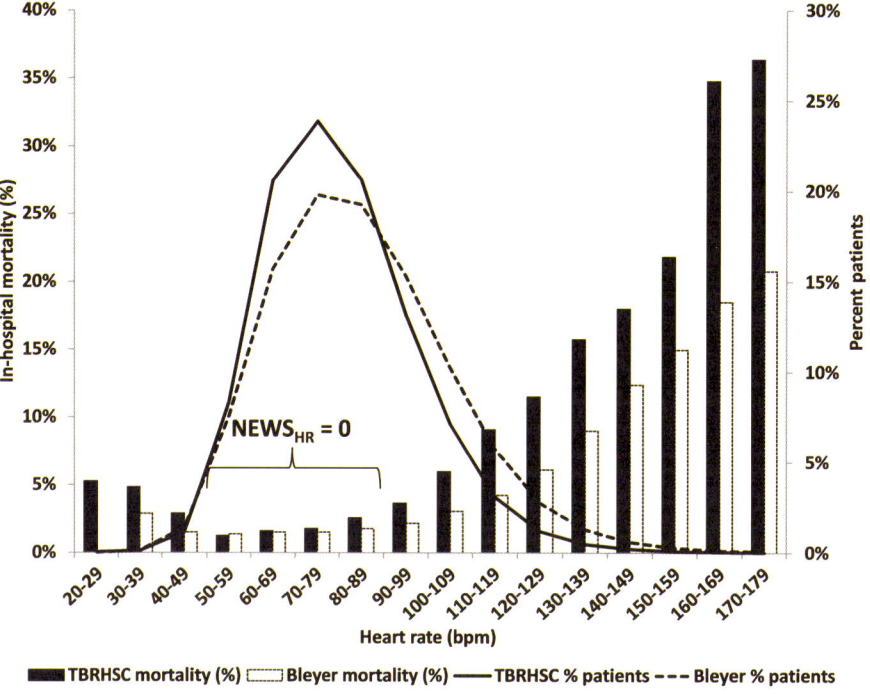

Fig. 8.1 In-hospital mortality according to heart rate in 42,430 patients admitted to hospital reported by Bleyer et al. (Ref. [16]) and 75,419 patients admitted to Thunder Bay Regional Health Sciences Center (TBRHSC) (Ref. [17]). $NEWS_{HR} = 0$—range of heart rate with a National Early Warning Score of zero (Ref [15]). bpm = beats per minute. *Bars* show mortality, and *lines* show percentage of patients

Blood Pressure

Although low diastolic pressure has been reported to be a better predictor of cardiac arrest than systolic pressure [28], hypotension has been mostly studied in terms of systolic pressure and has been defined as a systolic blood pressure below 90 mmHg or a reduction of more than 40 mmHg from the patient's usual pressure [29]. The obvious problem with this definition is determining the patient's "usual" blood pressure in an emergency. In a study of 815 healthy subjects, the two standard deviation lower limits of systolic blood pressure over 24 h were 102 mmHg in men and 95 mmHg in women; overnight this fell to 90 mmHg in men and 84 mmHg in women [30]. Low blood pressure, therefore, is not a reliable indicator of severe illness and on its own does not indicate inadequate cardiac output, intravascular volume, or peripheral perfusion unless other symptoms and signs are present. However, for "sick" patients requir-

ing hospitalization, even a transient reduction of systolic blood pressure below 100 mmHg increases the risk of death [12]. This does not necessarily mean that hypotension should always be corrected immediately. The rapid treatment of hypotension after major trauma, for example, is controversial as there is concern that too rapid and large increase in pressure may be associated with worse outcomes [31].

Ironically, once systolic blood pressure drops below 100 mmHg, it may be difficult to detect manually both by auscultation and palpation, and detection by automated devices is unreliable. Most of these automated devices rely on a piezoelectric crystal that detects pressure oscillations. Systolic blood pressure is taken at the appearance of a pulsatile signal, mean pressures are taken as the peak oscillations, while diastolic blood pressure is calculated using a proprietary formula [32]. Many such devices have been found to be inaccurate at systolic blood pressures below 120 mmHg [33]. Therefore, all low

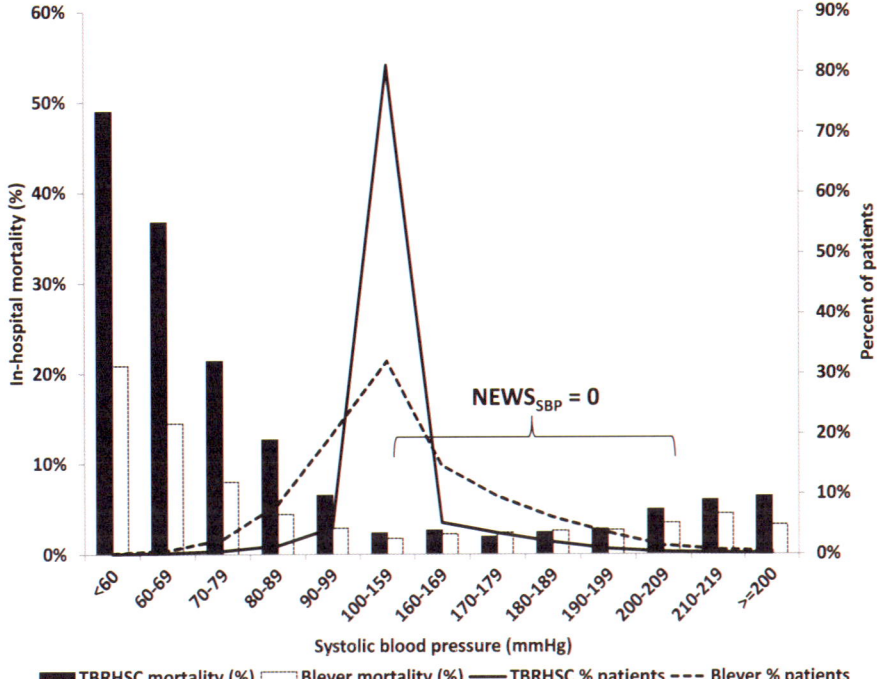

Fig. 8.2 In-hospital mortality according to systolic blood pressure in 42,430 hospitalized patients reported by Bleyer et al. (Ref. [16]) and 75,419 patients admitted to Thunder Bay Regional Health Sciences Center (TBRHSC) [Ref 17]. NEWS$_{SBP}$ = 0 indicates the range of systolic blood pressures that would not receive any points (i.e., considered largely normal) by the National Early Warning Score (NEWS) (Ref. [15]). *Bars* show mortality, and *lines* show percentage of patients

blood pressure readings (i.e., systolic blood pressure below 120 mmHg) should be carefully verified. Indeed, once the pulse can no longer be felt at the wrist, the systolic blood pressure probably cannot be measured accurately noninvasively [34].

Although several severity of illness scores [10, 35–39] consider hypertension a risk factor, for both TBRHSC and Bleyer et al.'s patients, elevated blood pressure was not associated with an increased risk of death, except possibly for the 2.0% of patients with a blood pressure above 200 mmHg (Fig. 8.2). This may not be the case for patients with altered mental status. Ikeda et al. reported that an intracranial lesion was more likely if patients with impaired consciousness had a systolic blood pressure over 170 mmHg [40]. Moreover, the Cushing response of bradycardia with hypertension is a well-recognized clinical manifestation of increased intracranial pressure [41].

Temperature

There was only a modest increase in mortality associated with temperatures above 38°C in both TBRHSC and Bleyer et al.'s patients. In contrast, a low temperature was much more ominous (Fig. 8.3). More than 120 years ago, Wunderlich's million observations on 25,000 subjects defined the "normal" human temperature as 37 °C. Unfortunately recent tests suggest that his thermometers may have been calibrated as much as 1.4 °C–2.2 °C higher than today's instruments [42]. More recently Mackowiak et al. reported that 36.8 °C +/− 0.4°C was the normal range of oral temperature and the 37.2 °C and 37.7 °C were the upper limits of normal morning and evening temperature, respectively [9]. Body temperature varies at different parts of the body. In 2002 Sund-Levander et al. defined a wide normal range of oral temperature from 33.2°C to 38.2°C [43]. Tympanic

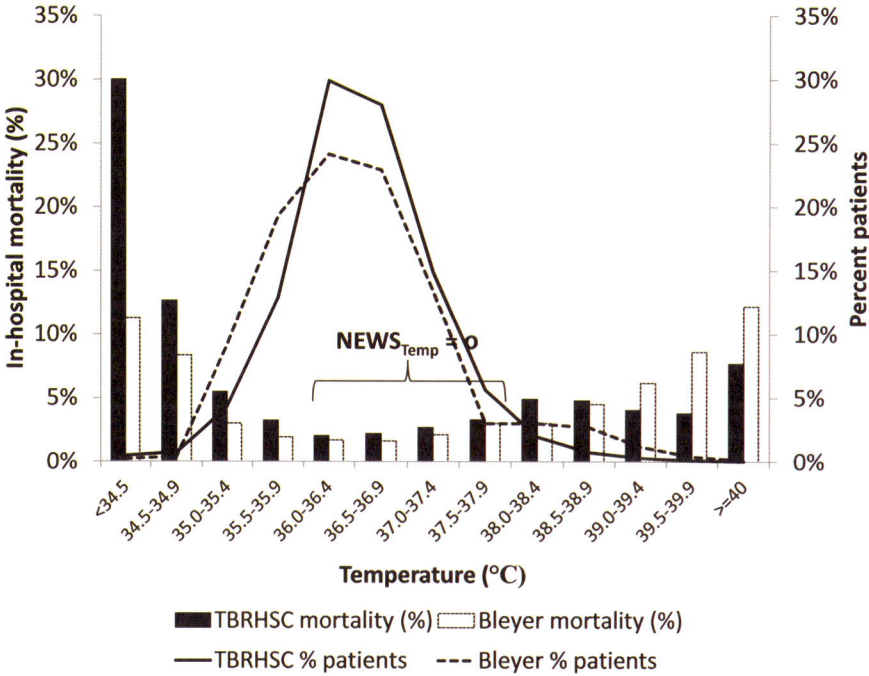

Fig. 8.3 In-hospital mortality according to body temperature in 42,430 hospitalized patients reported by Bleyer et al. (Ref. [16]) and 75,419 patients admitted to Thunder Bay Regional Health Sciences Center (TBRHSC) (Ref. [17]). $NEWS_{Temp} = 0$ indicates the range of temperatures that would not receive any points (i.e., considered largely normal) by the National Early Warning Score (NEWS) (Ref. [15]). *Bars* show mortality, and *lines* show percentage of patients

temperature, however, had a narrow normal range from 35.4 °C to 37.8 °C.

Temperature changes both heart and breathing rate [9, 44–46]. In a recent study of 4493 Danish patients, these changes have been shown to vary according to the patient's temperature. If the patient's temperature was below 36.4 °C, then the heart rate changed by 2.7 SD 1.9 beats per minute per °C and breathing rate by 0.5 SD 0.5 breaths per minute per °C; if the temperature was between 36.4 °C and 37.2 °C, then the heart rate changed by 6.9 SD 1.9 beats per minute per °C and breathing rate by 1.5 SD 0.5 breaths per minute per °C, and at a temperature above 37.2 °C, heart rate changed by 7.4 SD 0.9 beats per minute per °C and breathing rate by 2.3 SD 0.3 breaths per minute per °C [47].

Since the time of Florence Nightingale, doctors and nurses have feared fever and responded to it energetically. However, the benefits of reducing fever have been recently questioned [48, 49]. Infected patients with an increased temperature have been reported to have a better outcome than those without fever, and infected hypothermic patients are twice as likely to die. Out of 1901 patients with infection treated with antibiotics within 24 h of arrival to a large Danish hospital, those without fever (i.e., 36.0–38.0 °C) were twice as likely to die as those with a temperature over 38 °C (i.e., 18.1% versus 9.3%) [50]. In a related study of 3563 patients presenting with severe infections, the 30-day mortality for patients admitted with a temperature below 36 °C was 27.9% versus 14.4% for those with a higher temperature; the hazard ratio for mortality adjusted for sex, age, comorbidity, and number of organ failures was 2.1 (95% CI, 1.4–3.2) [51].

Respiratory Rate

Respiratory rate is a powerful predictor of disease severity and of a poor outcome [52], and, since it is increased by both hypoxia and metabolic acidosis, it can indicate severe derangement in many body systems [53]. It has been called the vexatious clinical sign because it requires patience and diligence to measure accurately [54]. Although currently there is no widely used convenient, cheap, reliable method of monitoring respiratory rate, these are in development and may soon be available for widespread use [55]. Respiratory rate measurements by nursing staff correlate poorly with those of prototype machine systems and, unlike machine measurements, did not predict patient outcome [56]. Only a few studies have examined the interobserver reliability of respiratory rate measurements, and these depended upon a few observers assessing the same patients, but not necessarily at exactly the same time [52, 57, 58]. Since respiratory rate fluctuates over time, it is not certain that these observers were all witnessing the same rate. This problem has been avoided by using video recordings of seven acutely ill medical patients to assess the interobserver reliability of respiratory rate measurement by trained nurses with a median experience of 15.2 years. The respiratory rates reported for each video ranged from 22 to 36, 24 to 32, 14 to 32, 12 to 30, 22 to 32, 20 to 30, and 19 to 30 breaths per minute, respectively; the individual intra-class coefficient was only 0.13 (95% CI, 0.00–0.56) [59].

Although many authors have defined the "normal" respiratory rate to be from 8 to 18 breaths per minute, there are few studies to support their conclusions. In the studies that are available, the mean respiratory rate is between 16 and 20.5 breaths per minute, and only one of these studies was performed on emergency patients [60]. The largest published study was probably that of Hutchinson in 1846 [8] who reported a mean respiratory rate in 1714 adult males of 20.2 with a range of 6 to 40 breaths per minute—patients with pneumonia had a mean rate of 28 breaths per minute [61]. In 1959 Mead measured the respiratory rate in 75 adults seated at a public gathering and found the mean to be 16 with a range between 11 and 26 [62]. In 1982 McFadden found the normal respiratory rate in 82 hospitalized elderly adults to be 20.5 breaths per minute [63]. In 1988 Hooker et al. [60] reported the "normal" respiratory rates in 110 emergency department patients as 20.1 +/− 4.0 breaths per minute—almost identical to other reports [64]. For any given level of alveolar ventilation, there is an

optimum respiratory rate at which the muscular work of breathing is minimal [65, 66]. In normal subjects this "theoretical" optimum frequency was predicted by Otis et al. to be 15 breaths per minute [67]. However, when diseases such as pneumonia modify the elastic and airway properties of the lung, the respiratory frequency at which minimum work is performed for the required level of alveolar ventilation changes [67].

Several respiratory rates have been suggested as triggers for emergency response teams, ranging from 14 to over 36 breaths per minute [68, 69]. The current evidence-based consensus is that an adult with a respiratory rate over 20 breaths/minute is unwell, and a rate over 24 breaths/minute indicates critical illness [52, 69–74]. Just over half of all patients suffering a serious adverse event on the general wards (such as a cardiac arrest or ICU admission) have been reported to have a respiratory rate greater than 24 breaths per minute. These patients could have been identified as high risk up to 24 hours before the event with a specificity of over 95% [52]. Goldhill and colleagues reported that 21% of ward patients with a respiratory rate of 25–29 breaths/minute assessed by a critical care outreach service died in hospital [72]. These results are worse than those of the Bleyer et al.'s and TBRHSC cohorts. Mortality rate increased in TBRHSC patients when respiratory rate was 22 or more breaths per minute and 24 breaths per minute for Bleyer et al.'s patient cohort. Although TBRHSC and Bleyer et al.'s patients with a breathing rate below 10 breaths per minute had an in-hospital mortality rate of 9%, they represented less than 0.2% of patients. Similarly only 2.7% of patients had breathing rates over 28 breaths per minute, which were associated with a 14.7% mortality rate (Fig. 8.4). The rarity of extremely slow and fast breathing rates is probably explained by the fact that neither can be tolerated for prolonged periods, and both require an emergency intervention.

The Shock Index

The ratio between pulse rate and blood pressure (i.e., the Shock Index) was first described by Allgower and Buri in 1967 [13] and has a normal range from 0.5 to

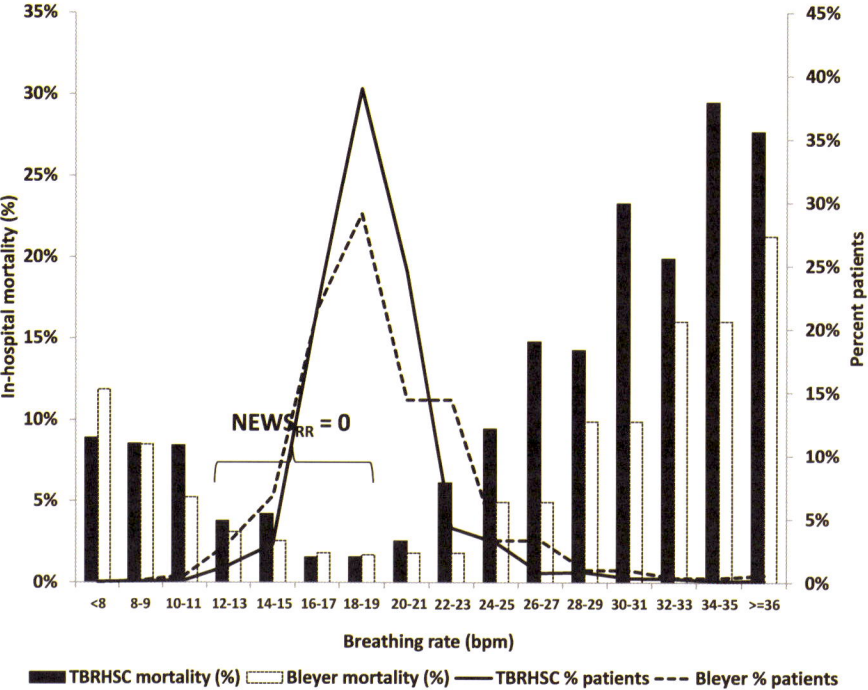

Fig. 8.4 In-hospital mortality according to breathing rate in 42,430 patients admitted to hospital reported by Bleyer et al. (Ref. [16]) and 75,419 patients admitted to Thunder Bay Regional Health Sciences Center (TBRHSC) (Ref. [17]). NEWS$_{RR}$ = 0 indicates the range of respiratory rates that would not receive any points (i.e., considered largely normal) by the National Early Warning Score (NEWS) (Ref. [15]). *Bars* show mortality, and *lines* show percentage of patients

0.7 in healthy adults. The in-hospital mortality of acutely ill medical patients admitted to TBRHSC increased from 1.3% for those with a Shock Index of 0.3 to 25% for those admitted with an index of ≥1.5 (Fig. 8.6). The Shock Index is elevated in acute hypovolemia and left ventricular dysfunction and correlates with left ventricular end-diastolic pressure [75–77]. Hypotension and tachycardia are common in metabolic brain dysfunction caused by, for example, intoxication, endocrine disease, and sepsis [78]. The Shock Index has been used to predict the outcome of ectopic pregnancy [79], traumatic injury [80], sepsis, gastrointestinal hemorrhage [81], and pulmonary embolus [82]. Persistent elevation of the Shock Index over 1.0 for several hours following trauma or acute circulatory failure has been related to a poor outcome [83]. While a pulse rate below 100 beats per minute with a systolic blood over 110 mmHg and a respiratory rate of 16 breaths per minute indicates a blood loss of less than 750 ml, a pulse rate over 140 beats per minute in association with a systolic

blood pressure below 90 mmHg and a respiratory rate over 26 breaths per minute indicates Class IV shock or a blood loss of over 2000 ml [84].

The ratio between pulse pressure and systolic blood pressure (i.e., the pulse pressure index) has also been proposed a predictor of cardiovascular outcomes [85]. Recently this has been reported, along with respiratory rate, heart rate, and diastolic blood pressure, to be an accurate predictor of cardiac arrest [28].

Oximetry

Although developed in 1974 [86], many newly qualified doctors are still unaware of the normal range of oxygen saturation and do not know how to investigate or adequately manage patients with low values [87]. Patients cannot by an act of will lower their oxygen saturation below 95% at sea level, and mortality rises dramatically once oxygen saturation

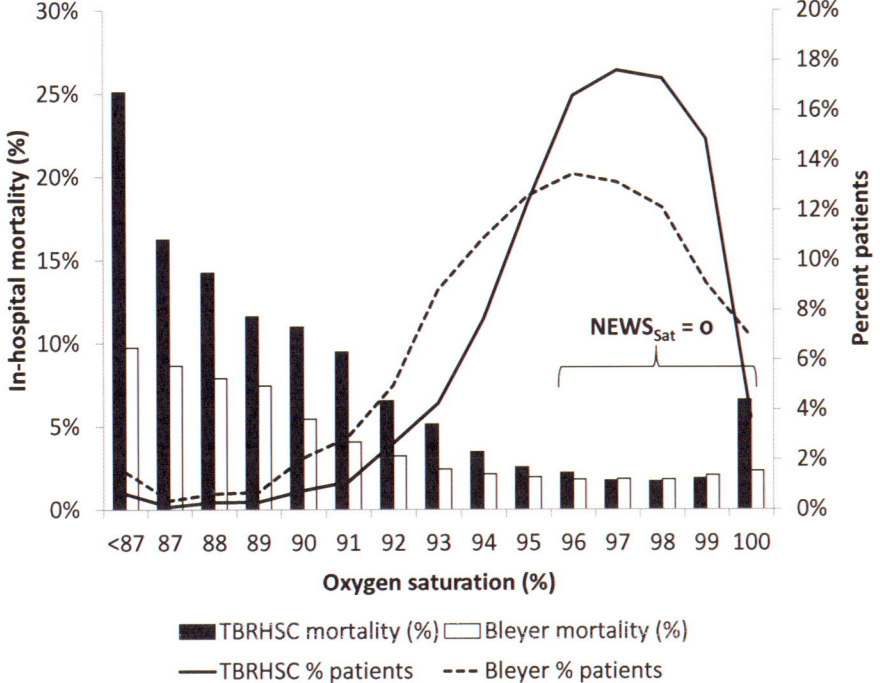

Fig. 8.5 In-hospital mortality according to oxygen saturation in 42,430 patients admitted to hospital reported by Bleyer et al. (Ref. [16]) and 75,419 patients admitted to Thunder Bay Regional Health Sciences Center (TBRHSC) (Ref. [17]). NEWS$_{Sat}$ = 0 indicates the range of oxyhemoglobin saturation that would not receive any points (i.e., considered largely normal) by the National Early Warning Score (NEWS) (Ref. [15]). *Bars* show mortality, and *lines* show percentage of patients

falls below this level. The high mortality rate of TBRHSC patients with an oxygen saturation of 100% is probably explained by the use of supplemental oxygen in seriously ill patients (Fig. 8.5). Oximetry requires little skill or training and rapidly measures both oxygen saturation and pulse rate—if neither is detectable it is likely that the patient has poor peripheral circulation and is either suffering from hypovolemia or some other form of low cardiac output. In addition the response of both oxygen saturation and pulse rate to exercise and change in posture can be quickly assessed. A rise in heart rate of more than 30 beats per minute on standing indicates the presence of hypovolemia [88], while a fall in oxygen saturation with exercise indicates a likelihood for serious lung or heart disease [89–92], especially in the elderly [89].

Pain

Pain is one of the most common reasons for seeking medical care, and the proposal that it be considered the fifth vital sign in 1995 [1] has been widely adopted. This has produced a number of unfortunate unintended consequences because pain assessment and treatment have been poorly taught [93–95] and, in particular, the fundamental differences between acute and chronic pain have not been recognized [96, 97]. While pain has been reported to produce physiological changes in the autonomic nervous system leading to cardiovascular changes, there is little or no correlation between the severity of pain experienced and other vital sign changes or the degree of injury [98]. Hypertension associated with acute chest

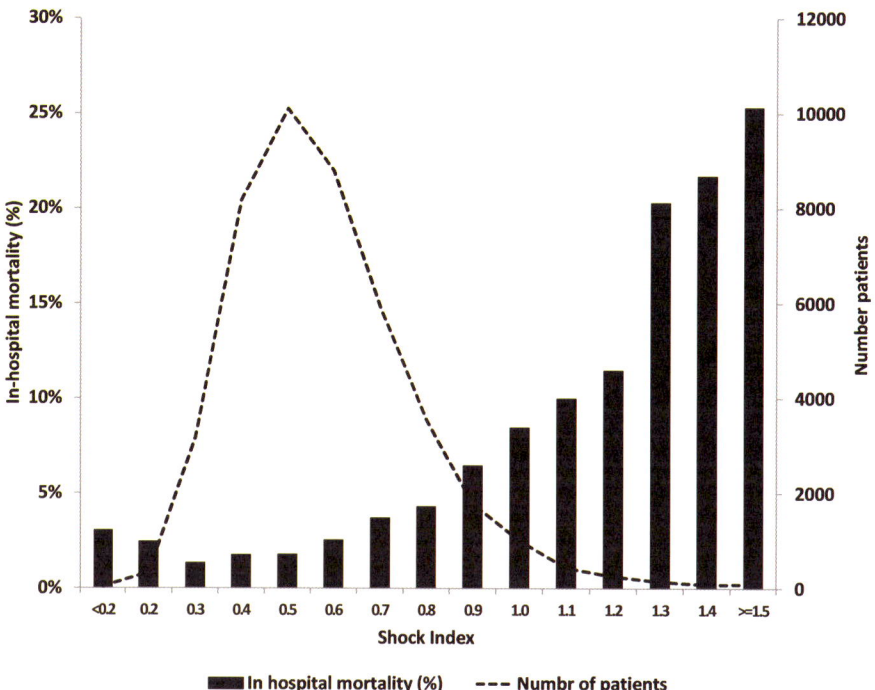

Fig. 8.6 In-hospital mortality by Shock Index (i.e., pulse rate in beats per minute divided by systolic blood pressure in mmHg) in 43,693 consecutive unselected acute medical patients admitted to Thunder Bay Regional Health Sciences Center (TBRHSC) (Ref. [17]). *Bars* show mortality, and *lines* show number of patients

pain improves its outcome [99, 100], and some pains, such as nonspecific chest pain, are associated with reduced, rather than increased, in-hospital mortality [64]. Physiological responses, therefore, are often not specific enough to serve as pain indicators [101, 102].

The rationale behind making pain a vital sign is that pain is injurious to the patient and that its control is of benefit. Even though the relationship between the tissue damage of battlefield injuries and the amount of pain experienced has been shown to be statistically significant, it is surprisingly small [103]. Acute pain and injury of various types are inevitably interrelated, and the associated complex neurohumoral and immune injury response may become counterproductive and have adverse effects [104, 105]. However, it may be difficult to determine if the adverse events associated with pain are caused by the pain itself or its treatment. It is not clear, for example, if postoperative ileus is caused by pain or its treatment with opiates [106]. Yet when pain is produced without any tis-

sue injury (e.g., by electrical stimulation of the abdominal wall), it still evokes such an injury response with an increase in cortisol, catecholamines, and glucagon and decreased insulin sensitivity [107], and this response is reduced by effective pain relief [108]. Moreover, there is increasing evidence that effective pain relief, at least by some treatments, reduces the complications of surgery and improves outcomes [109].

It has been argued that recording pain routinely does not change management or greatly influence outcomes [110]. The explanation for this is that the assessment and treatment of pain is complex and requires a combination of experience, skill, and knowledge that may not be consistently applied. Pain is an individual, multifactorial experience influenced by culture, previous pain events, beliefs, mood, and ability to cope [111, 112]. Therefore, pain measured on scales based on the patients' subjective assessments is inevitably unreliable and may not agree with those of their caregivers [113]. Although good inter-rater agreement on the assessment of pain has been reported [114–116], this is not the case in practice [117]. Prescription rates for long-acting opiates are increasing and, according to geographical location and other factors, vary considerably [118, 119]. Data from the USA, where the use of pain medication is dramatically increasing and currently 3% of the Americans are receiving long-acting or extended-release opiates each year [120], suggests that pain assessment by health-care professionals is highly variable and prone to a large variety of influences and perverse incentives.

Pain assessment includes evaluation of the type of pain, its intensity, its functional impact, and its response to treatment using tools that are consistent, valid, and reliable [121]. There are three common types of pain: somatic, visceral, and neuropathic. These can be distinguished by the patient's description and associated findings [122]. Various different scales are used to measure pain intensity. Categorical scales are quick and simple, using verbal descriptors (e.g., none, mild, moderate, severe, excruciating) that can be converted to numerical scales for clarity and easy comparison over time. Such verbal numerical scales when recalled over the previous 24 h have been shown to be a reasonable indicator of the average pain experienced by the patient during that time [123]. Visual analogue scales consist of a 100 mm horizontal line that starts with "no pain" and ends with "the worst pain imaginable" along which the patient marks the severity of their pain: a mark between 5 and 44 mm, between 45 and 70 mm, and more than 70 mm indicates mild, moderate, and severe pain, respectively [124], while a greater than 30 mm reduction in pain signifies a clinically meaningful response to treatment [125–129]. These scales correlate well with the less sensitive categorical and numerical rating scales [130–132] and have been shown to be linear for mild, moderate, and severe postoperative pain [133, 134]. The variance of visual analogue scales can be reduced by combining them with emoticon faces [135, 136], and computer programs are being developed that can automatically detect pain based on facial expressions [137]. For patients who cannot communicate (e.g., children, postoperative patients, ventilated patients, those with dementia, etc.), various behavioral and functional scales have also been developed [138, 139].

The WHO pain ladder for the treatment of cancer pain was introduced in 1987 [140] and coincided with promotion of long-acting opiate formulations amidst accusations that physicians, in particular, were poor at pain assessment and even had a sadistic reluctance to treat it [141]. While it might have been true that the medical profession was inappropriately "narcophobic" in the past, this is certainly no longer the case [142]. In the USA, narcotic prescriptions increased by an order of magnitude between 1990 and 2010, and drug overdoses are now the second leading cause of accidental death, with legally prescribed narcotics causing more deaths than heroin and cocaine combined [120]. This is the result of chronic pain being inappropriately considered and treated as a vital sign, so that an immediate treatment response is demanded at each assessment. Opiates are now prescribed inappropriately for many forms of chronic pain including chronic abdominal pain, chronic back pain, as well as the other multiple aches associated with aging. The opioid-tolerant patients that such treatment creates are more difficult to manage if and when they do develop, for whatever reason, severe acute pain [143]. The management of acute pain, in particular, is too complex to be captured by the simple WHO four-step ladder, and the poor management of acute postoperative pain is now known to greatly increase the risk of chronic postoperative pain [144, 145]. Instead each step increase in pain severity should represent a platform of multiple treatments (e.g., ketamine infusions, tricyclic antidepressants, anticonvulsants, etc.) [143, 146], which also incorporate non-pharmacological and supportive options that can be tailored to the individual patient's requirements.

Breathlessness

Breathlessness, respiratory rate, and oxygen saturation are all independent predictors of in-hospital mortality [64]. Dyspnea is a complex phenomenon. While a relationship between respiratory effort, chemoreceptors, and mechano-receptors has been suggested, the precise physical mechanism of dyspnea remains unclear [147]. Although there is an association between dyspnea and anxiety [148–150], the severity of breathlessness cannot be attributed to psychological factors alone [151].

In addition to vital signs and pulse oximetry the assessment of acute breathlessness should also determine: if the patient can complete a sentence, if there is cough or sputum, if there is peripheral oedema, and then observe the chest wall and accessory muscle movements and auscultate the chest. A number of tools are available to measure dyspnea including visual analogue, Likert, and numerical rating scales. The sensitivity and reproducibility of these scales are broadly similar, although the Borg scale may outperform the others in some cases. The Borg or Rating of Perceived Dyspnea (RPD) scale is a categorical scale consisting of numbers and a set of verbal qualifiers [152]. Originally it was developed to measure exertion and referred to as the Rating of Perceived Exertion (RPE) scale ranging from 6 to 20. A 10-point ratio scale was subsequently developed to quantify both dyspnea (RPD) and exertion (RPE) in COPD. The Medical Research Council Scale [153] is a quick, simple, and valid method of assessing the patient's usual disability produced by dyspnea [154, 155]. However, since it does not capture rapid changes in breathlessness, it is not useful for day-to-day monitoring of patients.

Mental and Functional Status

Overreliance on the traditional vital signs reduces the patient to a series of numbers that are deemed to be either normal or abnormal. Treatment is often simplistically directed at returning values to within the normal range, so that if a vital sign is "abnormal," efforts are made to either lower or raise it. This ignores the fact that changes in vital signs are compensatory and represent the body's attempt to restore circulatory homeostasis. The benefits of overaggressive correction of hypotension [156] and pyrexia [48, 49] have recently been questioned. The best

judge as to whether or not a vital sign value is appropriate for a clinical situation is to ask the patients how they feel or observe their mental and physical functions [157].

Mental Status

While florid dementia and delirium may be obvious, mild alteration of mental status is often not noticed, thought to be a normal part of the aging process, or, in the intoxicated young, not taken seriously [158]. Although most reports consider altered mental status to be largely confined to the elderly [158], it can occur in the young, as a consequence of alcohol and drug intoxication. Although such patients are disruptive and consume a considerable amount of time and attention, their mortality rates are low. On the other hand, any degree altered mental status is associated with death in older patients [159].

There are four components to mental status: alertness, memory, thought content, and behavior. Changes in alertness are the most frequently monitored, commonly using either the Glasgow Coma Scale or the AVPU scale (i.e., alert and calm, responds to voice, responds to pain, and unresponsive) [160]. Approximately 10% of acutely ill patients admitted to hospital in the developed world have impaired alertness (i.e., Glasgow Coma Scale less than 14), and 3% are in coma (i.e., only respond to pain or are unresponsive) (16,161). Any alteration in alertness has been shown to considerably increase in-hospital mortality. Agitation also increases the chance of death, both within 24 h [161] and after 1 year [159, 162], and has been reported to be twice as common in patients as sedation [161].

In delirium mental status fluctuates and often includes changes in thought content such as disorientation, delusions, and hallucinations. Delirium is a serious condition, especially in elderly hospitalized patients, and the Confusion Assessment Method (CAM score) and its modifications are becoming the standard method of assessment [163]. In contrast to delirium, dementia is a stable condition characterized by impaired short-term memory usually with normal alertness and, often, normal behavior. However, in some cases, such as vascular dementia, dementia can be associated with major behavioral changes, such as aggression and wandering, which makes its management problematic. The cardinal features of delirium are inattention and altered level of consciousness (i.e., agitation, lethargy, stupor, and coma), which can be quickly assessed [163]. However, fluctuations in confusion or disorganized thinking require prolonged observation and may, therefore, not be appreciated during the initial emergency room encounter.

Functional Status

The prognostic importance of frailty and reduced mobility is well documented [164]. Rylance et al. reported an increased mortality in patients admitted to a Tanzanian hospital depending on whether they walked into the hospital unaided, required help to walk, or were brought in by stretcher [165]. His findings have been confirmed in young patients elsewhere in Africa [166, 167] and in elderly Irish [64, 168, 169] as well as in a large group of Danish [170] patients. Moreover, several well-validated early warning scores include a mobility component [164–166, 171, 172]. Adding mobility to NEWS has been show to increase its discrimination both in African patients [167] and Danish patients [173]. Mobility may be particularly important for patients presenting with a low NEWS—only 0.8% of a Danish patient cohort with an initial NEWS score of 0–2 who were not bedridden died within 30 days compared with 7.6% of bedridden patients, $p < 0.001$ [173]. The inability to walk is common in patients, occurring in as many as 11% of patients and carrying a similar odds ratio for in-hospital mortality in patients in both developed and developing countries (i.e., odds ratio 4.6) [64, 165–170]. In these studies all that was recorded was whether the patient was walking freely around the ward without assistance, required help to walk, or was bedridden. The inability of the patient to walk is, therefore, a simple observation that can be rapidly assessed. It has been incorporated into the Cape Triage Score, which has recently been introduced in many centers in South Africa, and has been shown to reduce both patient waiting time and mortality [174, 175].

In addition to delaying death, the prime objective of health care, especially of the elderly, should be to maintain independence, prevent functional decline, and improve the quality of life. Traditionally, none of these objectives are accurately or reliably recorded as functional status is often poorly documented and may show little agreement with the opinions expressed by patients when they are subsequently interviewed [176]. A minimum data set on the functional status of all residents of certified nursing homes is now required in the USA and has been tested elsewhere [177]. However, these assessments are complex and time-consuming and not easily suited to acute hospital care. In contrast a brief battery of physical performance assessments, which include gait speed, can be quickly and easily performed and predict the risk of future hospitalization and decline in health and function in the elderly [178]. A four-item scale based on whether the patients had a stable gait and unstable gait, needed help to walk, or was bedridden (i.e., SUHB scale) strongly correlates with 30-day in-hospital mortality, mental status, history of falls, manual handling requirements, and the presence of pressure sores, dementia, and incontinence. The c statistics of the SUHB scale for 30-day in-hospital mortality, mental status, history of falls, manual handling requirements, and the presence of pressure sores, dementia, and incontinence were 0.85, 0.79, 0.79, 0.94, 0.80, 0.86, and 0.88, respectively [179]. Currently methods that use accelerometers to measure mobility and assess frailty and falls risk are under development [180]. These hold the promise of cheaply continuously monitoring and assessing the movement of all acutely ill patients both in and out of hospital.

Age and Vital Signs

The mortality associated with all vital sign abnormalities is greatly influenced by age. Patients aged ≥ 80 years with a breathing rate of 24–25 breaths per minute have been reported to have four times the mortality of those in the age between 40 and 64 years, and those aged ≥ 80

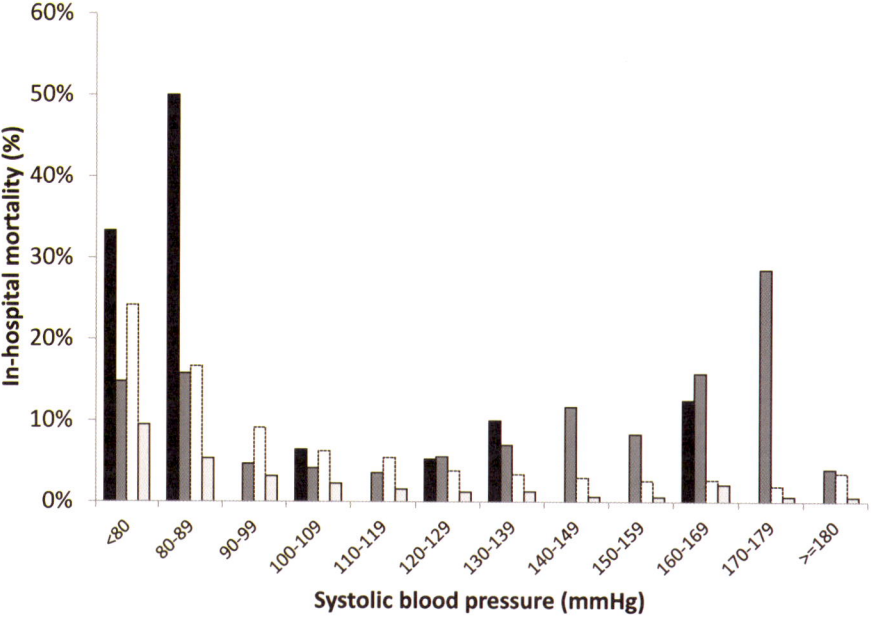

Fig. 8.7 In-hospital mortality according to systolic blood pressure and age in 43,693 acute medical patients admitted to Thunder Bay Regional Health Sciences Center (TBRHSC) (Ref. [17]) and 1,350 acutely ill medical patients admitted to St. Joseph's Kitovu Health Care Complex, Masaka, Uganda (Kitovu)

years with a systolic blood pressure from 90 to 94 mmHg have ten times the mortality of those between 40 and 64 years [181]. These differences may be attributable to the natural physiology of illness in the elderly, or it may be that older patients require more rapid correction of vital sign abnormalities than is currently provided.

It has often been assumed that the physiology of the sick elderly must be different from the sick young [181] as, at least in the developed world, older patients are far more likely to die than younger ones. However, age has been reported to make no difference to the in-hospital mortality of Ugandan patients [182]. The in-hospital mortality of TBRHSC patients over 70 years of age was much higher than younger patients for all levels of systolic blood pressure. However, in those with a systolic blood pressure over 110 mmHg, the mortality rate of patients admitted to an Ugandan mission hospital was substantially higher than that of TBRHSC patients regardless of their age. Unlike TBRHSC patients, in these African patients mor-

tality increased at the same rate in younger and older patients as blood pressure increased (Fig. 8.7). The differences in mortality between older and younger patients, therefore, are not present in all patient populations and, therefore, may be explained by factors other than age, such as differences in the causes and nature of illness and quality of care. Furthermore, when vital signs are combined into an early warning score, depending on how the thresholds are selected, the impact of age on the score's discrimination can be largely eliminated [183].

Vital Sign Trends

Outside of intensive care units, clinical practice currently relies on the periodic, manual observation of vital signs, which typically occurs every 4–6 h in most hospital wards. In the near future, wearable devices are likely to become available that will provide continuous streams of vital sign information on all patients. This will generate massive requirements for both their storage and analysis, with potential dangers associated with the availability of too much information [184] such as information overload, false alarms, alarm fatigue, etc. Since it is not known how often, to what extent, and over what time frame vital signs change and what the implications of those changes are, it is impossible to know how to respond to them or develop rational management protocols [185].

The temperature chart pattern is of diagnostic value; a rising pulse rate with a falling blood pressure identifies hypovolemia and shock, and a slow pulse and rising blood pressure is caused by raised intracranial pressure. However, little else is known about the changes and trends of individual vital signs during the entire course of acute illness in hospital. Recent studies have started to explore the trends in vital signs during hospitalization. Patients who suffered a cardiac arrest in hospital had increases both in their respiratory and heart rates prior to arrest. In contrast in control patients, these vital signs remained more or less stable throughout their hospital stay. Although blood pressure also fell in patients who arrested, these changes were not significantly different from controls [28]. A retrospective study of all the vital signs recorded during the hospitalization of TBRHSC patients showed that in patients who died, temperature changed very little throughout their time in hospital and their blood pressure only fell a few hours before death. Although heart rate started to increase and oxygen saturation fell sometime before death, respiratory rate was the vital sign that changed the most before death, and these changes occurred well before changes in other vital signs were detected. Even so, for all vital signs these differences were modest and only became apparent when they were amplified by applying the NEWS weighting system to them [186].

Vital signs are constantly changing, so that they are better expressed by their trends rather than their precise value at any one point in time. Since the technology to measure them continuously is only becoming available, we have very little knowledge on the clinical significance of their changes over time, such as the directions, rates, variability, or patterns of change. The physiologi-

cal response to illness is a complex adaptive system that we do not fully understand. Vital signs do not change in isolation, so that a change in one vital sign cannot be assumed to be an improvement or deterioration without taking into account what is happening to the other vital signs and the rest of the patient's physiology. Combining vital signs into early warning scores might be one simple method of taking multiple vital sign changes into account. However, so far studies on early warning score trends suggest that improving scores may not predict a better outcome, especially in the first few hours after treatment [187–189]. An alternative more sophisticated approach is to try to improve outcome predictions by manipulating vital signs using neural networks [190].

Laboratory Tests and Biomarkers

Although laboratory and biomarker results are not traditionally considered to be vital signs, they have become an integral part of the assessment of acute illness and are the main component of risk stratification scores such as APACHE and SOFA. Indeed it could be argued that in the minds of many clinicians, lab studies are awarded inappropriately more weight than traditional bedside vital signs. Nevertheless some tests, such as blood sugar, are so cheap and easy to perform at the bedside and provide such valuable information that it is hard to deny their importance. Routine evaluation of acutely ill patients now always includes an ECG, full blood count, urea and electrolytes, and increasingly the use of bedside biomarkers such as troponin and D-dimers. In addition to diagnosing cardiac disease, ECG abnormalities have been shown to predict mortality [64, 156, 191, 192]. A recent review has identified five novel biomarkers (i.e., fatty acid-binding protein, ischemia-modified albumin, B-type natriuretic peptide, copeptin, and matrix metalloproteinase-9) that, combined with troponin levels, have the potential to improve the speed and accuracy of acute coronary syndrome diagnosis [193]. The novel biomarkers copeptin and peroxiredoxin levels have also been used to identify the risk of deterioration of elderly patients presenting with nonspecific complaints [194]. Several scoring systems of combined laboratory results have been developed [195–199]. While four of these scores based on biochemical data were excellent predictor of mortality, their precision was low and required adjustment from local data to recalculate the scores [200].

Summary

Serious illness is more likely to be present when there is a combination of abnormal vital signs rather than a single abnormality. Both the magnitude and interrelationship between vital signs can provide valuable diagnostic and therapeutic information, and both should be considered as part of any patient evaluation (Fig. 8.8). Moreover, the vital signs, including mental status, are strongly influenced by pain, breathlessness, acute diagnoses, and medication. All of these factors together will determine the patient's functional status and sense of well-being. The first signs of illness are subjective changes in the patient's sense of well-being. In the elderly this is often followed by impairment of functional status, which may occur before changes in traditional vital signs are detected. Noninvasive monitoring technology will soon start to provide streams of continuous vital sign information that will improve our understanding of the evolution of critical illness. It remains to be seen if this sophisticated technology will be able to predict patient deterioration before subjective or objective signs of illness are apparent or at a time where therapeutic intervention can alter morbidity and mortality.

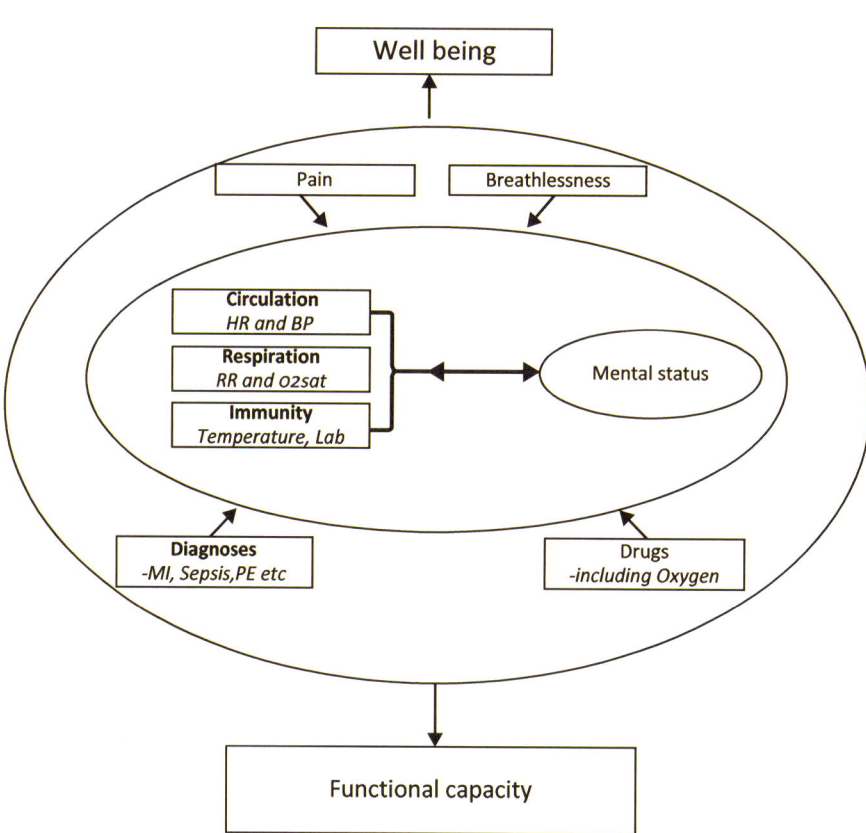

Fig. 8.8 Conceptual model of how vital signs influence and are related to each other. For explanation, *see* Summary. HR = heart rate, BP = blood pressure, RR = respiratory rate, O2sat = oxygen saturation, Lab = laboratory investigations and biomarkers, MI = myocardial infarction, PE = pulmonary embolus

Acknowledgment The author would like to acknowledge the assistance and cooperation of Kristi Taylor and Dawn Bubar of the Thunder Bay Regional Health Sciences Center information technology department. He would also like to thank Dr Martin Opio, Kitovu Hospital, Masaka, Uganda, and Dr Mikkel Brabrand, Department of Medicine, Sydvestjysk Sygehus, Esbjerg, Denmark, for their help and advice.

Conflict of interest Dr John Kellett is a director and chief medical officer of Tapa Healthcare DAC, Dundalk, Ireland.

References

1. Campbell JN. American pain society 1995 presidential address. Pain forum. J Pain. 1996;5:85–8.
2. Registered Nurses' Association of Ontario. Nursing care of dyspnea: the 6th vital sign in individuals with chronic obstructive pulmonary disease (COPD). Toronto, Canada: Registered Nurses' Association of Ontario; 2005.
3. Mower W, Myers G, Nicklin E, Kearin K, Baraff L, Sachs C. Pulse oximetry as a fifth vital sign in emergency geriatric assessment. Acad Emerg Med. 1998;5:858–65.
4. Neff T. Routine oximetry. A fifth vital sign? Chest. 1988;94:227.
5. Flaherty JH, Rudolph J, Shay K, Kamholz B, Bookvar KS, Shaughnessy M, Shapiro R, Stein J, Weir C, Edes T. Delirium is a serious and unrecognized problem: why assessment of mental status should be the sixth vital sign. J Am Med Dir Assoc. 2007;8:273–5.
6. Bierman AS. Functional status: the sixth vital sign. J Gen Intern Med. 2001;16:785–6.
7. Dellinger RP, Levy MM, Rhodes A, et al. Surviving sepsis campaign: international guidelines for management of severe sepsis and septic shock: 2012. Crit Care Med. 2013;41(2):580–637.
8. Hutchinson J. On the capacity of the lungs, and on the respiratory functions with a view to establishing a precise and easy method of detecting disease by the spirometer. Med Chir Trans. 1846;29:137–252.
9. Mackowiak PA, Wasserman SS, Levine MM. A critical appraisal of 98.6 degrees F, the upper limit of the normal body temperature and other legacies of Carl Reinhold August Wunderlich. JAMA. 1992;268:1578–80.
10. Subbe CP, Kruger M, Rutherford P, Gemmel L. Validation of a modified early warning score in medical admissions. Q J Med. 2001;94:521–6.
11. Duckitt RW, Buxton-Thomas R, Walker J, Cheek E, Bewick V, Venn R, Forni LG. Worthing physiological scoring system: derivation and validation of a physiological early-warning system for medical admissions. An observational, population-based single-centre study. Br. J. Anaesth. 2007;98:769–74.
12. Jones AE, Yiannibas V, Johnson C, Kline JA. Emergency department hypotension predicts sudden unexpected in-hospital mortality. Chest. 2006;130:941–6.
13. Allgower M, Buri C. Shockindex Deutsche Medizinische Wochenschrift 1967; 46:1–10.
14. Morgan RJ, Williams F, Wright MM. An early warning scoring system for detecting developing critical illness. Clin Intensive Care. 1997;8:100.
15. Royal College of Physicians; National early warning score (NEWS): standardising the assessment of acute illness severity in the NHS. Report of a working party. London: RCP 2012. <www.rcplondon.ac.uk/resources/nationalearlywarningscore-news>.
16. Bleyer AJ, Vidya S, Russell GB, et al. Longitudinal analysis of one million vital signs in patients in an academic medical center. Resuscitation. 2011;82:1387–92.
17. Kellett J, Kim A. Validation of an abbreviated Vitalpac TM early warning score (ViEWS) in 75, 419 consecutive admissions to a Canadian Regional Hospital. Resuscitation. 2011;83:297–302.
18. Smith GB, Prytherch DR, Schmidt PE, Featherstone PI, Higgins B. A review, and performance evaluation, of single-parameter "track and trigger" systems. Resuscitation. 2008;79:11–21.
19. Osler W. Neuroses of the heart. In: Osler W, editor. The principles and practice of medicine. Edinburgh and London: Young J. Pentland; 1901. p. 759.
20. Criteria Committee of the New York Heart Association. Nomenclature and criteria for diagnosis of diseases of the heart. 5th ed. New York: New York Heart Association; 1953.
21. Spodick DH, Raju P, Bishop RL, Rifkin RD. Operational definition of normal sinus heart rate. Am J Cardiol. 1992;69:1245–6.
22. Scott O, Williams GJ, Fiddler GI. Results of 24 hour ambulatory monitoring of electrocardiogram in 131 healthy boys aged 10 to 13 years. Br Heart J. 1980;44:304–8.
23. Brodsky M, Wu D, Denes P, et al. Arrhythmias documented by 24 hour continuous electrocardiographic monitoring in 50 male medical students without apparent heart disease. Am J Cardiol. 1977;39:390–5.
24. Bjerregaard P. Mean 24 hour heart rate, minimal heart rate, and pauses in healthy subjects 40-79 years of age. Eur Heart J. 1983;4:44–51.
25. Hilgard J, Ezri MD, Denes P. Significance of ventricular pauses of three seconds or more on 24 hour Holter recordings. Am J Cardiol. 1985;55:1005–8.
26. Agruss NS, Rosin EY, Adolph RJ, Fowler NO. Significance of chronic sinus bradycardia in elderly people. Circulation. 1972;46:924–30.
27. Tresch DD, Fleg JL. Unexplained sinus bradycardia: clinical significance and long term prognosis in apparently healthy persons older than 40 years. Am J Cardiol. 1986;58:1009–12.
28. Churpek MM, Yuen TC, Huber MT, Park SY, Hall JB, Edelson DP. Predicting cardiac arrest on the wards a nested case-control study. Chest. 2012;141:1170–6.
29. Bone RC, Balk RA, Cerra FB, Dellinger RP, Fein AM, Knaus WA, Schein RM, Sibbald WJ. Definitions

for sepsis and organ failure and guidelines for the use of innovative therapies in sepsis. The ACCP/SCCM consensus conference committee. American college of chest physicians/society of critical care medicine. Chest. 1992;101:1644–55.

30. O'Brien E, Murphy J, Tyndall A, Atkins N, Mee F, McCarthy G, Staessen J, Cox J, O'Malley K. Twenty-four-hour ambulatory blood pressure in men and women aged 17 to 80 years: the allied Irish bank study. J Hypertens. 1991;9:355–60.

31. Stern SA, Dronen SC, Birrer P, Wang X. Effect of blood pressure on hemorrhage volume and survival in a near-fatal hemorrhage model incorporating a vascular injury. Ann Emerg Med. 1993;22:155.

32. Wonka F. Oscillometric blood pressure measurement: description of the method used. Z Kardiol. 1996;85:1–7.

33. Beaubien ER, Card CM, Card SE, Biem HJ, Wilson TW. Accuracy of the dinamap 1846 XT automated blood pressure monitor. J Hum Hypertens. 2002;16:647–52.

34. Deakin CD, Low JL. Accuracy of the advanced trauma support guidelines for predicting systolic blood pressure using carotid, femoral and radial pulses: observational study. BMJ. 2000;321:673–4.

35. Knaus WA, Draper EA, Wagner DP, et al. APACHE II: a severity of disease classification system. Crit Care Med. 1985;12:818–29.

36. Olsson T, Lind L. Comparison of the rapid emergency medicine score and APACHE II in non-surgical emergency department patients. Acad Emerg Med. 2003;10:1040–8.

37. Rhee K, Fisher C, Willitis N. The rapid acute physiology score. Am J Emerg Med. 1987;5:278–86.

38. Le Gall J-R, Lemeshow S, Saulnier F. A new simplified acute physiology score (SAPS II) based on a European/North American multicenter study. JAMA. 1993;270:2957–63.

39. Lemeshow S, Teres D, Klar J, Avrunin JS, Gehlbach SH, Rapoport J. Mortality probability models (MPM II) based on an international cohort of intensive care patients. JAMA. 1993;270:2478–86.

40. Ikeda M, Matsunaga T, Irabu N, Yoshida S. Using vital signs to diagnose impaired consciousness: cross sectional observational study. BMJ. 2002;325:800–5.

41. Guyton AC, Hall JE. Textbook of medical physiology. 9th ed. Philadelphia: W.B. Saunders; 1996. p. 209–20.

42. Mackowiak PA. Concepts of fever. Arch Intern Med. 1998;158:1870–81.

43. Sund-Levander M, Forsberg C, Wahren LK. Normal oral, rectal, tympanic and axillary body temperature in adult men and women: a systematic literature review. Scand J Caring Sci. 2002;16:122–8.

44. Tanner JM. Relation of heart rate and body temperature in man at rest. J Physiol. 1951;114:9–10p.

45. Lyon D. The relation of pulse-rate to temperature in febrile conditions. Q J Med. 1927;20:205–18.

46. Davies P, Maconochie I. The relationship between body temperature, heart rate and respiratory rate in children. Emerg Med J. 2009;26:641–3.

47. Jensen MM, Brabrand M. The relationship between body temperature, heart rate and respiratory rate in acute patients at admission to a medical care unit. 6th Danish emergency medicine conference, Odense 2014. Abstracts. Scandinavian Journal of Trauma, Resuscitation and Emergency Medicine 2015 23(Suppl 1):A12.

48. Young PJ, Saxena M. Fever management in intensive care patients with infections. Crit Care. 2014;18:206.

49. Kushimoto S, Yamanouchi S, Endo T, Sato T, Nomura R, Fujita M, Kudo D, Omura T, Miyagawa N, Sato T. Body temperature abnormalities in non-neurological critically ill patients: a review of the literature. J Intensive Care. 2014;2:14.

50. Henriksen DP, Jensen HCK, Laursen CB, Lassen AT. Increased short-term mortality among normothermic patients presenting to a medical emergency department with infection - a cohort study. 6th Danish Emergency Medicine Conference, Odense 2014. Abstracts. Scandinavian Journal of Trauma, Resuscitation and Emergency Medicine 2015 23(Suppl 1): A26.

51. Henriksen DP, Laursen CB, Lassen AT. Patients hospitalized with severe infections and hypothermia, a cohort study of mortality and prognostic factors. 6th Danish emergency medicine conference, Odense 2014. Abstracts. Scand J Trauma, Resusc Emerg Med. 2015;23(Suppl 1):A27.

52. Cretikos M, Chen J, Hillman K, Bellomo R, Finfer S, Flabouris A. The MERIT study investigators. The objective medical emergency team activation criteria: a case-control study. Resuscitation. 2007;73:62–72.

53. Cretikos MA, Bellomo R, Hillman K, Chen J, Finfer S, Flabouris A. Respiratory rate: the neglected vital sign. Med J Aust. 2008;188:657–9.

54. Lovett PB, Buchwald JM, Sturmann K, Bijur P. The vexatious vital: neither clinical measurements by nurses nor electronic monitor provides accurate measurements of respiratory rate in triage. Ann Emerg Med. 2005;45:68–76.

55. Tarassenko L, Villarroel M, Guazzi A, Jorge J, Clfton DA, Pugh C. Non-contact video-based vital sign monitoring using ambient light and autoregressive models. Physiol Meas. 2014;35:807–31.

56. Kellett J, Li M, Rasool S, Green GC, Seely A. Comparison of the heart and breathing rate of acutely ill medical patients recorded by nursing staff with those measured over 5 min by a piezoelectric belt and ECG monitor at the time of admission to hospital. Resuscitation. 2011;82:1381–6.

57. Lim WS, Carty SM, Macfarlane JT, et al. Respiratory rate measurement in adults – how reliable is it? Respir Med. 2002;96:31–3.

58. Lui LL, Gallaher MM, Davis RL, et al. Use of a respiratory clinical score among different providers. Pediatr Pulmonol. 2004;37:243–8.

59. Brodersen JB, Hallas P, Brabrand M. Respiratory rate – interobserver reliability study. 6th Danish Emergency Medicine Conference, Odense 2014.

Abstracts. Scand J Trauma, Resusc Emerg Med. 2015;23(Suppl 1):A14.

60. Hooker EA, O'Brien DJ, Danzel DF, Barefoot JAC, Brown JE. Respiratory rates in emergency department patients. J Emerg Med. 1989;7:129–32.

61. Hutchinson J. Thorax. In: Todd RB. editor. Cyclopaedia of anatomy and physiology. London: Longman, Brown, Green, Congmans, and Roberts; 1849:IV. p. 1079–87.

62. Mead JH. Control of respiratory frequency. J Appl Physiol. 1960;15:325–36.

63. McFadden JP, Price RC, Eastwood HD, Briggs RS. Raised respiratory rate in elderly patients: a valuable physical sign. BMJ. 1982;284:626–7.

64. Kellett J, Deane B. The simple clinical score predicts mortality for 30 days after admission to an acute medical unit. Q J Med. 2006;99:771–81.

65. Otis AB, Fenn WG, Rahn H. Mechanics of breathing in man. J Appl Physiol. 1950;2:592–607.

66. McIlroy MB, Marshall R, Christie RV. The work of breathing in normal subjects. Clin Sci. 1954;13:127–36.

67. Marshall R, Christie RV. The visco-elastic properties of the lungs in acute pneumonia. Clin Sci. 1954;13:403–8.

68. Hillman K, Chen J, Cretikos M, et al. MERIT study investigators. Introduction of the medical emergency team (MET) system: a cluster randomised controlled trial. Lancet. 2005;365:2091–7.

69. Subbe CP, Davies RG, Williams E, et al. Effect of introducing the modified early warning score on clinical outcomes, cardio-pulmonary arrests and intensive care utilisation in acute medical admissions. Anaesthesia. 2003;58:797–802.

70. Hodgetts TJ, Kenward G, Vlachonikalis IG, et al. The identification of risk factors for cardiac arrest and formulation of activation criteria to alert a medical emergency team. Resuscitation. 2002;54:125–31.

71. Fieselmann JF, Hendryx MS, Helms CM, et al. Respiratory rate predicts cardiopulmonary arrest for internal medicine patients. J Gen Intern Med. 1993;8:354–60.

72. Goldhill DR, McNarry AF, Mandersloot G, et al. A physiologically-based early warning score for ward patients: the association between score and outcome. Anaesthesia. 2005;60:547–53.

73. Goldhill DR, McNarry AF. Physiological abnormalities in early warning scores are related to mortality in adult inpatients. Br J Anaesth. 2004;92:882–4.

74. Harrison GA, Jacques TC, Kilborn G, et al. The prevalence of recordings of the signs of critical conditions and emergency responses in hospital wards — the SOCCER study. Resuscitation. 2005;65:149–57.

75. Rady MY, Nightingale P, Little RA, Edwards JD. Shock index: a re-evaluation in acute respiratory failure. Resuscitation. 1992;23:227–34.

76. Rady MY. The role of central venous oximetry, lactic acid concentration and shock index in the evaluation of clinical shock: a review. Resuscitation. 1992;24:55–60.

77. Rady MY, Rivers EP, Martin GB, Smithline H, Appelton T, Nowak RM. Continuous central venous oximetry and shock index in the emergency department: use in the evaluation of clinical shock. Am J Emerg Med. 1992;10:538–41.

78. Victor M, Ropper AH. Coma and related disorders of consciousness. In: Adams and Victor's principles of neurology. 7th ed. New York: McGraw-Hill; 2001. p. 366–89.

79. Birkhahn RH, Gaeta TJ, Bei R, Bove JJ. Shock index in the first trimester of pregnancy and its relationship to ruptured ectopic pregnancy. Acad Emerg Med. 2002;9:115–9.

80. King RW, Plewa MC, Buderer NM, Knotts FB. Shock index as a marker for significant injury in trauma patients. Acad Emerg Med. 1996;3:1041–5.

81. Rady MY, Smithline HA, Blake H, Nowak R, Rivers E. A comparison of the shock index and conventional vital signs to identify acute critical illness in the emergency department. Ann Emerg Med. 1994;24:685–90.

82. Kline JA, Nelson RD, Jackson RE, Courtney DM. Criteria for the safe use of d-dimer testing in emergency department patients with suspected pulmonary embolism: a multicenter US study. Ann Emerg Med. 2002;39:144–52.

83. Ostern HJ, Trentz O, Hemplemann G, Trentz OA, Sturm J. Cardiorespiratory and metabolic patterns in multiple trauma patients. Resuscitation. 1980;7: 169–84.

84. Fundamental Critical Care Support, 3rd Edition. In: Zimmerman JL. editor. Society of critical care medicine des plaines. Illinois; 2001, p. 9–4.

85. Yang P-L, Li Y-C. Pulse pressure index (pulse pressure/systolic pressure) may be better than pulse pressure for assessment of cardiovascular outcomes. Med Hypotheses. 2009;72:729–31.

86. Sinex JE. Pulse oximetry: principles and limitations. Am J Emerg Med. 1999;17:59–67.

87. Smith GB, Poplett N. Knowledge of aspects of acute care in trainee doctors. Postgrad Med J. 2002;78:335–8.

88. McGee S, Abernethy WB, Simel DL. Is this patient hypovolemic? JAMA. 1999;281:1022–9.

89. Pilling J, Cutaia M. Ambulatory oximetry monitoring in patients with severe COPD: a preliminary study. Chest. 1999;116:314–21.

90. Schenkel NS, Burdet L, de Muralt B, Fitting JW. Oxygen saturation during daily activities in chronic obstructive pulmonary disease. Eur Respir J. 1996;9:2584–9.

91. Rao V, Todd TRJ, Kuus A, Buth KJ, Pearson FG. Exercise oximetry versus spirometry in the assessment of risk prior to lung resection. Ann Thorac Surg. 1995;60:603–8.

92. Warner L, Bartlett KA, Charles SA, O'Brien LM. Use of pulse oximetry with exercise in the diagnosis of PCP. Int Conf AIDS. 1991;7:232.

93. Weiner DK, Turner GH, Hennon JG, Perera S, Hartmann S. The state of chronic pain education in geriatric medicine fellowship training programs: results of a national survey. J Am Geriatr Soc. 2005;53:1798–805.

94. Cayea D, Perera S, Weiner DK. Chronic low back pain in older adults: What physicians know, what they think they know, and what they should be taught. J Am Geriatr Soc. 2006;54:1772–7.

95. Mezei L, Murinson BB. Pain education in North American medical schools. J Pain. 2011;12:1199–208.

96. Morone NE, Weiner DK. Pain as the 5th vital sign: exposing the vital need for pain eduction. Clin Ther. 2013;35:1728–32.

97. Pergolizzi J. The development of chronic pain: physiological CHANGE necessitates a multidisciplinary approach to treatment. Curr Med Res Opin. 2013;29:1127–35.

98. Lord B, Woollard M. The reliability of vital signs in estimating pain severity among adult patients treated by paramedics. Emerg Med J. 2011;28:147e150.

99. Stenestrand U, Wijkman M, Fredrikson M, Nystrom FH. Association between admission supine systolic blood pressure and 1-year mortality in patients admitted to the intensive care unit for acute chest pain. JAMA. 2010;303:1167–72.

100. Irfan A, Haaf P, Meissner J, Twerenbold R, Reiter M, Reichlin T, Schaub N, Zbinden A, Heinisch C, Drexler B, Winkler K, Mueller C. Systolic blood pressure at emergency department presentation and 1-year mortality in acute chest pain patients. Eur J Intern Med. 2011;22:495–500.

101. Hadjistavropoulos T, Von Baeyer C, Craig KD. Pain assessment in persons with limited ability to communicate. In: Handbook of pain assessment. Turk DC, Melzack R. editors. New York-London: The Guilford Press; 2001. p. 134–50.

102. Arboura C, Gélinasa C. Are vital signs valid indicators for the assessment of pain in postoperative cardiac surgery ICU adults? Intensive and Critical Care. Nursing. 2010;26:83–90.

103. Fowler M, Slater TM, Garza TH, Maani CV, DeSocio PA, Hansen JJ, McGhee LL. Relationships between early acute pain scores, autonomic nervous system function, and injury severity in wounded soldiers. J Trauma. 2011;71:S87–90.

104. Kehlet H, Dahl JB. Anaesthesia, surgery, and challenges in postoperative recovery. Lancet. 2003;362:1921–8.

105. Chapman CR, Tuckett RP, Song CW. Pain and stress in a systems perspective: reciprocal neural, endocrine, and immune interactions. J Pain. 2008;9:122–45.

106. Lubawski J, Saclarides T. Postoperative ileus: strategies for reduction. Ther Clin Risk Manag. 2008;4:913–7.

107. Greisen J, Juhi CB, Grofte T, Vilstrup H, Jensen TS, Schmitz O. Acute pain induces insulin resistance in humans. Anesthesiology. 2001;95:578–84.

108. Desborough JP. The stress response to trauma and surgery. Br J Anaesth. 2000;85:109–17.

109. Kehlet H, Holte K. Effect of postoperative analgesia on surgical outcome. Br J Anaesth. 2001;87:62–72.

110. Mularski RA, White-Chu F, Overbay D, Miller L, Asch SM, Ganzini L. Measuring pain as the 5th vital sign does not improve quality of pain management. J Gen Intern Med. 2006;21:607–12.

111. George SZ, Dannecker EA, Robinson ME. Fear of pain, not pain catastrophizing, predicts acute pain intensity, but neither factor predicts tolerance or blood pressure reactivity: an experimental investigation in pain-free individuals. Eur J Pain. 2006;10:457–65.

112. Williams ACdeC, Davies HTO, Chadury Y. Simple pain rating scales hide complex idiosyncratic meanings. Pain 2000; 85:457–463.

113. Berg I, Sjostrom B. A comparative study of nurses' and elderly patients ratings of pain and pain tolerance. J Gerontol Nurs. 1999;5:30–6.

114. Aissaoui Y, Zeggwagh AA, Zekraoui A, Abidi K, Abouqal R. Validation of a behavioral pain scale in critically ill, sedated, and mechanically ventilated patients. Anesth Analg. 2005;101:1470–6.

115. Ahlers SJGM, van Gulik L, van der Veen AM, van Dogen HPA, Bruins P, Belitser SV, de Boer A, Tibboel D, Knibbe CAJ. Comparison of different pain scoring systems in critically ill patients in a general ICU. Crit Care. 2008;12:R15.

116. Ahlers SJGM, van der Veen AM, van Dijk M, Tibboel D, Knibbe CAJ. The use of the behavioral pain scale to assess pain in conscious sedated patients. Anesth Analg. 2010;110:127–33.

117. Lorenz KA, Sherbourne CD, Shugarman LR, Rubenstein LV, Wen L, Cohen A, Goebel JR, Hagenmeier E, Simon B, Lanto A, Asch SM. How reliable is pain as the fifth vital sign? J Am Board Fam Med. 2009;22:291–8.

118. Gomes T, Mamdani MM, Paterson JM, Dhalla IA, Juulink DN. Trends in high-dose opioid prescribing in Canada. Can Fam Physician. 2014;60:826–32.

119. Sehgal N, Manchikanti L, Smith HS. Prescription opioid abuse in chronic pain: a review of opioid abuse predictors and strategies to curb opioid abuse. Pain Physician. 2012;15:ES67–92.

120. Okie S. A flood of opioids, a rising tide of deaths. N Engl J Med. 2010;363(21):1981–5.

121. Macintyre PE, Schug SA, Scott DA, Visser EJ, Walker SM, APM:SE Working Group of the Australian and New Zealand College of Anaesthetists and Faculty of. Pain Medicine. Acute pain management: scientific evidence. 3rd ed. Melbourne: ANZCA & FPM; 2010.

122. Melzack R. The McGill Pain Questionnaire: Major properties and scoring methods. Pain. 1975;1:277–99.

123. Jensen MP, Mardekian J, Lakshminarayanan M, Boye ME. Validity of 24-h recall ratings of pain severity: biasing effects of "Peak" and "End" pain. Pain. 2008;137:422–7.

124. Aubrun G, Langeron O, Quesnel C, Coriat P, Riou B. Relationships between measurement of pain using visual analog score and morphine requirements during postoperative intravenous morphine titration. Anesthesiology. 2003;98:1415–21.

125. Cepeda MS, Africano JM, Polo R, Alcala R, Carr DB. What decline in pain intensity is meaningful to patients with acute pain? Pain. 2003;105:151–7.

126. Jensen MP, Chen C, Brugger AM. Interpretation of visual analog scale ratings and change scores: a reanalysis of two clinical trials of postoperative pain. J Pain. 2003;4:407–14.

127. Lee JS, Hobden E, Stiell IG, Wells GA. Clinically important change in the visual analog scale after adequate pain control. Acad Emerg Med. 2003;10:1128–30.

128. Farrar JT, Portenoy RK, Berlin JA, Kinman JL, Strom BL. Defining the clinically important difference in pain outcome measures. Pain. 2000;88:287–94.

129. Farrar JT, Young Jr JP, LaMoreaux L, Werth JL, Poole RM. Clinical importance of changes in chronic pain intensity measured on an 11-point numerical pain rating scale. Pain. 2001;94:149–58.

130. Murphy DF, McDonald A, Power C, Unwin A, MacSullivan R. Measurement of pain: a comparison of the visual analogue with a nonvisual analogue scale. Clin J Pain. 1987;3:191–7.

131. DeLoach LJ, Higgins MS, Caplan AB, Stiff JL. The visual analog scale in the immediate postoperative period: intrasubject variability and correlation with a numeric scale. Anesth Analg. 1998;86:102–6.

132. Breivik EK, Bjornsson GA, Skovlund E. A comparison of pain rating scales by sampling from clinical trial data. Clin J Pain. 2000;16:22–8.

133. Myles PS, Troedel S, Boquest M, Reeves M. The pain visual analog scale: is it linear or nonlinear? Anesth Analg. 1999;89:1517–20.

134. Myles PS, Urquhart N. The linearity of the visual analogue scale in patients with severe acute pain. Anaesth Intensive Care. 2005;33:54–8.

135. Machata AM, Kabon B, Willschke H, Fassler K, Gustoff B, Marhofer P, Curatolo M. A new instrument for pain assessment in the immediate postoperative period. Anasthesia. 2009;64:392–8.

136. Arif-Rahua M, Grap MJ. Facial expression and pain in the critically ill non-communicative patient: State of science review. Intensive Crit Care Nurs. 2010;26:343–52.

137. Lucey P, Cohn JF, Matthews I, Lucey S, Sridharan S, Howlett J, Prkachin KM. Automatically Detecting Pain in Video Through Facial Action Units Journal Institute of Electrical and Electronics Engineers (IEEE). http://www.cs.cmu.edu/~jeffcohn/pubs/IEEE_SMC_Pain_2010_final.pdf.

138. Zwakhalen SMG, Hamers JPH, Abu-Saad HH, Berger MPF. Pain in elderly people with severe dementia: a systematic review of behavioural pain assessment tools. BMC Geriatr. 2006;6:3. doi:10.1186/1471-2318-6-3.

139. Royal College of Physicians, British Geriatrics Society and British Pain Society. The assessment of pain in older people: national guidelines. Concise guidance to good practice series, No 8. London: RCP; 2007.

140. World Health Organization. Traitement de la douleur cancéreuse. Geneva, Switz: World Health. Organization; 1987.

141. Ruddick W. Do doctors undertreat pain? Bioethics. 1997;11:248–55.

142. Veysman BD. Prescriber's narcophobia syndrome: physicians' disease and patients' misfortune. BMJ. 2009;339:b4987.

143. MacIntyre PE, Walker S, Power I, Schug SA. Acute pain management: scientific evidence revisited. Br J Anaesth. 2006;96:1–4.

144. Perkins FM, Kehlet H. Chronic pain as an outcome of surgery — a review of predictive factors. Anesthesiology. 2000;93:1123–33.

145. Macrae WA. Chronic pain after surgery. Br J Anaesth. 2001;87:88–98.

146. Leung L. From ladder to platform: a new concept for pain management. J Prim Health Care. 2012;4(3):254–8.

147. Killian KJ. The objective measurement of breathlessness. Chest. 1985;88(2 Suppl):84S–90S.

148. Carrieri-Kohlman V, Douglas M, Murray Gormley J, Stulbarg M. Desensitization and guided mystery: treatment approaches for the management of dyspnea. Heart Lung. 1993;22:226–34.

149. Gift AG, Plaut SM, Jacox A. Psychologic and physiologic factors related to dyspnea in subjects with chronic obstructive pulmonary disease. Heart Lung. 1986;15:595–601.

150. Gift A, Cahill CA. Psychophysiologic aspects of dyspnea in chronic obstructive pulmonary disease: A pilot study. Heart Lung. 1990;19:252–7.

151. Bailey PH. Dyspnea-anxiety-dyspnea cycle. COPD patients stories of breathlessness: "It's scary when you can't breathe". Qual Health Res. 2004;14(6):760–78.

152. Borg G. Perceived exertion as an indicator of somatic stress. Scand J Rehabil Med. 1970;2(2):92–8.

153. Fletcher CM. (Chairman). Standardised questionnaire on respiratory symptoms: a statement prepared and approved by the MRC committee on the aetiology of chronic bronchitis (MRC breathlessness score). BMJ. 1960;2:1665.

154. Bestall JC, Paul EA, Garrod R, Garnham R, Jones PW, Wedzicha JA. Usefulness of the medical research council (MRC) dyspnoea scale as a measure of disability in patients with chronic obstructive pulmonary disease. Thorax. 1999;54(7):581–6.

155. O'Donnell DE, Aaron S, Bourbeau J, Hernandez P, Marciniuk D, Balter M, et al. Canadian thoracic society recommendations for management of chronic obstructive pulmonary disease – 2003. Can Respir J. 2003;10(Suppl.A):11A–65A.

156. Asfar P, Meziani F, Hamel J-F, Grelon F, Megarbane B, SEPSISPAM investigators, et al. High versus low

blood-pressure target in patients with septic shock. N Engl J Med. 2014;370:1583–93.

157. Jylhä M, Volpato S, Guralnik JM. Self-rated health showed a graded association with frequently used biomarkers in a large population sample. J Clin Epidemiol. 2006;59:465–71.

158. Meagher DJ. Delirium: optimising management. BMJ. 2001;322:144–9.

159. Kiely DK, Jones RN, Bergmann MA, Marcantonio ER. Association between psychomotor activity delirium subtypes and mortality among newly admitted post-acute facility patients. J Gerontol A Biol Sci Med Sci. 2007;62:174–9.

160. McNarry AF, Goldhill DR. Simple bedside assessment of level of consciousness: comparison of two simple assessment scales with the Glasgow Coma scale. Anaesthesia. 2004;59:34–7.

161. Clifford M, Ridley A, Gleeson M, Kellett J. The early mortality associated with agitation and sedation in acutely ill medical patients. Eur J Intern Med. 2013;24:e85.

162. Bellelli G, Speciale S, Barisione E, Trabucchi M. Delirium subtypes and 1-year mortality among elderly patients discharged from a post-acute rehabilitation facility. J Gerontol A Biol Sci Med Sci. 2007;62:1182–3.

163. Inouye S, van Dyck C, Alessi C, Balkin S, Siegal A, Horwitz R. Clarifying confusion: the confusion assessment method. Ann Intern Med. 1990;113:941–8.

164. Hogan DB, MacKnight C, Bergman H. Steering Committee, Canadian initiative on frailty and aging. Models, definitions, and criteria of frailty [review]. Aging Clin Exp Res. 2003;15(3 Suppl):1–29.

165. Rylance J, Baker T, Mushi E, Mashaga D. Use of an early warning score and ability to walk predicts mortality in medical patients admitted to hospitals in Tanzania. Trans R Soc Trop Med Hyg. 2009;103:790–4.

166. Wheeler I, Price C, Sitch A, et al. Early warning scores generated in developed healthcare settings are not sufficient at predicting early mortality in blantyre, malawi: a prospective cohort study. PLoS One. 2013;8(3):e59830. doi:10.1371/journal. pone.0059830.

167. Opio MO, Nansubuga G, Kellett J. Validation of the VitalPACTM Early Warning Score (ViEWS) in acutely ill medical patients attending a resource-poor hospital in sub-Saharan Africa. Resuscitation. 2013;84:743–6.

168. Opio MO, Nansubuga G, Kellett J, Clifford M, Murray A. Performance of TOTAL, in medical patients attending a resource-poor hospital in sub-Saharan Africa and a small Irish rural hospital. Acute Med. 2013;12:135–40.

169. Kellett J, Deane B, Gleeson M. Derivation and validation of a score based on hypotension, oxygen saturation, low temperature, ECG changes and loss of independence (HOTEL) that predicts early mortality between 15 minutes and 24 hours after admission to an acute medical unit. Resuscitation. 2008;78:52–8.

170. Brabrand M, Hallas J, Knudsen T. Loss of independence: a novel but important global marker of illness. Scandinavian J Trauma, Resuscitation Emerg Med. 2013;21(Suppl 2):A34. doi:10.1186/ 1757-7241-21-S2-A34.

171. Brabrand M, Folkestad L, Clausen NG, Knudsen T, Hallas J. Risk scoring systems for adults admitted to the emergency department: a systematic review. Scandinavian J Trauma, Resuscitation and Emerg Med.

172. Rockwood K, Song X, MacKnight CA, et al. A global clinical measure of fitness and frailty in elderly people. CMAJ. 2005;173(5):489–95.

173. Brabrand M, Kellett J. Mobility measures should be added to the national early warning score (NEWS). Resuscitation. 2014;85:e151.

174. Wallis PA, Gottschalk SB, Wood D, et al. The cape triage score - a triage system for South Africa. S Afr Med J. 2006;96:53–6.

175. Wallis LA, Balfour CH. Triage in emergency departments. S Afr Med J. 2007;97:13.

176. Bogardus ST, Towle V, Williams CS, Desai MM, Inouye SK. What does the medical record reveal about functional status? J Gen Intern Med. 2001;16:728–36.

177. Hirdes JP, Ljunggren G, Morris JN, Frijters DHM, Soveri HF, Gray L, Björkgren M, Gilgen R. Reliability of the interRAI suite of assessment instruments: a 12-country study of an integrated health information system. BMC Health Serv Res. 2008;8:277. doi:10.1186/1472-6963-8-277.

178. Studenski S, Perera S, Wallace D, et al. Physical performance measures in the clinical setting. J Am Geriatr Soc. 2003;51:314–22.

179. Kellett J, Clifford M, Ridley A, Murray A, Gleeson M. A four item scale based on gait for the immediate global assessment of acutely ill medical patients – one look is more than 1000 words. Eur Geriatr Med. 2014;5:92–6.

180. Karnik K, Mazzatti DJ. Review of tools and technologies to assess multi-system functional impairment and frailty. Clin Medicine: Geriatric. 2009;31–8.

181. Smith GB, Prytherch DR, Schmidt PE, Featherstone PI, Kellett J, Deane B, Higgins B. Should age be included as a component of track and trigger systems used to identify sick adult patients? Resuscitation. 2008;78:109–15.

182. Opio MO, Nansubuga G, Kellett J. In-hospital mortality of acutely ill medical patients admitted to a resource poor hospital in sub-Saharan Africa and to a Canadian regional hospital compared using the abbreviated VitalPAC™ early warning score. Eur J Intern Med. 2014;25:142–6.

183. Prytherch DR, Smith GB, Schmidt PE, Featherstone PI. ViEWS—towards a national early warning score for detecting adult inpatient deterioration. Resuscitation. 2010;81:932–7.

184. Latré B et al. A survey on wireless body area networks. Wireless Networks. 2011;17(1):1–18.

185. Kellett J. Will continuous surveillance monitoring of vital signs provide cheaper, safer, and better hospital care for all? Jt Comm J Qual Patient Saf. 2012;38:426–7.

186. Kellett J, Murray A, Woodworth S, Huang W. Trends in weighted vital signs and the clinical course of 44,531 acutely ill medical patients while in hospital. Acute Med. 2015;14:4–10.

187. Kellett J, Woodworth S, Wang F, Huang W. Changes and their prognostic implications in the abbreviated VitalPAC™ early warning score (ViEWS) after admission to hospital of 18,853 acutely ill medical patients. Resuscitation. 2013;84:13–20.

188. Murray A, Kellett J, Huang W, Woodworth S, Wang F. Trajectories of the averaged abbreviated VitalpacTM early warning score (AbEWS) and clinical course of 44,531 consecutive admissions hospitalized for acute medical illness. Resuscitation. 2014;85:544–8.

189. Kellett J, Murray A. How to follow the NEWS. Acute Med. 2014;13:104–7.

190. Hravnak M, Edwards L, Clontz A, Valenta C, DeVita MA, Pinsky MR. Defining the incidence of cardiore-spiratory instability in patients in step-down units using an electronic integrated monitoring system. Arch Intern Med. 2008;168:1300–8.

191. Kellett J, Rasool S. The prediction of the in-hospital mortality of acutely ill medical patients by electro-cardiogram (ECG) dispersion mapping compared with established risk factors and predictive scores — A pilot study. Eur J Intern Med. 2011;22:394–8.

192. Kellett J, Emmanuel A, Rasool S. The prediction by ECG dispersion mapping of clinical deterioration, as measured by increase in the simple clinical score. Acute Med. 2012;11:8–12.

193. Lin S, Yokoyama H, Rac VE, Brooks SC. Novel biomarkers in diagnosing cardiac ischemia in the emergency department: a systematic review. Resuscitation. 2012;83:684–91.

194. Nickel CH, Messmer AS, Geigy N, Misch F, Mueller B, Dusemund F, Hertel S, Hartmann O, Giersdorf S, Bingisser R. Stress markers predict mortality in patients with nonspecific complaints presenting to the emergency department and may be a useful risk stratification tool to support disposition planning. Acad Emerg Med. 2013;20:670–9.

195. Prytherch DR, Sirl JS, Schmidt P, et al. The use of routine laboratory data to predict in-hospital death in medical admissions. Resuscitation. 2005;66:203–7.

196. Froom P, Shimoni Z. Prediction of hospital mortality rates by admission laboratory tests. Clin Chem. 2006;52:325–8.

197. Asadollahi K, Hastings IM, Gill GV, et al. Prediction of hospital mortality from admission laboratory data and patient age: a simple model. Emerg Med Aust. 2011;23:354–63.

198. Loekito E, Bailey J, Bellomo R, Hart GK, Hegarty C, Davey P, Bain C, Pilcher D, Schneider H. Common laboratory tests predict imminent death in ward patients. Resuscitation. 2013;84:280–5.

199. Silke B, Kellett J, Rooney T, Bennett K, O'Riordan D. An improved medical admissions risk system using multivariable fractional polynomial logistic regression modelling. QJM. 2010;103:23–32.

200. Brabrand M, Knudsen T, Hallas J. Identifying admitted patients at risk of dying: a prospective observational validation of four biochemical scoring systems. BMJ Open. 2013;3:e002890.

Multiple Parameter Track and Trigger Systems

John Asger Petersen

Background

Track and trigger systems (TTS) are an essential part of the afferent limb of rapid response systems [1]. They are designed to detect on the ward deteriorating patients on the general floor of an acute hospital and activate an appropriate response from the staff. Most instances of clinical deterioration are preceded by a period of unstable physiology and could potentially be prevented if recognized early and responded to in a timely and competent manner [2]. This has proved to be a complex task and the aim of TTS is to facilitate the process [3, 4].

In general, TTS can be divided into two parts: a crisis detection component and a response algorithm. A variety of different systems exist and vary according to the number of different vital signs and observations analyzed, monitoring frequencies, trigger thresholds, and clinical responses. In general, they can be categorized as single parameter track and trigger systems (SPTTS) and multiparameter track and trigger systems (MPTTS) [5]. In the former, the clinical response is triggered by a single aberrant vital sign or observation and usually consists of a call to the medical emergency team (MET). In MPTTS, triggering depends on deviations of several physiological parameters and the derivation of a composite score. Different responses can be attached to different numeric values of the severity scale. The most widely distributed MPTTS is the aggregated weighted track and trigger system (AWTTS); other forms of MPTTS are rarely used and will not be discussed further.

In AWTTS, points are allocated for each measured physiological parameter according to how much it deviates from a predefined normal range and are aggregated to a single score—originally termed the early warning score (EWS). The EWS reflects the degree of deterioration, with higher scores indicating greater severity [6]. In this way, it is theoretically possible to adapt the urgency of the clinical response as well as the provider's level of expertise to patients' needs. The overall performance of a given AWTTS depends on its ability to detect early deterioration and to trigger a timely appropriate clinical response [7]. This requires efficient crisis detection through monitoring of relevant physiological parameters at the right intervals and proper trigger thresholds for escalating care. Furthermore, the system must be simple to use in order to routinely achieve reliable scores on busy hospital wards and ensure adherence to monitoring frequency and responses [4].

J.A. Petersen, EDIC (✉)
Department of Anesthesia and Intensive Care,
Bispebjerg and Frederiksberg University Hospital,
Bispebjerg Bakke 23, 2400 Copenhagen, Nordvest,
Denmark
e-mail: john.asger.petersen@regionh.dk

© Springer International Publishing Switzerland 2017
M.A. DeVita et al. (eds.), *Textbook of Rapid Response Systems*, DOI 10.1007/978-3-319-39391-9_9

Crisis Detection

Until recently, most hospitals used AWTTS that were based on the original EWS by Morgan et al. with minor local adjustments—few of which were validated with respect to their ability to predict serious adverse events [6]. In 2008, Smith et al. found no less than 56 different AWTTS, of which 33 were based on physiological parameters and 23 had additional parameters such as the presence of pain and need for respiratory support [8]. Of the 33 physiologically based AWTTS, all included respiratory rate (RR), heart rate (HR), systolic blood pressure (BP), and level of consciousness (LOC); 17 included urine output and 26 temperature. The authors found 19 different weightings for temperature, 15 for respiratory rate and blood pressure, 12 for heart rate, and six for LOC. The performance of the AWTTS to predict hospital mortality differed widely and ranged from 0.567 to 0.782 in the area under the receiver operating characteristic curve (AUROC). Subsequent work led to the VitalPAC™ Early Warning Score (ViEWS) which was found to be the best performing AWTTS [9]. ViEWS was developed to predict death within 24 h in acutely admitted medical patients, and its performance in an abbreviated version (AbEWS), without values for level of consciousness (LOC), was confirmed in a mixed medical and surgical population [10]. A slightly modified version, the National Early Warning Score (NEWS), is recommended for use across the UK [7]. The ability of NEWS to predict the combined outcome of cardiac arrest, unanticipated admission to the ICU, and death was recently found to be superior to other forms of EWS [11].

The crisis detection component of NEWS (Table 9.1) consists of a scoring system that includes the following routinely measured physiological parameters:

- Respiratory rate (RR).
- Peripheral oxygen saturation (SAT).
- Heart rate (HR).
- Systolic blood pressure (BP).
- Temperature (Tp).
- Level of consciousness (LOC).

In addition, patients who require oxygen supplementation are allocated a weighting score of 2. As shown in Table 9.1, each physiological parameter contains weighted scores between 0 and 3 points. The more a physiological parameter deviates from the normal range, the higher the assigned score. The sum of points from each parameter determines the total score, termed NEWS, which has a maximum of 20 points [7].

It is important to keep in mind that both the individual parameters included in NEWS and its weighting are calibrated to achieve the highest discriminative power in predicting in-hospital mortality. Although this may be a strength of a scoring system, the rapid response system is aimed at minimizing other clinical end points such as organ failures, severity of illness, hospital costs, delays in recovery, and loss of independent function. Reliance on numerical values as the sole

Table 9.1 The National Early Warning Score (NEWS)

Vital sign	3	2	1	0	1	2	3
Respiratory rate/min	<9		9–11	12–20		21–24	>24
Oxygen saturation	<92%	92–93%	94–95%	>95%			
Supplemental oxygen		Yes		No			
Temperature	<35.1		35.1–36.0	36.1–38.0	38.1–39.0	>39	
Systolic blood pressure	<91	91–100	101–110	111–219			>219
Heart rate	<41		41–50	51–90	91–110	111–130	>130
Level of consciousness				A			V, P, U

Legend: Derivation of NEWS is shown with physiological parameters and corresponding score given for deviation from the normal range. The scores in the "0" column are considered normal (Adapted from [7])

source of assessing deterioration exposes one to a number of systematic errors. The limits for elevated blood pressure and LOC are especially problematic in this regard. For the former, an upper limit of 220 mmHg is well above the current recommendations for treating hypertension, and for the latter, the recommended use of the Alert, Voice, Pain, Unresponsive (AVPU) scale to assess neurologic status ignores the relevance of delirium, which in its own right warrants urgent clinical evaluation [7]. Further, over-reliance on numerical scores ignores the complexity of the human condition and the ability of intuition and experience (e.g. nurses) to integrate situational variables and develop concern.

How Often Should Vital Signs Be Assessed?

Detecting at-risk patients early in their disease course requires a regular and systematic assessment of physiologic parameters. Accordingly, monitoring can be defined as: "the ongoing assessment of a patient with the intention of (1) detecting abnormality, and (2) triggering a response if an abnormality is detected" [4]. The purpose of monitoring can either be *to detect* or *to predict* clinical deterioration. This puts different demands on the monitoring system. Detective monitoring is usually reserved for unstable, high-risk patients in need of continuous surveillance with staff being alerted automatically when abnormalities are detected. The purpose of AWTTS is primarily predictive monitoring, i.e. to identify at-risk patients in advance of manifest clinical deterioration and to alert staff in a manner that allows for early intervention and triaging to higher level care if necessary.

The optimum monitoring interval is unknown and should ideally be frequent enough to identify at-risk patients at a time when intervention can make a clinical difference. Creating a balance between frequency of observation and disruptions in work flow is a key concern. Theoretically, automated, continuous surveillance would be best suited for this purpose, but current technology is not advanced enough to reliably measure all required parameters in ambulatory patients on general wards. Furthermore, there is no evidence of positive effect of continuous surveillance of general ward patients. In fact, an observational study found an increased rate of afferent limb failure in continuously monitored vs. unmonitored ward patients (81 vs. 53%, $p < 0.001$) despite better documentation of vital signs (96 vs. 74%, $p < 0.001$) in the 6 h prior to MET activation [12]. A randomized controlled trial of 402 high-risk patients in medical and surgical wards showed no effect of continuous surveillance between intervention and control group in regard to morbidity and mortality [13].

While there is a lack of evidence for the benefit of continuous surveillance, another study recently showed a doubling of MET calls on wards randomized to use mandatory *intermittent* monitoring (three times daily) compared to control wards, where monitoring was based on indication. However, the increased MET activity did not translate to differences in serious adverse event rates, which decreased equally in both groups during the study period [14].

Present recommendations on monitoring frequency are based on expert opinion with little convincing scientific evidence. Using the NEWS system, patients are stratified into low, medium, or high risk, based on their aggregate score, with cutoff intervals of 0–4, 5–6, or ≥7, respectively, with an additional recommendation that if a single parameter generates a score of 3, a patient should be regarded as a medium risk. Monitoring frequencies are also supposed to increase according to NEWS as shown in Table 9.2 [7]. The recommended intervals constitute minimum requirements, and individual monitoring plans should also take patient-specific factors into account, such as severity of illness, types and severity of comorbidities, and the acuity and nature of the presenting disease. It is also important to remember that intermittent measurements only give a "snapshot" of the clinical state; the trend and rate of changes of vital signs are presumably just as important as the degree of deviation when assessing a patient's need for escalation in care.

Table 9.2 Suggested clinical responses triggered by specific NEWS (Adapted from [7])

NEWS score	Frequency of monitoring	Clinical response
0	Minimum 12 hourly	Continue routine NEWS monitoring with every set of observations
Total: 1–4	Minimum 4–6 hourly	Inform registered nurse who must assess the patient Registered nurse to decide if increased frequency of monitoring and/or escalation of clinical care is required
Total: 5 or more or 3 in 1 parameter	Increased frequency to a minimum of 1 hourly	Registered nurse to urgently inform the medical team caring for the patient Urgent assessment by a clinician with core competencies to assess acutely ill patients Clinical care in an environment with monitoring facilities
Total: 7 or more	Continuous monitoring of vital signs	Registered nurse to immediately inform the medical team caring for the patient—this should be at least at specialist registrar level Emergency assessment by a clinical team with critical care competencies, which also includes a practitioner(s) with advanced airway skills Consider transfer of clinical care to a level 2 or 3 care facility, i.e. higher dependency or ITU

Legend: Composite scores derived from the weighted parameter score in Table 9.1 are used to determine an appropriate clinical response. One suggested for the NEWS [7] is provided here

In one of the few studies that investigate the dynamic aspects of EWS, Kellett et al. used the AbEWS to estimate the extent and time frame of changes in the score [15]. Paradoxically, they found higher in-hospital mortality among patients who showed initial "improvement" reflected by a decrease in the average score during the first 6 h of hospitalization compared to the initial score measured on admission. This finding applied to all risk groups independent of the admission score. After the initial 6-h period, changes in score correlated directly with mortality and doubled among patients with an increase in scores compared to those with a decrease. A possible explanation for this paradox could be that the initial treatment of acutely admitted patients is aimed at correcting physiology through fluid resuscitation, supplemental oxygen, and similar resuscitative measures, but these interventions might be without lasting benefit or give a false sense of security leading to mis-triage. This has important clinical implications and underlines the importance of maintaining a high level of care. Another important finding of the study was that 4.7% of all deaths occurred in patients with scores below 3 during in the preceding 24 h, most of

whom also had a low admission score. So there appears to exist a subset of patients in whom the ability to respond to life-threatening illness with a physiological response is reduced.

The Response Algorithm

The response algorithm prescribes the thresholds at which different clinical interventions should be triggered and defines both its urgency and the level of expertise of the providers. However, little evidence exists regarding optimum trigger thresholds, response times, or composition of the response team [16–19]. Prytherch et al. showed in the original study of ViEWS™ that 20% of all observations had a score of ≥ 5 and that this threshold would detect 82% of all 24-h mortality in the study population [9]. In a similar study, it was shown that adding the additional trigger of 3 for a single component score would increase detection rates from 2.99 to 3.08 per day (3% increase), but at the expense of increasing doctors' workload by 40% [20]. It is intuitively clear that further threshold reductions increase detection rates, but do so at the expense of increased workload. The ideal cutoff point must strike a balance between patient safety and available resources.

It is generally agreed that response times should be kept as short as possible; however, the optimum response time has not been defined and is also dependent on the availability and location of care providers. A number of descriptive studies have investigated the effect of delayed interventions, and these studies generally set the upper limit at 24 h with the lower limit varying widely and set as low as 15 min prior to an event [12, 21–23]. A consistent finding is that delays are common and that delays of more than an hour are independent predictors of increased mortality [23, 24]. Most of these studies however employed single parameter triggers, which make inferences to the graded response algorithm of AWTTS difficult. It is clear that both the urgency of the response and the expertise level of the care providers must correspond both to the severity and rate of deterioration to be successful. One of the postulated advantages of AWTTS is their ability to deliver a graded response depending on these factors. This approach can be classified as a "ramp-up" approach, where clinical care is escalated in a stepwise fashion depending on the patient's condition. There exists no high-quality evidence to the effect of this approach, and while it arguably holds high face value, the question to its effectiveness compared to other systems remains to be determined [19].

Performance of AWTTS

Despite the wide dissemination of AWTTS, serious adverse events still occur frequently and prompt one to consider whether this is a failure of the system or whether other factors are involved [3]. They may result from intrinsic shortcomings of the TTS, i.e. lack of sensitivity to detect at-risk patients or non-adherence to monitoring or care escalation protocols. While the original study showed good discriminative power for the outcome in question (death after 24 h), it failed to describe situations where the afferent limb failed and whether this was related to non-adherence to the escalation protocol or due to suboptimal care

[9–11]. ViEWS is derived from a large database of nearly 200,000 observation sets with values for RR, systolic and diastolic BP, HR, SAT, Tp, LOC, and the use of supplemental oxygen. These data were obtained from more than 35,000 acute medical admissions during 2006–2008 in the UK. The parameters included and their weightings were calibrated so ViEWS could yield the highest discriminative power to distinguish between survivors and non-survivors at 24 h following the initial observations. Subsequently, ViEWS was tested against 33 previously described AWTTS and was found to be best at predicting short-term in-hospital mortality with an AUROC of 0.888 (0.880–0.895, 95% CI) and AUROC's spanning from 0.803 to 0.850 for the remaining systems. NEWS is a modified version of ViEWS, with reduced weighting for supplemental oxygen from 3 to 2 points and reduced threshold for elevated systolic blood pressure from 250 to 220 mmHg. The ability of NEWS to predict short-term in-hospital mortality, cardiac arrest, and unplanned ICU admissions was tested with the ViEWS derivation cohort and compared to the previous 33 AWTTS. The AUROC for the composite outcome was 0.873 (0.866–0.879, 95% CI) and is still superior to the other systems (0.736–0.834). However, its ability to predict cardiac arrest was only moderate with an AUROC of 0.722 (0.685–0.745, 95% CI), but good for predicting ICU admissions and death, 0.857 (0.847–868) and 0.894 (0.887–0.902), respectively. These results are hardly surprising considering that validation was performed on the same dataset it was derived from. But it raises the issue whether mortality is a pertinent outcome, since most in-hospital deaths are expected and preceded by limitations in treatment, i.e. do not resuscitate orders. Likewise cardiac arrest and unexpected death are variably defined in different studies and are also highly influenced by the number of limitations in treatment issued by the MET. Admission to the ICU is not necessarily a negative outcome, and further, the physiologic makeup of patients admitted to the ICU is not at all heterogeneous and is highly institution dependent. So while most AWTTS have the ability to identify patients at risk of clinical deterioration, their impact on patient outcomes remains to be established. In general, they are regarded as an improvement upon single parameter systems that along with implementation of comprehensive rapid response systems have improved actual patient outcomes [19, 25–27].

Strengths and Weaknesses of AWTTS

Despite the lack of high-level evidence on positive patient outcome, AWTTS hold a number of promises for safer patient care. The systems have fairly good predictive power for short-term mortality among hospitalized patients, and especially at low scores, where 0–2 is associated with very low mortality [10]. Generation of early warning scores can be helpful at allocating staff resources effectively to those patients most in need of acute care. Also the crisis detection component together with the response algorithm can be helpful in enforcing an institution's monitoring and treatment plan. The latter may provide valuable assistance to inexperienced staff and junior doctors who may lack the experience to detect clinical deterioration and formulate an action plan. EWS also seems to facilitate communication both between nurses and doctors and the MET, which again has a positive influence on patient safety and resource allocation [28, 29].

Despite its good ability to predict outcomes for cohorts of patients, the discriminative power of AWTTS to distinguish between deteriorating and non-deteriorating patients is inadequate to form the basis for clinical decisions for individual patients. The dynamic nature of many disease processes, patient factors including frailty, the presence of comorbidities, and response to treatment are all important aspects that AWTTS do not take into account. So there is an inherent risk in AWTTS to disregard clinical context and reduce complex situations to a single number. Especially, critical observations like obstructed airway and seizures, or general concern for the patient are not weighted adequately. The latter accounts for one half of MET calls in mature RRS based on single parameter triggers. Particularly subtle changes in a

patient's condition could give rise to staff concern before they are reflected in vital sign changes and lead to delay in review by more experienced staff. Patients with a moderately increased EWS also constitute a problem. A number of these patients might actually be the ones that benefit the most from MET review, especially the ones belonging to the subgroup unable to mount a sufficient physiological response to severe disease processes.

Overall, it is important for clinicians to remember that the systems are meant to function as a safety net, to identify and direct attention to vulnerable patients on the ward, and that further care must be individualized. Warning scores are intended to complement, rather than substitute experience and good judgment. It is equally important that ward staff continue to use their clinical acumen and respond to clinical situations where deterioration is suspected, even when there are only subtle changes in vital signs [30].

Conclusion

The aim of AWTTS is to identify deteriorating ward patients as early as possible, alert staff, and trigger a clinical response that matches the severity of the underlying condition. Most AWTTS have good discriminative power to distinguish between deteriorating and non-deteriorating patients, but their predictive capacity is inadequate to form the sole basis for clinical decisions. Therefore, it is important to keep in mind that it is impossible to reduce a complex situation to a single number and evaluate the patient according to the clinical context and individual risk factors. Further work on track and trigger systems will likely focus on the impact of their implementation on patient care and outcomes.

References

1. Devita MA, Bellomo R, Hillman K, Kellum J, Rotondi A, Teres D, et al. Findings of the first consensus conference on medical emergency teams. Crit Care Med. 2006;34(9):2463–78.
2. Kause J, Smith G, Prytherch D, Parr M, Flabouris A, Hillman K. A comparison of antecedents to cardiac

arrests, deaths and emergency intensive care admissions in Australia and New Zealand, and the United Kingdom—the ACADEMIA study. Resuscitation. 2004;62(3):275–82.

3. Petersen JA, Mackel R, Antonsen K, Simon RL. Serious adverse events in a hospital using early warning score—what went wrong? Resuscitation. 2014;85(12):1699–703.

4. DeVita MA, Smith GB, Adam SK, Adams-Pizarro I, Buist M, Bellomo R, et al. "Identifying the hospitalised patient in crisis"—a consensus conference on the afferent limb of rapid response systems. Resuscitation. 2010;81(4):375–82.

5. Jones DA, DeVita MA, Bellomo R. Rapid-response teams. N Engl J Med. 2011;365(2):139–46.

6. Morgan R, Williams F, Wright M. An early warning scoring system for detecting developing critical illness. Clin Intensive Care. 1997;8:100.

7. Royal College of Physicians. National Early Warning Score (NEWS): standardising the assessment of acute-illness severity in the NHS. 2012. https://www.rcplondon.ac.uk/sites/default/files/documents/national-early-warning-score-standardising-assessment-acute-illness-severity-nhs.pdf.

8. Smith GB, Prytherch DR, Schmidt PE, Featherstone PI. Review and performance evaluation of aggregate weighted "track and trigger" systems. Resuscitation. 2008;77(2):170–9.

9. Prytherch DR, Smith GB, Schmidt PE, Featherstone PI. ViEWS-towards a national early warning score for detecting adult inpatient deterioration. Resuscitation. 2010;81(8):932–7.

10. Kellett J, Kim A. Validation of an abbreviated Vitalpac™ Early Warning Score (ViEWS) in 75,419 consecutive admissions to a Canadian Regional Hospital. Resuscitation. 2012;83(3):297–302.

11. Smith GB, Prytherch DR, Meredith P, Schmidt PE, Featherstone PI. The ability of the National Early Warning Score (NEWS) to discriminate patients at risk of early cardiac arrest, unanticipated intensive care unit admission, and death. Resuscitation. 2013;84(4):465–70.

12. Tirkkonen J, Ylä-Mattila J, Olkkola KT, Huhtala H, Tenhunen J, Hoppu S. Factors associated with delayed activation of medical emergency team and excess mortality: an Utstein-style analysis. Resuscitation. 2013;84(2):173–8.

13. Watkinson PJ, Barber VS, Price JD, Hann A, Tarassenko L, Young JD. A randomised controlled trial of the effect of continuous electronic physiological monitoring on the adverse event rate in high risk medical and surgical patients. Anaesthesia. 2006;61(11):1031–9.

14. Ludikhuize J, Borgert M, Binnekade J, Subbe C, Dongelmans D, Goossens A. Standardized measurement of the Modified Early Warning Score results in enhanced implementation of a Rapid Response System: a quasi-experimental study. Resuscitation. 2014;85(5):676–82.

15. Murray A, Kellett J, Huang W, Woodworth S, Wang F. Trajectories of the averaged abbreviated Vitalpac early warning score (AbEWS) and clinical course of 44,531 consecutive admissions hospitalized for acute medical illness. Resuscitation. 2014;85(4):544–8.

16. Alam N, Hobbelink EL, van Tienhoven AJ, van de Ven PM, Jansma EP, Nanayakkara PWB. The impact of the use of the Early Warning Score (EWS) on patient outcomes: a systematic review. Resuscitation. 2014;85(5):587–94.

17. McGaughey J, Alderdice F, Fowler R, Kapila A, Mayhew A, Moutray M. Outreach and Early Warning Systems (EWS) for the prevention of intensive care admission and death of critically ill adult patients on general hospital wards. Cochrane database Syst Rev. 2007;18(3):CD005529.

18. McNeill G, Bryden D. Do either early warning systems or emergency response teams improve hospital patient survival? A systematic review. Resuscitation. 2013;84(12):1652–67.

19. Smith MEB, Chiovaro JC, O'Neil M, Kansagara D, Quiñones AR, Freeman M, et al. Early warning system scores for clinical deterioration in hospitalized patients: a systematic review. Ann Am Thorac Soc. 2014;11(9):1454–65.

20. Jarvis S, Kovacs C, Briggs J, Meredith P, Schmidt PE, Featherstone PI, et al. Aggregate National Early Warning Score (NEWS) values are more important than high scores for a single vital signs parameter for discriminating the risk of adverse outcomes. Resuscitation. 2015;87:75–80.

21. Trinkle RM, Flabouris A. Documenting Rapid Response System afferent limb failure and associated patient outcomes. Resuscitation. 2011;82(7):810–4.

22. Boniatti MM, Azzolini N, Viana MV, Ribeiro BSP, Coelho RS, Castilho RK, et al. Delayed medical emergency team calls and associated outcomes. Crit Care Med. 2014;42(1):26–30.

23. Calzavacca P, Licari E, Tee A, Egi M, Downey A, Quach J, et al. The impact of Rapid Response System on delayed emergency team activation patient characteristics and outcomes—a follow-up study. Resuscitation. 2010;81(1):31–5.

24. Downey AW, Quach JL, Haase M, Haase-Fielitz A, Jones D, Bellomo R. Characteristics and outcomes of patients receiving a medical emergency team review for acute change in conscious state or arrhythmias. Crit Care Med. 2008;36(2):477–81.

25. Chen J, Bellomo R, Flabouris A, Hillman K, Finfer S. The relationship between early emergency team calls and serious adverse events. Crit Care Med. 2009;37(1):148–53.

26. Hillman K, Chen J, Cretikos M, Bellomo R, Brown D, Doig G, et al. Introduction of the medical emergency team (MET) system: a cluster-randomised controlled trial. Lancet. 2005;365(9477):2091–7.

27. Priestley G, Watson W, Rashidian A, Mozley C, Russell D, Wilson J, et al. Introducing Critical Care Outreach: a ward-randomised trial of phased introduction in a

general hospital. Intensive Care Med. 2004;30(7):1398–404.

28. Brady PW, Goldenhar LM. A qualitative study examining the influences on situation awareness and the identification, mitigation and escalation of recognised patient risk. BMJ Qual Saf. 2014;23(2):153–61.

29. Bunkenborg G, Samuelson K, Poulsen I, Ladelund S, Keson J. Lower incidence of unexpected in-hospital death after interprofessional implementation of a bedside track-and-trigger system. Resuscitation. 2014;85(3):424–30.

30. Morgan RJM, Wright MM. In defence of early warning scores. Br J Anaesth. 2007;99(5):747–8.

Causes of Failure to Rescue

10

Marilyn Hravnak, Andrea Mazzoccoli, Eliezer Bose, and Michael R. Pinsky

Introduction

Failure to rescue (FTR) is a term first coined by Silber in 1992 [1]. FTR has been used increasingly as a measure of hospital quality of care and has been named by the US Agency for Healthcare Research and Quality as one of the 20 patient safety indicators [2]. It refers to patient death attributable to a complication while hospitalized [1–3]. Patient-level, hospital-level, or system-level factors can influence a facility's FTR rate. The risk of FTR is lowered when complications and adverse occurrences are recognized quickly and treated aggressively [3]. Likewise, the risk of FTR increases when deleterious changes in patient status occur and steps to reverse the change are not taken [4, 5]. The FTR literature relates several models which define "complications" in different ways [3, 6–8].

The most comprehensive list of complications in the hospitalized patient used in the traditional FTR analysis was first developed by Silber and includes 14 categories [3] (Table 10.1).

The occurrence of a complication, however, does not necessarily imply wrongdoing. Although some complications may be hospital acquired, others may be present as admission comorbidities. Nevertheless, the premise is that failure to identify these complications quickly and treat them aggressively in order to prevent death during hospitalization should be regarded as FTR [4]. Thus, it is the "rescue capability" of a hospital in recognizing and then responding to complications and adverse occurrence which denotes quality [9]. In the past decade, FTR is emerging as an important and quantifiable measure for hospitalized patient care quality and safety and a framework within which to improve medical, trauma, and surgical care [10–13]. FTR causation is of particular interest in the surgical community as it attempts to define those complications that are surgeon or procedure related versus those that may be due to failure in care processes or infrastructure [14].

M. Hravnak, RN, PhD, ACNP-BC, FCCM, FAAN (✉)
E. Bose, RN, PhD, ACNP-BC
Department of Acute and Tertiary Care,
School of Nursing, University of Pittsburgh,
336 Victoria Hall, 3500 Victoria Street, Pittsburgh,
PA 15261, USA
e-mail: mhra@pitt.edu

A. Mazzoccoli, MSN, MBA, RN, PhD, FAAN
Bon Secours Health System Inc., 1505 Marriottsville
Rd., Marriottsville, MD 21104, USA

M.R. Pinsky, MD, Dr hc, FCCP, FCCM
Department of Critical Care Medicine,
University of Pittsburgh, 606 Scaife Hall,
3550 Terrace Street, Pittsburgh, PA 15261, USA

Table 10.1 Complications developed by hospitalized patients which can lead to death and failure to rescue. Sequela common to all complications before death is cardiorespiratory instability

Categories of complications	Examples and sequelae
Cardiac	Arrhythmias, cardiac arrest, infarction, congestive heart failure
Respiratory	Pneumonia, pneumothorax, bronchospasm, respiratory compromise, aspiration pneumonia
Hypotension	Shock, hypovolemia
Neurologic	Stroke, transient ischemic attack, seizure, psychosis, coma
Deep vein thrombosis	Pulmonary embolus, arterial clot, phlebitis
Internal organ damage, return to surgery	
Infection	Deep wound infection, sepsis
Gangrene	Amputation
Gastrointestinal bleeding	Blood loss
Peritonitis, intestinal obstruction	
Renal dysfunction	
Hepatitis	
Pancreatitis	
Decubitus ulcers	
Orthopedic complications and compartment syndromes	

Adapted from Silber et al., 2007

The concept of FTR only recognizes the problem, not what to do about it. When it is linked to a rapid response system, we begin to see not only the measurement of a problem, but the problem is linked to a solution. No matter what the individual or system nature of the failure to rescue, a deteriorating patient as a result of the complication will trigger pathophysiological signs, which should result in a rapid response call by appropriately trained staff.

Usually there are a number of opportunities between the initial development of a complication and eventual death resulting from that complication wherein the complication can be identified and treated. The earlier the complication is recognized and acted upon, the lesser the negative impact that the complication will have on patient outcome. Examples from Table 10.1 serve as illustrations. Although complications have varied causation, the common end manifestation prior to death is the eventual development of physiologic instability manifested by abnormalities in vital signs evolving to compromise of end-organ perfusion and associated metabolic derangement due to tissue hypoperfusion. At the present time, vital sign monitoring and surveillance of easily discernible physiologic and behavioral changes are the key to first detecting instability, identifying it as such appropriately, and then applying appropriate interventions in order to prevent adverse outcomes [15]. For the purposes of this discussion, vital signs include not only the basic intermittently measured blood pressure (BP), temperature, heart rate (HR), and respiratory rate (RR) but also noninvasively measured pulse oximetry (SpO$_2$). In fact, all these vital signs can be measured continuously using readily available bedside monitoring devices.

Even so, numerous studies demonstrate both the development and even documentation of abnormal vital signs many hours before unplanned death in hospitalized patients [16, 17], even within electronic health records [18]. The failure to rescue is related not to the failure to recognize deterioration but the failure to appropriately respond.

Expecting that access to a medical emergency team (MET) alone can prevent FTR is likely overly simplistic [19]. Medical emergency teams (METs) can only impact FTR if the important initial step of instability detection is followed by recognition, which in turn translates into a supportive or rescue action [20, 21]. Detection means that signs and symptoms of the unstable state are noted, while recognition means that there is awareness that these noted signs and symptoms represent a patient at risk and in need of care escalation. Finally, action must be based on knowing which action to take and being both empowered and encouraged to do so. All of these steps in human cognition must be backed by organizational processes and structures [22, 23]. It can be argued that knowing and empowerment are just as important as the availability of rescue resources [24]. Therefore, the other complex factors which lead to FTR can be present and must be addressed in order for the full potential of the rescue capability of rapid response systems and METs to be realized [25]. Although there are several different models which denote those factors and characteristics which influence FTR [9, 15], the most simplistic approach put forth by Silber specifies that causes of FTR can be attributed to patient-level factors and hospital- or system-level factors.

Causes of FTR: Patient-Level Factors

Static Patient-Level Factors

Patient-level factors contributing to FTR can be static or dynamic. The traditional static patient-level factors that are present upon hospital admission but which contribute to death due to complications are age, race, gender, and health risk factors such as obesity and smoking [1]. Comorbid disease states also contribute to FTR and are not only associated with increased mortality [26], but with increased risk to develop instability. Patients with even one comorbid condition are more likely to become unstable than those without comorbidities, and each 1-unit increase on the Charlson comorbidity index increases the odds of becoming unstable by 1.7-fold [27]. Thus, demographic risk factors, the complexity of the patient's health problem, and the presence of comorbidities are important attributes in targeting those patients who are most at risk for the development of complications and therefore in need of a higher level of surveillance [28]. These static patient-level factors, long known to contribute to the mortality of hospitalized patients, are incorporated in a variety of illness acuity scoring systems. More recently, frailty has also emerged as a demonstrable FTR risk present upon admission [29].

Dynamic Physiologic Patient Data and Surveillance

Dynamic patient-level factors contributing to FTR are those variable signs of physiologic deterioration which precede cardiac arrest, death, or emergency intensive care unit (ICU) admission. The ultimate goal is to both identify and quantify these dynamic monitoring variables and their thresholds which precede such events [30, 31] in a manner that is sensitive and specific. Such information is essential to first detect the instability and then recognize its importance, in order to intervene or escalate care. However, the efficacy of METs is dependent upon the two components of the MET: the ability to "track," meaning to detect instability using periodic or continuous observation of the dynamic physiologic signals, and "trigger," meaning to appropriately respond to the instability:

1. *Some types of instability are harder to detect and recognize than others.* Instability can be a manifestation of a large number of pathophysiologic underpinnings, but the rapid response literature suggests that reasons for MET calls aggregate into a limited number of clusters or "MET syndromes" [32]. They are (1) hypotension, (2) dysrhythmias, (3) respiratory distress [any or all of dyspnea, tachypnea, hypopnea, or hypoxemia], (4) neurologic derangements, and (5) oliguria, with finally (6) "worried" or concern by any member of staff or even by visitors [33]. Although the literature suggests that MET calls are mainly associated with a respiratory cause [32], these are also more likely to be delayed [33, 34]. Quach et al. [34] related that delayed MET calls occurred in 50% of patients with a call for the MET syndrome of respiratory distress, as compared to 39% of those with hypotension and that the median delay duration was 13 h for respiratory syndrome calls vs 5 h for hypotension syndrome ($p = 0.016$). The delay in making a call was associated with increased mortality (odds ratio 2.10; 95% CI 1.01–4.34, $p = 0.045$). Santiano et al. [35] retrospectively

analyzed the charts of patients for whom "worried" was the reason for the MET call and evaluated notes and other data to characterize etiology according to a so-called MET syndrome. They found that staff concern for the patients' "breathing" status was by far the most common syndrome associated with a subjective "worried" call. Thus, it appears that respiratory causation, although the most common MET syndrome, is also the syndrome clinicians feel less sure about, resulting in delayed calls. Further research needs to be conducted in this important area. For example, we don't understand why respiratory rate is the vital sign most likely to be missing from vital sign documentation charted vitals [36, 37], even in systems requiring early warning scoring systems for which respiratory rate is needed for calculation [38, 39]. In one study by Mok et al. [40], nurses indicated that they had less confidence in respiratory rate as an indicator of respiratory distress than in pulse oximetry, thereby missing the importance of tachypnea as an early distress indicator prior to overt hypoxemia. In another study, Ansell [41] found that respiratory rate measures were not highly valued by nurses as an indicator of instability. Nevertheless, a systematic review examining the clinical relevance of measured vital signs in relation to mortality, shock, and ICU admission indicated that respiratory rate was the vital sign most highly associated with these negative outcomes [42]. It may be that refocusing bedside caregivers on assessment of a patient's respiratory status (rate, depth, pattern, dyspnea, use of accessory muscles, etc.) and its importance as an instability indicator [43, 44] and the need for calling the MET in a timely manner may be beneficial in addressing improvement in FTR rates.

2. *Instability is a process that usually evolves continuously over time, making its quantification difficult until late in its course.* Dynamic physiologic data are traditionally measured via the periodic observation of vital signs. Bell et al. [45] demonstrated that patients who exhibited even one episode of single-parameter vital sign abnormality during hospitalization had a higher 30-day mortality rate (25%) as compared to patients who did not (3.5%). However, it is difficult to determine which vital sign parameters, and which threshold values, can demonstrate MET efficacy when being used for track and trigger functions. DeVita et al. showed that using some predefined numeric trigger thresholds for HR, RR, BP, and SpO_2 was superior to an open-ended clinician judgment call alone [46]. However, which parameters and which threshold trigger for these vital signs remain debatable. There are many reports published using single-parameter track and trigger criteria, but there is variability in which parameters and thresholds should be used [47].

In attempt to improve the triggering levels, so-called early warning scores (EWS) which aggregate and weight scores are assigned to multiple vital signs. Increasing levels of abnormality are aggregated to a single index score, which in turn has a different trigger threshold [47–49]. Smith et al. [50] conducted a systematic review of 33 unique aggregate weighted track and trigger systems. Although most were poor at discriminating between survivors and non-survivors, 12 had area under the receiver operating characteristics (AUROC) curve between 0.700 and 0.799, with the top four methods incorporating age and the top two methods incorporating temperature. However, none had AUROC ≥ 0.8 which would indicate good discrimination. More recent iterations demonstrate improved metrics, with the National Early Warning Score (NEWS) demonstrating area AUROC 0.722 (0.685–0.759) for cardiac arrest, 0.857 (0.847–0.868) for unanticipated cardiac arrest, 0.894 (0.887–0.902) for death, and 0.873 (0.866–0.879) for any outcomes [51]. Similar efficacy has been demonstrated by the decision-tree early warning score (DTEWS) which determines values and weighting via machine learning [51]. In their current iterations, most EWS track and trigger systems still require intermittent clinician presence at the bedside to gather the data and develop the score by hand, with personal digital assistant (PDA) calculation at the bedside [52] or through linkage of the PDA or electronic medical record to a local area network and centralized evaluation [53] to determine the aggregated threshold value and make a call decision.

However, EWS systems can only work to their full benefit if they are populated accurately and completely and then used as calling protocols recommend. Odell [19] noted in one study of 214 cardiorespiratory arrests that the EWS was completed in 84% of the time but was done so inaccurately in nearly 25 percent of cases. Further, even when trigger thresholds were reached, adherence to referral was substandard, suggesting that other mechanisms or processes contributed to lack of adherence. Several systematic reviews have been conducted for the ability of EWS to improve patient survival [54, 55]. Although they conclude that these aggregated scoring systems are likely more sensitive and specific than single-parameter systems, there is still inability to demonstrate unequivocal benefit based on scoring system alone, since ultimately such scores must be coupled with a clinical decision to make the call so as to impact outcome. Moreover, concentrating on numbers ignores the obvious clinical impressions of experienced bedside clinicians and overlooks what is arguably the important trigger—staff concern.

In addition to the difficulty in identifying which vital sign parameters and thresholds, either singly or in weighted combination, should serve as activation criteria, the frequency with which the surveillance occurs presents another barrier. Galhotra et al. demonstrated that even mature RRSs with track and trigger mechanisms based upon intermittent patient evaluation may still miss potentially avoidable cardiac arrests [56]. Parameters and triggers aside, this can be partly explained by the fact that instability, when it occurs, is not a static phenomenon. Rather, it is characterized by patient's cyclically moving above and below abnormality thresholds as their compensatory mechanisms first correct and then fail to correct the physiologic cause for instability [57]. An example is shown in Fig. 10.1. This patient first demonstrates hypoxemia with low SpO_2. In compensation, RR and HR increase to improve oxygen uptake and transport, which is effective—SpO_2 improves for a brief period, and RR and HR lower. Shortly, however, the cycle repeats itself, with 4 cycles of deterioration, compensation, and improvement over a 5-h period which increase in intensity and duration. Intermittent observation and recording of vital signs for this patient between cycles would have missed the instability.

Even continuous monitoring of vital signs provides no guarantee that instability will not be missed. And in fact, continuous monitoring brings with it the real and present danger of alarm fatigue. Fatigue occurs when so many monitoring alarms are false or not acted on and they are ignored and no longer "heard" [58]. Although alarm fatigue has been a known entity for some time, it advanced in public consciousness, when a highly publicized patient death occurred at a prestigious medical center, despite multiple low heart rate alarms sounding on a patient prior to cardiac arrest. No one working on the unit that day recalled hearing an alarm [59, 60]. This represents a serious patient safety concern. The ideal alarm system would never miss a clinically important event (100% sensitivity) and would never go off if there is no clinically important event (100% specificity) [60]. The literature reports than anywhere from 72–95% of single-parameter monitor alarms are false [61–64]. This is because alarms are designed to err on the side of high sensitivity but at the expense of low specificity [60]. As a result, clinicians begin to consider alarms as a nuisance rather than a helpful alert, leading to such alarms being ignored, disabled, or silenced [65]. In one survey, 18% of nurses reported patients experiencing adverse events related to alarms at their institutions [58]. Several reviews have been conducted on the problem of alarm fatigue [58, 66]. Some approaches to addressing the problem include connecting alarms with escalation protocols to pagers [67], adjusting alarm thresholds and delays [68, 69], tailoring

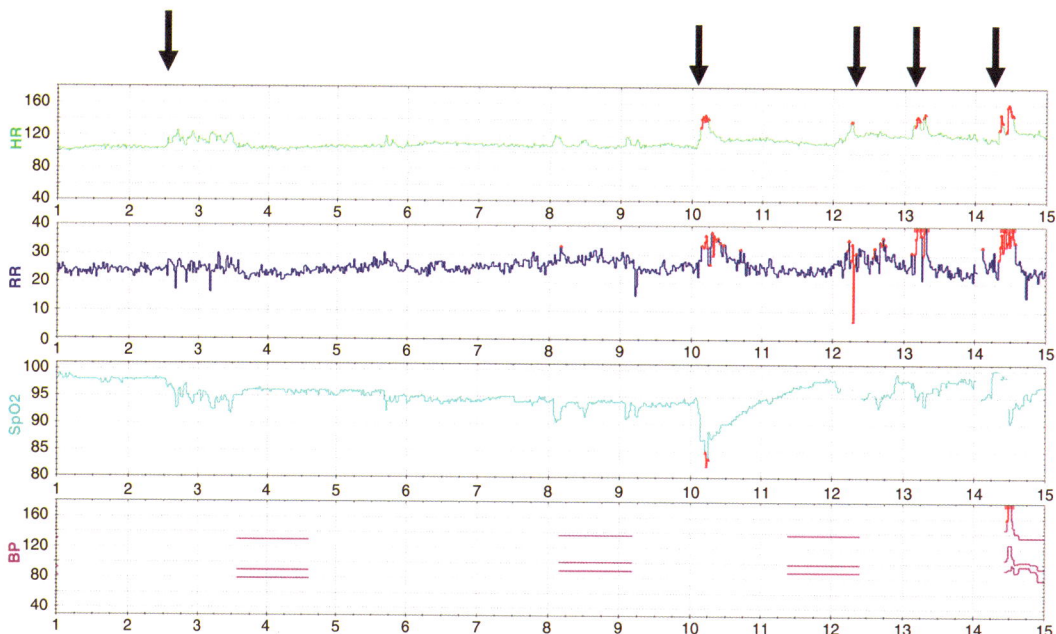

Fig. 10.1 Illustration of the cyclic nature of typical cardiorespiratory instability. Oxygen saturation (SpO$_2$) begins to trend downward beginning at 02:30, with gradual rise in respiratory rate (RR). At shortly after 10:00, abrupt drop in SpO$_2$ triggers compensatory mechanisms of tachypnea and tachycardia, resulting in transiently improved oxygen saturation. At 12:30 the cycles begin again. At the fourth cycle at 14:30, hypertension occurs as well. Although the patient is unstable for 5 h beginning at 10:00 onward, intermittent observation not timed to the vital sign nadirs and apices would have not recognized the patient as being across track and trigger threshold

thresholds to the individual patient [59, 70], and scaling alerts to severity [71].

Additional approaches to increase the sensitivity and specificity of alerting mechanisms to instability, while reducing false alerts and thereby reducing alarm fatigue, lie in data fusion methods. "Smart alarm systems" use technology to review incoming data streams from multiple sources, analyze these data to reject artifact, use multiple inputs to determine clinical conditions worthy of alarms, and then pass that information to the best person to address the problem [72]. These systems utilize multiple parameters, parameter features, rate of parameter change, interactions between multiple parameters, and signal quality to inform alarms [73–75]. These systems have not yet been developed to the extent of widespread clinical use and acceptance, but information about them is passing into the literature, and in one survey, 77% of nurses felt that such systems held promise for reducing false alerts [58].

In the context of FTR, such smart alarm systems can also "marry" weighted aggregate scoring with continuous monitoring. Such systems can continuously evaluate multiple physiologic parameters for subtle departure from normality [76]. In one example, the ability of an IMS (Visensia™, OBS Medical, Carmel, IN) to detect instability on a single step-down unit (SDU) was made [77]. The IMS used the standard noninvasive hardwired monitoring variables of HR, RR, BP, and SpO$_2$ to develop a single neural networked signal. In the first phase, the IMS was connected but the index values were not visible to the clinicians. In patients for whom a MET was called, the IMS detected instability with a mean advance time of 6.3 h [77]. In a later phase, index values were available to the staff, who responded to audible alerts when the IMS crossed an instability threshold. In this phase, both the incidence and duration of patient instability were reduced, presumably due to earlier instability recognition and treatment [78]. Thus, the use of data fusion approaches which aggregate and weight physiologic data within a continuous monitoring environment, coupled with an alerting system and algorithm for clinician action, has shown promise in permitting clinicians to reduce patient instability.

The future in assessing dynamic patient-level factors contributing to FTR may lie in perfecting track and trigger systems which utilize wireless technology to continuously and non-invasively monitored patients for early subtle departures from normality and utilize aggregate data to both screen out artifact [79] and develop dynamic index scores which can alert the clinician to attend to the patient for further evaluation and early intervention [80]. Detection will be further improved with ability to measure metabolic markers of tissue wellness noninvasively and continuously [81, 82]. Nevertheless, improvements in detection of the dynamic patient-level factors contributing to FTR can only be fully realized when the system-level factors as indicated below are also addressed, since improved detection can only positively impact patient outcomes when coupled with appropriate recognition, timely therapy [83], and empowerment to act.

As yet we do not know what affect a RRS has on the culture of an organization. It could be that just the presence of such a system is important and the exact levels of triggering as less important.

Causes of FTR: Hospital- or System-Level Factors

Acute care hospitals are highly complex environments in which many factors contribute to the achievement of quality patient outcomes. Care delivered within such environments is an interdependent and interactive process that is influenced by nurses, physicians, support staff, and the infrastructure and technology designed to support patient care. Providing clinically effective care has been defined as doing the right thing in the right way for the right patient at the right time [84]. Silber and other colleagues who introduced FTR as an outcome measurement found it to be influenced by characteristics other than patient

acuity, such as whether anesthesia care was provided by a board-certified anesthesiologist, or the level of registered nurse staffing. Their assumption was that development of a complication is most strongly influenced by patient-level characteristics but that once a complication develops, provider and organizational characteristics are more strongly linked to patient survival [1, 85]. Hospital characteristics originally determined by Silber as contributory to FTR are level of technology, number of beds, average daily census, total number of physicians, physician specialties and board certification, nurse-to-patient ratio, and nurse-to-bed ratio [1]. Additional system-level factors that are described by others, especially within the nursing literature, are system factors which inhibit recognition of instability and a call for help, such as inadequate nurse staffing or education [86–88].

Staffing and Education

Using the same surgical patient population as Silber and colleagues, Aiken and colleagues reported that, after adjusting for patient and hospital characteristics, an assignment of one additional patient per nurse was associated with a 7% increase in the likelihood of FTR [7]. Both Aiken et al. and Needleman et al. [7, 9] found significant differences in FTR rates that were directly related to nurse education and the number of patients assigned. Senior nursing staff, certified nurses, and lower nurse/patient ratios all were associated with lower FTR rates. Even though the effect of higher nurse staffing levels associated with lower FTR has been corroborated by others [89], both patient acuity [90] and the rate of patient throughput are also implicated as factors contributing to FTR [91]. Park et al. [91] demonstrated that higher nurse staffing was associated with decreased FTR, but when patient turnover (the percentage of patients on a unit or hospital changing over [admissions, discharges, and transfers] in a 24-h period) increased from 48.6% to 60.7% in non-ICUs, the beneficial effect of staffing on FTR was reduced by 11.5%.

Kendall-Gallagher et al. [92] demonstrated nurse educational preparation as significantly related to inpatient mortality and FTR, and each 10% increase in hospital proportion of baccalaureate and certified baccalaureate staff nurses decreased odds of adjusted 30-day inpatient mortality by 6% and 2%, respectively, with identical results for FTR. Common features of system-level factors hinge on the ability of the healthcare facility to provide both adequate personnel as defined by numbers, education and training, and experience of bedside nurses, as well as sufficient resources to permit opportunities for evaluative encounters, process the evaluative information accurately, and implement the correct interventions in a timely manner. Linking those common system-level factors and the role of nursing to FTR, Aiken's conceptual model demonstrates the relationship between patient outcomes and nursing outcomes: burnout, retention, and nurse-rated quality of care [7]. Nurse-assessed quality of care was directly related to effective organizational support provided to the nursing staff, and nurse job satisfaction and retention of experienced nurses improved patient outcomes [93]. Magnet and magnet-like hospitals experiencing adequate nurse resources, nurse autonomy, and improved nurse-physician relations reported higher nurse satisfaction and retention, with lower FTR [7, 94]. Aiken's work has emphasized the importance of the adequacy of clinical staff—both in numbers and education—in improving patient outcomes and decreasing FTR.

Varying Staffing Levels Over Time of Day and Day of Week

A variety of other system-level factors contributory to FTR have also been identified. While it is assumed that overall instability prevalence should be relatively constant over a 24-h day, staffing and surveillance levels temporally vary, and the common finding of diurnal variation of MET activation strongly suggests that this system factor relates to delayed MET activation and ultimately FTR. Presently, the interaction of these factors and FTR is not well understood. Several studies have reported a pattern characterized by more MET activations during the day shift, compared with the night shift, as well as clustering of MET activations at times associated with routine observations and nursing handover [95–97]. Nevertheless, it has been shown that the rate at which patients become unstable is not related to time of day or day of week once time of admission is accounted for. Patients are more likely to become unstable in the hours immediately following admission to a unit, but not more likely at nights or weekends [98]. One explanation for the increased number of MET calls during daylight hours and weekday, in spite of lack of a corroborating fluctuation in patient instability at those times, is that nonclinical or support staff availability is typically greater during the day shift, which would increase the number of people supporting the registered nurse and visits to patient rooms. Accordingly, it is possible that we are "seeing" the patient with more vigilance during the weekday. A corollary to this is that patients are equally unstable during the night hours but that this instability is missed because of fewer patient encounters by the staff. This is corroborated by data demonstrating that survival rates for in-hospital cardiac arrest are lower during nights and weekends, even when adjusting for potentially confounding patient and hospital characteristics, suggesting that these patients are not discovered until later in their event period [99]. Staff fatigue may be another factor contributing to FTR rates [100]. Equality in staffing levels around the clock and across the week has the potential to decrease FTR.

Lack of Clinician Exposure to Instability Events on a Consistent Basis

Another factor that can contribute to FTR is that staff may be unsure in how to assess and respond to instability if they are not exposed to such cases on a consistent basis [101]. Although bedside clinicians may advance from novice to expert in instability detection, recognition, and care as they become more experienced, the learning curve may be lengthy and steep, at the expense of patient safety. Potentially, high-fidelity human simulation (HFHS) education can provide for increased exposure and education in low-frequency high-risk events in order to improve both technical and cognitive skills [102]. Education using HFHS can be used to teach, practice, and remediate skills without harm to patients, thereby increasing experience and correcting problem areas in a safe environment [103]. HFHS education has demonstrated the ability to increase the knowledge and confidence of nurses on hospital wards in identifying deteriorating patients, as well as improve communication between nurses and healthcare providers in relaying key information regarding the patients' deteriorating state [104]. In one study, HFHS education was able to demonstrate decreased time to application of critical interventions and time to escalation of care [105]. HFHS education is also being used to improve recognition of patient deterioration within nursing education programs prior to those nurses' entry into practice [106, 107]. It will be important to determine if such efforts translate into changes in practice in the dynamic clinical setting, resulting in decreased FTR.

Lack of Situation Awareness

Another contributor to FTR is lack of clinician awareness of the patient's situation and unstable state. Situation awareness (SA) is the perception of data elements in the environment, comprehension of their meaning, and projection of their status in the near future [108]. Clearly, if the bedside nurse does not perceive that the patient's condition is deteriorating even though it is, having higher nurse-to-patient ratios cannot be expected to decrease FTR. SA can be measured on three levels: perception, understanding, and prediction. SA is a skill that can be used to help clinicians "think ahead" by improving awareness of what is happening, understanding what is happening, and anticipating what might occur next. Improving SA is becoming part of a reasoned and systematic approach to teaching clinicians about the compo-

nents of detecting, recognizing, and managing deteriorating patients—both as individuals and as teams [109, 110]—or as a way of exploring patterns of error [111]. Importantly, there are tools to evaluate SA, making it quantifiable. As such, it can also be used to complement HFHS education to assess education effectiveness [110]. Using a SA framework for education regarding deteriorating patients has been demonstrated to provide valuable metrics in understanding areas needing improvement as well as measuring improvement [112–114] and has potential to decrease FTR.

Lack of Human Factors Awareness

While situation awareness concentrates on an individual's understanding of the situation, human factors awareness is more closely related to team function and communication. Human factors that can contribute to poor performance include breakdowns in communication, poor teamwork, lack of leadership, and lack of a safety culture [115, 116]. Crew resource management (CRM), long utilized in aviation safety, is a system approach to improve human factors awareness and safety culture and as such aims to use standardized communication tools to improve process effectiveness and safety. Aspects of CRM in the dynamic clinical setting include situation awareness, recognition of adverse situations, human errors and non-putative response, communication and briefing and debriefing techniques, providing and receiving performance feedback, management of stress, workload and fatigue, creating and managing team structure and climate, leadership in a flat hierarchy environment, and risk management and decision-making [116, 117]. CRM adoption has demonstrated positive results. In a prospective 3-year cohort study in an ICU, adoption of CRM resulted in a significant decrease in serious complications, the incidence of cardiopulmonary arrests, and mortality [116]. There are also reports on the effect of CRM training and adoption on step-down or high-density units [118] and wards [113]. In one study, CRM resulted in an increase in the number of patients achieving MET trigger criteria for whom the team was called (improved from 4% to 22%, $p < 0.0001$) and decreased the percentage of patients achieving MET trigger criteria for whom the team was not called (fell from 25% to 12%, $p = 0.03$) [118].

Barriers Are Present to Escalating Care

A number of barriers may exist to escalation of care (EOC). In one qualitative study by Johnston et al. [119], two main themes as EOC barriers emerged: failure to recognize patient deterioration and failure to communicate concerns to a senior colleague. For the latter, fear of a negative response was identified as a key reason why a nurse or junior physician would not communicate their concerns to a senior. These findings were corroborated in another qualitative study targeting barriers to calling for the MET in a system where the MET was well established [120]. Themes in barriers to EOC in that study were lack of self-efficacy in detecting and recognizing instability (i.e., perception that one has the skills and abilities to perform a behavior), hierarchical barriers (i.e., fear of or actual negative response to EOC), expectation of a negative outcome such as loss of patient care control when they are up-transferred, or even fear of resistance and criticism from the MET team themselves (e.g., MET team feels the patient is stable, and clinicians have to use excessive time and energy to provide strong justification for their decision to call). Information overload has also been cited as a barrier to EOC [121]. Similarly, allegiance to the primary team often inhibits MET activation [122]. However, when nurses activate the MET directly, patients are more likely to be stabilized and remain on the ward or step-down unit and not require transfer to a higher-intensity unit, than when they first consult with physicians who in turn activate the call [123]. It has proven difficult to overcome these barriers relative to fear of negative responses on a variety of levels. In response to this barrier, some institutions are implement-

ing a more "bundled" approach to the rapid response system, such as adding charge nurse rounding to seek out at-risk patients proactively and concentrated education of both nurses and physicians on patient surveillance and deterioration recognition [124]. The use of "ramp-up" approaches has also been reported, which provides clinicians with an opportunity to first obtain consultation with a single skilled nurse or physician before full MET activation [125, 126].

Conclusion

FTR is a serious patient safety concern that is due to a complex chain of both static and dynamic patient-level and system-level factors, and there is interplay and likely even synergism between factors. Evaluation of the impact of METs and their variants has provided both positive [127–130] and ambivalent [131–133] results. As the push to minimize hospitalizations for the treatment of acute illness increases and the time of acute care hospitalization decreases with greater pressure to move more potentially unstable patients out of intensive monitoring units into less well-monitored sites, the risk of FTR will only increase. We provide a model which incorporates Aiken's conceptual model for hospital-level factors, Silber's patient and hospital characteristics, the FTR literature in general, and our own observations regarding the static and dynamic patient-level factors for FTR in Fig. 10.2. Such a model may help to guide the understanding of the complexity of the interrelationships impacting FTR in the context of METs.

The often observed inconsistency in the effectiveness of the MET approach across different healthcare systems might be explained by the many other patient- and system-level factors which also impact FTR beyond the scope of the MET. Developing mechanisms to improve the acquisition of continuous, sensitive, and specific physiologic data to predict future instability likelihood or detect present instability accurately and support the bedside caregiver's decision to call for help; eliminating system barriers that inhibit recognition of and response to instability, such as

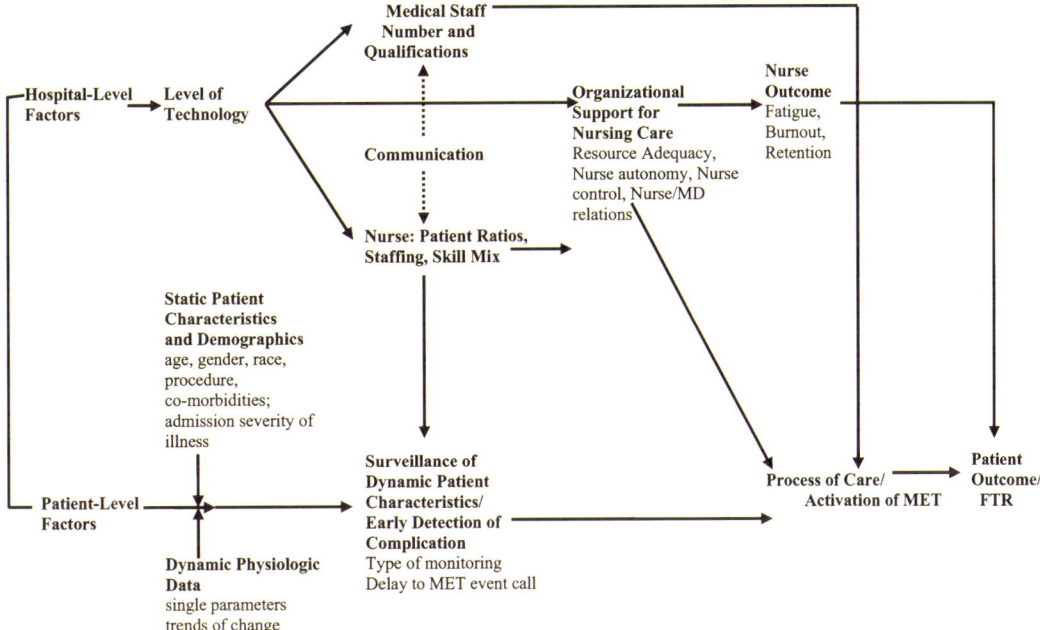

Fig. 10.2 Conceptual model for causes of failure to rescue incorporating medical emergency team availability

staff availability, education, and experience; and employing a culture of safety and teamwork are necessary for a successful comprehensive approach to FTR reduction.

References

1. Silber JH, Williams SV, Krakauer H, Schwartz JS. Hospital and patient characteristics associated with death after surgery. A study of adverse occurrence and failure to rescue. Med Care. 1992;30:615–29.
2. AHRQ. Patient safety indicators. AHRQ quality indicators. Rockville, MD: Agency for Healthcare Research and Quality; February 2006.
3. Silber JH, Romano PS, Rosen AK, Wang Y, Even-Shoshan O, Volpp KG. Failure-to-rescue: comparing definitions to measure quality care. Med Care. 2007;45:918–25.
4. Schmid A, Hoffman LA, Happ MB, Wolf GA, DeVita MA. Failure to rescue: a literature review. J Nurs Adm. 2007;4:188–98.
5. Aiken LH, Clarke SP, Sloane DM, Lake ET, Cheney T. Effects of Hospital care environment and patient mortality and nurse outcomes. J Nurs Adm. 2008;38:223–9.
6. Needleman J, Buerhaus P, Mattke S. Nurse staffing and quality of care in hospitals. NEJM. 2002;346:1415–22.

7. Aiken LH, Clarke SP, Sloane DM, Sochalski J, Silber JH. Hospital nurse staffing and patient mortality, nurse burnout, and job dissatisfaction. JAMA. 2002;288:1987–93.
8. National Quality Forum (NQF). National voluntary consensus standards for nursing-sensitive care: an initial performance measure set. Washington, DC: National Quality Forum; 2004.
9. Needleman J, Buerhaus PI. Failure-to-rescue: comparing definitions to measure quality of care. Med Care. 2007;45:913–5.
10. Bail K, Berry H, Grealish L, et al. Potentially preventable complications of urinary tract infections, pressure areas, pneumonia, and delirium in hospitalised dementia patients: retrospective cohort study. BMJ Open. 2013;3:e002770.
11. Sammon JD, Pucheril D, Abdollah F, et al. Preventable mortality after common urological surgery: failing to rescue? BJU Int. 2015;115:666–74.
12. Ilonzo N, Egorova NN, McKinsey JF, Nowygrod R. Failure to rescue trends in elective abdominal aortic aneurysm repair between 1995 and 2011. J Vasc Surg. 2014;60:1473–80.
13. Joseph B, Zangbar B, Khalil M, et al. Factors associated with failure-to-rescue in patients undergoing trauma laparotomy. Surgery. 2015;158(2):393–8. doi:10.1016/j.surg.2015.03.047.
14. Westaby S, De Silva R, Petrou M, Bond S, Taggart D. Surgeon-specific mortality data disguise wider failings in delivery of safe surgical services. Eur J Cardiothorac Surg. 2014;ezu380.

15. Aiken LH, Clarke SP, Chueng RB, Sloan DM, Silber JH. Educational levels of hospital nurses and surgical patient mortality. JAMA. 2003;290:1617–23.

16. Nurmi J, Harjola VP, Nolan J, Castren M. Observations and warning signs prior to cardiac arrest: should medical emergency teams intervene earlier? Acta Anesthesiol Scand. 2005;49:702–6.

17. Vetro J, Natarajan DK, Mercer I, Buckmaster JN, Heland M, Hart GK, Bellomo R, Jones DA. Antecedents to cardiac arrests in a hospital equipped with a medical emergency team. Crit Care Resusc. 2011;13:162–6.

18. Stevenson JE, Israelsson J, Nilsson GC, Petersson GI, Bath PA. Recording signs of deterioration in acute patients: the documentation of vital signs within electronic health records in patients who suffered in-hospital cardiac arrest. Health Informatics J. 2014;22(1):21–33.

19. Odell M. Detection and management of the deteriorating ward patient: an evaluation of nursing practice. J Clin Nurs. 2015;24:173–82.

20. Devita MA, Bellomo R, Hillman K, et al. Findings of the first consensus conference on medical emergency teams. Crit Care Med. 2006;34:2463–78.

21. DeVita MA, Smith GB. Rapid response systems: is it the team or the system that is working? Crit Care Med. 2007;35:2218–9.

22. Acquaviva K, Haskell H, Johnson J. Human cognition and the dynamics of failure to rescue: the Lewis Blackman case. J Prof Nurs. 2013;29:95–101.

23. Ghaferi AA, Dimick JB. Understanding failure to rescue and improving safety culture. Ann Surg. 2015;261:839–40.

24. Wakeam E, Hevelone ND, Maine R, et al. Failure to rescue in safety-net hospitals: availability of hospital resources and differences in performance. JAMA Surg. 2014;149:229–35.

25. Mackintosh N, Humphrey C, Sandall J. The habitus of 'rescue' and its significance for implementation of rapid response systems in acute health care. Soc Sci Med. 2014;120:233–42.

26. Smith GB, Prytherch DR, Schmidt PE, Featherstone PI, Kellett J, Deane B, Higgins B. Should age be included as a component of track and trigger systems used to identify sick adult patients? Resuscitation. 2008;78:109–15.

27. Yousef KM, Pinsky MR, DeVita MA, Sereika S, Hravnak M. Characteristics of patients with cardiorespiratory instability in a step-down unit. Am J Crit Care. 2012;21:344–0.

28. Talsma AN, Bahl V, Campbell DA. Exploratory analyses of the "failure to rescue" measure. J Nurs Care Qual. 2008;23(3):202–10.

29. Arya S, Sim SI, Duwayri Y, Brewster LP, Veeraswamy R, Salam A, Dodson TF. Frailty increases the risk of 30-day mortality, morbidity, and failure-to-rescue after elective abdominal aortic aneurysm repair independent of age and comorbidities. J Vasc Surg. 2015;61:324–31.

30. Cuthbertson BH, Boroujerdi M, McKie L, Aucott A, Prescott G. Can physiological variables and early warning scoring systems allow early recognition of the deteriorating surgical patient? Crit Care Med. 2007;35:402–9.

31. Bobay KL, Fiorelli KL, Anderson AJ. Failure to rescue: a preliminary study of patient level factors. J Nurs Care Qual. 2008;23:211–5.

32. Jones D, Duke G, Green J, et al. Medical emergency team syndromes and an approach to their management. Crit Care. 2006;10:R30.

33. Calzavacca P, Licari E, Tee A, et al. A prospective study of factors influencing the outcome of patients after a medical emergency team review. Intensive Care Med. 2008;34:2112–6.

34. Quach JL, Downey AW, Haase M, Haase-Fielitz A, Jones D, Bellomo R. Characteristics and outcomes of patients receiving a medical emergency team review for respiratory distress or hypotension. J Crit Care. 2008;23:325–31.

35. Santiano N, Young L, Hillman K, et al. Analysis of medical emergency team calls comparing subjective to "objective" call criteria. Resuscitation. 2009;80:44–9.

36. Chen J, Hillman K, Bellomo R, et al. The impact of introducing medical emergency team system on the documentations of vital signs. Resuscitation. 2009;80:35–43.

37. Tirkkonen J, Ylä-Mattila J, Olkkola KT, Huhtala H, Tenhunen J, Hoppu S. Factors associated with delayed activation of medical emergency team and excess mortality: an Utstein-style analysis. Resuscitation. 2013;84:173–8.

38. Kyriacos U, Jelsma J, Jordan S. Record review to explore the adequacy of post-operative vital signs monitoring using a local modified early warning score (mews) chart to evaluate outcomes. PLoS One. 2014;9(1):e87320. doi:10.1371/journal.pone.0087320.eCollection 2014.

39. Jonsson T, Jonsdottir H, Möller AD, Baldursdottir L. Nursing documentation prior to emergency admissions to the intensive care unit. Nurs Crit Care. 2011;16:164–9.

40. Mok W, Wang W, Cooper S, Ang ENK, Liaw SY. Attitudes towards vital signs monitoring in the detection of clinical deterioration: scale development and survey of ward nurses. International J Qual Health Care. 2015;27(3):mzv019.

41. Ansell H, Meyer A, Thompson S. Why don't nurses consistently take patient respiratory rates? Br J Nurs. 2014;23(8):414–8.

42. Storm-Versloot MN, Verweij L, Lucas C, et al. Clinical relevance of routinely measured vital signs in hospitalized patients: a systematic review. J Nurs Scholarsh. 2014;46:39–49.

43. Ludikhuize J, Smorenburg SM, de Rooij SE, de Jonge E. Identification of deteriorating patients on general wards; measurement of vital parameters and potential effectiveness of the modified early warning score. J Crit Care. 2012;27(4):424.e7–13. doi:10.1016/j.jcrc.2012.01.003.

44. Lynn LA, Curry JP. Patterns of unexpected in-hospital deaths: a root cause analysis. Patient Saf Surg. 2011;5(1):3. doi:10.1186/1754-9493-5-3.

45. Bell MB, Konrad D, Granath F, Ekbom A, Martline CR. Prevalence and sensitivity of MET-criteria in a Scandinavian-University Hospital. Resuscitation. 2006;70:66–73.

46. DeVita MA, Braithwaite RS, Mahidhara R, et al. Use of medical emergency team responses to reduce cardiopulmonary arrests. Qual Saf Health Care. 2004;13:251–4.

47. Gao H, McDonnell A, Harrison DA, Moore T, Adam S, Daly K, Esmonde L, Goldhill DR, Parry GJ, Rashidan A, Subbe CP, Harvey S. Systematic review and evaluation of physiological track and trigger warning systems for identifying at risk patients on the ward. Intensive Care Med. 2007;33:667–79.

48. Subbe CP. Validation of a modified early warning score in medical admissions. QJM. 2001;94:521–6.

49. Subbe CP, Gao H, Harrison DA. Reproducibility of physiological track-and-trigger warning systems for identifying at-risk patients on the ward. Intensive Care Med. 2007;33:667–79.

50. Smith GB, Prytherch DR, Schmidt PE, Featherstone PI. Review and performance evaluation of aggregate weighted "track and trigger" systems. Resuscitation. 2008;77:170–9.

51. Badriyah T, Briggs JS, Meredith P, et al. Decision-tree early warning score (DTEWS) validates the design of the National Early Warning Score (NEWS). Resuscitation. 2014;85:418–23.

52. Prytherch DR, Smith GB, Schmidt P, Featherstone PI, Stewart K, Knight D, Higgins B. Calculating early warning scores—a classroom comparison of pen and paper and hand-held computer methods. Resuscitation. 2006;70:173–8.

53. Smith GB, Prytherch DR, Schmidt P, Featherstone PI, Knight D, Clement G, Mohammed MA. Hospital-wide surveillance—a new approach to the early identification and management of the sick patient. Resuscitation. 2006;71:19–28.

54. Alam N, Hobbelink E, van Tienhoven A, van de Ven P, Jansma E, Nanayakkara P. The impact of the use of the Early Warning Score (EWS) on patient outcomes: a systematic review. Resuscitation. 2014;85(5):587–94.

55. McNeill G, Bryden D. Do either early warning systems or emergency response teams improve hospital patient survival? A systematic review. Resuscitation. 2013;84(12):1652–67.

56. Galhotra D, DeVita MA, Simmons RL, Dew MA, Members of the Medical Emergency Response Improvement Team (MERIT) Committee. Mature rapid response system and potentially avoidable cardiopulmonary arrests in hospital. Qual Saf Health Care. 2007;16:260–5.

57. Bose EL, Hravnak M, Pinsky MR. The interface between monitoring and physiology at the bedside. Crit Care Clin. 2015;31(1):1–24. doi:10.1016/j.ccc.2014.08.001.

58. Funk M, Clark JT, Bauld TJ, Ott JC, Coss P. Attitudes and practices related to clinical alarms. Am J Crit Care. 2014;23(3):e9–e18.

59. Drew BJ, Harris P, Zègre-Hemsey JK, et al. Insights into the problem of alarm fatigue with physiologic monitor devices: a comprehensive observational study of consecutive intensive care unit patients. PLoS One. 2014;9(10):e110274. doi:10.1371/journal.pone.0110274.

60. Sendelbach S, Funk M. Alarm fatigue: a patient safety concern. AACN Adv Crit Care. 2013;24:378–86.

61. Atzema C, Schull MJ, Borgundvaag B, Slaughter GR, Lee CK. ALARMED: adverse events in low-risk patients with chest pain receiving continuous electrocardiographic monitoring in the emergency department: a pilot study. Am J Emerg Med. 2006;24:62–7.

62. Gorges M, Markewitz BA, Westenskow DR. Improving alarm performance in the medical intensive care unit using delays and clinical context. Anesth Analg. 2009;108:1546–52.

63. Siebig S, Kuhls S, Imhoff M, Gather U, Schölmerich J, Wrede CE. Intensive care unit alarms—how many do we need? Crit Care Med. 2010;38:451–6.

64. Tsein CL, Fackler JC. Poor prognosis for existing monitors in the intensive care unit. Crit Care Med. 1997;25:614–9.

65. Cvach M. Monitor alarm fatigue: an integrative review. Biomed Instrum Technol. 2012;46(4):268–77.

66. Curry JP, Jungquist CR. A critical assessment of monitoring practices, patient deterioration, and alarm fatigue on inpatient wards: a review. Patient Saf Surg. 2014;8:29.

67. Cvach MM, Frank RJ, Doyle P, Stevens ZK. Use of pagers with an alarm escalation system to reduce cardiac monitor alarm signals. J Nurs Care Qual. 2014;29(1):9–18.

68. Graham KC, Cvach M. Monitor alarm fatigue: standardizing use of physiological monitors and decreasing nuisance alarms. Am J Crit Care. 2010;19(1):28–34.

69. Dandoy CE, Davies SM, Flesch L, et al. A team-based approach to reducing cardiac monitor alarms. Pediatrics. 2014;134:e1686–94.

70. Kokani A, Oakley B, Bauld TJ. Reducing hospital noise: a review of medical device alarm management. Biomed Instrum Technol. 2012;46:478–87.

71. Whalen DA, Covelle PM, Piepenbrink JC, Villanova KL, Cuneo CL, Awtry EH. Novel approach to cardiac alarm management on telemetry units. J Cardiovasc Nurs. 2014;29(5):E13–22.

72. Block FE. Why we do not have—and will not have—the integrated and "smart" alarm systems that technology would allow us to have today. J Electrocardiol. 2012;45:592–5.

73. Li Q, Clifford GD. Signal quality and data fusion for false alarm reduction in the intensive care unit. J Electrocardiol. 2012;45:596–603.

74. King A, Fortino K, Stevens N, Shah S, Fortino-Mullen M, Lee I. Evaluation of a smart alarm for intensive care using clinical data. Paper presented at Engineering in Medicine and Biology Society (EMBC), 2012 Annual International Conference of the IEEE2012.

75. Scalzo F, Hu X. Semi-supervised detection of intracranial pressure alarms using waveform dynamics. Physiol Meas. 2013;34:465–78.

76. Tarassenko L, Hann A, Young D. Integrated monitoring and analysis for early warning of patient deterioration. Br J Anaesth. 2006;97:64–8.

77. Hravnak M, Edwards L, Clontz A, Valenta C, DeVita M, Pinsky M. Defining the incidence of cardiorespiratory instability in step-down unit patients using an electronic integrated monitoring system. Arch Intern Med. 2008;168:300–1308.

78. Hravnak M, DeVita MA, Edwards L, Clontz A, Valenta C, Pinsky MR. Cardiorespiratory instability before and after implementing an integrated monitoring system. Am J Respir Crit Care Med. 2008;177:A842.

79. Fiterau M, Dubrawski A, Chen L, Clermont G, Pinsky MR. Automatic identification of artifacts in monitoring critically ill patients. Intensive Care Med. 2013;39(Suppl 2):S470.

80. Guillame-Bert M, Dubrawski A, Chen L, Hravnak M, Pinsky M, Clermont G. Learning temporal rules to forecast instability in intensive care patients. Intensive Care Med. 2013;39(Suppl 2):S470.

81. Hadrian J, Pinsky MR. Functional hemodynamic monitoring. Curr Opin Crit Care. 2007;13:318–23.

82. Puyana JC, Pinsky MR. Searching for non-invasive markers of tissue hypoxia. Crit Care. 2007;116. doi:10.1186/cc5691.

83. Pinsky MR. Hemodynamic evaluation and monitoring in the ICU. Chest. 2007;132:2020–9.

84. Anon. Clinical effectiveness: Royal College of Nursing Guide. London: Royal College of Nursing; 1996.

85. Silber J, Rosenbaum P, Schwartz JS, Ross RN, Williams V. Evaluation of the complication rate as a measure of quality of care in coronary artery bypass surgery. JAMA. 1995;274:317–23.

86. Hinshaw AS. Navigating the perfect storm: Balancing a culture of safety with workforce challenges. Nurs Res. 2008;57:S4–10.

87. Rafferty AM, Clarke SP, Coles J, Ball J, James P, McKee M, Aiken L. Outcomes of variation in hospital nurse staffing in English hospitals: cross-sectional analysis of survey data and discharge records. Int J Nurs Stud. 2007;44:175–82.

88. Seago JA, Williamson A, Atwood C. Longitudinal analyses of nurse staffing and patient outcomes. J Nurs Adm. 2006;36:13–21.

89. Unruh LY, Zhang NJ. Nurse staffing and patient safety in hospitals: new variable and longitudinal approaches. Nurs Res. 2012;61:3–12.

90. Talsma AN, Jones K, Guo Y, Wilson D, Campbell DA. The relationship between nurse staffing and failure to rescue: where does it matter most? J Patient Saf. 2014;10:133–9.

91. Park SH, Blegen MA, Spetz J, Chapman SA, De Groot H. Patient turnover and relationship between nurse staffing and patient outcomes. Res Nurs Health. 2012;35:277–88.

92. Kendall-Gallagher D, Aiken LH, Sloane DM, Comiotti JP. Nurse specialty certification, inpatient mortality, and failure to rescue. J Nurs Scholarsh. 2011;43:189–94.

93. Aiken LH, Clarke SP, Sloane DM, International Hospital Outcomes Research Consortium. Hospital staffing, organization, and quality of care: cross national findings. International J Qual Health Care. 2002;14:5–13.

94. Aiken LH, Sloane DM, Lake ET, Sochalski J, Weber AL. Organization and outcomes of inpatient AIDS care. Med Care. 1999;37:760–72.

95. Jones D, Bellomo R, Bates S, Warrillow S, Goldsmith D, Hart G, Opdam H. Patient monitoring and the timing of cardiac arrests and medical emergency team calls in a teaching hospital. Intensive Care Med. 2006;32:1352–6.

96. Galhotra S, DeVita MA, Simmons RL, Schmid A, Members of the Medical Emergency Response Improvement Team (MERIT) Committee. Impact of patient monitoring on the diurnal pattern of medical emergency team activation. Crit Care Med. 2006;34:1700–6.

97. Schmid A. Frequency and pattern of medical emergency team activation among medical cardiology patient care units. Crit Care Nurs Q. 2007;30:81–4.

98. Hravnak M, Chen L, Dubrawski A, Bose E, Pinsky MR. Temporal distribution of instability events in continuously monitored step-down unit patients: implications for rapid response systems. Resuscitation. 2015;89:99–105.

99. Perberdy MA, Ornato JP, Larkin GL, Braithwaite RS, Kashner TM, Carey SM, Meaney PA, Cen L, Nadkarni VM, Praestgaard AH, Berg RA, National Registry of Cardiopulmonary Resuscitation Investigators. Survival for in-hospital cardiac arrest during nights and weekends. JAMA. 2008;299:785–92.

100. Manojlovich M, Talsma A. Identifying nursing processes to reduce failure to rescue. J Nurs Adm. 2007;11:504–9.

101. Smith GB, Welch J, DeVita MA, Hillman KM, Jones D. Education for cardiac arrest: treatment or prevention? Resuscitation. 2015;92:59–62.

102. Hravnak M, Tuite P, Baldisseri M. Expanding acute care nurse practitioner and clinical nurse specialist education: invasive procedure training and human simulation in critical care. AACN Clin Issues. 2005;16:89–104.

103. Hravnak M, Beach M, Tuite M. Simulator technology as a tool for education in cardiac care. J Cardiovasc Nurs. 2007;22:16–24.

104. Liaw AY, Zhou WT, Lau TC, Siau C, Chan SW. An interprofessional communication trailing using sim-

ulation to enhance safe care for a deteriorating patient. Nurse Educ Today. 2014;34:259–64.

105. Ozekcin LR, Tuite P, Willner K, Hravnak M. Simulation education: early identification of patient physiologic deterioration by acute care nurses. Clin Nurs Spec. 2015;29:166–73.

106. Kelly MA, Forber J, Conlon L, Roche M, Stasa H. Empowering the registered nurses of tomorrow: student's perspectives of a simulation experience for recognising and managing a deteriorating patient. Nurse Educ Today. 2014;34:724–9.

107. Lindsey PL, Jenkins S. Nursing student's clinical judgment regarding rapid response: the influence of a clinical simulation education intervention. Nurs Forum. 2013;48:61–70.

108. Brady PW, Goldenhar LM. A qualitative study examining the influences on situation awareness and the identification, mitigation and escalation of recognised patient risk. BMJ Qual Saf. 2014;23:153–61.

109. Cooper S, Cant J, Missen K, Sparkes L, McConnell-Henry T, Endacott R. Managing patient deterioration: assessing teamwork and individual performance. Emerg Med. 2013;30:377–81.

110. Cooper S, Kinsman L, Buykx P, McConnell-Henry T, Endacott R, Scholes J. Managing the deteriorating patient in a simulated environment: nursing student's knowledge, skill and situation awareness. J Clin Nurs. 2010;19:2309–18.

111. Tallentire VR, Smith SE, Skinner J, Cameron HS. Exploring patterns in error in acute care using framework analysis. BMC Med Educ. 2015;15:3. doi:10.1186/s12909-015-0285-6.

112. McKenna L, Missen K, Cooper S, Bogossian F, Bucknall T, Cant R. Situation awareness in undergraduate nursing students managing simulated patient deterioration. Nurse Educ Today. 2014;34:e27–31.

113. Scuilli GL, Fore AM, West P, Neily J, Mills PD, Paull DE. Nursing crew resource management. JONA. 2013;43:122–6.

114. Bogossian F, Cooper S, Cant R, Beauchamp A, Porter J, Kain V, Bucknall T, Phillips NM, The FIRSTACT Research Team. Undergraduate nursing students' performance in recognising and responding to sudden patient deterioration in high physiological fidelity simulated environments: an Australian multi-center study. Nurse Educ Today. 2014;34:691–6.

115. O'Dea A, O'Connor P, Keough I. A meta-analysis of the effectiveness of crew resource management training in acute care domains. Postgrad Med J. 2014;90:699–708.

116. Haerkens MH, Knox M, Lemson J, Houterman S, van der Hoeven JG, Pickers P. Crew resource management in the intensive care unit: a prospective 3-year cohort study. Acta Anesthesiol Scand. 2015. doi:10.1111/aas.12573. [Epub ahead of print].

117. Haerkens MH, Jenkins DH, van der Hoeven JG. Crew resource management in the ICU: the need for culture change. Ann Intensive Care. 2012 Aug 22;2(1):39. doi:10.1186/2110-5820-2-39.

118. Young-Xu Y, Fore AM, Metcalf A, Payne K, Neily J, Scuilli GL. Using crew resource management and a "read-and-do checklist" to reduce failure to rescue on a stepdown unit. AJN. 2013;113:51–7.

119. Johnston M, Arora S, King D, Stroman L, Darzi A. Escalation of care and failure to rescue: a multi-center, multiprofessional qualitative study. Surgery. 2014;155:989–94.

120. Roberts KE, Bonafide CP, Paine CW, Paciotti B, Tibbetts KM, Keren R, Barg FK, Holmes JH. Barriers to calling for urgent assistance despite a comprehensive pediatric rapid response system. Am J Crit Care. 2014;23:223–9.

121. Swartz C. Recognition of clinical deterioration: a clinical leadership opportunity for nurse executives. JONA. 2013;43:377–81.

122. Jones D, Baldwin I, McIntyre T, Story D, Mercer I, Miglic A, Goldsmith D, Bellomo R. Qual Saf Health Care. 2006;15:427–32.

123. Lobos AR, Fernendes R, Ramsay T, McNally JD. Patient characteristics and disposition after pediatric medical emergency team (MET) activation: disposition depends on who activates the team. Hosp Pediatr. 2:99–105.

124. Davis DP, Aguilar SA, Graham PG, Lawrence B, Sell R, Minodadeh A, Husa R. A novel configuration of a traditional rapid response team decreases nonintensive care unit arrests and overall hospital mortality. J Hosp Med. 2015;10:352–7.

125. Pirret AM, Takerwi SF, Kazula LM. The effectiveness of a patient at risk team comprised of predominantly experienced nurses: a before and after study. Intensive Crit Care Nurs. 2015. doi:10.1111/aas.12573.

126. Massey D, Aitken LM, Chaboyer W. The impact of a nurse led rapid response system on adverse, major adverse events and activation of the medical emergency team. Intensive Crit Care Nurs. 2015;31:83–90.

127. Bucknall TK, Jones D, Bellomo R, Staples M, The RESCUE Investigators. Responding to medical emergencies: system characteristics under examination (RESCUE). A prospective multi-site point prevalence study. Resuscitation. 2013;84:179–83.

128. Jones D, Bellomo R, Bates S, Warrillow S, Goldsmith D, Hart G, Opdam H, Gutteridge G. Long term effect of a medical emergency team on cardiac arrests in a teaching hospital. Crit Care. 2005;9:R808–15.

129. Jones D, Egi M, Bellomo R, Goldsmith D. Effect of the medical emergency team on long-term mortality following major surgery. Crit Care. 2007;11:R12. doi:10.1186/cc5673.

130. Buist M, Harrison J, Abaloz E, Van Dyke S. Six-year audit of cardiac arrests and medical emergency

team calls in an Australian teaching hospital. Br Med J. 2007;335:1210–2.

131. Hillman K, Chen J, Creitkos M, Bellomo R, Brown D, Doig G, Finfer S, Flabouris A, MERIT Investigators. Introduction of the medical emergency team (MET) system: a cluster-randomized controlled trial. Lancet. 2005;365:2091–7.

132. Winters BD, Pham JC, Hunt EA, et al. Rapid response systems: a systematic review. Crit Care Med. 2007;35:1238–43.

133. Chan PS, Khalid A, Longmore LS, Berg RA, Kosiborod M, Spertus JA. Hospital-wide code rates and mortality before and after implementation of a rapid response team. JAMA. 2008;300:2506–13.

Bradford Winters

Introduction

Patients rarely deteriorate suddenly; however, their deterioration is often recognized only at the last minute. In the late 1980s and early 1990s, retrospective chart review studies demonstrated that it was quite clear patient deterioration toward arrest on general hospital wards was heralded by premonitory signs and symptoms, and that there was time to intervene to prevent the patient from going on to a respiratory and/or cardiac arrest. Forward-thinking clinicians took this knowledge and went on to develop the patient safety intervention we now call the Rapid Response System. This System merges an approach to better identify deteriorating patients on general wards with an activation process that brings additional resources to the patient's bedside, usually in the form of a Medical Emergency Team or Rapid Response Team.

Over the last two decades, systems have diversified from the early Medical Emergency Teams (METs) piloted in Australia and in Pittsburgh, Pennsylvania to an array of systems that include Rapid Response Teams (RRTs), Critical Care Outreach Teams (CCOTs), and other strategies to bring additional resources to the bedside of a deteriorating and/or arresting patient. While the rapid response strategy makes intuitive sense and has strong face validity, all patient safety and quality initiatives including RRSs should be put to the test with appropriately rigorous metrics. In this chapter, we will review the published literature for RRSs to try and answer the questions, "do RRS improve patient safety and quality?"

Evaluating the Evidence

Evidence may come from a wide range of sources and vary significantly in quality and quantity. When we weigh the evidence for an intervention, we must be sure to consider these factors. While a thorough review of evidence-based medicine is beyond the scope of this chapter, we will address some guiding principles. First, we should always seek the highest possible quality of evidence when designing studies and reviewing the data to inform our decision-making. Evidence may be categorized based on level of quality (Table 11.1) [1]. At the very top (Level 1) are systematic reviews and meta-analyses of randomized controlled trials (RCTs) that exhibit a high degree of homogeneity; these are followed by individual RCTs with narrow confidence intervals. Level 2 studies include historical or concurrent cohort trials. Level 3 includes case-controlled studies.

B. Winters (✉)
Departments of Anesthesiology, Critical Care
Medicine and The Johns Hopkins University School
of Medicine, Zayed 9127, 1800 Orleans Street,
Baltimore, MD 21298, USA
e-mail: bwinters@jhmi.edu

Table 11.1 Levels of evidence

Evidence level	Types of included studies
Level 1a	Meta-analysis and systematic reviews of RCTS
Level 1b	RCTs (single and multiple institution)
Level 2a	Cluster randomized trials, concurrent cohort controlled trials, step-wise trials
Level 2b	Historically (before/after) controlled trials
Level 3	Case controlled studies
Level 4	Case studies, case series without controls
Level 5	Expert opinion, experience, pathophysiological reasoning, basic science data

Level 4 evidence consists primarily of case series and case studies and Level 5 data is based on expert opinion, physiological principles, bench-top basic science data, or experience. Level 1 trials are able to establish "cause and effect" while studies that do not actively control the intervention in their design can only establish an association.

We should always seek Level 1 evidence as the goal; however, it may not always be available to answer a particular question or may be impractical to carry out in a research setting or may be possibly unethical. There are many situations where the "best" attainable evidence may only be Level 2 quality or lower, leaving us to rely on such evidence to guide decisions. While we should not be dogmatic on insisting on Level 1 or even 2 data when it is not practical or possible, we must be very critical in our appraisals especially if the intervention carries great cost or risk.

How we balance quantity of evidence with quality is more problematic. Do numerous lower quality studies trump a single high quality study with conflicting results? How many lower quality studies does it take? What if the aggregate number of patients in the lower quality study(s) is vastly larger than the higher quality study(s)? Finally, how do we reconcile or own biases toward the results? Clearly, the answers are difficult, especially when study quality varies significantly. It is no wonder that different reviewers often come to very different conclusions. These issues will become important as we review the RRS literature.

The Rapid Response System: Is It Effective?

The effectiveness of RRSs has been examined using a variety of outcome measurements including in-hospital mortality, unanticipated ICU admission, incidence of cardiorespiratory arrest, ICU mortality, and hospital and ICU length of stay (LOS). Recently, research has also evaluated the impact of the RRS on the institution of not for resuscitation (NFR) status and the timing of goal-directed resuscitation and administration of broad-spectrum antibiotics in patients with sepsis. Outcome measures such as mortality are often more attractive methodologically, and are often sought by hospital administrators and regulatory agencies. Hard outcomes such as mortality resonate with the public and are generally readily available in hospital administrative databases. In the United States, there is even a specific patient safety indicator called "Failure to Rescue" that is identified with free software from the Agency for Healthcare Research and Quality (AHRQ) that scours administrative databases for patient safety events [2]. The alternative is for us to use process measures such as "how many pages were sent to the primary service before a response," but these are often more difficult to obtain despite the fact that they are potentially more important in understanding the function and failure of complex systems. Unfortunately, process measures and some relevant outcomes are either not collected with good fidelity, or tend to be buried in patients' medical charts making data collection laborious and expensive.

Success stories of Rapid Response Systems are abundant. In the two decades since the inception of the RRS, there has been a steady stream of primary research reports [3–45] as well as several systematic reviews and meta-analyses of this literature [46–51]. While the data is not homogeneous, the overwhelming conclusion is that the RRS intervention has been successful in reducing the incidence of cardiorespiratory arrests and mortality. The quality of evidence is generally considered moderate since no study has used a true randomized methodology. This is not surprising given the logistical as well as ethical considerations in conducting such a study. Maintaining a randomized methodology without bias from influences such as the Hawthorne effect would be nearly impossible. Additionally, how would we randomize such a study? Would one deteriorating patient get "usual" care while another get the MET/RRT intervention? As such, only two studies to date have attempted to use a randomized methodology [8, 9]. The randomization methodology chosen was cluster randomization. In Priestley et al., 2004 [8], the randomization scheme introduced the RRS in blocks into a large district hospital in Great Britain comparing blocks with and without the RRS as the introduction occurred step-wise. They also were able to historically compare each block to itself prior to the introduction of the RRS. In the MERIT trial [9] in Australia, whole hospitals were randomized to either have an RRS or not, and then compared to each other as a group (no RRS vs. RRS) as well as to themselves individually in a pre- postintervention comparison. The single institution study [8] found a statistically significant benefit for total hospital mortality (the only outcomes studied) in both types of comparisons. The large multi-center study (MERIT) found no changes in mortality, cardiac arrest, or unplanned ICU admission in the analysis of control vs. RRS hospitals. However, the data also showed a significant improvement in all three outcomes in the pre vs. postintervention comparison of all participating hospitals.

The seemingly contradictory result may be in part explained by the finding that during the study control hospitals changed their behavior and used existing "code" teams as MET/RRTs, and activated them for patients who had not yet arrested ("MET-like" activities) [52, 53]. This strong Hawthorne effect (the hospitals obviously knew they were or were not a RRS hospital since blinding the study was impossible) led to all of the hospitals improving their outcomes while likely obscuring the impact of the intervention. While evidence-based medicine purists may reject this notion since it is based on post-hoc analysis, the data does have logical and historical support.

Another argument made is that the Priestley study and MERIT trial were not randomized but rather concurrent cohort trials, and therefore

there is no Level 1 evidence for RRSs. In fact, several of the more recent systematic reviews [48, 49, 51] have assumed this view, and have considered all RRS trials to be observational in nature (concurrent cohort controlled or pre-postintervention design). Accordingly, the best evidence for the efficacy of rapid response systems would be Level 2. At this point, we are not likely to ever be able to develop truly randomized trials for this intervention since it has become ubiquitous in many places and it would be methodologically unfeasible and possibly unethical to attempt to do so. Even cluster-randomized methodologies are difficult to implement, and controlling for the Hawthorne effect is extremely problematic. We simply need to realize that this is the best evidence we are likely to have and move forward from here.

So what does the current state of the literature show? Figure 11.1 shows a forest plot of all studies up to 2012 that are included in one meta-analysis. The pooled effect for non-ICU adult cardiorespiratory arrest using the random effects model is an odds ratio (OR) of 0.62, with 95 % confidence intervals (CI) 0.53–0.73. This is a statistically significant 38 % reduction in arrests. The pooled effect for adult total in-hospital mortality is shown in Fig. 11.2. The pooled results using the random effects model are an OR of 0.88 (95 % CI 0.82–0.96) providing statistically significant mortality reduction of 12 %. In the pediatric population similar results are seen; for non-ICU arrest (Fig. 11.3), the OR is 0.55, 95 % CI 0.40–0.75 (statistically significant), and 0.82 95 % CI 0.67–1.0 for in-hospital mortality (Fig. 11.4). A very recent systematic review and meta-analysis [51] corroborated prior studies by finding that RRSs are associated with statistically significant reduction in hospital mortality in both the adult (RR 0.87, 95 % CI 0.81–0.95, $p < 0.001$) and pediatric (RR = 0.82, 95 % CI 0.76–0.89) populations as well as a statistically significant reduction in cardiopulmonary arrests in adults (RR 0.65, 95 % CI 0.61–0.70, $p < 0.001$) and children (RR = 0.64, 95 % CI 0.55–0.74).

Additional studies also point to the ability of RRSs to improve outcomes but do not provide adequate statistics or uniformity in definitions to

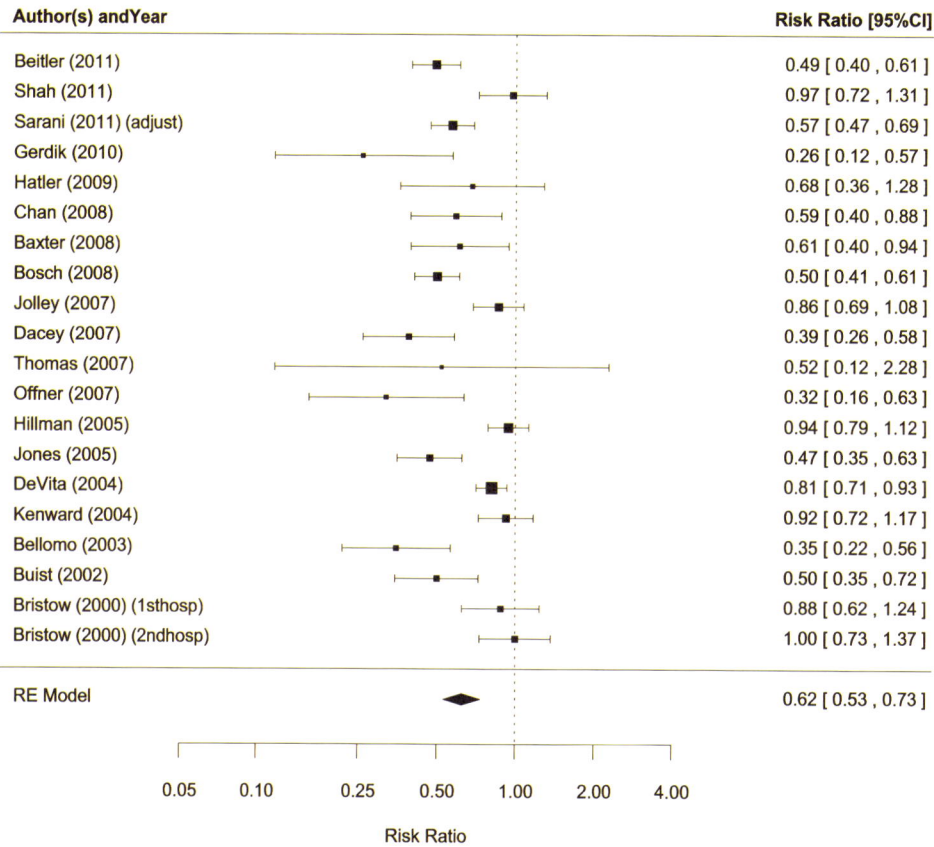

Author(s) andYear	Risk Ratio [95%CI]
Beitler (2011)	0.49 [0.40 , 0.61]
Shah (2011)	0.97 [0.72 , 1.31]
Sarani (2011) (adjust)	0.57 [0.47 , 0.69]
Gerdik (2010)	0.26 [0.12 , 0.57]
Hatler (2009)	0.68 [0.36 , 1.28]
Chan (2008)	0.59 [0.40 , 0.88]
Baxter (2008)	0.61 [0.40 , 0.94]
Bosch (2008)	0.50 [0.41 , 0.61]
Jolley (2007)	0.86 [0.69 , 1.08]
Dacey (2007)	0.39 [0.26 , 0.58]
Thomas (2007)	0.52 [0.12 , 2.28]
Offner (2007)	0.32 [0.16 , 0.63]
Hillman (2005)	0.94 [0.79 , 1.12]
Jones (2005)	0.47 [0.35 , 0.63]
DeVita (2004)	0.81 [0.71 , 0.93]
Kenward (2004)	0.92 [0.72 , 1.17]
Bellomo (2003)	0.35 [0.22 , 0.56]
Buist (2002)	0.50 [0.35 , 0.72]
Bristow (2000) (1sthosp)	0.88 [0.62 , 1.24]
Bristow (2000) (2ndhosp)	1.00 [0.73 , 1.37]
RE Model	0.62 [0.53 , 0.73]

Risk Ratio

Fig. 11.1 Aggregate analysis of RRS effect on the incidence of adult non-ICU cardiorespiratory arrest

include in a pooled result. Leach et al. (2011) [19] found a nonsignificant drop in adult hospital mortality from 18 to 15 % over the first two years of their RRS intervention. Karvellas et al. (2012) [43] also found a downward trend in mortality (not significant; OR = 0.73 95 % CI 0.51–1.03, $p = 0.08$). Rothberg et al. (2012) [20] reported that cardiorespiratory arrests as defined by "code" calls, declined statistically from 4.70/1000admits to 3.11. Simmes et al. (2012) [44] found a 50 % reduction in both cardiorespiratory arrests and unexpected death (different from total in-hospital mortality) though the result did not reach statistical significance secondary to a very low baseline arrest and unexpected death rates at the study hospital. Al-Qahtani et al. (2013) [45] found that their RRS intervention reduced both non-ICU cardiorespiratory arrest with a relative risk reduction (RR) of 0.68, 95 % CI 0.53–0.86, and

in-hospital mortality with RR of 0.90, 95 %, and CI 0.85–0.95).

Long-term studies also suggest that these benefits are sustained over time. Buist et al. [54] have reported data over a 6-year time frame that shows sustained reductions in cardio-respiratory arrest [54]. This result is echoed by Jones et al. [55], who also found a sustained reduction in the incidence of cardio-respiratory arrest over a four-year period. In Jones' study, surgical patients had reductions in hospital mortality with the RRS program with two of those years being statistically significant though this did not occur with medical patients. It is unclear why medical patients did not receive the same mortality benefit. Perhaps their problems are different from surgical patients, and RRSs are more effective at intervening with the deteriorations that kill surgical patients. It is also interesting that the effect on

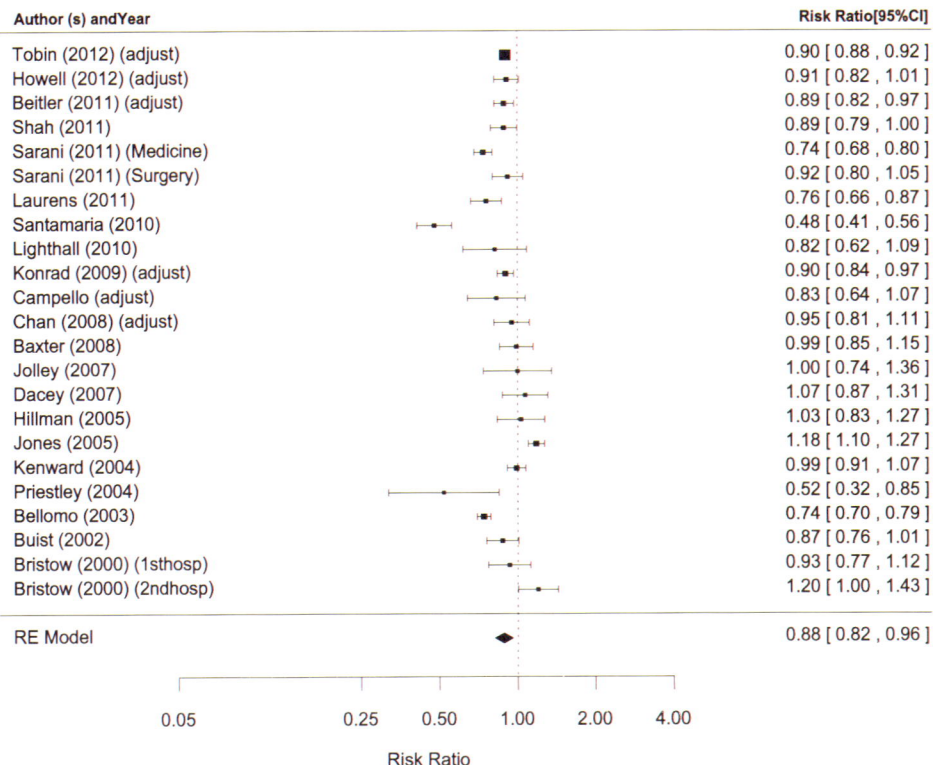

Fig. 11.2 Aggregate analysis of RRS effect on adult total in-hospital mortality

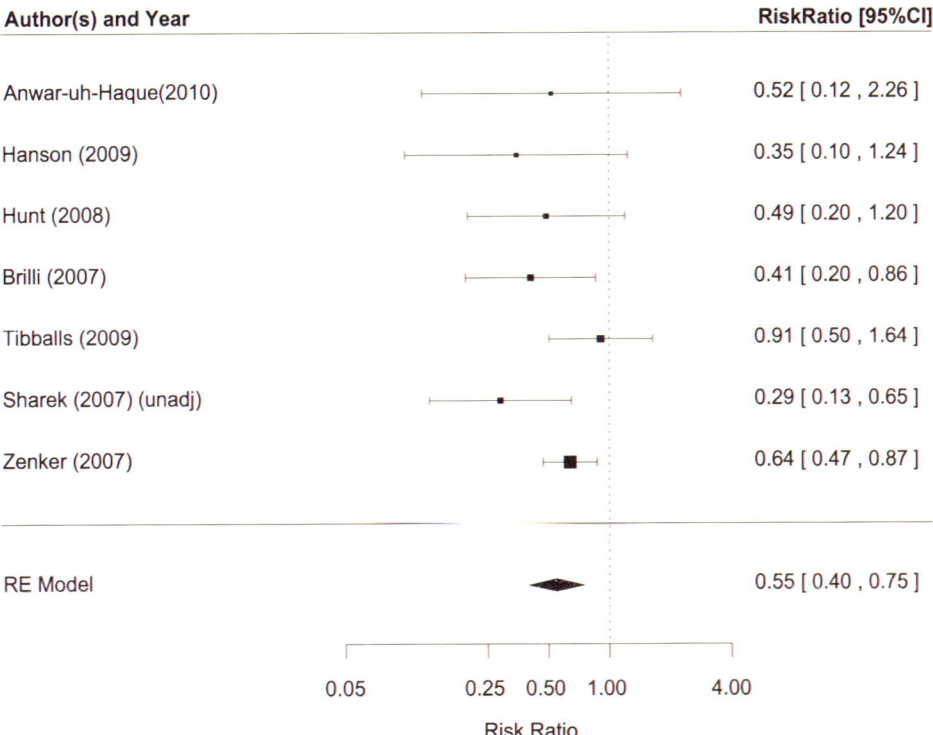

Fig. 11.3 Aggregate analysis of RRS effect on incidence of pediatric non-ICU cardiorespiratory arrest

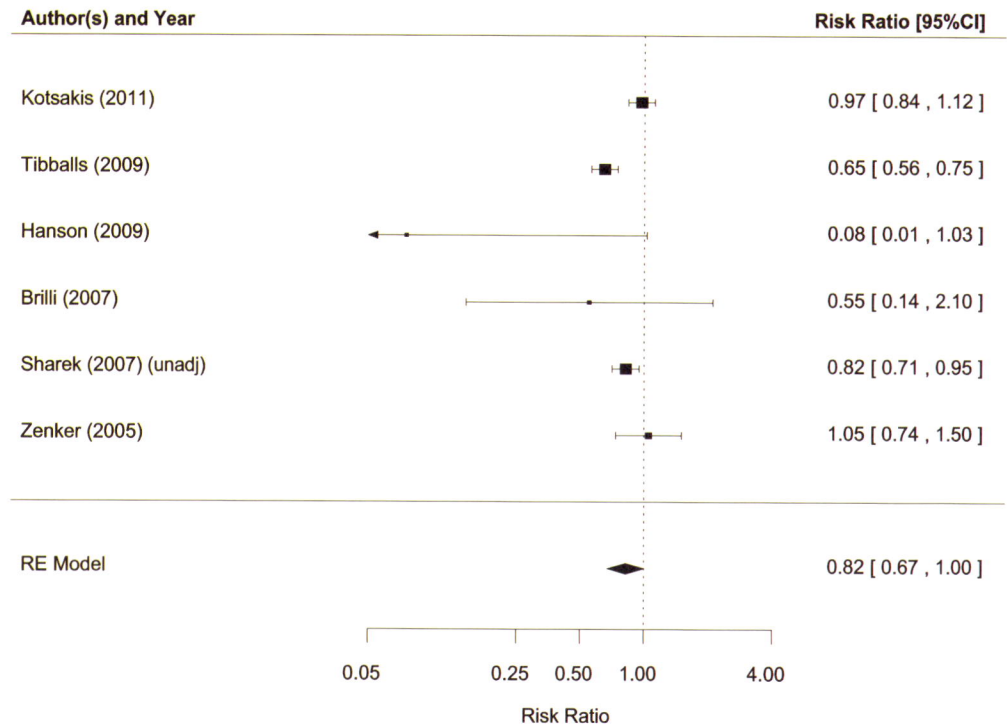

Fig. 11.4 Aggregate analysis of RRS effect on pediatric total in-hospital mortality

arrest rates seems more powerful than the effect on mortality here and in other studies. This, along with the differential effect seen by Jones's group, may suggest that while RRSs can prevent arrests, their ability to prevent eventual death is more limited especially in certain patient groups. Chan et al. [49] also noted this potential limitation of RRSs—that is, while we can prevent more floor arrests, we also move more pre-arresting patients to the ICU where they may eventually die from their underlying condition. Thus, we reduce arrests but may have no net impact on mortality.

Many patients admitted to hospital have very severe or terminal illnesses and are unlikely to survive their hospital stay. We should not expect RRSs to affect the inevitability of such death, but trying to control for this is nearly impossible. Accordingly, some have suggested that the ideal mortality outcome should be unexpected mortality. While this is the true mortality outcome we would expect RRS could improve (the true exposure group for the intervention) as opposed to total mortality, collecting this outcome would be

difficult and introduce its own biases (what criteria do we use to determine what is or is not an unexpected in-hospital death?). Certainly most "full resuscitation status" deaths should be worrisome. Likewise, we need to be careful of what other outcomes we report. Some studies have reported whole hospital cardiorespiratory arrest rates though, with possible rare exceptions, RRS do not respond to ICU patients. The exposure groups that can benefit are only non-ICU patients and reporting all cardiorespiratory arrests includes a group of patients not exposed to the intervention. This may skew the results toward a neutral effect.

Jones et al. [55] also examined the effect a RRS has on the long-term mortality of surgical patients finding a benefit extending well beyond hospital discharge. Again, we find early effective interventions in the types of problems surgical patients tend to have may explain this extended benefit as well as the in-hospital benefit.

The effect of RRSs on unanticipated ICU admission is quite variable. Earlier studies by

Bristow et al. (2002) [3] and Bellomo et al. (2004) [5] found statistically significant reductions but one by Buist et al. (2002) [4] found a statistically significant increase. The MERIT study found no benefit in the primary comparison but did in the pre-post comparison. This variability is not surprising given the effect that individual hospital systems, resources, and culture have on which patients get admitted to the ICU and under what circumstance. There is no consensus on whether an increase in unanticipated ICU admissions necessarily represents a positive or negative outcome. This statistic should be interpreted in terms of patient care needs and in the context of the institution's culture. When admission rates go up but mortality and arrest rates go down, it is inappropriate for us to consider this a failure.

Two studies have examined RRSs in combination with other patient safety initiatives and reported favorable results [56, 57]. Both studies found reductions in mortality but the component attributable to the RRS is unknown. One of the studies [56] also found a reduction in cardiorespiratory arrest rate, which was most likely attributable to the RRS. The US Institute of Healthcare Improvement's (IHI) 100,000 Lives Campaign likewise reports a mortality reduction across its participating hospitals [57], however the RRS was only one of six interventions that were part of the program. Nonetheless, the IHI suggested that RRSs were responsible for the majority of the improvements.

Other outcomes such as ICU mortality and LOS either have too few reports and/or unclear denominators make interpretation difficult. Like ICU admission, it is unclear whether LOS should go up or down with a RRS since patients who are rescued may have much longer LOS than those who died. Additionally, there are many local factors that affect LOS making generalizability of the data difficult.

The effect of RRSs on the process of care is an area for great potential that has only been explored in a limited fashion. Sebat et al. [58] studied septic and hypovolemic shock patients over a five-year period and found that having a RRS significantly improved process measures such as institution of appropriate goal-directed

fluid therapy. These improvements were associated with reductions in mortality especially for those with septic shock. Not for Resuscitation orders (NFR or DNR) and better institution of End-of-life care (EOLC) [59] are increasingly being examined as a process of care that RRS can improve. While it has not been studied in a rigorous manner yet, many papers have alluded to the number of patients appropriately made NFR with palliative care becoming central to the patient's care plan after a RRS activation. Perhaps the need to activate the RRS underscores the patient's severe condition and creates a forum in which these discussions may begin.

RRSs may also have a positive impact on nursing satisfaction, nurse retention, physician and nurse education, and patient and family satisfaction. Unfortunately, much of the evidence in support of these remains anecdotal. Where family RRS activation is available, families report tremendous support of the system. Nurses are generally quite positive with some finding the idea of stopping such programs abhorrent. More qualitative reports are needed and this is an active area for investigation.

Identifying the Deteriorating Patient, the RRS Afferent Limb

It is important to note that the previously discussed pooled results for the effectiveness of RRSs on relevant outcomes such as mortality and cardiorespiratory arrest have changed little since the publication of the first systematic review [46] to most recent [51]. The point estimates of efficacy have shifted slightly over time settling in the range of about a 40 % reduction in cardiorespiratory arrest for adults and children, and reduction in hospital mortality of 12–18 %. As the numbers of patients exposed to the intervention have increased the confidence intervals have tightened but we have been unable to change absolute risk reduction or odds ratios. Our current model seems to have reached a limit. Why is this so? Two interdependent explanations seem likely. One is the continuing maladaptive culture that sustains the rigid hierarchal system among physicians and

Table 11.2 National Health Service Early Warning Score

NHS Early Warning Score (NEWS)							
Physiological parameters	3	2	1	0	1	2	3
Pulse	≤40		41–50	51–90	91–110	111–130	≥131
Temperature	≤35.0		35.1–36.0	36.1–38.0	38.1–39.0	≥39.1	
Systolic BP	≤90	91–100	91–110	111–219			≥220
Respiration rate	≤8		9–11	12–20		21–24	≥25
Consciousness level				A			V, P, or U
Oxygen saturations	≤91	92–93	94–95	≥96			
Any supplemental oxygen		Yes		No			

between physicians and nurses as well as a mentality of "patient ownership" and the perception that to seek help is an indication of incompetence on part of the provider. This includes both doctors and nurses. The other is the process by which we monitor patients on general hospital wards; a process that has changed almost not at all in over 100 years. We will focus on the evidence regarding the Afferent limb of the RRS.

In the late 1980s and 1990s, several studies published the results of chart reviews of patients who had experienced a cardio-respiratory arrest. These reviews showed clear physiologic abnormalities in variables such as heart rate, respiratory rate, and mental status in the hours to days prior to the arrest event [60–74]. These signs and symptoms were often present for many hours if not days [60] and often went unrecognized even when health care professionals visited the patients [60]. Most agreed that tachycardia, bradycardia, tachypnea, desaturation, low systolic blood pressure, respiratory distress, and mental status changes were the clearest signs. While difficult to quantify, concern or worry on part of the nursing staff was also considered predictive of progression to arrest. These retrospective results led to the widespread use of these physiological limits and "worry or concern" being used as "alert" or "activation" criteria for RRSs.

Unfortunately, the sensitivity and specificity of physiological limits for preventing arrest are unclear since these early chart review studies were necessarily retrospective in nature. Throughout the development of the RRS intervention, clinician researchers have tried to determine if better use can be made of these discretely measured physiological triggers. Several have proposed early warning scoring (EWSs) systems such as the United Kingdom's NHS Early Warning Score (Table 11.2) instead of single vital sign triggers [67–73]. Multi-parameter systems assign numerical values to degrees of abnormality such as one point for a heart rate >110, two points for a heart rate >125 etc; all scores are then summed to create a composite score. Success in predicting outcomes has been reported for the Modified Early Warning Score (MEWS) [67], ASSIST score [68] and Soccer Scores, [69] but some have found poor inter-rater reliability on assigning and calculating these scores [72]. On average though, simpler scores have been found to work better but not necessarily better than specific vital signs [67]. The Soccer score study concluded that use of more extended criteria would catch abnormalities earlier allowing for earlier intervention. Bell et al., 2006 [71] found similar results when comparing restricted to extended criteria, but concluded that while extended criteria would identify problems earlier, their lower sensitivity would lead to a larger number of "false alerts," resulting in a heavy workload on the responding MET/RRT members. This can be especially problematic since most RRSs are staffed with ICU providers as discussed below. On the other hand, Bell's study also concluded that as you restricted the criteria for activation, you were more likely to miss opportunities to intervene and this could lead to an increase in the incidence of failure to rescue. Cretikos et al., 2007 [72] also noted this tendency for low sensitivity (53.6 %) and low positive predictive value (a disappointing 15.7 %) but did find high specificity for a combination of heart rate, respiratory rate, systolic blood pressure, and change in mental status. Attempts to modify the cutoffs for these triggers, however, did not improve the results. Maurice and Simpson, 2007 [73] found that standard physiological measurements, such as heart rate, were unable to identify at-risk patients with any reasonable validity. A systematic review [74] of 36 studies found that no scoring system was adequate to prevent failure to rescue while at the same time not creating an unsustainable number of false alerts.

Why do physiological variables and scoring systems seem to do so poorly in telling us when a patient is deteriorating? One possible consideration is the frequency with which patients are monitored. Even if physiological limits are predictive of deterioration, general ward patients are infrequently monitored, allowing for significant deteriorations to occur before they may even have the chance to be recognized. Buist et al. [60] noted that the median time between the recording of vital sign abnormalities in general ward patients and their arrest was about 6–7 h. If vital signs are only taken every 8 h, which is common in hospitals in the United States, there are significant opportunities to miss a serious problem. This is compounded by the frequent lack of realization that the signs are worrisome. All of the evaluations discussed previously used manually collected intermittent vital signs. An inherent weakness of the Afferent limb is the way we collect vital sign on general wards. In addition to the manual and intermittent nature of vital signs collection the data is sparse and there is lack of integration with other data such as labs and patient history.

Earlier and earlier recognition is crucial. It has been noted by several studies that delays in activation or absence of activation of the RRS has serious consequences for the patient. Calzavacca et al. (2008) [27] noted that early recognition was the most robust component of the RRS in terms of predicting success. Jones et al. [75] found that to achieve a measureable reduction in arrests, there is needed to be a utilization rate ("dose") of approximately 17 activations per 1000 admissions. Fydshou and Gillesberg (2013) [76] found

that RRS activations were less frequent than predicted when they implemented their system and that one half of their ICU admissions continued to occur through the traditional hierarchy as opposed to the RRS. Guinane et al. (2013) [77] reported that while 14 % of a patient sample exhibited RRS trigger criteria, only 40 % had an activation. Those who exhibited RRS criteria had twice the length of stay of those who did not. Boniatti et al. (2013) [78] found that activations were delayed 21.4 % of the time, despite documented instability resulting in a statistically higher mortality (61.8 vs. 41.9 %, $p < 0.001$). Simmes et al. (2012) [44] also found 16 % of activations were delayed for up to 2 days. Vetro et al. (2011) [79] reported 20 % of patients who met objective criteria for activation had no RRS call and Shearer, et al. (2012) [80] found that while 4.04 % of their adult population had clear evidence of clinical instability, 42 % did not receive an RRS activation and this was despite nearly 70 % of the staff acknowledging that they knew their patient met RRS activation criteria. Bucknall et al. (2013) [81] found that the majority of patients meeting criteria never had an activation and that this was associated with increased hospital mortality. Adelstein et al. (2011) [82] attempted to correct this afferent limb failure mode by implementing policy changes designed to reduce delayed and non-activations. They were only able to improve the delayed activation incidence from 30 % before instituting the changes to 26 % afterward. With this degree of continued failure to recognize and/or activate the RRS, it is no wonder we seem to be have difficulty realizing further improvements in RRS outcomes.

How can we move forward? If manually intermittently collected physiologic vital sign criteria (individual or aggregated into a score) is less than adequate to optimize opportunities for intervention, can we develop electronic continuous systems, like those used in the ICU, and successfully apply them to general ward patients? Several barriers exist including the need for greatly increased patient mobility, high fidelity uninterrupted monitoring for these mobile patients, and most especially an acceptable signal-to-noise ratio so that all patients' deteriorations are recognized with minimal false alarms. Many technologies are rapidly developing to address the need for wireless high fidelity monitors. Controlling the signal-to-noise problem is much more difficult.

Recent evidence suggests that we may be able successfully engage in what is referred to as surveillance monitoring on general hospital wards and transform the way patients are monitored. Additionally, these systems may provide the evidence to nurses to support their making an RRS activation as well as provide the accountability showing when the patient began to deteriorate allowing for more directed root cause analysis so as to drive quality improvement. Taenzar et al. (2014) [83] found that manually collected oxygen saturation data on a high-risk group of post-surgical obstructive sleep apnea patients, over-estimated their actual saturation by about 6.5 %. A prior pilot study [84] using continuous pulse oximetry, heart rate, and respiratory rate monitoring lowered the number of deaths of general ward patients from 4 pre-intervention to 2 post-intervention. Rescue events dropped from 3.4 to 1.2 ($p = 0.01$) and unanticipated ICU transfers dropped from 5.6 to 2.9 ($p = 0.02$) between the pre and post-implementation time periods; the average alarm rate was 4 per patient per day. Concurrent cohort comparison wards (other surgical services) exhibited no similar changes.

While some older reports show no improvementsd [85], (they do not always meet the criteria for surveillance monitoring), these results are encouraging. As we move forward developing strategies that merge vital sign data with laboratory and comorbidity data may allow us to better predict who is at risk of deterioration, and allow us to create escalation protocols directly to staff and/or the RRS. These kinds of future possibilities may allow us to further improve outcomes relevant to the RRS intervention.

The Efferent Limb: The Responding Team

Unlike the afferent limb there is less evidence evaluating the team that responds to a deteriorating patient. This efferent limb may be staffed in a myriad of ways depending on the human resources available. Many programs use METs, which include physicians as well as nurses, respiratory therapists, and others on the team, while RRTs are typically nurse-led teams without physician staffing. While most of these clinicians are based out of the ICU or are critical care trained, some programs use other providers such as Hospitalists to staff their team. Some programs do not even create a separate team but rather use the primary service as the responders though their response must be immediate when activation criteria are met. Still others use their code teams but with a different functionality when it is a noncode rather than a true code call. To date, there are no head to head comparisons of these different models of team staffing. All models have been associated with improved outcomes and there is no evidence to support the superiority of one model over another. In the absence of clear data for guidance, choosing a staffing model for an RRS still depends on local resources and culture.

Understanding and improving team function has become the subject of interest in a variety of fields including RRSs [86–90]. Jones et al. have suggested that commonly encountered modes of patient deterioration such as respiratory distress deserve standardization and protocols.

Simulation is a powerful tool for understanding how teams function, identifying opportunities for teamwork and self-improvement, and for developing and testing protocols for care in urgent/emergent situations such as those frequently encountered by emergency teams. The University of Pittsburgh has been particularly active in using this strategy to assess and develop RRS team performance. They have shown that team performance can be significantly enhanced through simulator education and training [89]. Wallin et al. [91] have found similar results related to teamwork skills. However, while they found improved performance, they also found that this type of education did not help improve attitudes toward "safe" teamwork. Although performance is essential, there is also much value in cultivating the "culture of safety." However, to expect that simulation education alone can change culture is shortsighted. Changing culture and attitudes requires a multi-pronged approach that includes and engages stakeholders and front-line staff together through teamwork tools and a shared vision of patient safety.

Conclusion

It is time to stop asking whether RRS "work." Overall, the balance of evidence indicates that RRS are effective at reducing cardiorespiratory arrest and mortality. However, we seem to have reached a limit in driving down cardiorespiratory arrests rates and reducing mortality. This may reflect inherent limitations but more likely is a reflection of our continued inability to identify the patient at risk early and with high fidelity, and to translate detection into activation of the Efferent limb. In addition to emphasizing the focus on process measures such as early sepsis recognition and management, institution of appropriate EOLC discussions, and other markers of high quality care, we need to focus on how we can improve the Afferent Limb and the culture that allows patients to continue to deteriorate toward death in our hospitals.

References

1. Owens DK, Lohr KN, Atkins D, Treadwell JR, Reston JT, Bass EB, et al. AHRQ series paper 5: grading the strength of a body of evidence when comparing medical interventions—Agency for Healthcare Research and Quality and the Effective Health-Care Program. J Clin Epidemiol. 2010;63:513–23 [PMID:19595577].
2. http://www.ahrq.gov/ Last Accessed 1 Aug 2015.
3. Bristow PJ, Hillman KM, Chey T, Daffurn K, Jacques TC, Norman SL, et al. Rates of in-hospital arrests, deaths and intensive care admissions: the effect of a medical emergency team. Med J Aust. 2000;173:236–40 [PMID:11130346].
4. Buist MD, Moore GE, Bernard SA, Waxman BP, Anderson JN, Nguyen TV. Effects of a medical emergency team on reduction of incidence of and mortality from unexpected cardiac arrests in hospital: preliminary study. BMJ. 2002;324:387–90 [PMID: 11850367].
5. Bellomo R, Goldsmith D, Uchino S, Buckmaster J, Hart GK, Opdam H, et al. A prospective before-and-after trial of a medical emergency team. Med J Aust. 2003;179:283–7 [PMID: 12964909].
6. DeVita MA, Braithwaite RS, Mahidhara R, Stuart S, Foraida M, Simmons RL, Medical Emergency Response Improvement Team (MERIT). Use of medical emergency team responses to reduce hospital cardiopulmonary arrests. Qual Saf Health Care. 2004;13:251–4 [PMID: 15289626].
7. Kenward G, Castle N, Hodgetts T, Shaikh L. Evaluation of a medical emergency team one year after implementation. Resuscitation. 2004;61:257–63 [PMID: 15172703].
8. Priestley G, Watson W, Rashidian A, Mozley C, Russell D, Wilson J, et al. Introducing Critical Care Outreach: a ward-randomised trial of phased Introduction in a general hospital. Intensive Care Med. 2004;30:1398–404 [PMID:15112033].
9. Hillman K, Chen J, Cretikos M, Bellomo R, Brown D, Doig G, MERIT study investigators, et al. Introduction of the medical emergency team (MET) system: a cluster-randomised controlled trial. Lancet. 2005;365:2091–7 [PMID: 15964445].
10. Chan PS, Khalid A, Longmore LS, Berg RA, Kosiborod M, Spertus JA. Hospital-wide code rates and mortality before and after implementation of a rapid response team. JAMA. 2008;300:2506–13 [PMID: 19050194].
11. Zenker P, Schlesinger A, Hauck M, Spencer S, Hellmich T, Finkelstein M, et al. Implementation and impact of a rapid response team in a children's hospital. Jt Comm J Qual Patient Saf. 2007;33:418–25 [PMID: 17711144].
12. Dacey MJ, Mirza ER, Wilcox V, Doherty M, Mello J, Boyer A, et al. The effect of a rapid response team on major clinical outcome measures in a community hospital. Crit Care Med. 2007;35:2076–82 [PMID: 17855821].
13. Baxter AD, Cardinal P, Hooper J, Patel R. Medical emergency teams at The Ottawa Hospital: the first two years. Can J Anaesth. 2008;55:223–31 [PMID: 18378967].
14. Sharek PJ, Parast LM, Leong K, Coombs J, Earnest K, Sullivan J, et al. Effect of a rapid response team on hospital-wide mortality and code rates outside the ICU in a children's hospital. JAMA. 2007;298:2267–74 [PMID: 18029830].
15. Brilli RJ, Gibson R, Luria JW, Wheeler TA, Shaw J, Linam M, et al. Implementation of a medical emergency team in a large pediatric teaching hospital prevents respiratory and cardiopulmonary arrests outside the intensive care unit. Pediatr Crit Care Med. 2007;8:236–46 [PMID: 17417113].
16. Tibballs J, Kinney S. Reduction of hospital mortality and of preventable cardiac arrest and death on introduction of a pediatric medical emergency team. Pediatr Crit Care Med. 2009;10:306–12 [PMID: 19307806].
17. Hunt EA, Zimmer KP, Rinke ML, Shilkofski NA, Matlin C, Garger C, et al. Transition from a traditional code team to a medical emergency team and categorization of cardiopulmonary arrests in a children's center. Arch Pediatr Adolesc Med. 2008;162:117–22 [PMID: 18250234].

18. Medina-Rivera B, Campos-Santiago Z, Palacios AT, Rodriguez-Cintron W. The effect of the medical emergency team on unexpected cardiac arrest and death at the VA Caribbean Healthcare System: a retrospective study. Crit Care and Shock. 2010;13:98–105.

19. Leach LS, Mayo A, O'Rourke M. How RNs rescue patients: a qualitative study of RNs' perceived involvement in rapid response teams. Qual Saf Health Care. 2010;19(5):e13.Epub 2010 Apr 8. [PMID:20378624]

20. Rothberg MB, Belforti R, Fitzgerald J, Friderici J, Keyes M. Four years' experience with a hospitalist-led medical emergency team: an interrupted time series. J Hosp Med. 2012;7:98–103 [PMID: 21998088].

21. Scherr K, Wilson DM, Wagner J, Haughian M. Evaluating a new rapid response team: NP-led versus intensivist-led comparisons. AACN Adv Crit Care. 2012;23:32–42 [PMID: 22290088].

22. Scott SS, Elliott S. Implementation of a rapid response team: a success story. Crit Care Nurse. 2009;29:66–75 [PMID: 19487782].

23. Jolley J, Bendyk H, Holaday B, Lombardozzi KA, Harmon C. Rapid response teams: do they make a difference? Dimens Crit Care Nurs. 2007;26:253–60 [PMID: 18090145].

24. Offner PJ, Heit J, Roberts R. Implementation of a rapid response team decreases cardiac arrest outside of the intensive care unit. J Trauma. 2007;62:1223–7 [PMID: 17495728].

25. Thomas K, VanOyen Force M, Rasmussen D, Dodd D, Whildin S. Rapid response team: challenges, solutions, benefits. Crit Care Nurse. 2007;27:20–7 [PMID: 17244856].

26. Bosch FH, de Jager CPC. Number of resuscitations for in-hospital cardiopulmonary arrests decreases after introduction of a medical emergency team. "The Arnhem experience". Neth J Crit Care. 2008;12:256–9.

27. Calzavacca P, Licari E, Tee A, Egi M, Downey A, Quach J, et al. The impact of Rapid Response System on delayed emergency team activation patient characteristics and outcomes — a follow-up study. Resuscitation. 2010;81:31–5 [PMID: 19854557].

28. Anwar-ul-Haque, Saleem AF, Zaidi S, Haider SR. Experience of pediatric rapid response team in a tertiary care hospital in Pakistan. Indian J Pediatr. 2010;77:273–6 [PMID: 20177830].

29. Beitler JR, Link N, Bails DB, Hurdle K, Chong DH. Reduction in hospital wide mortality after implementation of a rapid response team: a long-term cohort study. Crit Care. 2011;15:R269 [PMID: 22085785].

30. Campello G, Granja C, Carvalho F, Dias C, Azevedo LF, Costa-Pereira A. Immediate and long-term impact of medical emergency teams on cardiac arrest prevalence and mortality: a plea for periodic basic life-support training programs. Crit Care Med. 2009;37:3054–61 [PMID: 19770754].

31. Gerdik C, Vallish RO, Miles K, Godwin SA, Wludyka PS, Panni MK. Successful implementation of a family and patient activated rapid response Team in an adult level 1 trauma center. Resuscitation. 2010;81:1676–81 [PMID:20655645].

32. Hanson CC, Randolph GD, Erickson JA, Mayer CM, Bruckel JT, Harris BD, et al. A reduction in cardiac arrests and duration of clinical instability after implementation of a paediatric rapid response system. Qual Saf Health Care. 2009;18:500–4 [PMID: 19955465].

33. Hatler C, Mast D, Bedker D, Johnson R, Corderella J, Torres J, et al. Implementing a rapid response team to decrease emergencies outside the ICU: one hospital's experience. Medsurg Nurs. 2009;18:84–90 .126. [PMID: 19489205]

34. Howell MD, Ngo L, Folcarelli P, Yang J, Mottley L, Marcantonio ER, et al. Sustained effectiveness of a primary-team-based rapid response system. Crit Care Med. 2012;40:2562–8 [PMID: 22732285].

35. Konrad D, Jäderling G, Bell M, Granath F, Ekbom A, Martling CR. Reducing in-hospital cardiac arrests and hospital mortality by introducing a Medical emergency team. Intensive Care Med. 2010;36:100–6 [PMID: 19760206].

36. Kotsakis A, Lobos AT, Parshuram C, Gilleland J, Gaiteiro R, Mohseni-Bod H, Ontario Pediatric Critical Care Response Team Collaborative, et al. Implementation of a multicenter rapid response system in pediatric academic hospitals is effective. Pediatrics. 2011;128:72–8 [PMID: 21690113].

37. Laurens N, Dwyer T. The impact of medical emergency teams on ICU admission rates, cardiopulmonary arrests and mortality in a regional hospital. Resuscitation. 2011;82:707–12 [PMID: 21411218].

38. Lighthall GK, Parast LM, Rapoport L, Wagner TH. Introduction of a rapid response system at a United States veterans affairs hospital reduced cardiac arrests. Anesth Analg. 2010;111:679–86 [PMID: 20624835].

39. Santamaria J, Tobin A, Holmes J. Changing cardiac arrest and hospital mortality rates through a medical emergency team takes time and constant review. Crit Care Med. 2010;38:445–50 [PMID: 20029341].

40. Sarani B, Palilonis E, Sonnad S, Bergey M, Sims C, Pascual JL, et al. Clinical emergencies and outcomes in patients admitted to a surgical versus medical service. Resuscitation. 2011;82:415–8 [PMID: 21242020].

41. Shah SK, Cardenas Jr VJ, Kuo YF, Sharma G. Rapid response team in an academic institution: does it make a difference? Chest. 2011;139:1361–7 [PMID: 20864618].

42. Tobin AE, Santamaria JD. Medical emergency teams are associated with reduced mortality across a major metropolitan health network after two years service: a retrospective study using government administrative data. Crit Care. 2012;16:R210 [PMID: 23107123].

43. Karvellas CJ, de Souza IA, Gibney RT, Bagshaw SM. Association between implementation of an intensivist-led medical emergency team and mortality. BMJ Qual Saf. 2012;21:152–9 [PMID: 22190540].

44. Simmes FM, Schoonhoven L, Mintjes J, Fikkers BG, van der Hoeven JG. Incidence of cardiac arrests and unexpected deaths in surgical patients before and after implementation of a rapid response system. Ann Intensive Care. 2012;2(1):2 [PMID: 22716308].

45. Al-Qahtani S, Al-Dorzi HM, Tamim HM, Hussain S, Fong L, Taher S, Al-Knawy BA, Arabi Y. Impact of an intensivist-led multidisciplinary extended rapid response team on hospital-wide cardiopulmonary arrests and mortality. Crit Care Med. 2013;41(2):506–17 [PMID:23263618].

46. Winters BD, Pham JC, Hunt EA, Guallar E, Berenholtz S, Pronovost PJ. Rapid response systems: a systematic review. Crit Care Med. 2007;35(5):1238–43 .Review [PMID:17414079]

47. Ranji SR, Auerbach AD, Hurd CJ, O'Rourke K, Shojania KG. Effects of rapid response systems on clinical outcomes: systematic review and meta-analysis. J Hosp Med. 2007;2(6):422–32 [PMID:18081187].

48. Jones DA, DeVita MA, Bellomo R. Rapid-response teams. N Engl J Med. 2011;365:139–46 [PMID: 21751906].

49. Chan PS, Jain R, Nallmothu BK, Berg RA, Sasson C. Rapid response teams: a systematic review and meta-analysis. Arch Intern Med. 2010;170:18–26 [PMID: 20065195].

50. Winters BD, Weaver SJ, Pfoh ER, Yang T, Pham JC, Dy SM. Rapid-response systems as a patient safety strategy: a systematic review. Ann Intern Med. 2013;158(5 Pt 2):417–25.

51. Maharaj R, Raffaele I, Wendon J. Rapid response systems: a systematic review and meta-analysis. Crit Care. 2015;19:254 [PMID:26070457].

52. Chen J, Bellomo R, Hillman K, Flabouris A, Finfer S, MERIT Study Investigators for the Simpson Centre and the ANZICS Clinical Trials Group. Triggers for emergency team activation: a multicenter assessment. J Crit Care. 2010;25:359.e1–7 [PMID: 20189754].

53. Cretikos MA, Chen J, Hillman KM, Bellomo R, Finfer SR, Flabouris A, MERIT Study Investigators. The effectiveness of implementation of the Medical emergency team (MET) system and factors associated with use during the MERIT study. Crit Care Resusc. 2007;9:206–12 [PMID: 17536993].

54. Buist M, Harrison J, Abaloz E, Van Dyke S. Six year audit of cardiac arrests and medical emergency team calls in an Australian outer metropolitan teaching hospital. BMJ. 2007;335:1210–2 [PMID: 18048504].

55. Jones D, Bellomo R, Bates S, Warrillow S, Goldsmith D, Hart G, et al. Long term effect of a medical emergency team on cardiac arrests in a Teaching hospital. Crit Care. 2005;9:R808–15 [PMID: 16356230].

56. Tolchin S, Brush R, Lange P, Bates P, Garbo JJ. Eliminating preventable death at Ascension Health. Jt Comm J Qual Patient Saf. 2007;33(3):145–54 [PMID:17425236].

57. Institute for Healthcare Improvement. 5 Million Lives Campaign: Overview. Accessed at www.ihi.org/offerings/Initiatives/PastStrategicInitiatives/5MillionLives Campaign/Pages/default.aspx on. Last Accessed 3 Aug 2015.

58. Sebat F, Musthafa AA, Johnson D, Kramer AA, Shoffner D, Eliason M, Henry K, Spurlock B. Effect of a rapid response system for patients in shock on time to treatment and mortality during 5 years. Crit Care Med. 2007;35:2568–75 [PMID:17901831].

59. Jones D, Moran J, Winters B, Welch J. The rapid response system and end-of-life care. Curr Opin Crit Care. 2013;19(6):616–23 .Review.[PMID: 23799463]

60. Buist MD, Jarmolowski E, Burton PR, Bernard SA, Waxman BP, Anderson J. Recognising clinical instability in hospital patients before cardiac arrest or unplanned admission to intensive care. A pilot study in a tertiary-care hospital. Med J Aust. 1999;171:22–5 [PMID: 10451667].

61. Schein RM, Hazday N, Pena M, Ruben BH, Sprung CL. Clinical antecedents to in-hospital cardiopulmonary arrest. Chest. 1990;98(6):1388–92 [PMID:2245680].

62. Hillman KM. Recognising and preventing serious in-hospital events. Med J Aust. 1999;171(1):8–9 [PMID 10451662].

63. Matthew Franklin C, Mathew J. Developing strategies to prevent in-hospital cardiac arrest: analyzing responses of physicians and nurses in the hours before the event. Crit Care Med. 1994;22:244–7 [PMID:8306682].

64. Smith AF, Wood J. Can some in-hospital cardio-respiratory arrests be prevented? A prospective survey. Resuscitation. 1998;37:133–7 [PMID:9715771].

65. McQuillan P, Pilkington S, Allan A, et al. Confidential inquiry into quality of care before admission to intensive care. BMJ. 1998;316:1853–8 [PMID:9632403].

66. Goldhill DR, White SA, Sumner A. Physiological values and procedures in the 24 h before ICU admission from the ward. Anaesthesia. 1999;54(6):529–34 [PMID:10403864].

67. Subbe CP, Kruger M, Rutherford P, Gemmel L. Validation of a modified Early Warning Score in medical admissions. QJM. 2001;94(10):521–6 [PMID:11588210].

68. Subbe CP, Gao H, Harrison DA. Reproducibility of physiological track-and-trigger warning systems for identifying at-risk patients on the ward. Intensive Care Med. 2007;33(4):619–24 [PMID:17235508].

69. Jacques T, Harrison GA, McLaws ML, Kilborn G. Signs of critical conditions and emergency responses (SOCCER): a model for predicting adverse events in the inpatient setting. Resuscitation. 2006;69(2):175–83 [PMID:16497427].

70. Smith GB, Prytherch DR, Schmidt PE, Featherstone PI. Review and performance evaluation of aggregate weighted 'track and trigger' systems. Resuscitation. 2008;77(2):170–9 [PMID:18249483].

71. Bell MB, Konrad D, Granath F, Ekbom A, Martling CR. Prevalence and sensitivity of MET-criteria in a Scandinavian University Hospital. Resuscitation. 2006;70(1):66–73 [PMID:16757089].

72. Cretikos M, Chen J, Hillman K, Bellomo R, Finfer S. Flabouris A; MERIT study investigators. The objec-

tive medical emergency team activation criteria: a case-control study. Resuscitation. 2007;73(1):62–72 [PMID:17241732].

73. Morrice A, Simpson HJ. Identifying level one patients. A cross-sectional survey on an in-patient hospital population. Intensive Crit Care Nurs. 2007;23(1):23–32 [PMID:16973361].

74. Gao H, McDonnell A, Harrison DA, Moore T, Adam S, Daly K, Esmonde L, Goldhill DR, Parry GJ, Rashidian A, Subbe CP, Harvey S. Systematic review and evaluation of physiological track and trigger warning systems for identifying at-risk patients on the ward. Intensive Care Med. 2007;33(4):667–79 [PMID:17318499].

75. Jones DA, Mitra B, Barbetti J, Choate K, Leong T, Bellomo R. Increasing the use of an existing medical emergency team in a teaching hospital. Anaesth Intensive Care. 2006;34:731–5 [PMID: 17183890].

76. Frydshou A, Gillesberg I. Medical emergency teams are activated less than expected. Ugeskr Laeger. 2013;175(8):488–90 [PMID:23428262].

77. Guinane JL, Bucknall TK, Currey J, Jones DA. Missed medical emergency team activations: tracking decisions and outcomes in practice. Crit Care Resusc. 2013;15(4):266–72 [PMID:24289507].

78. Boniatti MM, Azzolini N, Viana MV, Ribeiro BS, Coelho RS, Castilho RK, Guimarães MR, Zorzi L, Schulz LF, Filho EM. Delayed medical emergency team calls and associated outcomes. Crit Care Med. 2014;42(1):26–30 [PMID:23989173].

79. Vetro J, Natarajan DK, Mercer I, Buckmaster JN, Heland M, Hart GK, Bellomo R, Jones DA. Antecedents to cardiac arrests in a hospital equipped with a medical emergency team. Crit Care Resusc. 2011;13(3):162–6 [PMID:21880003].

80. Shearer B, Marshall S, Buist MD, Finnigan M, Kitto S, Hore T, et al. What stops hospital clinical staff from following protocols? An analysis of the incidence and factors behind the failure of bedside clinical staff to activate the rapid response system in a multi-campus Australian metropolitan healthcare service. BMJ Qual Saf. 2012;21:569–75 [PMID: 22626737].

81. Bucknall TK, Jones D, Barrett J, Bellomo R, Botti M, Considine J, Currey J, Dunning TL, Green D, Levinson M, Livingston PM, O'Connell B, Ruseckaite R, Staples M. Point prevalence of patients fulfilling MET criteria in ten MET equipped hospitals. The methodology of the RESCUE study. Resuscitation. 2011;82(5):529–34 [PMID:21345573].

82. Adelstein BA, Piza MA, Nayyar V, Mudaliar Y, Klineberg PL, Rubin G. Rapid response systems: a prospective study of response times. J Crit Care. 2011;26:635.e11–8 [PMID: 21703813].

83. Taenzer AH, Pyke J, Herrick MD, Dodds TM, McGrath SP. A comparison of oxygen saturation data in inpatients with low oxygen saturation using automated continuous monitoring and intermittent manual data charting. Anesth Analg. 2014;118(2):326–31 [PMID:24361847].

84. Taenzer AH, Pyke JB, McGrath SP, Blike GT. Impact of pulse oximetry surveillance on rescue events and intensive care unit transfers: a before-and-after concurrence study. Anesthesiology. 2010;112(2):282–7 [PMID:20098128].

85. Watkinson PJ, Barber VS, Price JD, Hann A, Tarassenko L, Young JD. Randomised controlled trial of the effect of continuous electronic physiological monitoring on the adverse event rate in high risk medical and surgical patients. Anaesthesia. 2006;61(11):1031–9 [PMID:17042839].

86. Genardi ME, Cronin SN, Thomas L. Revitalizing an established rapid response team. Dimens Crit Care Nurs. 2008;27:104–9 [PMID: 18434864].

87. Jones CM, Bleyer AJ, Petree B. Evolution of a rapid response system from voluntary to mandatory activation. Jt Comm J Qual Patient Saf. 2010;36:266–70 .241. [PMID: 20564888]

88. Peebles E, Subbe CP, Hughes P, Gemmell L. Timing and teamwork—an observational pilot study of patients referred to a rapid response team with the aim of identifying factors amenable to re-design of a rapid response system. Resuscitation. 2012;83:782–7 [PMID: 22209834].

89. Foraida MI, DeVita MA, Braithwaite RS, Stuart SA, Brooks MM, Simmons RL. Improving the utilization of medical crisis teams (Condition C) at an urban tertiary care hospital. J Crit Care. 2003;18:87–94 [PMID: 12800118].

90. Jones D, Bates S, Warrillow S, Goldsmith D, Kattula A, Way M, et al. Effect of an education programme on the utilization of a medical emergency team in a teaching hospital. Intern Med J. 2006;36:231–6 [PMID: 16640740].

91. Wallin CJ, Meurling L, Hedman L, Hedegård J, Felländer-Tsai L. Target-focused medical emergency team training using a human patient simulator: effects on behaviour and attitude. Med Educ. 2007;41(2):173–80 [PMID:17269951].

Shane C. Townsend

Why Write a Business Plan?

Rapid Response Systems have been introduced widely. How often without writing a business plan? Historically, this may have led to slow adoption. Turf wars may have been avoided by better marketing of the concept to sceptical clinicians and hospital executives. The consequences today may be underfunding, neglect of essential elements, and a poor appreciation of financial and clinical risks.

Writing a Business Plan allows better definition of the innovation and associated opportunity costs. While many health services are not-for-profit organisations and are therefore primarily motivated by service delivery to patients, they are equally "not-for-loss" and must remain financially viable to deliver their mission. Constructing a Business Case is an important step to secure funding for the service in a competitive environment.

An operational plan is essential to avoid constant "fire-fighting". Foresight at the planning stage may save a lot of time later. Implementation of a new service requires ready solutions to such issues as communication pathways and supporting information technology, way-finding within

S.C. Townsend, MBBS, FANZCA, FCICM, MBA (✉)
Complex-Wide Adult Intensive Care, Mater Health Services, Raymond Terrace, South Brisbane, QLD 4101, Australia
e-mail: Shane.Townsend@mater.org.au

facilities, handling concurrent emergencies, and coverage of specialized areas such as the Radiology Department and Post-anaesthesia Care Unit.

Risk needs to be managed. This issue falls within the Governance "limb" of the Rapid Response System. It includes a consideration of medico-legal indemnity, clinical credentialing of practitioners, and governing policies. Data will need to be collected for audit and Quality Assurance purposes.

Finally, the marketing plan is crucial, not only in "selling" the benefits of a Rapid Response System to hospital administrators, but also in approaching the diffusion strategy. Adoption of a seemingly radical new innovation throughout a conservative healthcare organisation requires advocacy, education and persistence.

The Business Model Canvas

A Business Model Canvas is useful to display the outline of the plan in a semi-graphical format all on one page ([1]) (Refer Fig. 12.1). This allows capture of important elements and relationships in a way that is visually easy to understand and convey to others. This step facilitates brainstorming and can be helpful in testing the viability of the service plan.

Key partners in a Rapid Response System include ward-based clinicians, critical care units (ICU, CCU, ED), specialties such as anaesthesia, hospital administration and of course the patient

© Springer International Publishing Switzerland 2017
M.A. DeVita et al. (eds.), *Textbook of Rapid Response Systems*, DOI 10.1007/978-3-319-39391-9_12

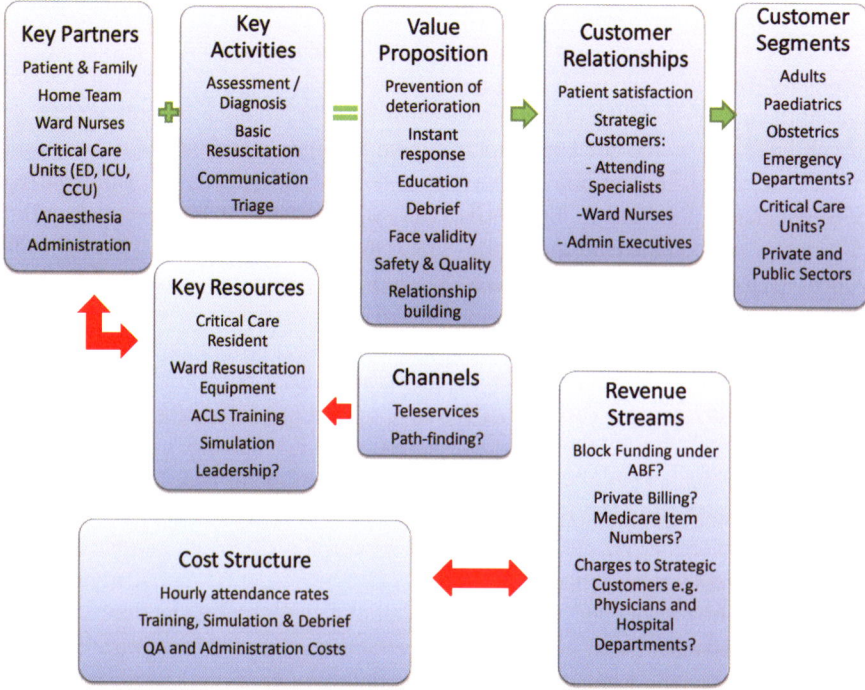

Fig. 12.1 The business model canvas for the rapid response system

and his or her family. Patient-centred care demands that the plan is designed around the needs of the deteriorating patient as distinct from the convenience of clinicians. At this stage, it is imperative to describe how the patient and family members can directly activate the afferent limb and achieve an escalation in care.

Will the Track and Trigger System be based on a weighted score or single variable threshold? To what extent will clinicians be empowered to raise concerns independent of the Track and Trigger System? How will emerging technology in vital signs telemetry [2, 3, 4] be incorporated to enhance the sensitivity and specificity of the afferent limb?

What will the attending team actually do—will they assess and triage or undertake more complex and prolonged resuscitation? What are the implications, particularly in terms of resources? The decision may depend upon availability of ICU beds, proximity of the patient to ICU or CCU, distances encountered in retrieving patients from remote locations within the hospital complex,

response times and the expertise of the clinicians responding.

Relationships are important to capture especially with strategic customers such as the admitting medical or surgical specialists. Rapid Response Systems operate on behalf of the treating specialist or home unit. They also operate on behalf of the hospital that shares a duty of care to the patient. It is imperative that all stakeholders caring for the patient share in open communication and are made aware by the Rapid Response System that a patient is in fact deteriorating. They must have confidence that the patient is receiving satisfactory attention.

Are we going to provide a comprehensive service to all patients or will we fragment the service to provide specialised responses according to case-mix? There may be merit in differentiating the afferent and efferent limbs to respond specifically to obstetric patients, paediatric patients, and surgical and medical patients.

Capturing all the costs including those pertaining to education and data collection is essential.

What expertise and clinical resources do we already have at our disposal? What additional training will be required and how will the investment in education be retained given the reality of an itinerant medical and nursing workforce in many hospitals? How will the Rapid Response System be funded—fee for service, block funding under Activity Based Funding [5] , Bundled Payments for Care Improvement [6] or a levy imposed on clinical units? The answer will largely depend on the public and private models of remuneration dictated by State and Federal jurisdictions.

Once the Canvas is complete it is worthwhile garnering broad feedback from all stakeholders. At this stage "critics" are your allies in determining weaknesses of the proposed system and may help in planning a better, more sustainable service.

Gap Analysis

When approaching this task a useful starting point is a Gap Analysis between the realities of what we have and compliance with the National Standards [7, 8, 9] or Guidelines [10] and Best Practice as described in the literature [11].

The traditional emphasis of hospital Resuscitation Committees has been focused on Cardiac Arrest. However in-hospital cardiac arrest still carries a high mortality, whereas mortality gains will likely derive from earlier intervention [12–14] (Refer Fig. 12.2). The dramatic

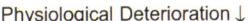

Physiological Deterioration ↓

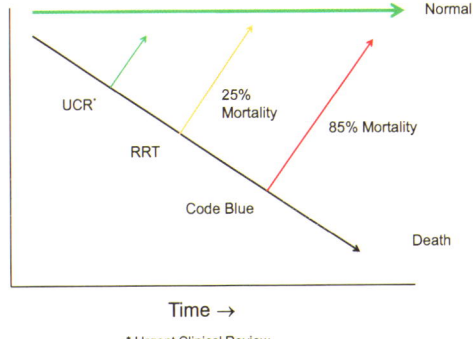

* Urgent Clinical Review

Fig. 12.2 Clinical pathway of the deteriorating patient

reduction in reported rates of in-hospital cardiac arrest has been accompanied by disproportionately modest declines in adult hospital mortality [15, 16]. Perhaps the system needs to intervene earlier?

Considerable resources are devoted to ACLS Training. Comparatively little educational resource is expended on training doctors and nurses to respond to patients who are becoming critically ill in the pre-arrest phase [17]. Simulation of a broad range of clinical scenarios may hold the answer. A change in focus beginning with the clinical leadership of the resuscitation Committee is needed.

There is still to be defined a minimum data set for measuring performance of Rapid Response Systems, although a consensus is evolving [18]. Key Performance Indicators are difficult to define for a service that must respond to a broad array of patients and range of conditions. Collection of data will not occur without allocation of resources and appropriate information technology infrastructure to underpin the incident reporting system. Thankfully, many hospitals are implementing real-time on-line electronic reporting systems to facilitate this aim [19].

Reliability of Vital Signs recording and interpretation is still in the domain of humans. Accordingly it is prone to human error. An appreciation of human factors science [20] is valuable in planning a Rapid Response System. For example, the weighted score Track and Trigger System requires careful calculation of an aggregate score from multiple vital signs observations and has been shown to suffer from inaccuracy [21, 22]. Simpler single variable systems may lack sensitivity and specificity. Technological solutions relying upon new telemetry devices integrated with an Electronic Medical Record (EMR) may offer a way forward. However, barriers to adoption may include cost and clinician resistance.

Multi-disciplinary teams would seem intuitively more appropriate. They replicate the model of how care is delivered to patients in hospitals and allow training of doctors and nurses in non-technical team skills (NTS) [23] or crisis resource management (CRM) [24, 25]. Many systems in Australia and New Zealand are medical based [26]. The UK has adopted a nurse-led Critical Care Outreach System. Neither approach has proven superior [27]. Local resources may dictate the optimal model.

Critical Care Outreach and follow-up of patients after discharge from ICU may offer additional benefit to an at-risk group of patients [28–30]. Defining high-risk groups of patients and rounding by critical care nurses may constitute a more proactive approach to Rapid Response Systems. Most existing Rapid Response Systems are reactive.

Notification of treating specialists should be mandatory. Apart from the obvious medico-legal implications, early involvement of the primary clinicians responsible for the patient in the event of clinical deterioration may lead to better outcomes [31]. Many existing systems suffer from a communication block at this critical juncture and fail to observe and maintain the principle of continuity of care. Clinician disengagement can be an unintended by-product.

Rapid Response Systems were initially intended to provide education and debrief to the staff members working on hospital wards [32]. It was envisaged that they would be supportive, enlightening and empowering. The frequent reality has been a failure to provide education and support post incident owing to a lack of resources and the imperative for the Rapid Response Team to return to other pressing duties. The result may be further clinician disengagement and disempowerment.

Standardisation is difficult when best practice remains to be defined. Nevertheless, it is desirable that unwarranted variation in the delivery of care should be avoided. Supporting protocols for the management of many predictable clinical emergencies are essential to underpin the operation of an effective Rapid Response System. Examples would include seizure, chest pain and sepsis protocols. This policy work cannot be overlooked and gaps need to be addressed in the planning stage.

Finally, many Rapid Response Systems are under-resourced or receive no dedicated resources whatsoever. In Australia only 25% of Rapid Response Systems received additional funding [33]. It is implausible that a clinical system could be expected to deliver dramatic improvements in patient outcomes at no cost. How should resources be allocated efficiently?

Hospitals are not free markets and do not subscribe to the principles of allocative efficiency. More likely, resources are distributed according to traditional models of care and medical hierarchies. The point is that good patient care need not cost more and may in fact cost less. However, paying for a service twice by grafting a Rapid Response System on top of a traditional model of service delivery (home units composed of ward nurses, physician/surgeon, advanced trainee, resident and intern) inevitably leads to duplication and waste.

Many of these issues would be endemic to RRS's throughout the US, UK, Australia and New Zealand.

The Financial Plan

Perhaps the most neglected area in planning for a Rapid Response System is a detailed financial plan. The starting point should be to build a comprehensive model of how the system will operate. It is important to be inclusive. Costs can be broken down per Rapid Response Team attendance, and according to system costs and establishment costs. System costs include training, research, data collection, quality assurance, governance and administration.

With the introduction of any new service there will be learning curve effects over time. Rapid Response Systems must change with the rapid pace of innovation in hospitals. They are dynamic systems. As the service grows economies and eventually diseconomies of scale can become apparent.

Various financial inputs can be considered for inclusion in the model. My suggestion is be inclusive. Underselling the cost will guarantee that the Rapid Response System is underfunded. Refer to Table 12.1 that details establishment costs, salaries and wages, team composition and governance positions for a typical 400-bed general hospital.

Money has a time value. Services should be costed over 5 years by employing an appropriate deflator for healthcare. In Australia between 2000 and 2011 the Government Final Consumption Expenditure (GFCE) Deflator for Hospitals and Nursing Homes has historically tracked from 2.7 to 4.4% per annum [34]. From 2008 to 2013 the average growth in recurrent expenditure by Australian public hospitals was 5.1% (adjusted for inflation) [35]. The long-term average US healthcare inflation rate is 5.44%, although by 2014 it had fallen to 2.61% per annum [36]. These figures are influenced by innovation in medical technology and pharmacotherapy.

Rapid Response Systems are principally dependent upon labour costs. An alternative approach may be to project increases based on the average rate of salary growth. This treatment would result in a more modest estimate of recurrent costs. It should be born in mind that in the near term it is likely that there will be broader implementation of new telemetry and central monitoring systems integrated with hospital-wide Electronic Medical Records. Technology costs at establishment of the Rapid Response System and depreciation of equipment over time will then assume a greater component of overall expenditure.

Businesses have a lifecycle that includes early investment and sunk costs before eventually maturing and paying a dividend (Refer Fig. 12.3). A problem with how Rapid Response Systems have been implemented is that often the upfront investment in training and governance has not been made. Neither has there been acknowledgement of the ongoing costs of operation over time.

Benefits may not be immediately apparent. Evidence suggests that approximately 2 years may be required for maturation of the service after which an improvement in hospital mortality may be observed [16]. This may be due to achieving efficiencies of scale, overcoming cultural barriers and the learning curve effect.

A sensitivity analysis allows prediction of costs by varying basic assumptions in the elements of the model from simple to more sophisticated. The more inclusive we can be at this stage the less likely we are to be confronted in the fullness

Table 12.1 Assumptions and inputs to a hypothetical model for a Rapid Response System

Salaries & Inflation[a]	
GFCE hospitals & nursing homes	0.04
Annual growth in RRT Calls	0.02
Total RRT Calls 2013	445
Training time per week (hours)	1
Post grad Y2 salary per fortnight (PFN)	$2826.62
Advanced trainee Y3 salary PFN	$3968.02
Registered nurse salary PFN	$3,762.55
AWARD annual increment	0.025
Team composition	
Registrars/advanced trainees	4
Residents	1
RRT nurse	1
Time per RRT call (Hours)	0.5
Governance positions	
Medical director salary PFN (MO2.1)	$10,920.51
Nurse practitioner salary PFN	$3762.55
Director full time equivalent (FTE)	0.25
Nurse practitioner FTE	1

[a] Salaries and Wages quoted from Queensland Health Nursing and Medical Officers AWARDs 2012

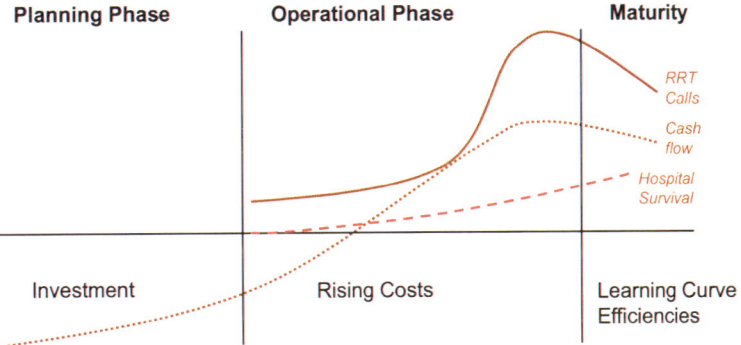

Fig. 12.3 Cash lifecycle for the rapid response system

of time by hidden costs. Scenario planning should test assumptions pertaining to the worst case, best case and most likely outcomes.

The Lean Model

A lean model has no funded governance or training positions and is purely medical in its composition. Patient caseloads for Registered Nurses are more strictly defined and regulated. Medical staff based in the ICU, Emergency Department and general wards can be temporarily redeployed to the Rapid Response Team.

The efferent limb may consist of only one junior medical officer based in the ICU. Nursing assistance is co-opted from the hospital medical or surgical ward where the patient is located. The average time spent at the patient bedside can be estimated to be 30 min [37]. This is consistent with a rapid assessment and triage model of care.

Conservatively, we may assume a 2% per annum growth in the number of calls, provided that the hospital is not expanding the inpatient bed platform and acuity remains stable.

Since the Global Financial Crisis, wages and salaries have grown at a more modest pace of 2.3% per annum [38].

Hospitals must comply with ILCOR Guidelines [39] for managing cardiac arrest and maintain appropriate resuscitation equipment in close proximity to inpatient areas. Accordingly, there may be little need for investment in specialised resuscitation equipment beyond what is already available.

The system may receive oversight from the hospital Resuscitation Committee. Training for medical responders may be confined to Advanced Cardiac Life Support. High-fidelity simulation training is not provided in this model. Debrief of clinical incidents is by exception.

Even this anaemic model still attracts a cost over 5 years (Refer Table 12.2). The key determinants of cost are the number of calls per annum, time spent per call and hourly rates of pay for junior medical staff.

This model is inexpensive and feasible to implement in smaller institutions and private hospitals that do not employ many senior medical staff. Its viability is critically dependent on a low rate of medical emergency calls since the medical officer may also be responsible for supervising the intensive care unit, especially after-hours.

The response relies on accurate and timely medical assessment with escalation to other services if more complex and sustained intervention is required. Clearly, this is not a team-based approach and either additional personnel will need to be summoned to the bedside of a critically ill patient or the patient will require expeditious transfer to a Coronary Care Unit, High Dependency Unit or Intensive Care Unit. The junior doctor who responds to medical emergencies must be supervised and supported by senior medical staff possessing advanced airway management and resuscitation skills.

Specialised training, research and collection of detailed data for Quality Assurance purposes are not funded components of this model. The focus of the service is clinical. Performance of the

Table 12.2 Cost projections for a lean hypothetical Rapid Response System

	2014	2015	2016	2017	2018
RRT calls	454	463	472	482	491
Hours	227.0	231.5	236.1	240.8	245.7
Team hourly rate[a]	$52.21	$ 53.52	$ 54.85	$ 56.23	$57.63
Cost of attendance per annum	$11,849	$12,388	$12,952	$13,541	$14,157
Cost of training time per annum	$	$	$	$	$
Cost of governance positions per annum	$	$	$	$	$
Total cost per annum	$11,849	$12,388	$12,952	$13,541	$14,157
Establishment Costs (Equipment)	$ Nil				
5 year total outlay					$64,888

[a] Salaries and wages based on 2012 AWARD rates and indexed according to Consumer Price Index.

system depends less upon the first responder and more critically upon the escalation to and coordination of hospital-wide expertise.

While a figure of AUD $13,000 (US $10,000) per annum to cover operational costs is very low, it is essential that the unfunded system costs including training, governance and Quality Assurance are supplemented in some way. This may require recruitment of more experienced (and expensive) medical personnel who are responsible for their own medical education and professional development. The goodwill of dedicated clinicians and administrators may be harnessed to provide a measure of oversight, reporting and quality control.

The Optimum Model

A more robust model consists of a multidisciplinary team of doctors and nurses possessing specialised skills and training in responding to medical emergencies. This team could include an Intensivist. The team may be tasked principally with the responsibility of responding to deteriorating patients outside the ICU. In this model greater emphasis is placed upon the performance of the dedicated (possibly stand-alone) first responders and their more definitive management of the patient at the bedside. The broader resources and expertise of the hospital are accessed only by exception when necessary.

The governance of the system assumes a higher priority with the provision of a dedicated Medical Director and Quality Assurance Officer. Data is routinely collected for benchmarking against Key Performance Indicators (KPI's). Training in technical and non-technical skills is well resourced and relies heavily upon high-fidelity simulation. Weekly dedicated training time is funded.

The growth in medical emergency calls may be increasing at higher rates than previously expected [40–42]. It is likely that this call rate will plateau as local Rapid Response Systems mature. However, increasing patient acuity, aggressive intervention and an aging population make it more likely that many institutions are still on the steep part of the growth curve. An annual increment in medical emergency calls of 10–15% may be more applicable to some healthcare services [43].

Expert team-based responses offer greater scope to manage the deteriorating patient for longer periods on the hospital ward. This may prevent the need for transfer of the patient to a higher acuity service such as the ICU. More complex management may require an hour or more time spent at the patient bedside. Obviously, the Rapid Response Team must be free of other duties to devote greater time exclusively to the deteriorating patient on the hospital ward.

Establishment costs could include a dedicated resuscitation equipment trolley. The team would have the facility of bringing to the bedside procedural equipment and a broader range of pharmaceuticals than would normally be maintained on the ward cardiac arrest trolley.

The Rapid Response System could avail new technology in remote telemetry and central monitoring of vital signs. This offers the promise of improved reliability of Track and Trigger Systems from automated collection of near continuous observations [44]. It does represent an additional sunk cost in setting up the telemetry and depreciation of equipment.

This more complex model is not dependent on labour costs alone, although they still account for the greatest proportion of recurrent spending. Provided there are enough calls to justify the service it is less sensitive to the absolute number of calls per annum or the time spent at the bedside. By contrast, the principle costs are fixed and relate to leadership positions, a stand-alone team who do not have alternate duties, investment in training and technology.

Since we are not dealing with labour costs alone, it may be more appropriate to apply a general measure of healthcare inflation to this elaborate model. The costs of a fully fledged model over 5 years can be quite confronting (Refer Table 12.3). We should not shy away from presenting this reality to hospital administrators. Rather, we should make them aware of the real costs, and the real deficiencies in existing services.

Table 12.3 Cost projections for optimal hypothetical rapid response system

	2014	2015	2016	2017	2018
RRT calls	467	491	515	541	568
Hours	350.4	368.0	386.4	405.7	426.0
Team hourly rate[a]	$295.54	$295.54	$295.54	$295.54	$295.54
Cost of attendance per annum	$103,569	$108,747	$114,185	$119,894	$125,889
Cost of training time per annum	$15,368	$15,368	$15,368	$15,368	$15,368
Cost of governance positions per annum	$168,809	$168,809	$168,809	$168,809	$168,809
Total cost per annum	$287,747	$292,925	$298,362	$304,072	$310,066
After application of GFCE deflator	$287,747	$299,257	$311,227	$323,676	$336,623
Establishment costs (equipment)	$10,000				
5 year total outlay					$1,568,531

[a] Wages based on 2012 AWARD.

Cost Benefit Analysis

We are not at the point where we can confidently bank the cost savings from improved patient outcomes due to implementation of the Rapid Response System.

Prevention of critical deterioration in paediatric patients has been shown to result in cost savings that can plausibly offset the operation of a multi-disciplinary medical emergency team [45]. There is some evidence that Rapid Response Teams that share personnel with traditional cardiac arrest teams are most cost effective [46]. Ideal team composition and overlap of personnel with the Code Blue Team remains an area for further research.

The alternative to implementing a Rapid Response System is to rely upon the traditional cardiac arrest (Code Blue) team to salvage deteriorating patients. The health system costs of in-hospital cardiac arrest are high for paediatric [47] and adult patients [48]. The cost per Quality Adjusted Life Year (QALY) saved following cardiopulmonary resuscitation adjusted to 2011 US Dollars is approximately $100000 [46, 49]. This figure does not take into account the average costs of training the Rapid Response Team (US $118000) [50] versus the Code Blue Team (US $279000) [51] adjusted to today's prices [46], respectively.

Perhaps a case can be made for improved staff retention rates, reduced parent medical unit overtime, more efficient use of our ICU's [52] and avoidance of litigation. But we must acknowledge the propensity for cost shifting and possibly an increase in admission rates to Intensive Care [53] and high dependency units.

Consider an estimated cost of AUD $1.5 million (US $1.05 million) for a fully fledged Rapid Response System over 5 years. Based on a benchmark of $50000 US per QALY saved [54], even a service that rescues 30 people, extending their quality of life by just one year, would represent acceptable value.

Recent meta-analyses have demonstrated an overall reduction in paediatric and adult hospital mortality since the advent of Rapid Response Systems that may be attributable to their effect [15, 16, 55, 56]. The point estimate for adult hospital mortality in the meta-analysis performed by Winters et al [55] was 0.88 (CI 0.82–0.96).

Medium sized hospitals average 5900 patient separations per annum, while large institutions exceed 15,000 separations per annum [57]. Mortality in US Hospitals has fallen gradually from 2.5% to 2.0% over the decade from 2000 to 2010 [58]. A 10–12% reduction in mortality over the last decade deriving from the implementation of Rapid Response Systems suggests that the number of lives saved in our worked example could be as many as 90 over 5 years. When compared to the cost-benefit analyses for ECMO [59] and solid organ transplantation [60], the Rapid Response System can be argued to be value for money.

Fig. 12.4 Operating costs versus frequency of RRT calls

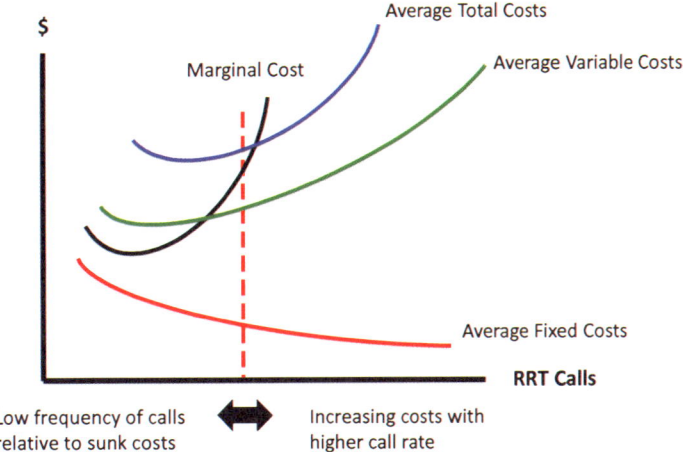

In the discipline of Economics there is a "sweet point" at which a service or production line is most efficient [61] (Refer Fig. 12.4). This frequency of Rapid Response Team calls needs to be defined for each institution relative to size and resources. Too few calls may be ineffective. Endless growth may result in cost blowouts and degradation of overall clinical performance. In the final analysis, it may be that safety and quality cannot readily be reduced to a dollar value.

Risk Management

Just because Rapid Response Systems enjoy strong face validity and seem like a good idea does not mean that they cannot do harm. Any Business Plan must include a treatment of risk. Indemnity for the Rapid Response Team particularly in the private sector is a controversial subject. Without a strong governance framework how can there be accountability? Most of these risks attract cost and can have a dollar value set beside them in a comprehensive plan.

These systems should be corporately owned. That is to say they should be regarded as essential infrastructure underpinning hospital safety and quality of care. They need strong identifiable leadership and should report to the Hospital Executive. It is imperative in the design phase that the "followership" among rank and file clinicians

not be given an opt-out. A fundamental question to ask is; *who is the team*?

Does the responsibility for responding to deteriorating patients reside solely with the members of the Rapid Response Team? What contribution should be made by ward-based clinical teams? How should Anaesthetists, Intensivists, Emergency Physicians and treating medical specialists be engaged? The choice is between many hands and just a few.

The implications of this decision are profound (Refer Fig. 12.5). Hospitals can adopt an approach to patient safety that makes it everyone's responsibility and incur relatively few emergency calls. Or we can delegate the sick and inconvenient to be cared for by the Intensive Care Unit doctors and nurses.

Marketing and Implementation

Today we are not in the position of having to "sell" a Rapid Response System to the Hospital Executive. They have already bought the concept. Compliance with National Standards means that implementation of a Rapid Response System is part of business as usual.

Introducing any new product or service has a characteristic Diffusion Curve [62]. Today, we are way over to the right of this curve. The majority conservatives have accepted the place of Rapid Response Systems. Stakeholders want solutions and convenience (Refer Fig. 12.6). Clinicians, administrators and patients want a mature service that works seamlessly. In other words, free from bugs!

At the other end of the bell curve medical sceptics will resist acceptance of the Rapid Response System while awaiting further proof of efficacy or optimal design.

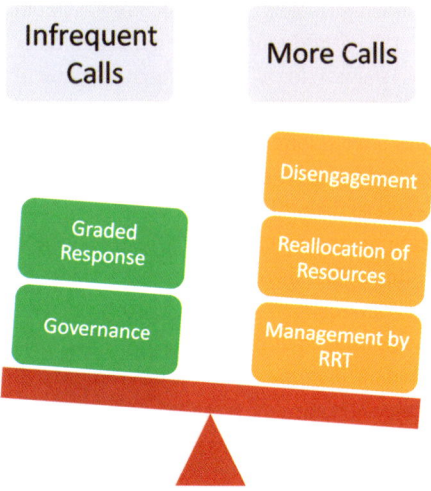

Fig. 12.5 The balance between governance and physician engagement

Pitching the Plan to Executive

At the completion of the Business Plan a crucial step will be "pitching" the proposal to the administration for the first time. Hospital Executives are not "Angel Investors" looking to donate funds to an enthusiastic entrepreneur with a great idea. Care should be exercised in offering a compromise model because that is probably what will be seized upon as a cheaper option. Thereafter, the journey towards better outcomes for deteriorating patients will be fixed on a lesser path.

The temptation to make ambit claims should also be avoided. Maintaining credibility is essential in winning support for a service innovation. A comprehensive Business Plan including an Executive Summary and supporting appendices is a firm foundation for arguing the case in favour of Rapid Response Systems.

References

1. Osterwalder A, Pigneur Y. Business model generation. A handbook for visionaries, game changers, and challengers. Hoboken: John Wiley & Sons, Inc.; 2010.
2. Orphanidou C, Clifton D, Khan S, Smith M, Feldmar J, Tarassenko L. Telemetry-based vital sign monitoring for ambulatory hospital patients. Conf Proc IEEE Eng Med Biol Soc. 2009;2009:4650–3 .Annual International Conference of the IEEE

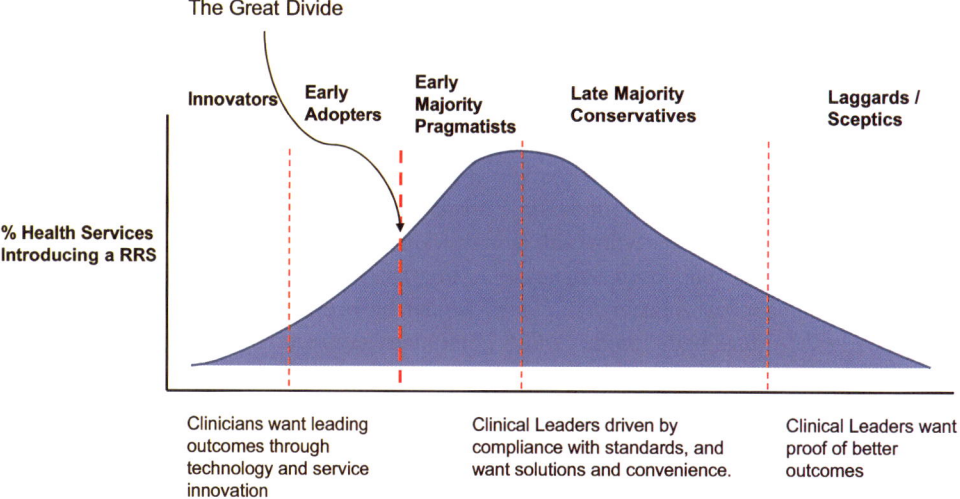

Fig. 12.6 Diffusion curve for introduction of rapid response systems

3. Smith GB, Prytherch DR, Schmidt P, Featherstone PI, Knight D, Clements G, Mohammed MA. Hospital-wide physiological surveillance – a new approach to the early identification and management of the sick patient. Resuscitation. 2006;71:19–28.

4. Tarassenko L, Hann A, Young D. Integrated monitoring and analysis for early warning of patient deterioration. Br J Anaesth. 2006;97:64–8.

5. Independent Hospital Pricing Authority. Activity based funding , [cited 2015 July 31] Available from: http://www.ihpa.gov.au/internet/ihpa/publishing.nsf/content/funding.

6. Centers for medicare & medicaid services. Bundled payments for care improvement (BPCI) initiative: general information\center for medicare & medicaid innovation. [cited 2013 December 19] Available from: http://innovation.cms.gov/initiatives/bundled- payments/.

7. Australian Commission on Safety and Quality in Health Care (ACSQHC). National safety and quality health service standards. Sydney: ACSQHC; 2011.

8. Australian Commission on Safety and Quality in Health Care. National consensus statement: essential elements for recognising and responding to clinical deterioration. Sydney: ACSQHC; 2010.

9. Berwick DM, Calkins DR, McCannon CJ, Hackbarth AD. The 100,000 lives campaign: setting a goal and a deadline for improving health care quality. JAMA. 2006;295:324–7.

10. How-to guide: deploy rapid response teams. Institute for Healthcare Improvement. Cambridge, Massachusetts, USA. 2012. [cited 2015 August 26] Available from: http://www.ihi.org/resources/Pages/Tools/HowtoGuideDeployRapidResponseTeams.aspx.

11. DeVita MA, Bellomo R, Hillman K, Kellum J, Rotondi A, Teres D, et al. Findings of the first consensus conference on medical emergency teams. Crit Care Med. 2006;34(9):2463–78.

12. Santamaria J. Crises and accountability, RRT from the director. Proceedings of the ANZICS Safety & Quality Conference: the role of intensive care with Rapid Response Teams. 2014; Melbourne, Australia

13. McGrath RB. In-house cardiopulmonary resuscitation – after a quarter of a century. Ann Emerg Med. 1987;16:1365–8.

14. Peberdy MA, Ornato JP, Larkin GL, Braithwaite RS, Kashner TM, Carey SM, et al. Survival from in-hospital cardiac arrest during nights and weekends. JAMA. 2008;299:785–92.

15. Chan PS, Jain R, Nallmothu BK, Berg RA, Sasson C. Rapid response teams. A systematic review and meta-analysis. Arch Intern Med. 2010;170(1):18–26.

16. Tobin A, Santamaria J. Medical emergency teams are associated with reduced mortality across a major metropolitan health network after two years' service: a retrospective study using government administrative data. Crit Care. 2012;16:R210.

17. Smith C, Perkins G, Bullock I, Bion J. Undergraduate training in the care of the acutely ill patient: a literature review. Intensive Care Med. 2007;33:901–7.

18. Hillman K. How to do post-hoc response reviews. 6th International symposium on rapid response systems and medical emergency teams. Pittsburgh, USA, 11, 12th May 2010.

19. Westbrook JI, Ling L, Lehnbom EC, Baysari MT, Braithwaite J, Burke R, Conn C, Day RO. What are incident reports telling us? A comparative study at two Australian hospitals of medication errors identified at audit, detected by staff and reported to an incident system. International J Qual Health Care. 2015;27:1–9.

20. Russ AL, Fairbanks RJ, Karsh BT, Militello LG, Saleem JJ, Wears RL. The science of human factors: separating fact from fiction. BMJ Quality and Safety. doi: 10.1136/bmjqs-2012-001450

21. Subbe CP, Welch JR. Failure to rescue: using rapid response systems to improve care of the deteriorating patient in hospital. Clinical Risk. 2013;19:6–11.

22. Cuthbertson BH, Sith GB. A warning on early-warning scores! Br J Anaesth. 2007;98:704–6.

23. Chalwin R, Flabouris A. Utility and assessment of non-technical skills for rapid response systems and medical emergency teams. Intern Med J. 2013;43(9):962–9.

24. Helmreich RL, Merritt AC, Wilhelm JA. The evolution of crew resource management training in commercial aviation. Int J Aviat Psychol. 1999;9:19–32.

25. Gillon S, Radford S, Chalwin R, DeVita M, Endacott R, Jones D. Crisis resource management, simulation training and the medical emergency team. Crit Care Resusc. 2012;14:227–35.

26. Jones D, Hicks P, Currey J, Holmes J, Fennessy GJ, Hillman K, et al. Findings of the first ANZICS conference on the role of intensive care in rapid response teams. Anaesth Intensive Care. 2015;43:369–79.

27. Outreach and Early Warning Systems (EWS) for the prevention of Intensive Care admission and death of critically ill adult patients on general hospital wards (Review) Copyright © 2009 The Cochrane Collaboration. Published by JohnWiley & Sons, Ltd.

28. Priestley G, Watson W, Rashidian A, Mozley C, Russell D, Wilson J, et al. Introducing critical care outreach: a ward-randomised trial of phased introduction in a general hospital. Intensive Care Med. 2004;30:1398–404.

29. Gao H, Harrison DA, Parry GJ, Daly K, Subbe CP, Rowan K. The impact of the introduction of CCOS in England: a multicentre interrupted time series analysis. Crit Care. 2007;11:R113.

30. Harrison D, Gao H, Welch CA, Rowan KM. The effects of critical care outreach services before and after critical care: a matched cohort analysis. J Crit Care. 2010;25:196–204.

31. O'Horo JC, Sevilla Berrios RA, Elmer JL, Velagapudi V, Caples SM, Kashyap R, Jensen JB. The role of the primary care team in the rapid response system. J Crit Care. 2015;30:353–7.

32. Benin AL, Borgstrom CP, Jenq GY, Roumanis SA, Horwitz LI. Defining impact of a rapid response team:

qualitative study with nurses, physicians and hospital administrators. BMJ Qual Saf. 2012;21:391–8.

33. The ANZICS-CORE MET. Dose investigators. rapid response team composition, resourcing and calling criteria in Australia. Resuscitation. 2012;83:563–7.

34. AIHW 2012. Health expenditure Australia 2010-11. Health and welfare expenditure series no. 47. Cat. no. HWE 56. Canberra: AIHW. [cited 2014 August 26] Available from: http://www.aihw.gov.au/publication-detail/?id=10737423009.

35. AIHW 2014. Australian hospital statistics 2012-13. Health services series no. 54. Cat. no. HSE 145. Canberra: AIHW. [cited 2015 August 26] Available from: http://www.aihw.gov.au/publication-detail/?id=60129546922.

36. Y Charts. US Health Care Inflation Rate. Bureau of Labor Statistics. [cited 2015 August 21] Available from http://ycharts.com/indicators/us_health_care_inflation_rate

37. Bellomo R, Goldsmith D, Uchino S, Buckmaster J, Hart GK, Opdam H, et al. A prospective before-and-after trial of a medical emergency team. Med J Aust. 2003;179:283–7.

38. Australian Bureau of Statistics, Wage Price Index Australia March 2015. [cited 2015 August 9] Available from: http://www.abs.gov.au/ausstats/abs@.nsf/mf/6345.0/.

39. Nolan JP, Hazinski MF, Billi JE, Boettiger BW, Bossaert L, de Caen AR, et al. Part 1: Executive summary 2010 international consensus on cardiopulmonary resuscitation and emergency cardiovascular care science with treatment recommendations. Resuscitation. 2010;81S:e1–e25.

40. Jones D, Bates S, Warrillow S, Goldsmith D, Kattula A, Way M, et al. Effect of an education program on the utilization of a medical emergency team in a teaching hospital. Intern Med J. 2006;36:231–6.

41. Jones D, Mitra B, Barbetti J, Choate K, Leong T, Bellomo R. Increasing the use of an existing medical emergency team in a teaching hospital. Anaesth Intensive Care. 2006;34:731–5.

42. DeVita MA, Braithwaite RS, Mahidhara R, Stuart S, Foraida M, Simmons RL, MERIT. Use of medical emergency team responses to reduce hospital cardiopulmonary arrests. Qual Saf Health Care. 2004;13:251–4.

43. Jones DA, Drennan K, Bailey M, Hart GK, Bellomo R, Webb SAR. ANZICS-CORE MET dose investigators. Mortality of rapid response team patients in Australia: a multicentre study. Crit Care Resusc. 2013;15:273–8.

44. Bassily-Marcus A. Early detection of deteriorating patients: leveraging clinical informatics to improve outcome. Crit Care Med. 2014;42:976–8.

45. Bonafide CP, Localio AR, Song L, Roberts KE, Nadkarni VM, Priestley M, et al. Cost-benefit analysis of a medical emergency team in a children's hospital. Pediatrics. 2014;134:235–41.

46. Spaulding A, Ohsfeldt R. Rapid response teams and team composition: a cost-effectiveness analysis. Nursing Economics. 2014;32:194–203.

47. Duncan HP, Frew E. Short-term health system costs of paediatric in-hospital acute life-threatening events including cardiac arrest. Resuscitation. 2009;80:529–34.

48. Gage H, Kenward G, Hodgetts TJ, Castle N, Ineson N, Shaikh L. Health system costs of in-hospital cardiac arrest. Resuscitation. 2002;54:139–46.

49. Ebell MH, Kruse JA. A proposed model for the cost of cardiopulmonary resuscitation. Med Care. 1994;32:640–9.

50. Dacey MJ, Mirza ER, Wilcox V, Doherty M, Mello J, Boyer A, Baute R. The effect of a rapid response team on major clinical outcome measures in a community hospital. Crit Care Med. 2007;35:2076–82.

51. Vrtis MC. Cost/benefit analysis of cardiopulmonary resuscitation: a comprehensive study—Part II. Nurs Manage. 1992;23:44–6 .50-41

52. Goldhill DR, Worthington L, Mulcahy A, Tarling M, Sumner A. The patient-at-risk team: identifying and managing seriously ill ward patients. Anesthesia. 1999;54:853–60.

53. Simmes F, Schoonhoven L, Mintjes J, Adang E, van der Hoeven JG. Financial consequences of the implementation of a rapid response system on a surgical ward. J Eval Clin Pract. 2014;20:342–7.

54. Weinstein MC. How much are americans willing to pay for a quality-adjusted life year? Med Care. 2008;46(4):343–5.

55. Winters BD, Weaver SJ, Pfoh ER, Yang T, Pham JC, Dy SM. Rapid-response systems as a patient safety strategy: a systematic review. Ann Intern Med. 2013;158:417–25.

56. Maharaj R, Raffaele I, Wendon J. Rapid response systems: a systematic review and meta-analysis. Crit Care. 2015;19:254. doi: 10.1186/s13054-015-0973-y.

57. Australian Hospital Statistics 2009-1010. [cited 2015 August 21] Available from: http://www.aihw.gov.au/WorkArea/DownloadAsset.aspx?id=10737419061.

58. Centers for Disease Control and Prevention. Trends in inpatient hospital deaths: National hospital discharge survey, 2000–2010. NCHS Data Brief 118, March 2013. [cited 2015 August 21] Available from: http://www.cdc.gov/nchs/data/databriefs/db118.pdf.

59. Crow S, Fischer AC, Schears RM. Extracorporeal life support: utilization, cost, controversy, and ethics of trying to save lives. Semin Cardiothorac Vasc Anesth. 2009;13:183–91.

60. Rana A, Gruessner A, Agopian V, Khalpey Z, Riaz IB, Kaplan B, et al. Survival benefit of solid-organ transplant in the United States. JAMA Surg. 2015;150:252–9.

61. Layton A, Robinson T, Tucker IB. Economics for today. 3rd ed. South Melbourne: Cengage Learning; 2009.

62. Rogers EM. Diffusion of innovations. 5th ed. New York: Simon and Schuster; 2003.

Part II

Creating an RRS

Hospital Size and Location and Feasibility of the Rapid Response System

13

Daryl A. Jones and Rinaldo Bellomo

Change is not made without inconvenience, even from worse to better

Samuel Johnson

We do not experience and thus we have no measure of the disasters we prevent

J.K. Galbraith

Introduction

Modern hospitals are complex institutions that treat increasingly unwell patients with multiple comorbidities. The aim of such institutions is obviously to improve the outcome of the patients they treat. Studies in the United States conducted more than 30 years ago reported that patients admitted to hospitals suffer serious adverse events unrelated to their admission diagnosis or underlying medical condition [1, 2]. Subsequently, similar findings have been reported from Australia [3], Canada [4], and New Zealand [5, 6].

The frequency and nature of serious adverse events and unexpected deaths is likely to be affected by factors such as the number of patients treated by the institution, the general health status of the patients, the nature of the services provided (e.g., trauma and cardiac surgery versus elective day surgery), as well as the presence of quality improvement initiatives and hospital governance mechanisms. Thus, it is likely that university-affiliated teaching hospitals will experience a greater burden of serious adverse events or unexpected deaths than smaller regional hospitals.

On the other hand, reports from the United States suggest that the risk of operative death is related to the total number of procedures that the hospital performs each year [7]. Thus, smaller or medium-sized regional hospitals may have a higher *rate* of postoperative complications for any given procedure, even if the *total number* of events is lower. Hence, serious adverse events and unexpected deaths are likely to be a ubiquitous phenomenon that all hospitals must somehow aim to prevent. Many hospitals have implemented Rapid Response Systems (RRS) to identify, review, and treat acutely ill ward patients. This chapter outlines the various approaches from the early warning systems that have been employed to prevent serious adverse events and unexpected deaths and to how RRSs can be implemented in different locations and in hospitals of different size.

D.A. Jones (✉) • R. Bellomo, MD
Department of Intensive Care, Austin Hospital,
Studley Rd, Heidelberg, Melbourne,
VIC 3084, Australia
e-mail: daryl.jones@austin.org.au;
Rinaldo.bellomo@austin.org.au

© Springer International Publishing Switzerland 2017
M.A. DeVita et al. (eds.), *Textbook of Rapid Response Systems*, DOI 10.1007/978-3-319-39391-9_13

Universal Requirements for Recognition and Response to Deteriorating Patients

Irrespective of the size and location of the hospital, there is a need to have systems and processes whereby patient deterioration can be reliably detected, recognized, and responded to (Table 13.1). Staff should receive education about the importance of vital signs [8], and how to provide an initial response to clinical deterioration [9, 10]. When a patient's condition is deteriorating, their care should be escalated until a point where the intensity of care provided and experience of the clinicians needed to provide it is reached [11]. In some instances, this may involve transfer of the patient from the area where they are currently being treated to a higher level of care, including transfer to another health care facility. All hospitals should have written protocols outlining the conditions under which escalation of care should occur, and the expected response that occurs when care is escalated [11].

Antecedents to Serious Adverse Events and Cardiac Arrests and Criteria for RRS Activation

The logic behind the conception of the RRSs and their role in identifying and treating acutely unwell hospital patients has been outlined in detail in other chapters in this book. In brief, a number of studies have demonstrated that serious adverse events and unexpected deaths are preceded by a period of physiological instability [12–14] manifesting in derangements of commonly measured observations and vital signs. These derangements in physiology are often present for some time before deterioration occurs, thus allowing time for appropriate intervention (Table 13.2). Accordingly, criteria for the activation of Rapid Response Systems are typically based on acute changes in heart rate, respiratory rate, blood pressure, conscious state, urine output and oxygen saturation derived from pulse oximetry [15].

In our institution, 82% of the Medical Emergency Team (MET) reviews are initiated by a nurse [15]. It is perhaps not surprising that analysis of the timing of 2568 MET reviews that occurred in the 3.5 years after the introduction of the MET service at our institution revealed that activation of the MET is more likely around periods of routine nursing observation and nursing shift handovers (Fig. 13.1) [16]. In areas where there is continuous patient monitoring, the detection of deranged vital signs may be less variable over a 24 h period [17]. These findings emphasize the need for creating simple criteria for activating review of unwell ward patient, regardless of the personnel that comprise the team that perform the review.

Table 13.1 Universal requirements for recognition and response to clinical deterioration

1. Detection: Deranged vital signs and other clinical abnormalities are reliably and promptly detected
2. Recognition: Staff reliably and promptly recognize that the patient's clinical condition is deteriorating
3. Escalation: that appropriate staff are notified of the deteriorating in a timely manner
4. Response: that the responding staff attend in a timely manner
5. Resuscitation: appropriate derangement of physiological deterioration occurs
6. Definitive care: the underlying diagnosis is recognized and treated and the patient is treated in the location most appropriate for their needs

Table 13.2 Principles underlying the Rapid Response System

1. Serious adverse events (SAEs) are seen in up to 17% of admissions
2. SAEs are preceded by derangements in commonly measured vital signs in up to 80% of cases
3. Development of such derangements predict an increased risk of in-hospital death
4. RRS calling criteria are usually simple and based on derangements in vital signs
5. The response of ward doctors and nurses leading up to an SAE may be suboptimal
6. Early intervention in the course of deterioration improves outcome
7. Clinicians can be trained to be experts in the management of deteriorating patients

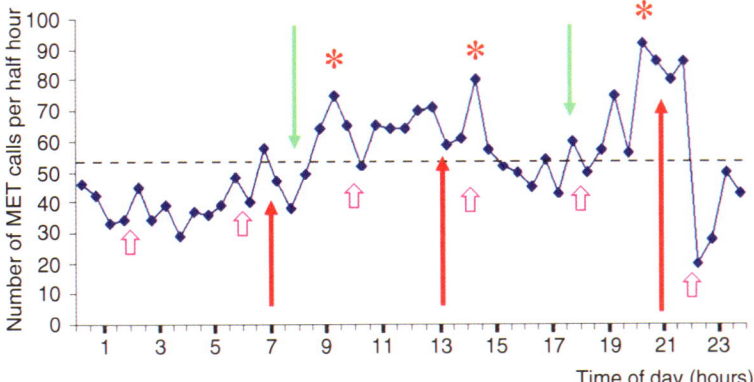

Fig. 13.1 Graph illustrating number of MET calls made per half hour over a 24-hour period in relation to aspects of daily nursing and medical routine for 2568 episodes of MET review. *Arrows* demonstrate periods of nursing handover (↑), beginning and end of daily medical shift (↓), as well as periods of routine nursing observations (⇑). The dotted line represents the average number of MET calls made per half hourly interval. Statistically significant ($p < 0.05$) levels of increased activity are also indicated (*)

Models, Location and Size

General Principles

The structure and personnel comprising the team that review acutely unwell ward patients must by necessity vary between hospitals. Multiple variables will influence the nature of the local hospital process of escalation [18] including:

1. Patient case-mix and acuity
2. The number and skill-mix of clinical staff in the hospital
3. The presence of critical care services
4. Hospital governance structures
5. Hospital culture
6. Other initiatives for deteriorating patients
7. Data indicating the nature, location and severity of problems related to deteriorating patients within the hospital
8. Available resources

In all instances there should be a combination of both proactive processes to prevent deterioration occurring, as well as reactive solutions that are activated once a patient breaches pre-defined criteria of clinical instability. In small country hospitals, the expert responders may not always be on site. Such

Table 13.3 Overview of models for recognition of, and response to clinical deterioration according to hospital size and location

Hospital type and resources	Recognition	Responding team & escalation
Small rural No HDU/ICU	Ward nurses ± local general practitioners (family physicians)	Local ambulance retrieval team aim = transfer out
Metropolitan general hospital has HDU/ICU few specialties	Ward nurses/ doctors ± CCO/ ICU LN	Nurse-led RRT Physician-led RRT
Tertiary referral hospital ICU (may be multiple) many specialties senior doctors	Ward nurses/ doctors Nurse consultants for specialty units Clinical nurse specialists ± CCO/ICU LN	Physician-led MET • parent unit • ICU-based

HDU high dependency unit. *ICU* intensive care unit. *CCO* critical care outreach. *ICU LN* Intensive care liaison nurse. *RRT* Rapid Response Team. *MET* medical emergency team

responders may include the local general practitioners (family physician) or ambulance service.

The ultimate disposition within the hospital will also vary according to its size, location, and in particular, the presence of absence of critical care facilities (Table 13.3). In hospitals without

Fig. 13.2 Figure
showing overlap and
relationship between
pro-active and reactive
approaches to the
recognition of, and
response to deteriorating
patients. *ICU LN*
Intensive care unit
liaison nurse

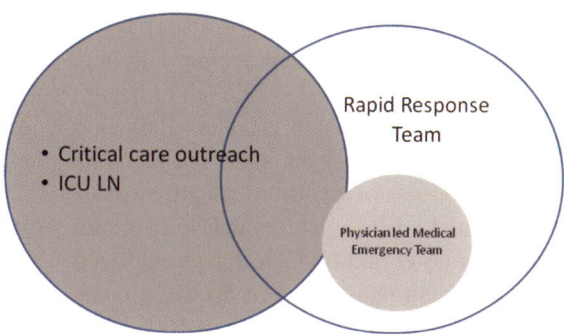

critical care services, it will often be necessary to transfer the patient to another facility. In such circumstances, a retrieval team may provide the treatment needed for stabilization. Because of this, escalation of care in such facilities should commence as early as possible.

In well-resourced university-affiliated teaching hospitals, the high degree of patient acuity and complexity will necessitate the requirement for an Intensive Care based team. In less well-resourced hospitals or district general hospitals servicing patients of lower acuity, alternative models may be adopted (Table 13.1). In addition to variations in the personnel comprising the team, the goals and objectives of the team may differ between models.

Ultimately, the aim of the system is to "improve recognition and response to changes in a patient's condition" [19]. Available evidence suggests that there is considerable heterogeneity in the composition of the responder teams throughout the world. [19, 20]. It may also be necessary to customize the threshold for the calling criteria that are used to activate the team.

In the United States there is wide variation in the reported team composition. Some centers utilize a nurse-led RRT [21–24], while others have implemented a physician-led MET [24, 25]. In Australia and New Zealand, the typical model is the MET, which is usually led by an Intensive care fellow (registrar) and nurse [20, 26, 27]. In the United Kingdom, nurse-led critical care outreach teams provide a surveillance service by routinely following up at-risk ward patients [28]. More recently, many hospitals in Australia have also introduced Intensive care liaison nurses who

assist ward nurses in "trouble-shooting" issues regarding aspects of nursing care and equipment related to high-acuity and complex ward patients [29–32].

At least one study has revealed that patient outcomes can be improved with a physician-led MET where the team leader is a responder from the usual treating team which appeared to be sustainable [33].

As discussed elsewhere in this book, these approaches can be categorized broadly into pro-active type approaches (critical care outreach/ICU liaison nurses) or reactive approaches (RRT/MET). There will frequently be some overlap in the nature of such responses (Fig. 13.2).

Teaching Hospitals and Academic Medical Centers

RRSs in teaching hospitals are frequently Medical Emergency Teams composed of intensive care based staff. In our institution the MET is composed of an intensive care fellow and nurse, as well as the admitting medical care fellow of the day [15, 27].

Teaching hospitals typically provide very frequent MET review for unwell ward patients. Reported studies in large teaching hospitals show a MET calling rate of between 25.8 [34] and 71.3 [35] calls per 1000 hospital admissions. This equates to MET reviews in 2.6–7.1% of all hospital admissions.

In the 3.5 years after the introduction of the MET service at the Austin hospital, 2568 review episodes occurred (average 734 calls per year).

The distribution of these calls was relatively even throughout the week indicating that the MET is an important mechanism for managing unwell ward patients in the periods not staffed by the parent unit doctors. Such information also makes it clear that a model created to service a teaching hospital must deliver the service with uniformity 24 h a day, 7 days a week. Although larger institutions have a greater need for a MET service resulting in a greater demand on resources, they are more likely to have a capacity to obtain more resources, making it possible to meet such demands.

The role of the MET in a university teaching hospital is to carry out advanced resuscitation of the patient, and to decide the location of their ongoing management after the MET review. If the patient is to remain on the ward, an ongoing management plan is communicated with the medical fellow and the parent unit caring for the patient. Each institution needs to develop protocols for intensive care medical handover of ward patients requiring MET review, as well as protocols for the management of patients receiving multiple MET reviews during a single admission episode.

In a University teaching hospital, the MET system may *reduce* the incidence of unplanned intensive care admissions [27]. In other institutions with less critical care personnel and resources, the MET may actually *facilitate* the process of intensive care referral and admission.

A recent review suggested that 13 of the 14 controlled studies that report a benefit in patient outcome associated with the introduction of a RRS, include a physician-led MET in the effector arm. This may suggest that medical presence in the efferent arm treatment may also affect outcomes of RRT review [36].

Secondary Referral Centers

Several different models of review have been adopted for patients fulfilling early warning system criteria in secondary referral centers. The MET may be implemented to supersede the existing cardiac arrest team [37] so that it reviews all medical emergencies in the hospital. In this model, the criteria for system activation are expanded to include MET criteria similar to those previously described. This approach is an effective way to meet the resource challenge by simply re-deploying those resources to intervene at an earlier time in the evolution of critical illness. As most hospitals have a cardiac arrest team, this is an easy initial way of allocating the necessary resources to provide a MET service.

In centers with limited critical care personnel, the MET can be divided into 2 levels or tiers (Table 13.4). The first tier ("*MET review—medical*") involves review by the medical fellow or the parent unit staff for patients who fulfill MET call criteria, but are not critically unwell. The second tier ("*MET review—intensive care*") is activated at the discretion of the nurse initiating the call, or following initial review by the medical fellow [38].

It is conceivable that the implementation of a MET could be initially restricted to a limited number of wards. In this model wards with the highest incidence of cardiac arrests and serious adverse events could be targeted to obtain maximum impact, with minimal outlay of resources. An alternative model is to use a different form of Rapid Response Team (RRT). Thus, the team leader may be an Intensive Care nurse who is specifically trained and can perform the initial review of the unwell ward patient [21, 22, 24]. Involvement of ICU medical staff is then at the discretion of the nurse team leader.

In all of these models, one of the aims of the review process is to improve the process of identification and referral for patients who require intensive care management.

If a cardiac arrest team is re-deployed to provide a RRT service, it is likely that its workload will increase as it attends more patients. This may require subsequent minor adjustments in resources. In addition, because the demands made by attendance to acute patient care under more complex circumstances require a wider array of interventions and knowledge, it may require a particular kind of nursing and medical expertise and training. These will have to be assessed in each institution on the basis of patient characteristics and acuity.

Table 13.4 Summary of various models of emergency teams for reviewing acutely unwell hospital patients.

Description of team	Personnel	Roles and objectives
Intensive Care Based Medical Emergency Team e.g., University teaching hospital [15, 25, 27]	Intensive Care fellow Intensive Care nurse Internal Medicine fellow Respiratory care practitioner	Advanced medical resuscitation Safe transfer to critical care environment if needed Formulate and coordinate ongoing management plan for patients remaining on the ward
Dual level medical emergency team e.g., Secondary referral center with limited critical care personnel [38]	**Level one** Internal Medical fellow and Hospital Medical Officer **Level two** Intensive Care fellow and nurse	Identification of patients requiring Intensive care fellow review Treatment and follow-up of acutely unwell ward patient not requiring Intensive care review or admission Activated at the discretion of ward staff or following review by medical fellow
Emergency department based MET e.g., district general hospital [39]	Emergency department hospital medical officer (Consultant/Attending and/or Registrar/Fellow attend if available)	Resuscitation conducted by emergency department doctor. Ongoing management carried out by ward doctors or visiting medical practitioner
Intensive care Liaison nurse e.g., District general hospital, In conjunction with MET [28–32]	Intensive care nurse	Review complex patients prior to MET criteria developing Follow-up of patients discharged from the ICU Consultation service

District General Hospitals

For institutions with very limited or no critical care facilities, the RRT can be comprised of emergency department staff, who review the ward patient and then communicate with the patient's visiting medical practitioner [39]. This system is appropriate for hospitals in which there are no dedicated ward medical staff, and in which the overall number of MET calls is not excessive. Daly and coworkers [39] reported on the implementation of such a model at the Swan District Hospital (Western Australia). Over a twelve-month period, there were 68 reviews in 63 patients. The system reduced the time delay for recognition of a life-threatening incident, and improved the process of communication with the visiting medical practitioner. This model required training of the emergency department staff in the skills of advanced resuscitation. The experience of these investigators provides proof of concept that an effective RRT service can be provided in a small hospital. It also emphasizes the need to use resources that are already available by re-engineering their use and also underlines the need to provide adequate training.

Small City Hospitals with an Intensive Care Unit

Increasingly, RRTs are being implemented into smaller privately operated hospitals in Australia. In 2004, we implemented a MET service in a small private city hospital in Melbourne containing a 6-bed ICU with 24-hour cover by an in-house ICU fellow. The hospital has 120 beds, and is located adjacent to a university teaching hospital with a well-established MET service. The hospital services a mixed population of surgical patients (including open heart surgery) and medical patients (mostly cardiology and oncology). It does not have an Emergency Department and patient care outside the ICU is provided by visiting specialists. In response to the occurrence of cardiac arrests (approximately 1 per month) and other serious adverse events, the medical advisory committee in conjunction with the ICU staff introduced a MET using the available resources. The ICU fellow and an ICU nurse became the medical emergency team and the hospital, nursing staff were educated to the benefits of the MET and the calling criteria were made known and available throughout the hospital. There was a rapid uptake of the system and over a 6-month period. Recently, the number of MET calls became stable at approximately 20 per month.

The service has proved sustainable and a preliminary data review that over a 6-month period there were only two cardiac arrests and an estimated six patients probably had their lives saved by the availability of the MET.

As the number of events is small, it is not possible to demonstrate a statistically significant reduction in cardiac arrests. However, the benefits of the MET service are already visible to nursing and visiting medical staff and the system is already fully supported by both groups of stakeholders.

Although the system is not perfect, and may require additional resources as well as better auditing, it is recognized by nurses and visiting physicians that it delivers a much better level of care than was previously available to acutely ill patients on the hospitals wards.

Summary

Despite the best efforts of hospital medical and nursing staff, serious adverse events and unexpected deaths are an unfortunate facet of medicine in the modern-day hospital. Although the overall burden of such events may be higher for teaching hospitals, all medical institutions can (and should) develop a system for the identification and management of unwell ward patients and are likely to benefit from its introduction. This system should be tailored to meet the burden of events and to incorporate the most appropriately trained personnel available within the hospital. The fact that a somewhat imperfect system may initially be deployed should not be a justification for inaction. Even an imperfect early intervention system is likely to be better than what is normally available in most institutions. The need for ongoing auditing and modification of the system cannot be overemphasized.

References

1. McGlynn EA, Asch SM, Adams J, et al. The quality of health care delivery to adults in the United States. N Engl J Med. 2003;348:2635–45.
2. Brennan TA, Leape LL, Laird NM, Hebert L, et al. Incidence of adverse events and negligence in hospitalized patients. Results of the Harvard Medical Practice Study I. N Engl J Med. 1991;324:70–6.
3. Wilson RM, Runciman WB, Gibberd RW, et al. The quality in Australian health care study. Med J Aust. 1995;163:458–71.
4. Baker GR, Norton PG, Flintoft V, Blais R, Brown A, et al. The Canadian adverse events study: the incidence of adverse events among hospital patients in Canada. CMAJ. 2004;170(11):1678–86.
5. Davis P, Lay-Yee R, Briant R, Ali W, Scott A, Schug S. Adverse events in New Zealand public hospitals I: occurrence and impact. N Z Med J. 2002; 115(1167):U271.
6. Davis P, Lay-Yee R, Briant R, Scott A. Adverse events in New Zealand public hospitals II: preventability and clinical context. N Z Med J. 2003;116(1183):U624.
7. Birkmyer JD, Siewers AE, Finlayson EVA, Stukel TA, et al. Hospital volume and surgical mortality in the United States. N Engl J Med. 2002;346:1128–37.
8. COMPASS. ACT Health, 2007. (Accessed 21 June 2010), at http://www.health.act.gov.au/c/health?a=da&did= 11025490.
9. Smith GB, Poplett N. Impact of attending a 1-day multi-professional course (ALERT) on the knowledge of acute care in trainee doctors. Resuscitation. 2004;61:117–22.
10. Zotti MG, Waxman BP. A qualitative evaluation of the care of the critically Ill surgical patient course. ANZ J Surg. 2009;79:693–6.
11. Australian commission on safety and quality in health care. National consensus statement: essential elements for recognising and responding to clinical deterioration. Sydney: ACSQHC; 2010.
12. Buist MD, Jarmaolowski E, Burton PR, et al. Recognising clinical instability in hospital patients before cardiac arrests or unplanned admissions to intensive care. Med J Aust. 1999;171:22–5.
13. Franklin C, Mathew J. Developing strategies to prevent in-hospital cardiac arrest: analyzing responses of physicians and nurses in the hours before the event. Crit Care Med. 1994;22:244–7.
14. Shein RMH, Hazday N, Pena M, et al. Clinical antecedents to in-hospital cardiopulmonary arrests. Chest. 1990;98:1388–92.
15. Bellomo R, Goldsmith D, Uchino S, Buckmaster J, et al. A prospective before-and-after trial of a medical emergency team. Med J Aust. 2003;179:283–7.
16. Jones D, Bates S, Warrillow S, Opdam H, Goldsmith D, Gutteridge G, Bellomo R. Circadian pattern of activation of the medical emergency team in a teaching hospital. Crit Care. 2005;9:R303–6.

17. Galhotra S, DeVita MA, Simmons RL, Schmid A, members of the Medical Emergency Response Improvement Team (MERIT) Committee. Impact of patient monitoring on the iurnal pattern of medical emergency team activation. Crit Care Med. 2006;24:1700–6.

18. Jones D, Hicks P, Currey J, Holmes J, Fennessy GJ, Hillman K, Psirides A, Rai S, Singh MY, Pilcher DV, Bhonagiri D, Hart GK, Fugaccia E. Findings of the first ANZICS conference on the role of intensive care in Rapid Response Teams. Anaesth Intensive Care. 2015;43:369–79.

19. Øvretveit J, Suffoletto J-A. Improving rapid response systems: progress, issues, and future directions. Jt Comm J Qual Patient Saf. 2007;33:512–9.

20. The ANZICS CORE MET dose Investigators. Rapid response team composition, resourcing and calling criteria in Australia. Resuscitation. 2012;83:563–7.

21. Chan PS, Khalid A, Longmore LS, Berg RA, Kosiborod M, Spertus JA. Hospital-wide code rates and mortality before and after implementation of a rapid response team. JAMA. 2008;300:2506–13.

22. Benson L, Mitchell C, Link M, Carlson G, Fisher J. Using an advanced practice nurse model for a rapid response team. Jt Comm J Qual Patient Saf. 2007; 33:512–9.

23. Steel AC, Reynolds SF. The growth of rapid response systems. Jt Comm J Qual Patient Saf. 2008;34:489–95.

24. Wood KA, Ranji SR, Ide B, Dracup K. Rapid response systems in adult academic medical centers. Jt Comm J Qual Patient Saf. 2009;35:475–82.

25. DeVita BS, Mahidhara R, et al. Use of medical emergency team responses to reduce hospital cardioplumonary arrests. Qual Saf Health Care. 2004; 13:251–425.

26. Jacques T, Harrison GA, McLaws ML. Attitudes towards and evaluation of medical emergency teams: a survey of trainees in intensive care medicine. Anaesth Intensive Care. 2008;36:90–5.

27. Bellomo R, Goldsmith D, Uchino S, Buckmaster J, et al. Prospective controlled trial of effect of medical emergency team postoperative morbidity and mortality rates. Crit Care Med. 2004;32:916–21.

28. Odell M, Forster A, Rudman K, Bass F. The critical care outreach service and the early warning system on surgical wards. Nurs Crit Care. 2002;7:132–5.

29. Green A. ICU liaison nurse clinical marker project. Aust Nurs J. 2004;11:27–30.

30. Chaboyer W, Foster MM, Foster M, Kendal E. The intensive care unit liaison nurse: towards a clear role description. Intensive Crit Care Nurs. 2004;20:77–86.

31. The Australian ICU Liaison Nurse Forum. Uptake and caseload of intensive care unit liaison nurse services in Australia. Crit Care Resusc. 2012;14:221–6.

32. Mcintyre T, Taylor C, Reade M, Jones D, Baldwin I. Characteristics and outcomes of patients subject to intensive care nurse consultant review in a teaching hospital. Crit Care Resusc. 2013;15:134–40.

33. Howell MD, Ngo L, Folcarelli P, Yang J, Mottley L, Marcantonio ER, Sands KE, Moorman D, Aronson MD. Sustained effectiveness of a primary team based rapid response system. Crit Care Med. 2012;40:2562–8.

34. Jones D, Mitra B, Barbetti J, Choate K, Leong T, Bellomo R. Increasing the use of an existing medical emergency team in a teaching hospital. Anaesth Intensive Care. 2006;34:731–5.

35. Santiano N, Young L, Hillman K, Parr M, Sanjay J, et al. Analysis of medical emergency team calls comparing subjective to "objective" call criteria. Resuscitation. 2009;80:44–9.

36. Jones D, Bellomo R, DeVita M. Effectiveness of the medical emergency team: the importance of dose. Crit Care. 2009;13:313.

37. Lee A, Bishop G, Hillman KM, Daffurn K. The medical emergency team. Anaesth Intensive Care. 1995;23:183–6.

38. Casamento AJ, Dunlop C, Jones DA, Duke G. Improving the documentation of medical emergency team reviews. Crit Care Resusc. 2008;10:24–9.

39. Daly FF, Sidney KL, Fatovich DM. The medical emergency team (MET): a model for the district general hospital. Aust N Z J Med. 1998;28:795–8.

Barriers to the Implementation of RRS

14

Oluwaseun Davies, Michael A. DeVita, and Ken Hillman

Introduction

While there is an abundance of literature on the success of simple medical interventions such as a new drug or procedure, there is considerably less in the way of evaluating system implementation. Certainly, a prospective, randomized, double-blinded, controlled trial is not possible for a system for a myriad of reasons that are beyond the scope of this chapter. Nevertheless, understanding the impact of system change is important, as are the facilitators and barriers to system change. The

O. Davies, MD
Critical Care Medicine—Internal Medicine, Adult Critical Care Internal Medicine/Emergency Medicine, University of Pittsburgh Medical Center, 3550 Terrace Street, Pittsburgh, PA 15261, USA

M.A. DeVita, MD, FCCM, FRCP
Department of Surgery, Critical Care, Harlem Hospital Center, 506 Lenox Avenue, New York, NY 10037, USA

Department of Internal Medicine,
Critical Care, Harlem Hospital Center, 506 Lenox Avenue, New York, NY 10037, USA
e-mail: michael.devita@NYCHHC.ORG

K. Hillman, MBBS, FRCA, FCICM, FRCP, MD (✉)
The Simpson Centre for Health Services Research, South Western Sydney Clinical School, UNSW Sydney, the Ingham Institute for Applied Medical Research and Intensive Care, Liverpool Hospital, Locked Bag 7103, Liverpool BC, NSW 1871, Australia
e-mail: k.hillman@unsw.edu.au

Rapid Response System (RRS) requires implementation across the whole organization as well as close cooperation between clinicians and administration [1]. This chapter will discuss potential obstacles as well as possible enhancement strategies for the implementation of an RRS across an organization. The major barriers and strategies for overcoming them are noted in Table 14.1.

Sources of Obstacles and Inertia

The Medical Emergency Team (MET) was first described in 1995 [1], but investigators are still attempting to quantify the types and magnitude of the benefits [2]. A cohort comparison study involving three hospitals demonstrated a reduction in case-mix-adjusted rates of unanticipated admissions to the intensive care unit (ICU) [3]. Another MET evaluation study demonstrated a significant reduction in the incidence of, and mortality from, unexpected hospital cardiac arrests [4]. An observational before-and-after study demonstrated a reduction in cardiac arrests and ICU admissions/readmissions [5] and a further prospective before-and-after trial demonstrated an impressive reduction of in-hospital cardiac arrests, deaths following cardiac arrest, and overall in-hospital mortality after the introduction of an MET [6]. Although these and other studies are preliminary in the sense that they are not randomized prospective placebo-controlled clinical trials, they nevertheless provide

Table 14.1 Barriers to MET implementation and methods to overcome them

Barrier	Suggested approach
Failure to view errors as products of the system rather than individual mistakes	Multidisciplinary event reviews of care antecedent to a crisis
Lack of data that METs are life-saving	Review current data; run focused trial; multidisciplinary crisis event reviews
Professional silos	Multidisciplinary event reviews; teach "system" of Care
Professional control	Emphasize METs to support, not supplant primary team's coverage; return patients to primary team immediately after event
Educational system	Emphasize benefit of better supervision of trainees by crisis team responders; track outcomes, delays in current system
Financial Lack of familiarity with criteria	Utilize current resources to staff MET response; identify frequency of avoiding ICU admission identify mortality benefit to offset cost Continuous education; hospital wide dissemination of criteria

considerable support for the concept of a planned system response to crises that would reliably rescue patients as they deteriorate. A larger cluster randomized study has demonstrated a reduction in mortality in the hospitals with a RRS using an MET as responders [7] as well as insight into factors such as the inadequacies of manual vital sign recording and the difficulty changing the culture of an organization [8, 9]. Many hospitals, quality improvement commissions, and even legislation, across North America, Australasia, and Europe have now implemented such Rapid Response Systems (RRS). However, why did it take so long, why is there heterogeneity in outcomes, and why do not all hospitals have such a fundamental and intuitively sound system to rapidly detect and respond to at-risk and deteriorating patients?

There is great variation in the success of organizations to implement an RRS [8]. The barriers to the introduction of an RRS may be related to cultural issues across organizations that are difficult to discern and overcome, and until recently they have not been well studied or described. This may be due in part because the very barriers to implementation that need description result in the failure of some organizations to implement system successfully. The fact that barriers may prevent successful implementation may lead organizations to conclude that the system itself is a failure, rather than being related to a failure to implement. Recently, there are publications that can provide some data rather than conjecture on what barriers exist, and their impact.

The first barrier is the failure to accept that many errors are a predictable result of the system of care that permits them to occur [10, 11]. While health care delivery may work well in providing individual patient clinical care, few systems function across existing health care "silos"—the professional groupings such as nursing or internal medicine physicians, or geographic groupings like emergency rooms or intensive care units (ICUs). Quality work within silos tends to be relatively easy to foster because members of a group tend to have common incentives and disincentives. Hospital-wide systems, however, are more difficult to effectively introduce and maintain in part because the framework for interdisciplinary systems improvement is relatively new to health care organizations and also because the members of diverse groups may have conflicting incentives. This perspective sometimes fosters the blaming of an individual rather than looking at it from a systematic perspective. Overcoming the perception that errors are not systematic is essential to creating an effective crisis response system.

The RRS is a hospital-wide patient safety system. It assumes errors will be made in a heterogenous fashion, and provides an important (and potentially life-saving) mechanism for the system to recover from this failure and prevent the further deterioration of a patient's condition, irrespective of whether the deterioration was due to an error of omission or commission, or even a natural consequence of disease. The successful implementation of an RRS requires interdisciplinary resources and teamwork. It presupposes that the system views these events as relatively common and preventable, as well as worth providing the necessary infrastructure and resources to ensure its effective operation. In other words, the hospital system of care must prioritize patient safety and view errors as a problem within the system, instead of an individual error. Failure to recognize the frequency of errors, the incidence of unrecognized and under-treated deterioration, as well as the failure to prioritize creating a systematic intervention are all a result of inadequate hospital leadership. Leaders must recognize that all "high reliability organizations" (HRO) have a system in place to not only reduce errors, but a recovery system to prevent errors from resulting in harm.

A second barrier may be the general reluctance of health to take up new interventions even when there is an evidence base. Interventions to reduce mortality, like low tidal volume ventilation for patients with Acute Respiratory Distress Syndrome, or preoperative surgical site infection prophylaxis are incompletely implemented many years after a consensus that the interventions should be used [12, 13]. The concept of an RRS is constructed around patient needs and, as such, seems to be becoming a more accepted and evidence-based intervention [3–9, 14–16]. However, none of these studies focus on other factors that may impact on the success or otherwise of implementing an organization-wide system, such as the culture of the organization. Some might argue that a conventional placebo-controlled trial for METs is impossible because withholding early intervention in half of the recruited seriously ill patients may be unethical. Thus, no trial will truly be controlled or be a "pure placebo." Furthermore, the MERIT study showed (among other things) that it is difficult to control an intervention that spans an entire healthcare system with individual hospitals as the randomized unit. In this study, the investigators found that both intervention and "control" hospitals had similarly varying degrees of MET intervention [8]. Although a post hoc analysis showed benefit correlated with degree of implementation of an RRS, there was little explanation about why there was such variation. A final consideration of the study of cultural barriers is that an interventional, prospective, randomized study of the influence of various cultural interventions on RRS implementation is difficult and has yet to be reported.

A third barrier is the existence of entrenched professional silos within hospitals and how they can create barriers to collaboration. The training of most hospital clinicians is specialty based. This creates cultural and intellectual isolation as well as increasing incompetence in areas not related to their own practice, or areas that require interdisciplinary cooperation for success. Specialist clinicians may become increasingly knowledgeable and confident in their own silo, but remain relatively ignorant of current practice outside that silo or of interactions between the professional silos. The intellectual and role isolationism sets up a system of ownership, competition, and egocentrism, and is perhaps the foundation for blame when things go wrong. Similarly, the "health care team" consisting of other health care workers is often deficient because they are rarely trained together and sometimes do not cooperate in system improvement activities.

Better models for teamwork exist in other industries. For example, the aviation industry sees itself as a global team continually striving to improve effectiveness and reduce error. A team learns and practices together before working as a team in "the real world." A prime example is in sports, where there is a long history of effective training to improve effectiveness and reduce error among those competing together as part of a team. In contrast, members of the health care professions tend to view themselves first as a physician, or nurse, rather than a team member [17, 18]. This cognitive "set" can prevent individuals from taking actions that are within their capability but outside the traditional boundaries of their position.

Another fundamental problem is that organizational competence of healthcare workers is not consistent. Health care education—while outstanding in training diagnosis and therapeutics—is often deficient in teaching system-based care. Instead, it focuses on diseases, diagnoses, and treatments, as well as procedural skills like setting up a ventilator, inserting a central line, or performing a dressing change. Training programs traditionally do not emphasize the "health care system": how a hospital works, including the hospital hierarchy; the roles and responsibilities of various staff; the interactions within the system; and the informatics infrastructure. Implementing systematic change is often left to health graduates to learn while on-the-job. This sets up system "blindness," where members of the health care professions may not trust the environment within which they are working, which in turn, leads them to set up their own methods for "getting around the system to get things done right." With this mindset, the system is the problem, not the solution.

Medicine is relatively resistant to change. For example, it took trauma systems 10 years before they demonstrated a decrease in mortality [19–21]. But there is also little acknowledgment or understanding of the complexity of health care and therefore little understanding of implementation strategies for any new process. The identification of facilitators and impeders is, for the most part, through personal experience, and only for those "trying to get something done" [22–25].

Finally, there are those who believe that the introduction of Rapid Response Systems can degrade the quality of care in hospitals. While they concede that a planned response may improve some outcomes, they express the concern that RRS may introduce a new burden on already overworked clinicians and negatively impact care elsewhere in the hospital. Indeed, one organization reported that there were 1.1 disruptive events per team activation. This led them to advise caution despite the fact that in the same report less than 1 % of the disruptions had clinical impact. Nevertheless, the other 99 % of disruptions to workflow certainly led to an unfavorable cultural environment even though lives were saved [27].

Foundations for System Change

Some recent social changes are laying the foundation for in-hospital transformations. First, scandals over potentially preventable deaths in the health care system have highlighted the frequency of errors and the harm that they cause [28]. *To Err Is Human* [10], a book published by the Institute of Medicine in the United States previously highlighted the under-publicized poor safety record of the US health care system. As a result, society now expects and is demanding more safety from the health care system. Demonstrating an improvement in this area will strengthen a fast eroding public confidence in health care institutions. However, despite enormous resources and effort there has been little overall improvement in acute hospital safety [29].

National healthcare policy is shifting, as constituencies demand safer care and greater accountability. This change is occurring globally. National safety bodies oversee strict standards for drugs and devices, but currently there is little in the way of evaluating and imposing standards around health systems. The Joint Commission on Accreditation of Healthcare Organizations (JCAHO) in the United States introduced tough new safety system audits [30] and mandated hospitals to have response systems by making it a national patient safety goal [31]. Their initiatives coincided with a tragic death in a hospital that had very recently been audited and accredited by the organization, which led some to conclude that the auditing system itself needed repair [32, 33]. The US Food and Drug Administration has altered its reporting mechanism and its methodology for notification of important drug error concerns. They now observe for sources of medication error and put pressure on manufacturers to alter packaging, labeling claims, and marketing approaches to prevent systematic sources of clinical errors and harm.

Health care marketing strategies have also changed. Health care buyers are working together to get the best value as well as the best cost. For example, the Leapfrog group in the United States has defined system standards and care goals that have prompted providers to alter their approach to care delivery, marketing, and data collection [34–36].

Senior health care officials are now attentive to safety as an important indicator of quality of care within a hospital. Thus, a number of agencies in the United States, Australia, and Europe are showing interest in the concept of RRS. For example, the Institute for Healthcare Improvement is providing courses on METs, and JCAHO has insisted that each accredited hospital must have a system to identify and respond to the seriously ill. Both the Federal and State governments in Australia are sponsoring implementation of the RRS concept and are advocating the MET model. One Australian state has implemented a standardized RRS in over 250 hospitals [29]. Because safety is a goal for all caregiver organizations, these forces are encouraging administrators and caregivers to recognize the possible benefit of the RRS for their institution and their patients. It would also demonstrate that they are practicing according to newly emerging practice patterns and safety initiatives.

Impediments Within the Hospital

There are a number of impediments within the hospital that may challenge the implementation of an MET system. The first is cost. For at least the last decade in the United States, there has been a huge focus on cutting costs. However, as noted above, there is now a shifting focus to safety. While cost is and will always remain an issue, the balance is changing from favoring cost considerations to a new concentration on quality.

There is limited data on the cost/cost effectiveness of the RRS. The RRS seems to increase cost because they appear to require new equipment and staffing. When an RRS is undertaken, one should expect a 3- to 5-fold rise in the frequency of calls to seriously ill patients [37], although the majority will not be for cardiac arrest events [1, 38]. Based on those numbers, it is easy to predict the staffing required for emergency stabilization [7].

Medical Emergency Teams often include one or more intensive care or emergency medicine physicians and nurses, an anesthesiologist or nurse anesthetist, and one or more respiratory therapists. In contrast, a Rapid Response Team (RRT), advocated by the Institute for Healthcare Improvement, does not utilize a physician, instead relying on senior critical care nurses to perform an assessment and triage. They may call in a physician as needed. This triaging system enables the hospital to utilize the costliest staff

only for situations where they are most needed. In addition, other members of staff who are not part of the team may respond and attempt to help manage the crisis. This activity is usually in addition to the other responsibilities they have. This perception of added work is a barrier to implementation and may stop discussion before accurate estimates of cost and benefit can be analyzed. It is estimated that training every staff member of a hospital to deal with cardiac arrests would cost over $500,000 per survivor [39]. Presumably, the cost to train every member of the hospital to care for their patients at the same level as someone trained in acute medicine would be many times that cost for each survivor.

On the other hand, an RRS aims to concentrate a small number of experts who respond to all hospital emergencies, rather than universal training for all staff in basic cardiopulmonary resuscitation. In this sense, RRSs can save costs and improve care. Newer studies show a decrease in healthcare delivery cost associated with RRS implementation as a result of reduced ICU admissions, shorter ICU length of stay, and earlier hospital discharge [40–42]. RRS can be a cost-effective and/or cost-saving intervention.

A second impediment is that crisis teams intervene for patients who are usually being cared for by other individuals. This raises two issues. The first is power: who is in "control" of the patient's care. If one group is already treating the patient, calling in a second group sets up a conflict regarding who is in charge, with the implied question of who is better? The second issue is based on historical perceptions that each team should give "total" care to its patients. In this model, calling for help may be perceived as a sign of weakness, perhaps both emotional and intellectual, implying that the caller is somehow not equipped to deal with the situation [43, 44]. A way around this barrier is to document all the skills, knowledge, and experience necessary to deal with deteriorating and seriously ill patients in a hospital and only allow those who conform with these requirements manage patients. This is similar to establishing the minimum training and expertise necessary before specific surgical or interventional procedures can be undertaken.

Because RRS require cultural as well as behavioral change, hospital nursing, physician, and administration leadership is required to make the system work. These leaders are needed for political support and for the required funding needed for the program. Without hospital leadership forcefully advocating for improved care of patients in crisis, and finding the resources needed to demonstrate both the need for and benefit of this service, the project is unlikely to succeed.

Senior colleagues in the allied health professions are key allies in culture change, in particular senior nurses and physician leaders. Nurses and doctors working in the hospital will not participate fully in the project without support from their leadership. The crisis response requires nursing and physician support; often the support arrives from other areas of the hospital. This shift of work responsibilities will be in addition to other responsibilities and so may be resisted. The leadership has to view the larger hospital perspective and be able to allocate resources that can both handle the added workload and have the skills necessary for the management of hospital crises. To protect these resources from added work, the leaders may balk at lending their support. Opting for the status quo—especially when it seems that individuals rather than systems are the cause of crisis events—is often the politically easier course to take.

Professional differences may create unanticipated barriers to implementation of an RRS. For example, nursing staff have a culture of recording patient vital signs and then reporting it to medical colleagues rather than acting on the findings directly [43–45]. This is due in part to a long history of not being empowered to translate concern into action. In this process, nurses who find hypotension will try to contact the physician responsible for that patient rather than immediately act. This may create unnecessary delays in responding to a change in patient status. Usually, this is not a problem, however, when the finding is critical, delays can lead to harm [46–48].

The exception to the rule of reporting along traditional lines before RRSs was when a patient had a cardiorespiratory arrest. A nurse could then commence CPR as well as activate a crisis response to deal with the patient. In contrast, an RRS empowers nurses to act much earlier in the patient's deterioration and activate a crisis response. Nurses (and physicians) may feel uncomfortable in participating in a new process that appears to change the traditional role of the nurse, and they may be reluctant to take on responsibilities that are not traditionally within their own boundaries. We have observed experienced individuals in our human simulator crisis team training course avoiding important tasks that are "not their jobs"—for example, no one may support respiration for a dyspneic patient because that is the job of anesthesia or critical care staff. Creating new processes for MET or RRT responses will challenge traditional roles and responsibilities, which is a potential barrier to the system's implementation.

Just as remaining mindful of one's profession may prove a barrier to the correct response, being aware that one's performance may be criticized will alter behavior. Junior medical staff, who are trying to learn and impress their seniors, are likely to see calling for help as a sign of weakness, laziness, or lack of knowledge. These perceptions may decrease the likelihood that a call will be triggered. Junior doctors traditionally look after their own patients no matter how sick they are and call for help only when they have insight into their own inadequacies and the potential consequence of this for patients. The problem is that until one is knowledgeable, one can neither appreciate these possibilities and dangers nor recognize when they are "in trouble." Medical trainees often do not possess the skills, knowledge, or experience necessary to recognize and resuscitate seriously ill patients [49, 50].

Physicians, nurses, and others in the hospital have operated in hierarchical and separate teams, creating an important barrier that needs to be acknowledged and understood. A nurse may recognize trouble and ask for input from other, more experienced nurses; when the situation is deemed to be beyond the capabilities of the nursing chain, they will call a physician. That physician will respond based on his or her skills and priorities. When that person finds the problem exceeds their skills, a second call is made, and a third or a fourth, until finally all the resources are assembled. This knowledge and skills ladder is hierarchical in nature and builds in delays. Even though there are well-recognized delays, caregivers may be reluctant to go outside the chain of command when a crisis occurs. For the RRS to work, that chain must be identified as a systematic barrier to rapid and effective care of a patient in crisis. This tacit statement that the current hierarchy is a source of error and harm could prove a barrier to accomplishing implementation of the system.

Traditional medical and nursing education is also a potential impediment to the RRS, since it teaches that learning is best when one thinks through a problem on one's own, and then learns from the successes and mistakes. Crisis response teams optimally intervene rapidly and with appropriate expertise. The response may be so fast that trainees may not have the opportunity to think it through and decide for themselves what are the most important considerations and best course of action. There may be a belief that not allowing mistakes somehow impedes learning. Since many advocate that education is an important component of medical and nursing care, creating a situation where teachers believe learning is not possible will cause concern.

The belief that an error results from an individual's actions, and not because of a failure of the "system" to prevent error, is a major barrier to RRS implementation [51]. Recognition that a faulty system permits error and harm to a patient is relatively advanced thinking in today's medical world. The Morbidity and Mortality (M&M) conference structure often concentrates on individual errors in judgment or skill rather than contextualizing it into "system thinking." The failure to recognize that a "system that permits errors" is a faulty system creates a fundamental barrier to implementing MET or RRTs. It seems to be easier to blame an individual than a system in such traditional M&M conferences because of the obvious connection between the caregiver and the patient, and so the need for a "system fix" can remain unrecognized. As long as this perception of "problem individuals" persists, there will be a significant barrier to creating a new process that threatens established hierarchy and current practice patterns.

It is well recognized that caregivers are not reliable in triggering the RRS when criteria are met [7]. In our experience, the barriers may be psychological: "If I call they may think I'm not smart/skilled/hard working," cognitive: "I am not sure if this patient meets the criteria," and/or cultural: "If I call others may criticize me." Each concern may require a different remediation technique. There is data on the likelihood of an individual provider triggering the RRS when activation criteria are met. In a study of physician trainees and ward nursing staff at an urban community hospital, caregivers were surveyed on their knowledge of the RRT triggering criteria, the perceived benefit of the RRT response, and finally, their perception of whether they will activate the RRS. The findings were as one might expect. As the level of familiarity with, agreement with and perceived benefit of the MET, and/or activation criteria increased, the self-reported adherence rates for triggering a response increased. Thus, failures to address these issues are key barriers to MET implementation [52].

Strategies to Overcome Hurdles

All the barriers seem to fall into the categories of knowledge gaps (what are the criteria?), cultural gaps (why should I call? Will I be blamed for calling?), and belief gaps (Do RRS really work? Does the response improve upon what I can do without it?). These gaps may lead to decisions resulting in a failure to act. Strategies to improve implementation of and sustaining the RRS should focus on these concerns. A staff questionnaire as done by Jones or Davies [43, 52] may highlight areas to target intervention.

The authors have noted a number of strategies to overcome a variety of hurdles. Some strategies may operate optimally during the implementation phase and others are more appropriate for systems maintenance. There is no data to support which barriers need to be overcome first, nor any to determine which strategies are most effective, easiest, or surest.

The authors have found that hospital "stories" of failures or near misses can become the basis for a forum where an alternative system approach can be discussed. There are two types of stories that tend to work. The first is the "cause celebre," in which some tragic event occurs, demanding analysis and action—for example, the wife of a staff physician who dies from an error involving an opioid overdose, after which careful analysis reveals that the death was due to both a life-threatening situation (the opioid dosing) but also to the hospital system's failure to respond to the event. The second is a compendium of smaller stories—for example, analysis of a series of people who had adverse events in a 6-month interval all due to opioid adverse events. The sheer number of events—whether near misses or actual harms—can be a powerful motivator to action. While it is easy to attribute a single adverse event to a single faulty practitioner, analysis of many events together will demonstrate a myriad of causes. We glibly call this "following the parade of the cadavers" to highlight how tracking similar events can lead to observations that may not be evident when singular events are scrutinized. This method makes it clear that the *system* is faulty if so many mistakes can occur, each mistake by a different individual, at a different step in the process, and at different times. This makes the need for a system response more evident. It is in this context that the person promoting an MET or RRT response must propose a *system* that may prevent serious adverse events no matter what their cause. Successes with one type of crisis tend to lead to the recognition by others that the system may work well for other types of problems. In this way, the MET and RRT response becomes the system's "goalkeeper" to rescue patients when other error-detection mechanisms have failed. A major selling point for the RRS is that they can prevent deaths and serious complications from myriad causes that result in patient deterioration.

A second method is to analyze and use data to promote motivating change: data is impersonal and unbiased, and can track harm and the benefits of process change. Possibly, the most important data to track is the frequency and duration of delays in care that occurred prior to a crisis event. Reviewing the 24 h prior to a crisis or cardiac arrest event for delays in delivery of appropriate treatment is possible once standards for response times and severity of illness are created. Crisis criteria enable reviewers to determine how long after the criteria were met that it takes to deliver the definitive treatment, or even get the responsible and capable person to the bedside of the patient in crisis [37, 46, 49]. Analysts can then graph delays by frequency, duration, location, service, day of week, time of day, etc. This data provides a powerful tool to recognize system deficiencies and motivate process change. We believe that delays in delivering definitive treatments are the hallmarks of hospital care systems without a RRS. Continued data collection and analysis will demonstrate effectiveness of process change in removing delays in care from an institution.

The authors have encountered individuals who remain resistant to group efforts to solve medical crisis situations. Data from the RRS can, in itself, facilitate the implementation and maintenance process [53], and may be processed and targeted to every level of the organization. Specific patient details are provided for individual clinicians, while departments, divisions, and the hospital would review aggregated, de-identified data. Data includes details of MET calls, number of deaths, cardiac arrests, and unplanned ICU admissions in which MET criteria had been met but no call made; these are called potentially preventable events. A graphic depiction of duration and frequency of delays from the onset of a crisis situation (determined by satisfying crisis criteria) can help target areas that need extra educational effort. Another important indicator is the number of MET calls/1000 hospital admissions as an increasing number of calls is strongly correlated with a significant reduction in deaths and cardiac arrests [6]. If caregivers accept the premise that an RRS is good, then this statistic can be very motivating. If they do not accept it, then of course less impact is expected.

Some clinicians or departments may not like having "unconsulted" doctors assume care of their patients, creating a political barrier to implementation of the RRS. One method to overcome this concern and facilitate the implementation of a hospital emergency system is to remind staff that calling for help in cases of complex acute medicine is no different from seeking consultations from colleagues in different specialties. Guarantees that the patient's care will remain under the control of the "primary" caregivers after the crisis is resolved (or even during it) can also foster an environment where an MET or RRT may be implemented successfully.

If all else fails, the admitting consultant can be reminded of the importance of them being ultimately responsible for their patient's care and convinced that because of the complex and serious nature of the patient's condition their urgent presence at any time of night or day would be ideal rather than leave such challenging management to trainees. Offers can also be made to upgrade the skills of the admitting physician in areas such as intubation, inotropes, and central line insertion.

One author discovered that the director of a residency education program did nothing to promote use of an MET, but permitted the use of METs with the caveat that it was the responsibility of the MET response organizers to "make sure my residents get taught." After the trainees reported decreased stress when caring for sick patients, and improved understanding of the management of suddenly critically ill patients—learned during observation of and working with the MET responders—the education director relented. With METs residents learn in a context where they have support, and become more comfortable in managing deteriorating patients [54]; on the other hand, they did feel that losing the opportunity to learn by doing detracted from their educational program.

The RRS can help to cost-effectively treat patients. For example, nursing infrastructure required to care for seriously ill patients on a general ward can detract from other routine activities. The MET and RRT response not only provides timely and expert care at all times but can decrease the burden on the rest of the staff having to care for the seriously ill in inappropriate environments. The average duration of an MET response is approximately 30 min [1]. Thus, a patient who is deteriorating can be assessed, treated, and if

necessary triaged in short order. This allows the nursing unit routine to remain relatively undisturbed despite the crisis event.

The RRS improves the safety of patients on general wards with patients in crisis. The authors have observed what we call "domino codes," where a second patient medical crisis occurs because staff either fail to deliver treatment or adequately monitor patients while they are coping with the first patient in crisis. We believe that an RRS decreases "domino codes" because they swiftly bring new critical care resources to the unit (which is suddenly understaffed to meet the workload), and they either rapidly resolve the crisis or triage the patient elsewhere. Identifying these unit-based resource issues and recognizing the successes that occur after RRS implementation are great motivators to overcome pockets of resistance. Highlighting the frequency of domino codes can provide impetus on ward staff to activate the RRS earlier.

Adding or increasing MET or RRT responses means increased work for the response team, because each response brings critical care workers from other areas to treat a single patient. It may seem a daunting task to marshal the resources to take on the task of responding to all patient medical crisis events. The authors' hospitals offer a service similar to the traditional cardiac arrest team: that is, resuscitate first, discuss after, and return the patient to the care of the primary doctor immediately after the crisis is resolved. By using the cardiac arrest team, no new resources need to be identified—the current resources are just taxed a bit more. Recognition that many emergency patients may go on to become cardiac arrest patients can help motivate responders to arrive early, before the heart stops. Early calls improve outcome and decrease the effort needed to restore homeostasis. Critical care admissions may be avoided, decreasing the downstream work of the ICU staff. On balance, responding to crises early and effectively reduces workload for hospital staff.

In hospitals, education is a continuous and essential activity needed to maintain quality care. To improve learning about the importance of an RRS and the behaviors needed to foster one, it helps to find opportunities to educate staff about the RRS. For example, new staff orientation should include a module on crisis management and appropriate use of MET or RRT capability. New staff will accept the process based on "accepted and expected" practice. In contrast, existing staff need to be re-educated in why a systematic approach makes more sense than ad hoc processes to build crisis intervention teams for each critical event. New systems of care must be perceived by existing staff to be both easier and more effective than current practice or the new process will fail. RRS rules must be made simple and objective. Any "interpretable" rules will not be consistently followed; the MET or RRT response should be viewed as "one-stop shopping" for management of any medical crisis. Buist et al. have found that "caregivers 'worried' about a patient" is a common trigger for an MET response [4]. Reliably rescuing staff members who have patient concerns will reinforce use of the response in the future.

For managers of the RRS, positive and negative reinforcement can foster culture change. Congratulate those who "call for help"; tell them, their bosses, and their colleagues how a life was saved. The University of Pittsburgh used email for this feedback to effect culture change [37]. Private notification of superiors about failure to trigger the MET or RRT response will demonstrate the impact of the failure. It is essential that RRS responders reinforce the call as well; it will do no good if superiors praise calling for help while the RRS responders criticize the same action. Every criticism of an RRS call must trigger re-education of those individuals. All members of the institution must view an RRS call as an act of heroism: it is putting patient care above ego. Even a call that does not meet criteria may mean the staff that activated the MET requires help even if the patient does not, and provides an opportunity for teaching and mentoring [26]. Other reinforcing educational strategies include placing team-triggering criteria in all parts of the hospital and on pocket cards for responders and staff, and notifying patients and families about the MET system to protect the patients.

As noted previously, "calling for help" can be perceived as a sign of weakness, and this perception is promoted when the criteria for what constitutes a crisis are subjective or ambiguous. As such, the request is an indirect measure of competency: the person perceiving the patient in crisis defines crisis by his or her inability to manage the situation alone. To prevent this barrier, objective and readily recognized crisis criteria must be adopted. With objective criteria, the person who finds the crisis is merely notifying others that the crisis exists (following hospital policy), and this does not imply that the person's ability to manage the situation is inadequate. Instead, the MET or RRT call becomes a mark of excellence in patient care and clinical judgment. Hospitals that have utilized crisis criteria have shown an increase in MET and RRT response frequency and a decrease in delays to treatment [4, 37]. In addition, creating a policy that "All RRS triggered events are good/reasonable" is important. If caregivers feel that they will be second guessed, a barrier is created. Caregivers must know that their decision will be respected as an act of trying to improve care.

Summary

Implementing a Rapid Response System in a hospital will likely alter the culture of care and threaten the status quo. There are many potential economic, social, cultural, and psychological barriers to bringing a new system of care to an environment. Nevertheless, strong data indicate that such a system of care will decrease morbidity and unexpected mortality in a variety of hospital settings. Therefore, the key question with which hospital leadership must grapple is how to implement the system, not whether to implement it. There is no strong data on how to overcome the barriers to implementing a Rapid Response System. Instead, in this chapter, we have proposed strategies that have been effective in our hospital environments and may benefit others as well.

References

1. Lee A, Bishop G, Hillman KM, Daffurn K. The medical emergency team. Anaesth Intensive Care. 1995;23:183–6.
2. Jones DA, DeVita MA, Bellomo R. Rapid-response teams. N Engl J Med. 2011;365:139–46.
3. Bristow PJ, Hillman KM, Chey T, et al. Rates of in-hospital arrests, deaths, and intensive care admissions: the effect of a medical emergency team. Med J Aust. 2000;173:236–40.
4. Buist MD, Moore GE, Bernard SA, Waxman BP, Anderson JN, Nguyen TV. Effects of a medical emergency team on reduction of incidence of and mortality from unexpected cardiac arrests in hospital: preliminary study. BMJ. 2002;324:387–90.
5. Baxter AD, Cardinal P, Hooper J, Patel R. Medical emergency teams at The Ottawa Hospital: the first two years. Can J Anaesth. 2008;55(4):223–31.
6. Bellomo R, Goldsmith D. Postoperative serious adverse events in a teaching hospital: a prospective study. Med J Aust. 2002;176:216–8.
7. Chen J, Flabouris A, Bellomo R, Hillman K, Finfer S, MERIT Study Investigators in the Simpson Centre and the ANZICS Clinical Trials Group. The relationship between early emergency team calls and serious adverse events. Crit Care Med. 2009;37:148–53.
8. MERIT Study Investigators. Introduction of the medical emergency team: a cluster-randomised controlled trial. Lancet. 2005;365:2091–7.
9. Chen J, Flabouris A, Bellomo R, Hillman K, Finfer S, MERIT Study Investigators in the Simpson Centre and the ANZICS Clinical Trials Group. The impact of introducing medical emergency teams on the documentation of vital signs. Resuscitation. 2009;80:35–43.
10. Institute of Medicine. To err is human: building a safer health system. In: Kohn LT, Corrigan JM, Donaldson MS, editors. Washtington, DC: National Academy Press; 2000.
11. Yourstone SA, Smith HL. Managing system errors and failures in health care organizations: suggestions for practice and research. Health Care Manage Rev. 2002;27(1):50–61.
12. Needham DM, Colantuoni E, Mendez-Tellez PA, Dinglas VD, Sevransky JE, Dennison Himmelfarb CR, Desai SV, Shanholtz C, Brower RG, Pronovost PJ. Lung protective mechanical ventilation and two year survival in patients with acute lung injury: prospective cohort study. BMJ. 2012;344:e2124.
13. Bratzler DW, Houck PM, Richards C, et al. Use of antimicrobial prophylaxis for major surgery: baseline results from the National Surgical Infection Prevention Project. Arch Surg. 2005;140(2):174–82.
14. Bellomo R, Goldsmith D, Uchino S, Buckmaster J, Hart G, Oppdam H, Silvester W, Doolan L, Gutteridge G. Prospective controlled trial of effects of medical emergency team on postoperative morbidity and mortality rates. Crit Care Med. 2004;32:916–21.
15. Bellomo R, Goldsmith D, Uchino S, Buckmaster J, Hart GK, Opdam H, Silvester W, Doolan L, Gutteridge G. A prospective before-and-after trial of a medical emergency team. Med J Aust. 2003;179(6):283–9.
16. Goldhill DR, Worthington L, Mulcahy A, Taring M, Sumner A. The patient-at-risk team: identifying and managing seriously ill ward patients. Anaesthesia. 1999;54:853–60.
17. Knox GE, Simpson KR. Teamwork: the fundamental building block of high-reliability organizations and patient safety. In: Youngberg BJ, Hatlie MJ, editors. Patient safety handbook. Boston: Jones & Bartlett; 2004. p. 379–415.
18. Baker DP, Day R, Salas E. Teamwork as an essential component of high-reliability organizations. Health Serv Res. 2006;41(4 Pt 2):1576–98.
19. Nathens AB, Jurkovich GJ, Cummings P, Rivara FP, Maier RV. The effect of organized systems of trauma care on motor vehicle crash mortality. JAMA. 2000;283:1990–4.
20. Lecky F, Woodford M, Yates DW. Trends in trauma care in England and Wales 1989–97. UK Trauma Audit Research Network. Lancet. 2000;355:1771–5.
21. Mullins RJ, Veum-Stone J, Helfand M, Zimmer-Gembeck M, Trunkey D. Outcome of hospitalized patients after institution of a trauma system in an urban area. JAMA. 1994;27:1919–24.
22. Plsek PE, Greenhalgh T. The challenge of complexity in health care. BMJ. 2001;323:625–8.
23. Eccles FR, Grimshaw J. Why does primary care need more implementation research? Fam Pract. 2001;18:353–5.
24. Dellinger RP. Fundamental critical care support: another merit badge or more? Crit Care Med. 1996;24:556–7.
25. Cook RI, Render M, Woods DD. Gaps in the continuity of care and progress on patient safety. BMJ. 2000;320:791–4.
26. Micthell A, Schatz M, Francis H. Designing a critical care nurse-led rapid response team using only available resources: 6 years later. Crit Care Nurse. 2014;34(3):41–55.
27. The Concord Medical Emergency Team (MET) incidents study investigators. Incidents resulting from staff leaving normal duties to attend medical emergency team calls. Med J Aust. 2014;201:528–31. doi:10.5694/mja14.00647.
28. Schneider EC, Lieberman T. Publicly disclosed information about the quality of health care: response of the US public. Qual Health Care. 2001;10:96–103.
29. Hillman KM, Lilford R, Braithwaite J. Patient safety and rapid response systems. Med J Aust. 2014;201:654–6.
30. Beyea SC. Implications of the 2004 National Patient Safety Goals. AORN J. 2003;78:834–6.
31. Joint Commission on Accreditation of Healthcare Organizations. 2008 National Patient Safety Goals. Jt Comm Persspect. 2007;27:10–22.
32. Griffith JR, Knutzen SR, Alexander JA. Structural versus outcomes measures in hospitals: a comparison

of joint commission and medicare outcomes scores in hospitals. Qual Manag Health Care. 2002;10:29–38.

33. Landis NT. Government finds fault with hospital quality review by joint commission and states. Am J Health Syst Pharm. 1999;56:1699–700.

34. Scanlon M. Computer physician order entry and the real world: we're only humans. Jt Comm J Qual Saf. 2004;30:342–6.

35. Pugliese G. In search of safety: an interview with Gina Pugliese. Interview by Alison P. Smith. Nurs Econ. 2002;20:6–12.

36. Cors WK. Physician executives must leap with the frog. Accountability for safety and quality ultimately lie with the doctors in charge. Physician Exec. 2001;27:14–6.

37. Foraida M, DeVita M, Braithwaite RS, Stuart S, Brooks MM, Simmons RL. Improving the utilization of medical crisis teams (Condition C) at an urban tertiary care hospital. J Crit Care. 2003;18:87–94.

38. Hourihan F, Bishop G, Hillman KM, Daffurn K, Lee A. The medical emergency team: a new strategy to identify and intervene in high-risk patients. Clin Intensive Care. 1995;6:269–72.

39. Lee KH, Angus DC, Abramson NS. Cardiopulmonary resuscitation: what cost to cheat death? Crit Care Med. 1996;24:2046–52.

40. Thomas K, VanOyen Force M, Rasmussen D, Dodd D, Whildin S. Rapid response team: challenges, solutions, benefits. Crit Care Nurse. 2007;27(1):20–7.

41. Bonafide CP, Localio AR, Song L, Roberts KE, Nadkarni VM, Priestley M, Paine CW, Zander M, Lutts M, Brady PW, Keren R. Cost-benefit analysis of a medical emergency team in a children's hospital. Pediatrics. 2014;134(2):235–41.

42. Dacey MJ, Mirza ER, Wilcox V, Doherty M, Mello J, Boyer A, Gates J, Brothers T, Baute R. The effect of a rapid response team on major clinical outcome measures in a community hospital. Crit Care Med. 2007;35(09):2076–82.

43. Jones D, Baldwin I, Mcintyre T, et al. Nurses' attitudes to a medical emergency team service in a teaching hospital. Qual Saf Health Care. 2006;15: 427–32.

44. Azzopardi P, Kinney S, Moulden A, Tibballs J. Attitudes and barriers to a Medical Emergency Team system at a tertiary paediatric hospital. Resuscitation. 2011;82(2):167–74.

45. Shearer B, Marshall S, Buist M, et al. What stops hospital clinical staff from following protocols? An analysis of the incidence and factors behind the failure of bedside clinical staff to activate the rapid response system I a multi-campus Australian healthcare service. BMJ Qual Saf. 2012;21:569–75.

46. Boniatti M, Azzolini N, Viana M, et al. Delayed medical emergency team calls and associated outcomes. Crit Care Med. 2014;42(1):26–30.

47. Trinkle RM, Flabouris A. Documenting rapid response system afferent limb failure and associated patient outcomes. Resuscitation. 2011;82(7):810–4.

48. Calzavacca P, Licari E, Tee A, et al. The impact of rapid response system on delayed emergency team activation patient characteristics and outcomes — a follow-up study. Resuscitation. 2010;81(1):31–5.

49. McQuillan P, Pilkington S, Alan A, et al. Confidential inquiry into quality of care before admission to intensive care. BMJ. 1998;316:1853–8.

50. Goldhill DR, White SA, Sumner A. Physiological values and procedures in the 24 hours before ICU admission from the ward. Anaesthesia. 1999;54:529–34.

51. Reason J. Combating omission errors through task analysis and good reminders. Qual Saf Health Care. 2002;11:40–4.

52. Davies O, DeVita MA, Ayinla R, Perez X. Barriers to activation of the rapid response system. Resuscitation. 2014;85(11):1557–61.

53. Hillman K, Alexandrou E, Flabouris M, et al. Clinical outcome indicators in acute hospital medicine. Clin Intensive Care. 2000;11:89–94.

54. Stevens J, Johansson A, Lennes I, Hsu D, Tess A, Howell M. Long-term culture change related to rapid response system implementation. Med Educ. 2014;48(12):1211–9.

Gary B. Smith, David R. Prytherch,
and Alex J. Psirides

Introduction

The afferent limb of a rapid response system (RRS) is responsible for monitoring the patient, detecting deterioration and triggering a response [1], i.e. three of the components of the 'Chain of Prevention' (Fig. 15.1) [2]. The provision of a fully functional, effective afferent limb seems simple, but failures in its individual components are common and frequently result in potentially avoidable, adverse clinical outcomes. Common failures include inadequate frequency of observations, incomplete observation sets, lack of knowl-edge of meaning of abnormal values and failure to call for assistance when required [3–36].

A UK 'National Confidential Enquiry into Patient Outcomes and Death' report found that the casenotes of 439 patients who died in an intensive care unit (ICU) after admission from general wards seldom contained written requests regarding the type and frequency of physiological observations to be measured [5]. Additionally, vital signs datasets were often incomplete. Pulse rate, blood pressure and temperature were the most frequently recorded variables; breathing rate the least [5]. Instructions regarding parameters that should trigger a patient review were rarely documented [5]. Similarly, in the Australian MERIT study, 81 % of patients without a documented 'Do Not Attempt Cardiopulmonary Resuscitation' order had an incomplete or absent record of heart rate, blood pressure and respiratory rate in the 15 min period before an unantici-pated cardiac arrest, unplanned ICU admission or an unexpected death [13]. Other studies show that the recording of physiological observations varies across different clinical areas [28] and through the day and night [27, 29]. The MERIT study also showed that a medical emergency team (MET) was only called in 41 % of cases where there were documented physiological MET criteria present >15 min before an unantici-pated cardiac arrest, unplanned ICU admission or an unexpected death [13]. Failure to call for assistance may be because of lack of recognition

G.B. Smith, BM, FRCP, FRCA (✉)
Faculty of Health and Social Sciences, Centre
of Postgraduate Medical Research and Education
(CoPMRE), University of Bournemouth,
Royal London House, Christchurch Road,
Bournemouth, Dorset BH1 3LT, UK
e-mail: gbsresearch@virginmedia.com

D.R. Prytherch, PhD, MIEPM, CSci
Centre for Healthcare Modelling and Informatics,
University of Portsmouth, Buckingham Building,
Lion Terrace, Portsmouth, Hampshire PO1 3HE, UK

A.J. Psirides
Department of Intensive Care Medicine, Wellington
Regional Hospital, Riddiford Street, Newtown,
Wellington, New Zealand

© Springer International Publishing Switzerland 2017
M.A. DeVita et al. (eds.), *Textbook of Rapid Response Systems*, DOI 10.1007/978-3-319-39391-9_15

Fig. 15.1 The Chain of Prevention [1] and the afferent limb of the Rapid Response System. Chain of Prevention [1] (copyright G B Smith)

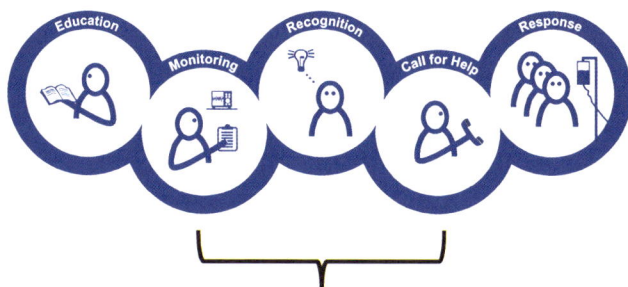

Afferent limb of the Rapid Response System

of patient deterioration, lack of knowledge of the escalation protocol, incorrect clinical judgement, lack of confidence in escalating or worry on the part of the caller that they might receive criticism [25, 26, 30–35].

Additionally, staff may not adequately inform each other regarding patients' care, particularly during handovers and transfers [6, 7, 36]. Andrews identified that quantifiable evidence is the most effective means of referring patients to doctors, and that using an early warning score (EWS), rather than reporting changes in individual vital signs, increases the chances of achieving good communication about a deteriorating patient [37].

The activation of RRTs shows a circadian pattern [38, 39], although this may merely reflect the time of patient admission [40]. Units with continuous monitoring of at least either pulse oximetry or electrocardiography have more activations than those without, but the pattern of activation is essentially identical [39].

Many of these problems, although well known, continue to occur. For example, in a recent report from the USA's Get With The Guidelines-Resuscitation registry of in-hospital cardiac arrests (IHCA), 55 % of patients having an IHCA had no documented vital signs recordings in the 4 h prior to the arrest. This was despite 65 % of patients being monitored at the time of the arrest; 43 % were also nursed in areas with telemetry [41].

Improving the Function of the Afferent Limb

Improving Regular Monitoring and Assessment

There should be a clear, documented vital signs measurement plan for each patient containing unambiguous instructions regarding the variables to be measured and the frequency of measurement [3, 42, 43]. This is most easily implemented by hospitals having an organisation-wide policy that emphasizes the minimum measurement plan for all patients. The plan should take account of the patient's diagnosis, co-morbidities, treatment plan and severity of illness, and should modify the frequency of measurement and level of care, accordingly [3, 42–45]. Whilst there is little research to guide the optimal frequency for monitoring vital signs [18, 19], it makes sense that it should adapt to changing clinical situations. In the UK, current recommendations suggest that the minimum frequency should be 12 hourly [42]; however, some attendees at a 2008 Consensus Conference preferred at least every 6 h [3] and others suggest every 2 h [45]. Whilst some advocate continuous monitoring, it is unknown whether continuous monitoring of all hospitalised patients is beneficial. However, the use of protocolised measurement (i.e. three times daily) of an EWS results in better detection of physiological abnormalities and more reliable activations of the RRT, compared with measurement on clinical indication [46].

Use of an EWS, the presence of an RRT, staff education, an observation protocol or the introduction of a new observation chart may all increase the frequency of vital signs measurements [16, 47–52]. However, electronic health records do not necessarily improve the documentation of vital signs [53]. Alterations to the monitoring frequency, especially reductions, should only be made by senior staff [3, 42].

Vital signs datasets should be complete every time, as physiological variables are inter-related, often by physiological compensatory mechanisms. When incomplete, physiological instability is often missed [29]. Current recommendations suggest that the dataset should include at least heart rate, breathing rate, systolic blood pressure, level of consciousness, S_pO_2 and temperature [3, 42, 44]. To give context to measurements of S_pO_2 the percentage oxygen concentration being delivered should also be recorded [43, 54].

Ensuring Vital Signs Measurements are Accurate

In the developed world, most vital signs are now measured by machine. It is obvious that these machines need to be properly calibrated and well maintained. Staff using them should have the appropriate training and should attain the necessary competence in monitoring, measurement and interpretation [55]. They should know the limits of accuracy and applicability of any machine that they use. Factors such as nail varnish influence the accuracy of pulse oximeters [56, 57]; the size of the blood pressure cuff in relation to the patient's arm influences the accuracy of BP measurements [58]. Measurements should be standardised— patients should be in the same position and, where a measurement is made in a particular limb, the same limb should always be used. Readings from automated oscillometric blood pressure monitors may differ markedly from those obtained with manual techniques if the patient has atrial fibrillation [59]. Breathing rate is generally not measured by machine outside of critical care areas, but rather by observation. There is considerable evidence that breathing rate is measured poorly and subject to poor inter-observer reliability [5, 10, 16, 20, 22, 23, 47, 60–65].

Ensuring Vital Signs Measurements are Accurately Recorded

Vital sign charts should allow the early recognition of patient deterioration. To do this, they must be immediately available, accurate, up to date and legible. These goals are often not met. It is common for many different versions of vital signs charts to exist within a single hospital. At least within a given institution, and perhaps within a whole health system, it would seem sensible to have a single format. There remains a requirement to define the optimal chart format, as their design can affect interpretation, the speed and accuracy of EWS calculations and the detection of deterioration [66–72]. If an EWS system is used, calculations and recording must also be accurate and legible.

Some hospitals have introduced colour-coded or colour-banded vital signs charts that are believed to assist in the recognition of patient deterioration [54, 66–69, 73, 74]. These use different colours to represent different levels of physiological abnormality linked to "track and trigger systems" (see below) or ghosted EWS values on the chart area to assist in calculations [73].

Systems for Identifying the Sick or Deteriorating Patient

In general, the clinical signs of acute illness are similar whatever the underlying process, as they usually reflect failing cardiovascular, respiratory and neurological systems. Abnormalities of vital signs are markers of impending critical events [1, 12, 15, 75–85]. Therefore, many hospitals now use a set of predetermined 'calling criteria' or 'track and trigger' systems, based upon vital signs, as indicators of the need to escalate monitoring or to call for more expert help (often in the form of an RRT).

The two most commonly used systems are the single-parameter track and trigger systems (SPTTS), more commonly known as MET criteria [86–91], and the aggregate weighted scoring systems (AWTTS), referred to as early warning scores (EWS) [86, 91–98]. The former predominate in the USA and Australia; the latter in the UK. MET criteria provide an all-or-nothing response (i.e. the calling of an RRT), whilst EWSs offer a graded escalation of care (Table 15.1).

MET Criteria

Lee first described MET criteria in 1995 [87]. Typically, they consist of specific physiological abnormalities (e.g. respiration rate <10 or >30/min and the non-specific criterion 'staff concern'). There is now a variety of different objective MET criteria in use, in which Lee's original calling criteria have been modified, often only subtly [13, 88–91]. The occurrence of at least one MET criterion indicates that the clinician should call for help, usually from an RRT. Typical MET calling criteria are shown in Table 15.2. The wide range of variables and trigger points extant in currently used METs underlines the arbitrary nature of the process by which they have been chosen, being based predominantly on expert clinical opinion and intuition. Most publications on the use of MET criteria do not report data about their sensitivity and specificity, as the studies contain no data regarding those patients who did not trigger an RRT response or had not developed a specific adverse outcome.

MET criteria are simple to teach and use but have the disadvantage that the objective components generally reflect extreme [13, 86–91, 99] vital sign values and so may detect deterioration late. Smith et al. compared the performance of 30 unique MET criteria, using a single, large vital signs dataset [90]. There was marked variation in sensitivity (7.3–52.8 %) and specificity (69.1–98.1 %) for mortality at hospital discharge. Choosing less extreme values generates additional workload due to additional false positives [99]. Cretikos et al. studied the impact of varying MET calling criteria and showed that all modifications provided positive predictive values of <16 %, indicating that ~84 % of resultant calls would be for patients who would not experience an adverse event [89]. They concluded that using these sets of activation criteria would result in a high proportion of false positive calls, and a substantial number of at-risk patients might remain unidentified [89].

Early Warning Scores (EWS)

It seems intuitive that combinations of abnormalities have greater predictive value than individual measures and that trends in values may contain further information; the reason for some hospitals

Table 15.1 The National Early Warning Score (NEWS)

Physiological parameters	3	2	1	0	1	2	3
Respiration rate (breaths per minute)	≤8		9–11	12–20		21–24	≥25
S$_p$O$_2$ %	≤91	92–93	94–95	≥96			
Any supplemental oxygen?		Yes		No			
Temperature (°C)	≤35.0		35.1–36.0	36.1–38.0	38.1–39.0	≥39.1	
Systolic BP (mmHg)	≤90	91–100	101–110	111–219			≥220
Heart/pulse rate (beats per minute)	≤40		41–50	51–90	91–110	111–130	≥131
Level of consciousness using the AVPU system				A			V, P or U

Level of consciousness: *A* alert; *V* responds to voice; *P* responds to pain; *U* unresponsive
Modified from National Early Warning Score (NEWS): Standardising the assessment of acute-illness severity in the NHS. Report of a working party. Royal College of Physicians, London, 2012 [54].

Table 15.2 Medical Emergency Team (MET) calling criteria (from Hillman et al. [13])

Airway
If threatened
Breathing
All respiratory arrests
Respiratory rate < 5 breaths per min
Respiratory rate > 36 breaths per min
Circulation
All cardiac arrests
Pulse rate < 40 beats per min
Pulse rate > 140 beats per min
Systolic blood pressure < 90 mmHg
Neurology
Sudden fall in level of consciousness (fall in GCS of >2 points)
Repeated or extended seizures
Other
Any patient you are seriously worried about that does not fit the above criteria

electing to use an EWS instead of MET criteria. EWSs allocate points in a weighted manner to reflect the derangement of physiology from predetermined 'normal' ranges [91–98]. The sum of the allocated points is used to direct care, e.g. to increase vital signs monitoring, involve more experienced staff or call an RRT [54, 86]. The constituent physiological variables typically include pulse rate, blood pressure, breathing rate and conscious level, but some also include other parameters. There is wide range of unique, but very similar, EWSs in clinical use [91–98], the majority differing only in minor variations in the weightings for physiological derangement and/or the cutoff points between physiological weighting bands. A typical EWS is shown in Table 15.1.

EWSs have the disadvantage of being relatively complex and requiring complete observations sets to allow calculation of a score. Obtaining the score involves looking up a weighting for each physiological parameter and summing the individual weighted scores; these tasks often introduce error [29, 100–104]. One study from Australia suggested that 86 % of calculations underestimated a computer-generated EWS value. Although EWS summation was usually correct, the assignment of EWS weightings was often inaccurate [102]. However, a single-centre UK study showed that errors of weighting and errors of summation featured equally, with the large majority of observation sets with errors showing both weight assignment and calculation mistakes [29]. Errors tend to increase with the degree of physiological abnormality [96, 101, 103]. Errors of calculation with EWS might be reduced if simplified binary EWSs, which can offer useful discrimination of a patient's risk of adverse outcomes, are used [105].

Of late, several groups have utilised large databases of vital signs to develop, or validate, a range of EWSs [97, 98, 106, 107] against a variety of clinical outcomes (death, cardiac arrest and unanticipated ICU admission) and time scales [108]. In EWSs, a high or rising score is considered premonitory of such adverse outcomes. A range of publications suggest that trends in EWS value add additional information [109–111]. Whilst some work has been done, further investigation is required to fully understand the relationship between EWS values, trends and adverse outcomes.

Efficiency of EWS and MET Criteria

The number of calls generated by any calling system has implications for resource utilisation. The aforementioned differences in performance of both EWSs and MET criteria lead to considerable differences in the number of calls generated by different systems. For example, for MET criteria, Smith et al demonstrated a 14-fold difference in the number of calls generated (i.e. workload) when applying 30 different published systems to the same physiological dataset [90]. The role of the EWS is to detect physiological derangement; the value to escalate care at is a decision for the institution [112]. The number of calls generated by a given EWS will depend upon the particular score chosen to trigger by any particular healthcare institution [112]. This allows the institution to fit its workload to its resource, something that cannot occur if the hospital uses a given set of MET criteria. EWS also appear to be better predictors of adverse outcomes than MET criteria [84, 113]. For EWSs, the relationship between workload (i.e. calls) and sensitivity is provided by the EWS efficiency curve [97].

Other Clinical Observations that May be Used to Trigger Rapid Response Systems

There are many other signs and symptoms that may be valid reasons to trigger an RRT that are not (usually) included in EWS or MET criteria, e.g. pallor, sweating, altered patient behaviour, prolonged capillary refill time, airway obstruction, uncontrolled bleeding, changes in functional capacity (e.g. a new inability to stand, loss of movement (or weakness) of face or limb, changes in speech or loss of ability to speak), reduced urine output and chest pain. While the use of physiologically based criteria is appealing as a method of identifying the need for increased monitoring and care, it is possible that a more subjective approach, based loosely on staff experience and expertise, may also be effective [114, 115]. MET criteria almost always contain the non-specific criterion 'staff concern' as a trigger for summoning help [13, 88, 90]. The National Early Warning Score (NEWS) documentation also makes it clear that '… concern about a patient's clinical condition should always override the …' score value [54]. This makes sense, even if staff are unable to identify the cause of their worry. Recent single-centre evidence suggests a reduction over time in the use of 'staff concern' as a trigger for calling an MET, compared to more physiologically based parameters [116].

In some hospitals, the patient's family and visitors are encouraged to form part of the calling process for RRTs as their intimate knowledge of the patient gives them a particular ability to recognise deterioration or subtle changes in the patient [117–120]. Family activation of the RRS is an important addition to an institution's ability to find all deteriorating patients as soon as possible.

Other clinical data have been used to estimate the risk of adverse clinical outcomes and so identify sick or deteriorating patients [121–124]. Recently Jarvis et al. published an EWS using solely clinical laboratory data [125]. Others have used various combinations of vital signs, clinical laboratory, clinical opinion and administrative data [126–132]. Such systems tend to be complex requiring the use of computers for their calculation. An important question when the detection system uses data such as biochemistry results is 'how long are the clinical laboratory data valid for?' as blood tests are usually taken far less frequently than vital signs. The results reported for these systems by their originators are superior to those for vital signs based EWSs [126–128, 130, 132] but external validation remains to be done.

The Need for Standardisation

It is common for many different versions of EWS/calling criteria to exist within a single hospital. However, it would seem sensible to use a single 'track and trigger' system within a given institution and perhaps across a whole health system, as both patients and staff move between wards and hospitals. To this end, the Royal College of Physicians of London advocates the use of NEWS across the UK National Health Service [54]. Wales has adopted NEWS nationwide. Ireland has adopted ViEWS (NEWS is a minor modification of ViEWS) as its national EWS [133]. Some authors have suggested adopting a different EWS for patients with chronic obstructive pulmonary disease [134, 135] or modifying MET trigger levels to take into account the clinical context [136].

Calling for Assistance

The failure of staff to follow protocols relating to care escalation is common [26, 27, 137]. Common reasons for failure to activate the RRS when the protocol demanded it include: staff feeling that the bedside clinical team were in control of the situation; a preference to call the covering doctor before the RRT; and poor communication and prioritisation [26, 30, 31, 35]. Other issues include nurses' fear of being reprimanded or criticised, lack of confidence, and misunderstanding of the purpose of the RRT and its activation criteria [32–34]. Several groups have shown that up to 57 % of patients with MET criteria have a delayed MET call of at least 30 m and that this is associated with higher incidence of hospital mortality, unanticipated ICU admission and morbidity, and longer hospital length of stay [138–143].

To ensure timely activation and an adequate response, there should be a universally known and understood, mandated, unambiguous, activation protocol. The culture of the organisation should be such that staff are never criticised for calling. Because of the need for speed and reliability, a pre-set calling system is preferred.

Hospitals should consider the use of standardised method of communication, such as RSVP, SBAR or ISBAR [144–146], as these may improve the communication of patient deterioration between staff. Whilst there is little evidence of the impact of using such systems in escalating care of deteriorating patients, one study has suggested improved patient outcomes following the use of SBAR [147].

The Role of Technology in Improving the Afferent Limb

Advances in technology may improve monitoring, recognition of deterioration and the triggering of an appropriate response. New monitoring sensors are being developed [148]. Existing vital signs monitoring techniques for general ward patients are being developed further, with improvements in wearability and patient mobility [149]. To date, there is insufficient data to recommend continuous monitoring for low-risk patients; however, logic would suggest that continuous monitoring would be required to identify every patient deterioration. The downside of continuous monitoring is alarm fatigue [150, 151].

The use of computerised point-of-care devices [43, 152–154] removes errors from the assignment of EWS weightings and their summation [100, 155] at worst being only vulnerable to only mistakes of transcription where the measurement devices do not enter the data automatically. There are also new methods of synthesising information from data [156].

The integration of computers with monitoring devices, communications devices, individual and population electronic repositories of clinical data (containing test results, symptoms, diagnoses, therapies, outcomes, etc.) offers the potential of greater assurance in both detecting deterioration and alerting responders. The computer could detect even subtle signs or trends sufficiently early to avert critical illness, contacting the responder without the involvement of the local carer [157–159]. It would be able to integrate and analyse more data than any one human, no matter how skilled or experienced, escalate care directly and suggest appropriate interventions to the responding team.

Most published research into technological solutions to improve the recognition of, and response to, patient deterioration are limited to small-scale implementations, studies in specific patient groups (e.g. patients receiving RRT calls) or focuses on process measures [148, 153, 154, 159–169]. However, one study has shown an association between the implementation of a computerised vital sign surveillance system and a significant reduction in hospital mortality in two hospitals across all major adult specialties [152].

Summary

A properly functioning afferent limb is essential to the workings of an effective Rapid Response System. However, considerable deficiencies exist in the three components of the afferent limb—the monitoring of patients, the detection of patient deterioration and the triggering of the efferent limb. Considerable improvements in the function of the afferent limb could be achieved by simple, obvious interventions such as regular, complete monitoring and assessment of patients and a monitoring plan for each patient. Organisations should consider the use of 'track and trigger' systems to assist in the detection of patient deterioration and the use of a standardised method of communicating patient illness between staff. Technology is also likely to provide solutions to improving the function of the afferent limb.

References

1. DeVita MA, Bellomo R, Hillman K, et al. Findings of the first consensus conference on medical emergency teams. Crit Care Med. 2006;34:2463–78.

2. Smith GB. In-hospital cardiac arrest: is it time for an in-hospital 'chain of prevention'? Resuscitation. 2010;81:1209–11.

3. DeVita MA, Smith GB, Adams SK, et al. "Identifying the hospitalised patient in crisis"—a consensus conference on the afferent limb of rapid response systems. Resuscitation. 2010;81:375–82.

4. McQuillan PJ, Pilkington S, Allan A, et al. Confidential inquiry into quality of care before admission to intensive care. BMJ. 1998;316:1853–8.

5. National Confidential Enquiry into Patient Outcomes and Death. An acute problem? London: National Confidential Enquiry into Patient Outcome and Death; 2005.

6. National Patient Safety Agency. Safer care for the acutely ill patient: learning from serious incidents. London: NPSA; 2007.

7. National Patient Safety Agency. Recognising and responding appropriately to early signs of deterioration in hospitalised patients. London: NPSA; 2007.

8. Chellel A, Fraser J, Fender V, et al. Nursing observations on ward patients at risk of critical illness. Nurs Times. 2002;98:36–9.

9. Smith S, Fraser J, Plowright C, et al. Nursing observations on ward patients—results of a five-year audit. Nurs Times. 2008;104:28–9.

10. Wheatley I. The nursing practice of taking level 1 patient observations. Intensive Crit Care Nurs. 2006;22:115–21.

11. Fuhrmann L, Lippert A, Perner A, Ostergaard D. Incidence, staff awareness and mortality of patients at risk on general wards. Resuscitation. 2008;77:325–30.

12. Hillman KM, Bristow PJ, Chey T, et al. Duration of life-threatening antecedents prior to intensive care admission. Intensive Care Med. 2002;28:1629–34.

13. Hillman K, Chen J, Cretikos M, et al. Introduction of the medical emergency team (MET) system: a cluster-randomised controlled trial. Lancet. 2005;365:2091–7.

14. Harrison GA, Jacques TC, Kilborn G, McLaws ML. The prevalence of recordings of the signs of critical conditions and emergency responses in hospital wards—the SOCCER study. Resuscitation. 2005;65:149–57.

15. Kause J, Smith G, Prytherch D, Parr M, Flabouris A, Hillman K. A comparison of antecedents to cardiac arrests, deaths and emergency intensive care admissions in Australia and New Zealand, and the United Kingdom—The ACADEMIA study. Resuscitation. 2004;62:275–82.

16. McBride J, Knight D, Piper J, Smith G. Long-term effect of introducing an early warning score on respiratory rate charting on general wards. Resuscitation. 2005;65:41–4.

17. Nurmi J, Harjola VP, Nolan J, Castrén M. Observations and warning signs prior to cardiac arrest. Should a medical emergency team intervene earlier? Acta Anaesthesiol Scand. 2005;49:702–6.

18. Zeitz K, McCutcheon H. Observations and vital signs: ritual or vital for the monitoring of postoperative patients? Appl Nurs Res. 2006;19:204–11.

19. Lockwood C, Conroy-Hiller T, Page T. Vital signs. JBI Libr Syst Rev. 2004;2:207–30.

20. Hogan J. Why don't nurses monitor the respiratory rates of patients? Br J Nurs. 2006;15:489–92.

21. Bristow PJ, Hillman KM, Chey T, et al. Rates of in-hospital arrests, deaths and intensive care admissions: the effect of a medical emergency team. Med J Aust. 2000;173:236–40.

22. Kenward G, Hodgetts T, Castle N. Time to put the R back in TPR. Nurs Times. 2001;97:32–3.

23. Subbe CP, Williams EM, Gemmell LW. Are medical emergency teams picking up enough patients with increased respiratory rate? Crit Care Med. 2004;32:1983–4.

24. Armstrong B, Walthall H, Clancy M, Mullee M, Simpson H. Recording of vital signs in a district general hospital emergency department. Emerg Med J. 2008;25:799–802.

25. Buist M. The rapid response team paradox: why doesn't anyone call for help? Crit Care Med. 2008;36:634–5.

26. Shearer B, Marshal S, Buist MD, et al. What stops hospital clinical staff from following protocols? An analysis of the incidence and factors behind the failure of bedside clinical staff to activate the rapid response system in a multi-campus Australian metropolitan healthcare service. BMJ Qual Saf. 2012;21:569–75.

27. Hands C, Reid E, Meredith P, et al. Patterns in the recording of vital signs and early warning scores: compliance with a clinical escalation protocol. BMJ Qual Saf. 2013;22:719–26.

28. Considine J, Trotter C, Currey J. Nurses' documentation of physiological observations in three acute care settings. J Clin Nurs. 2016;25:134–43. doi:10.1111/jocn.13010.

29. Clifton DA, Clifton L, Sandu D-M, et al. 'Errors' and omissions in paper based early warning scores: the association with changes in vital signs—a database analysis. BMJ Open. 2015;5:e007376.

30. Radeschi G, Urso F, Campagna S, et al. Factors affecting attitudes and barriers to a medical emergency team among nurses and medical doctors: a multi-centre survey. Resuscitation. 2015;88:92–8.

31. Jones D, Baldwin I, McIntrye T, et al. Nurses' attitudes to a medical emergency team service in a teaching hospital. Qual Saf Health Care. 2006;15:427–32.

32. Massey D, Chaboyer W, Aitken L. Nurses' perceptions of accessing a Medical Emergency Team: a qualitative study. Aust Crit Care. 2014;27:133–8.

33. Davies O, DeVita MA, Ayinla R, Perez X. Barriers to activation of the rapid response system. Resuscitation. 2014;85:1557–61.

34. Cioffi J. Nurses' experiences of making decisions to call emergency assistance to their patients. J Adv Nurs. 2000;32:108–14.

35. Bagshaw SM, Mondor EE, Scouten C, et al. A survey of nurses' beliefs about the Medical Emergency Team system in a Canadian tertiary hospital. Am J Crit Care. 2010;19:74–83.

36. Day BA. Early warning system scores and response times: an audit. Nurs Crit Care. 2003;8:156–64.

37. Andrews T, Waterman H. Packaging: a grounded theory of how to report physiological deterioration effectively. J Adv Nurs. 2005;52:473–81.

38. Jones D, Bates S, Warrillow S. Circadian pattern of activation of the medical emergency team in a teaching hospital. Crit Care. 2005;9:R303–6.

39. Galhotra S, DeVita MA, Simmons RL, Schmid A, et al. Impact of patient monitoring on the diurnal pattern of medical emergency team activation. Crit Care Med. 2006;34:1700–6.

40. Hravnak M, Chen L, Dubrawski A, et al. Temporal distribution of instability events in continuously monitored step-down unit patients: implications for Rapid Response Systems. Resuscitation. 2015;89:99–105.

41. Andersen LW, Kim WY, Chase M, et al. The prevalence and significance of abnormal vital signs prior to in-hospital cardiac arrest. Resuscitation. 2015;98: 112–7. doi:10.1016/j.resuscitation.2015.08.016. pii: S0300-9572(15)00389-5.

42. National Institute for Health and Clinical Excellence. NICE clinical guideline 50 acutely ill patients in hospital: recognition of and response to acute illness in adults in hospital. London: National Institute for Health and Clinical Excellence; 2007.

43. Smith GB, Prytherch DR, Schmidt P, et al. Hospital-wide physiological surveillance—a new approach to the early identification and management of the sick patient. Resuscitation. 2006;71:19–29.

44. Australian Commission on Safety and Quality in Health Care. National consensus statement: essential elements for recognizing and responding to clinical deterioration. Sydney: ACSQHC; 2010.

45. Schulman C, Staul L. Standards for frequency of measurement and documentation of vital signs and physical assessments. Crit Care Nurse. 2010;30:74–6.

46. Ludikhuize J, Borgert M, Binnekade J, Subbe C, Dongelmans D, Goossens A. Standardized measurement of the Modified Early Warning Score results in enhanced implementation of a Rapid Response System: a quasi-experimental study. Resuscitation. 2014;85:676–82.

47. Odell M, Rechner IJ, Kapila A, et al. The effect of a critical care outreach service and an early warning scoring system on respiratory rate recording on the general wards. Resuscitation. 2007;74:470–5.

48. Chen J, Bellomo R, Flabouris A, Hillman K, Finfer S. The impact of introducing medical emergency team system on the documentations of vital signs. Resuscitation. 2009;80:35–43.

49. Cahill H, Jones A, Herkes R, et al. Introduction of a new observation chart and education programme is associated with higher rates of vital sign ascertainment in hospital wards. BMJ Qual Saf. 2011; 20:791–6.

50. Hammond NE, Spooner AJ, Barnett AG, Corley A, Brown P, Fraser JF. The effect of implementing a modified early warning scoring (MEWS) system on the adequacy of vital sign documentation. Aust Crit Care. 2013;26:18–22.

51. De Meester K, Das T, Hellemans K, Verbrugghe W, Jorens PG, Verpooten GA, Van Bogaert P. Impact of a standardized nurse observation protocol including MEWS after Intensive Care Unit discharge. Resuscitation. 2013;84:184–8.

52. Bunkenborg G, Poulsen I, Samuelson K, Ladelund S, Åkeson J. Mandatory early warning scoring—implementation evaluated with a mixed methods approach. Appl Nurs Res. 2016;29:168–176. doi:10.1016/j. apnr.2015.06.012.

53. Stevenson JE, Israelsson J, Nilsson GC, Petersson GI, Bath PA. Recording signs of deterioration in acute patients: the documentation of vital signs within electronic health records in patients who suffered in-hospital cardiac arrest. Health Informatics J. 2016;22:21–33.

54. Royal College of Physicians London. National Early Warning Score (NEWS): standardising the assessment of acute-illness severity in the NHS. Report of a working party. 2012.

55. Department of Health. Competencies for recognising and responding to acutely ill patients in hospital. Clinical Guideline CG50. National Institute for Health and Care Excellence. London; 2009.

56. Kruger PS, Longden PJ. A study of a hospital staff's knowledge of pulse oximetry. Anaesth Intensive Care. 1997;25:38–41.

57. Stoneham MD, Saville GM, Wilson IH. Knowledge about pulse oximetry among medical and nursing staff. Lancet. 1994;344:1339–42.

58. Beevers G, Lip GYH, O'Brien E. Blood pressure measurement. Part II—conventional sphygmomanometry: technique of auscultatory blood pressure measurement. BMJ. 2001;322:1043–7.

59. Lamb T, Thakrar A, Ghosh M, et al. Comparison of two oscillometric blood pressure monitors in subjects with atrial fibrillation. Clin Invest Med. 2010;33:E54–62.

60. Edwards SM, Murdin L. Respiratory rate—an under-documented clinical assessment. Clin Med. 2001;1:85.

61. Helliwell VC, Hadfield JH, Gould T. Documentation of respiratory rate for acutely sick inpatients—an observational study. Intensive Care Med. 2002;28:S21.

62. Cretikos MA, Bellomo R, Hillman K, Chen J, Finfer S, Flabouris A. Respiratory rate: the neglected vital sign. Med J Aust. 2008;188:657–9.

63. Hudson A. Prevention of in hospital cardiac arrests—first steps in improving patient care. Resuscitation. 2004;60:113–5.

64. Lim WS, Carty SM, et al. Respiratory rate measurement in adults—how reliable is it? Respir Med. 2002;96:31–3.

65. Kellett J, Li M, Rasool S, Green GC, Seely A. Comparison of the heart and breathing rate of acutely ill medical patients recorded by nursing staff with those measured over 5 minutes by a piezoelectric belt and ECG monitor at the time of admission to hospital. Resuscitation. 2011;82:1381–6.

66. Preece MHW, Hill A, Horswill MS, Watson MO. Supporting the detection of patient deterioration: observation chart design affects the recognition of abnormal vital signs. Resuscitation. 2012;83:1111–8.

67. Preece MHW, Hill A, Horswill MS, Karamatic R, Hewett DG, Watson MO. Applying heuristic evaluation to observation chart design to improve the detection of patient deterioration. Appl Ergon. 2013;44:544–56.

68. Christofidis MJ, Hill A, Horswill MS, Watson MO. Observation charts with overlapping blood pressure and heart rate graphs do not yield the performance advantage that health professionals assume: an experimental study. J Adv Nurs. 2014;70:610–24.

69. Christofidis MJ, Hill A, Horswill MS, Watson MO. A human factors approach to observation chart design can trump health professionals' prior chart experience. Resuscitation. 2013;84:657–65.

70. Chatterjee MT, Moon JC, Murphy R, McCrea D. The "OBS" chart: an evidence based approach to re-design of the patient observation chart in a district general hospital setting. Postgrad Med J. 2005;81:663–6.

71. Christofidis MJ, Hill A, Horswill MS, Watson MO. Observation chart design features affect the detection of patient deterioration: a systematic experimental evaluation. J Adv Nurs. 2016;72:158–172. doi:10.1111/jan.12824.

72. Christofidis MJ, Hill A, Horswill MS, Watson MO. Less is more: the design of early-warning scoring systems affects the speed and accuracy of scoring. J Adv Nurs. 2015;71:1573–86.

73. Oakey RJ, Slade V. Physiological observation track and trigger system. Nurs Stand. 2006;20:48–54.

74. Patient safety first "how to guide' for reducing harm from deterioration. www.patientsafetyfirst.nhs.uk.

75. Buist M, Bernard S, Nguyen TV, Moore G, Anderson J. Association between clinically abnormal observations and subsequent in-hospital mortality: a prospective study. Resuscitation. 2004;62:137–41.

76. Lighthall GK, Markar S, Hsuing R. Abnormal vital signs are associated with an increased risk of critical events in US veteran inpatients. Resuscitation. 2009;80:1264–9.

77. Buist MD, Jarmolowski E, Burton PR, Bernard SA, Waxman BP, Anderson J. Recognising clinical instability in hospital patients before cardiac arrest or unplanned admission to intensive care. A pilot study in a tertiary-care hospital. Med J Aust. 1999;171:22–5.

78. Hillman KM, Bristow PJ, Chey T, et al. Antecedents to hospital deaths. Intern Med J. 2001;31:343–8.

79. Goldhill DR, McNarry AF. Physiological abnormalities in early warning scores are related to mortality in adult inpatients. Br J Anaesth. 2004;92:882–4.

80. Jacques T, Harrison GA, McLaws M-L, Kilborn G. Signs of critical conditions and emergency responses (SOCCER): a model for predicting adverse events in the inpatient setting. Resuscitation. 2006;69:175–83.

81. Hodgetts TJ, Kenward G, Vlachonikolis IG, Payne S, Castle N. The identification of risk factors for cardiac arrest and formulation of activation criteria to alert a medical emergency team. Resuscitation. 2002;54:125–31.

82. Fagan K, Sabel A, Mehler PS, MacKenzie TD. Vital sign abnormalities, rapid response, and adverse outcomes in hospitalized patients. Am J Med Qual. 2012;27:480–6.

83. Bleyer AJ, Vidya S, Russell G, et al. Longitudinal analysis of one million vital signs in patients in an academic medical center. Resuscitation. 2011;82:1387–92.

84. Churpek MM, Yuen TC, Edelson DP. Risk stratification of hospitalized patients on the wards. Chest. 2013;143:1758–65.

85. Smith GB, Prytherch DR, Schmidt P, Featherstone PI, Kellett J, Deane B, Higgins B. Should age be included as a component of track and trigger systems used to identify sick adult patients? Resuscitation. 2008;78:109–15.

86. Department of Health and NHS Modernisation Agency. The National Outreach Report. Department of Health, London; 2003.

87. Lee A, Bishop G, Hillman KM, Daffurn K. The Medical Emergency Team. Anaesth Intensive Care. 1995;23:183–6.

88. Hourihan F, Bishop G, Hillman K, Daffurn K, Lee A, et al. The Medical Emergency Team: a new strategy to identify and intervene in high-risk patients. Clin Intensive Care. 1995;6:269–72.

89. Cretikos J, Chen K, Hillman R, Bellomo S, Finfer A, Flabouris and the MERIT study investigators. The objective medical emergency team activation criteria: a case-control study. Resuscitation. 2007;73:62–72.

90. Smith GB, Prytherch DR, Schmidt PE, Featherstone PI, Higgins B. A review, and performance evaluation, of single-parameter "track and trigger" systems. Resuscitation. 2008;79:11–21.

91. Gao H, McDonnell A, Harrison DA, et al. Systematic review and evaluation of physiological track and trigger warning systems for identifying at-risk patients on the ward. Intensive Care Med. 2007;33:667–79.

92. Morgan R, Williams F, Wright M. An Early Warning Scoring System for detecting developing critical illness. Clin Intensive Care. 1997;8:100.

93. Duckitt RW, Buxton-Thomas R, Walker J, et al. Worthing physiological scoring system: derivation and validation of a physiological early-warning system for medical admissions. An observational,

population-based single-centre study. Br J Anaesth. 2007;98:769–74.

94. Goldhill DR, McNarry AF, Mandersloot G, McGinley A. A physiologically-based early warning score for ward patients: the association between score and outcome. Anaesthesia. 2005;60:547–53.

95. Smith GB, Prytherch DR, Schmidt PE, Featherstone PI. A review, and performance evaluation, of aggregate weighted "track and trigger" systems. Resuscitation. 2008;77:170–9.

96. Subbe CP, Kruger M, Rutherford P, Gemmel L. Validation of a modified Early Warning Score in medical admissions. QJM. 2001;94:521–6.

97. Prytherch D, Smith GB, Schmidt PE, Featherstone PI. ViEWS—towards a National Early Warning Score for detecting adult inpatient deterioration. Resuscitation. 2010;81:932–7.

98. Smith GB, Prytherch DR, Meredith P, Schmidt PE, Featherstone PI. The ability of the National Early Warning Score (NEWS) to discriminate patients at risk of early cardiac arrest, unanticipated intensive care unit admission, and death. Resuscitation. 2013;84:465–70.

99. Bell MB, Konrad D, Granath F, et al. Prevalence and sensitivity of MET-criteria in a Scandinavian University Hospital. Resuscitation. 2006;70:66–73.

100. Mohammed MA, Hayton R, Clements G, Smith G, Prytherch D. Improving accuracy and efficiency of early warning scores in acute care. Br J Nurs. 2009;18:18–24.

101. Smith AF, Oakey RJ. Incidence and significance of errors in a patient 'track and trigger' system during an epidemic of Legionnaires' disease: retrospective casenote analysis. Anaesthesia. 2006;61:222–8.

102. Edwards M, McKay H, Van Leuvan C, et al. Modified Early Warning Scores: inaccurate summation or inaccurate assignment of score? Crit Care. 2010;14:S88.

103. Kolic I, Crane S, McCartney S, Perkins Z, Taylor A. Factors affecting response to National Early Warning Score (NEWS). Resuscitation. 2015;90:85–90.

104. Subbe CP, Gao H, Harrison DA. Reproducibility of physiological track-and-trigger warning systems for identifying at-risk patients on the ward. Intensive Care Med. 2007;33:619–24.

105. Jarvis SW, Kovacs C, Briggs JS, et al. Can binary early warning scores perform as well as standard early warning scores for discriminating a patient's risk of cardiac arrest, death or unanticipated intensive care unit admission? Resuscitation. 2015;93:46–52.

106. Churpek MM, Yuen TC, Park SY, Meltzer DO, Hall JB, Edelson DP. Derivation of a cardiac arrest prediction model using ward vital signs. Crit Care Med. 2012;40:2102–8.

107. Tarassenko L, Clifton D, Pinsky M, et al. Centile-based early warning scores derived from statistical distributions of vital signs. Resuscitation. 2011;82:1013–8.

108. Smith MEB, Chiovaro J, O'Neil M, et al. Early warning system scores for clinical deterioration in hospitalized patients: a systematic review. Ann Am Thorac Soc. 2014;11:1454–65.

109. Kellett J, Emmanuael A, Deane B. Who will be sicker in the morning? Changes in the Simple Clinical Score the day after admission and the subsequent outcomes of acutely ill unselected medical patients. Eur J Intern Med. 2011;22:375–81.

110. Kellett J, Wang F, Woodworth S, Huang W. Changes and their prognostic implications in the abbreviated VitalPAC™ Early Warning Score (ViEWS) after admission to hospital of 18,827 surgical patients. Resuscitation. 2013;84:471–6.

111. Kellett J, Woodworth S, Wang F, Huang W. Changes and their prognostic implications in the abbreviated VitalPAC™ early warning score (ViEWS) after admission to hospital of 18,853 acutely ill medical patients. Resuscitation. 2013;84:13–20.

112. Smith GB, Prytherch DR, Schmidt PE, Meredith P. Early warning scores: unravelling detection and escalation. Int J Health Care Qual Assur. 2015;28:872–5.

113. Tirkkonen J, Olkkola KT, Huhtala H, et al. Medical emergency team activation: performance of conventional dichotomised criteria versus National Early Warning Score. Acta Anaesthesiol Scand. 2014;58:411–9.

114. Santiano N, Young L, Hillman K, et al. Analysis of medical emergency team calls comparing subjective to "objective" call criteria. Resuscitation. 2009;80:44–9.

115. Chen J, Bellomo R, Hillman K, et al. Triggers for emergency team activation: a multicenter assessment. J Crit Care. 2010;25:359.e1–7.

116. Herod R, Frost SA, Parr M, Hillman K, Aneman A. Long term trends in medical emergency team activations and outcomes. Resuscitation. 2014;85:1083–7.

117. http://www.ihi.org/IHI/Topics/CriticalCare/IntensiveCare/ Tools/ConditionHBrochureforPatientsandFamilies. htmAccessed 24/05.09.

118. Ray EM, Smith R, Massie S, et al. Family alert: implementing direct family activation of a pediatric rapid response team. Jt Comm J Qual Patient Saf. 2009;35:575–80.

119. Odell M, Gerber K, Gager M. Call 4 concern: patient and relative activated critical care outreach. Br J Nurs. 2010;19:1390–5.

120. Vorwerk J, King L. Consumer participation in early detection of the deteriorating patient and call activation to rapid response systems: a literature review. J Clin Nurs. 2016;1-2:38–52 doi:10.1111/jocn.12977.

121. Prytherch D, Sirl J, Schmidt P, Featherstone P, Weaver PC, Smith GB. The use of routine laboratory data to predict in-hospital death in medical admission. Resuscitation. 2005;66:203–7.

122. O'Sullivan E, Callely E, O'Riordan D, Bennett K, Silke B. Predicting outcomes in emergency medical admissions—role of laboratory data and comorbidity. Acute Med. 2012;11:59–65.

123. Loekito E, Bailey J, Bellomo R, et al. Common laboratory tests predict imminent medical emergency

team calls, intensive care unit admission or death in emergency department patients. Emerg Med Australia. 2013;25(2):132–9.

124. Loekito E, Bailey J, Bellomo R, et al. Common laboratory tests predict imminent death in ward patients. Resuscitation. 2013;84:280–5.

125. Jarvis SW, Kovacs C, Badriyah T, et al. Development and validation of a decision-tree early warning score based on routine laboratory result tests for the discrimination of hospital mortality. Resuscitation. 2013;84:1494–9.

126. Rothman MJ, Rothman SI, Beals J. Development and validation of a continuous measure of patient condition using the Electronic Medical Record. J Biomed Inform. 2013;46:837–48.

127. Churpek MM, Yuen TC, Park SY, Gibbons R, Edelson DP. Using electronic health record data to develop and validate a prediction model for adverse outcomes in the wards. Crit Care Med. 2014;42:841–8.

128. Churpek MM, Yuen TC, Winslow C, Robicsek AA, Meltzer DO, Gibbons RD, Edelson DP. Multicenter development and validation of a risk stratification tool for ward patients. Am J Respir Crit Care Med. 2014;190:649–55.

129. Mohammed MA, Rudge G, Watson D, et al. Index blood tests and National Early Warning Scores within 24 hours of emergency admission can predict the risk of in-hospital mortality: a model development and validation study. PLoS One. 2013;8:e64340.

130. Jo S, Lee JB, Jin YH, et al. Modified early warning score with rapid lactate level in critically ill medical patients: the ViEWS-L score. Emerg Med J. 2013;30:123–9.

131. Escobar GJ, LaGuardia JC, Turk BJ, Ragins A, Kipnis P, Draper D. Early detection of impending physiologic deterioration among patients who are not in intensive care: development of predictive models using data from an automated electronic medical record. J Hosp Med. 2012;7:388–95.

132. Alvarez CA, Clark CA, Song Z, et al. Predicting out of intensive care unit cardiopulmonary arrest or death using electronic medical record data. BMC Med Inform Decis Mak. 2013;13:28.

133. National Clinical Effectiveness Committee. National Early Warning Score. National Clinical Guideline No. 1. Department of Health, Dublin, Ireland; 2013.

134. Eccles SR, Subbe C, Hancock D, Thomson N. CREWS: improving specificity whilst maintaining sensitivity of the National Early Warning Score in patients with chronic hypoxaemia. Resuscitation. 2014;85:109–11.

135. O'Driscoll BR, Murphy P, Turkington PM. Acute monitoring of patients with chronic respiratory disease during hospital admission. Clin Med. 2012;12:79–81.

136. Davis T, Nogajski B. Alterations to calling criteria for Between the Flags (an early warning system). BMJ Qual Improv Rep. 2015;4. doi:10.1136/bmjquality.u206561.w2638.

137. Petersen JA, Mackel R, Antonsen K, Rasmussen LS. Serious adverse events in a hospital using early warning score—what went wrong? Resuscitation. 2014;85:1699–703.

138. Tirkkonen J, Ylä-Mattila J, Olkkola KT, Huhtala H, Tenhunen J, Hoppu S. Factors associated with delayed activation of medical emergency team and excess mortality: an Utstein-style analysis. Resuscitation. 2013;84:173–8.

139. Downey AW, Quach JL, Haase M, Haase-Fielitz A, Jones D, Bellomo R. Characteristics and outcomes of patients receiving a medical emergency team review for acute change in conscious state or arrhythmias. Crit Care Med. 2008;36:477–81.

140. Quach JL, Downey AW, Haase M, Haase-Fielitz A, Jones D, Bellomo R. Characteristics and outcomes of patients receiving a medical emergency team review for respiratory distress or hypotension. J Crit Care. 2008;23:325–31.

141. Calzavacca P, Licari E, Tee A, et al. The impact of Rapid Response System on delayed emergency team activation patient characteristics and outcomes—a follow-up study. Resuscitation. 2010;81:31–5.

142. Chen J, Bellomo R, Flabouris A, Hillman K, Assareh H, Ou L. Delayed emergency team calls and associated hospital mortality: a multicenter study. Crit Care Med. 2015;43:2059–65.

143. Barwise A, Thongprayoon C, Gajic O, Jensen J, Herasevich V, Pickering BW. Delayed rapid response team activation is associated with increased hospital mortality, morbidity, and length of stay in a tertiary care institution. Crit Care Med. 2016;44:54–63.

144. Featherstone P, Chalmers T, Smith GB. RSVP: a system for communication of deterioration in hospital patients. Br J Nurs. 2008;17:860–4.

145. Thomas CM, Bertram E, Johnson D. The SBAR communication technique: teaching nursing students professional communication skills. Nurse Educ. 2009;34:176–80.

146. Porteous JM, Stewart-Wynne EG, Connolly M, Crommelin PF. iSoBAR—a concept and handover checklist: the National Clinical Handover Initiative. Med J Aust. 2009;190:S152–6.

147. De Meester K, Verspuy M, Monsieurs KG, Van Bogaert P. SBAR improves nurse-physician communication and reduces unexpected death: a pre and post intervention study. Resuscitation. 2013;84:1192–6.

148. Brown H, Terrence J, Vasquez P, et al. Continuous monitoring in an inpatient medical-surgical unit: a controlled clinical trial. Am J Med. 2014;127:226–32.

149. Nangalia V, Prytherch DR, Smith GB. Health technology assessment review: remote monitoring of vital signs—current status and future challenges. Crit Care. 2010;14:233.

150. Gazarian PK. Nurses' response to frequency and types of electrocardiography alarms in a non-critical care setting: a descriptive study. Int J Nurs Stud. 2014;51:190–7.

151. Sendelbach S, Funk M. Alarm fatigue. A patient safety concern. AACN Adv Crit Care. 2013;24: 378–86.

152. Schmidt PE, Meredith P, Prytherch DR, et al. Impact of introducing an electronic physiological surveillance system on hospital mortality. BMJ Qual Saf. 2015;24:10–20.

153. Jones S, Mullaly M, Ingleby S, et al. Bedside electronic capture of clinical observations and automated clinical alerts to improve compliance with an Early Warning Score protocol. Crit Care Resusc. 2011;13:83–8.

154. Bannard-Smith J, Abbas S, Ingleby S, Fullwood C, Jones S, Eddleston J. Use of an electronic early warning score and mortality for patients admitted out of hours to a large teaching hospital. Crit Care. 2015;19:P408.

155. Prytherch DR, Smith GB, Schmidt P, Featherstone PI, Stewart K, Knight D, Higgins B. Calculating early warning scores—a classroom comparison of pen and paper and hand-held computer methods. Resuscitation. 2006;70:173–8.

156. Tarassenko L, Hann A, Young D. Integrated monitoring and analysis for early warning of patient deterioration. Br J Anaesth. 2006;97:64–8.

157. Evans RS, Kuttler KG, Simpson KJ, et al. Automated detection of physiologic deterioration in hospitalized patients. J Am Med Inform Assoc. 2015;22:350–60.

158. Whittington J, White R, Haig KM, Slock M. Using an automated risk assessment report to identify patients at risk for clinical deterioration. Jt Comm J Qual Patient Saf. 2007;33:569–74.

159. Huh JW, Lim C-M, Koh Y, et al. Activation of a medical emergency team using an electronic medical recording-based screening system. Crit Care Med. 2014;42:801–8.

160. Watkinson PJ, Barber VS, Price JD, et al. A randomized controlled trial of the effect of continuous electronic physiological monitoring on the adverse event rate in high risk medical and surgical patients. Anaesthesia. 2006;61:1031–9.

161. Hravnak M, Edwards L, Clontz A, et al. Defining the incidence of cardiorespiratory instability in patients instep-down units using an electronic integrated monitoring system. Arch Intern Med. 2008;168:1300–8.

162. Hravnak M, DeVita MA, Clontz A, et al. Cardiorespiratory instability before and after implementing an integrated monitoring system. Crit Care Med. 2011;39:65–72.

163. Taenzer AH, Pyke JB, McGrath SP, et al. Impact of pulse oximetry surveillance on rescue events and intensive care unit transfers: a before-and-after concurrence study. Anesthesiology. 2010;112:282–7.

164. Bellomo R, Ackerman M, Bailey M, et al. Vital signs to identify, target, and assess level of care study (VITAL Care Study) investigators. A controlled trial of electronic automated advisory vital signs monitoring in general hospital wards. Crit Care Med. 2012;40:2349–61.

165. Smith LB, Banner L, Lozano D, et al. Connected care: reducing errors through automated vital signs data upload. Comput Inform Nurs. 2009;27:318–23.

166. Gearing P, Olney CM, Davis K, et al. Enhancing patient safety through electronic medical record documentation of vital signs. J Healthc Inf Manag. 2006;20:40–5.

167. Meccariello M, Perkins D, Quigley LG, et al. Vital time savings. Evaluating the use of an automated vital signs documentation system on a medical/surgical unit. J Healthc Inf Manag. 2010;24:46–51.

168. Fieler VK, Jaglowski T, Richards K. Eliminating errors in vital signs documentation. Comput Inform Nurs. 2013;31:422–7.

169. Nwulu U, Westwood D, Edwards D, Kelliher F, Coleman JJ. Adoption of an electronic observation chart with an integrated early warning scoring system on pilot wards. A descriptive report. Comput Inform Nurs. 2012;30:371–9.

The Impact of Delayed Rapid Response System Activation

16

Daryl A. Jones, Christian Subbe, and Rinaldo Bellomo

Background—Principles of the Rapid Response System

Modern hospitals service patients of increasing complexity and co-morbidity [1]. Despite advances in technology and the best efforts of hospital staff, several studies have demonstrated that 6–17% of all hospital admissions are complicated by serious adverse events [2, 3, 4, 5–7]. These events are often unrelated to the patient's underlying medical condition and in approximately 10% of cases result in permanent disability and even death [7].

Other studies have shown that these events are not sudden or unpredictable. Instead, they are often preceded by signs of physiological instability that manifest as derangements in commonly measured vital signs [8–11, 12]. Most importantly, in many cases, the rate of deterioration is relatively slow, and occurs over 12–24 h [9].

One of the most important tenets underlying the Rapid Response System (RRS) concept is that early intervention in the course of critical illness improves outcome. This principle has been seen for the early management of severe trauma [13], resuscitation of patients presenting to the emergency department with sepsis [14], as well as for thrombolysis in the management of myocardial infarction [15] and selected cases of ischaemic stroke [16]. As stated by England and Bion, the principle of the RRS is to "take critical care expertise to the patient before, rather than after, multiple organ failure or cardiac arrest occurs" [17].

This chapter reviews the evidence for the prevalence, consequences and causes of delayed RRS activation. In addition, we suggest ways in which it might be prevented.

Definition, Measurement, Classification of Delayed MET Activation

How Should Delayed Activation Be Defined?

A delay in the activation of an MET is defined as the absence of timely action in response to the signs or symptoms of deterioration and/or the lack of anticipated improvement of a patient's condition in response to a treatment.

D.A. Jones (✉) • R. Bellomo, MD
Department of Intensive Care, Austin Hospital, Studley Rd, Heidelberg, Melbourne, VIC 3084, Australia
e-mail: daryl.jones@austin.org.au; Rinaldo.bellomo@austin.org.au

C. Subbe, DM, MRCP
Ysbyty Gwynedd, Penrhosgarnedd, Bangor, Wales, UK
e-mail: csubbe@hotmail.com

© Springer International Publishing Switzerland 2017
M.A. DeVita et al. (eds.), *Textbook of Rapid Response Systems*, DOI 10.1007/978-3-319-39391-9_16

How Should Delayed MET Activation Be Classified?

We propose that delayed MET activation should be described as "afferent limb failure". This should be further characterized as complete or partial. Complete afferent limb failure has occurred when a patient develops MET criteria, the MET is not activated, and the patient suffers a serious adverse event. Partial afferent limb failure has occurred when MET activation is delayed and the patient still suffers a serious adverse event. This chapter will focus predominately on partial afferent limb failure.

How Should We Measure Delayed Activation?

Delayed activation can be measured as a continuous variable or as a categorical parameter: Any abnormal vital-sign outside predefined limits that is not escalated within a predefined time frame is classified as a delay (delay yes/no). Alternatively, the time span between the abnormal vital-sign and the activation or arrival of the MET is the measure of the delay. In the literature delays have been defined for call-outs after physiological abnormalities for more than 15 min [18] or 30 min [19] or between 15 min and 24 h after criteria have been fulfilled [20].

In a context where the patient experience becomes the central unit of observation this measure can be seen as one or several milestones in the trajectory to an admission to Intensive Care: measurement of vital signs, calculation of an early warning or similar scoring tool (often a separate process in units operating electronic patient records), call to an MET, arrival of the MET, decision to admit to ICU, actual arrival in ICU. In this scenario, the measurement of an MET delay becomes part of a system measure that can be described as "score-to-door time" [21]. The latter seems to lead to worse outcomes for patients if it is more than four hours. An MET delay could thus be classified as significant or non-significant if it is more or less than 4 h.

What Are the Limitations in the Measurement of Afferent Limb Failure?

The measurement of delayed activation and its impact would on the face of it seem fairly straightforward: A patient develops sepsis, the blood pressure drops from 142/72 mmHg at 13:05 o'clock to 82/35 mmHg at 19:32 o'clock but treatment with antibiotics and intra-venous fluids starts only at 21:56 o'clock after handover between shifts and a call to the MET. In this case, the delay would seem to be 2 h and 24 min.

In real life things might however be more complicated: The measurement of delay requires a clear starting point for a process. This starting point might not always be obvious.

The patient could, for example, be a patient with chronic heart failure whose systolic blood pressure usually varies between 80 and 100 mmHg. In the absence of a sudden change of physiology or in the presence of chronic illness without a change in what can be regarded as normal values of physiology for a given patient, the recognition of deterioration and thus the measurement of delay can be next to impossible and might require techniques of process control to identify deviance. Process control statistics do however require more data-points [22] and are therefore only likely to be helpful in patients with very frequent or continuous measurements of vital signs [23].

Patients who are unwell have often more unstable physiology with frequent changes in vital signs: patients with Chronic Obstructive Pulmonary Disease (COPD) might reach abnormal values for respiratory rate of 35 breath per minute or more several times during the day: each time they return from the bathroom or after dressing and undressing. In an environment where they are well known this change will be acknowledged as a transient change that is likely to settle in a predictable time frame. Or they are foreseeably reversible with an additional dose of a bronchodilator. Interestingly, one of the papers coming from the MERIT study found it difficult to optimize call-out criteria by sampling the highest and lowest values for vital signs in a group of non-MET patients in a 24-h period [24]. It is possible that this was due to the presence of patients with chronically abnormal vital signs in the sample.

The measurement of delay does also assume that there are recordings of vital signs. In many health systems these might be infrequent (as low as once or twice per day) or incomplete (often not including the respiratory rate as the most sensitive sign of deterioration [25–27]). The delay in response is therefore often only quantifiable from the first measurement that is arbitrarily defined as abnormal according to local or national convention. It does not capture a failure to determine the right frequency of observations and usually does not capture non-numerical data about patients' aspect or their complaint of feeling uncomfortable or unwell.

In some instances, patients initially stabilize and then re-deteriorate adding further complexity to the measurement. It is arguable that this is part of natural variability but patients who do not stabilize after their first recovery have a worse prognosis: In a study of 410 hypotensive patients, 72 initially stabilized but had another MET event with ICU admission within 48-h. Mortality in the group with initial stabilization was 42% compared to 27% in those where the initial event leads to ICU admission and 7% in those who were stabilized on the ward by the MET in a single visit [28].

How Often Is RRS Activation Delayed?

There are a number of studies suggesting that activation of the RRS is delayed in a substantial proportion of cases. In one of the earliest comparative before and after studies of the Medical Emergency Team (MET), Buist and co-workers reported that there was a reluctance to call the MET because of adherence to the traditional model of calling the most junior member of medical staff first [29].

Four studies of the MET at the Austin hospital (Melbourne Australia) provide objective evidence of the prevalence of delayed MET activation. An assessment of the 162 cardiac arrests that occurred in the 4 years following the introduction of the MET reported that 45 (28%) of cardiac arrest calls occurred shortly after an initial MET activation [30]. This suggests that the MET call activation was excessively delayed and that there was insufficient time for MET intervention to prevent the cardiac arrest.

An assessment of the role of the MET in 105 consecutive deaths at the same hospital revealed that five of 105 deaths did not have a "Do Not Resuscitate (DNR)" order at the time of death. Three of these five patients suffered a cardiac arrest and did not receive an MET call despite the presence of MET criteria [31].

Two retrospective studies of patients subject to MET review identified a high incidence of delayed MET activation [32, 33]. These studies defined delayed MET activation as an interval of more than 30 min between the onset of MET criteria and subsequent MET review. They examined four "MET syndromes" which included altered conscious state, arrhythmia, respiratory distress, and hypotension. They reported that 24–39% of patients had a delayed activation of the MET, and that the median time of delay was between 5 and 13 h depending on the MET syndrome (Table 16.1) [32, 33].

A point prevalence study from 10 hospitals in Victoria (Australia) examined vital signs from 1688 patients. 55 patients had abnormal vital signs fulfilling MET criteria, not one was received an MET activation within 30 min and only two were eventually seen by an MET [34]. Similar results were seen in a study from New Zealand with a 70% rate of failure to escalate [35].

Table 16.1 Frequency, duration, and consequence of delayed RRT activation 32, 33

RRT activation criteria	Median duration of delayed activation	Delayed more than 30 min (%)	Risk of death associated with delay
Altered conscious state Arrhythmia	16 h 13 h	35% 24%	OR 3.1 (1.4–6.6)
Respiratory distress Hypotension	12 h 5 h	50% 39%	OR 2.1 (1.01–4.34)

The Medical Early Response Intervention and Therapy (MERIT) study reported a high incidence of delayed or failed activation in patients who suffered one of the composite outcomes. Thus, documented MET criteria were present for more than 15 min in 30% of cardiac arrests, 51% of unplanned ICU admissions, and 50% of unexpected deaths [18].

What Are the Consequences of Delayed MET Activation?

Delay in the review of deteriorating patients admitted to hospital wards undermines one of the most important principles on which the promotion of MET was founded; the notion that early intervention improves outcome. The impact of delayed MET activation can be described in several dimensions: Clinical outcomes and impact on organizational culture.

Impact on Clinical Outcomes

Studies by Downey et al. and Quach et al. suggest that delayed MET activation is associated with worse outcome. Downey and co-workers reported that the patients who experience delayed MET review for altered conscious state and arrhythmia, experienced an increased mortality with an odds ratio (OR) of 3.1 (p = 0.005) compared with reviews in which delay did not occur (Fig. 16.1) [32]. Similarly, Quach and co-workers revealed that delayed MET review for patients with respiratory distress or hypotension was associated with an increased risk of death with an OR of 2.1 (p = 0.045) (Fig. 16.2) [33]. Calzavacca showed unplanned ICU admission and hospital mortality with delayed activations [19] (O.R. 1.79, 95% C.I. 1.33–2.93, p = 0.003 and O.R. 2.18, 95% C.I. 1.42–3.33, p < 0.001, respectively). Mortality was also raised in another study from Brazil [36].

Indirect evidence from a retrospective chart review in two hospitals in Montreal showed higher mortality in patients with a delayed admission to ICU (odds ratio, 1.8; 95% confidence interval, 1.1–2.9; P = 0.01) and higher ICU length of stay in surgical patients fulfilling MET criteria at the time of the study in hospitals that did not use an MET [37].

Failure of adherence to escalation can result in cardio-pulmonary arrests [38]. Afferent limb failure increases the risk of cardio-pulmonary arrest and admission to ICU [20].

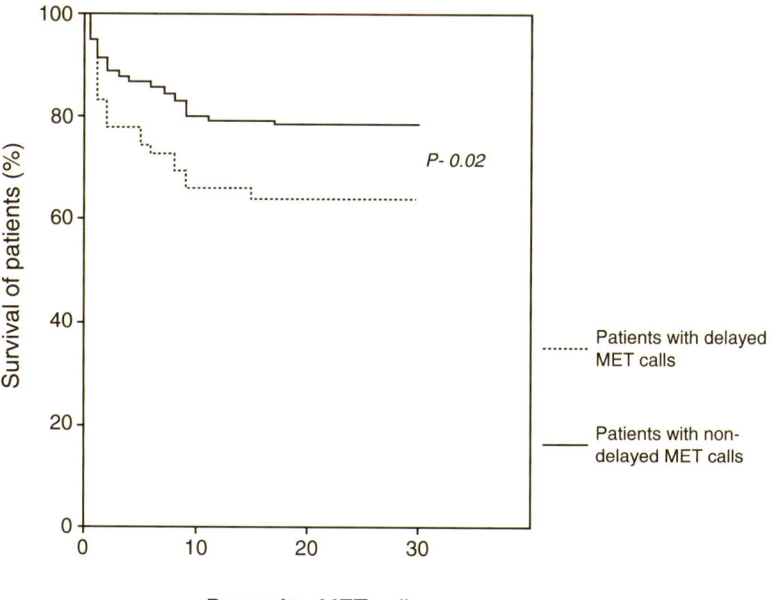

Fig. 16.1 Survival analysis for patient experiencing delayed versus non-delayed MET activation for low conscious state and tachycardia

Fig. 16.2 Survival analysis for patient experiencing delayed versus non-delayed MET activation for respiratory distress and hypotension

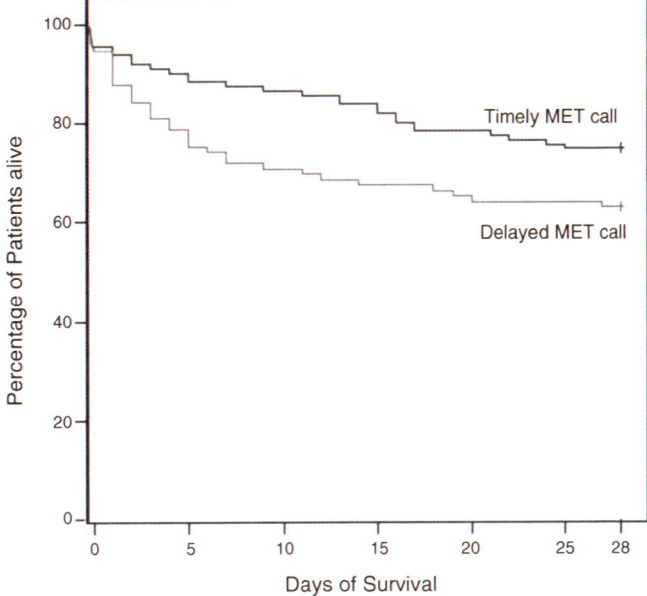

There are potential financial ramifications of delays in treatment. They might lead to a longer hospital stay [39] and in a more MET literate environment there is also a potential for increased litigation if due process for escalation of deteriorating patients is not followed.

Impact on Organizational Culture

RRS operate in a wider organizational culture. In order for healthcare providers to have faith in an RRS it requires face validity. This face validity includes the notion that the organization provides a framework of care that is evidence based, reliable and effective. If the MET activation is delayed because of complex activation criteria or an overworked MET team this bond of trust will weaken. At the same time, a delay of treatment that results in a reduced efficiency of the intervention will cause less impressive clinical improvements and thus deprive primary care teams and the MET of positive re-enforcement for their actions: Success breeds success, failure breeds failure.

What Are the Causes of Delayed MET Activation?

Existing evidence suggests that there are a number of causes of delayed or failed MET activation. Monitoring might be inadequate: A number of studies suggest that monitoring of acutely unwell patients may be inadequate to detect crisis early enough, especially at night. Cardiac arrest at the Austin hospital was most common overnight when MET call rates were lowest, and that arrest rates were lowest in the evening when MET call rates were highest [40]. Respiratory rate is infrequently monitored, despite the fact an elevated respiratory rate is shown to predict increased mortality [27].

Criteria might not have enough street-credibility. Ward staff may not appreciate the significance of a patient developing MET criteria. Many of the studies that preceded the development of the MET concept revealed that the management of acutely unwell ward patients by ward doctors and nurses is frequently sub-optimal in the period leading up to cardiac arrests and unplanned ICU admissions [9, 41]. A questionnaire of nurses at our hospital revealed that nurses frequently use discretion when confronted with a patient who has developed MET criteria, and frequently do not call the MET [42]. Foraida and co-workers reported that the introduction of objective calling criteria resulted in a near doubling of MET call activations in a university hospital in Pittsburgh [43]. A study at a teaching hospital in Melbourne revealed that altering the limits of the calling criteria, reducing the number of people in the MET, and making the mode of activation more subtle resulted in a marked increase in calling rate [44].

There is a culture of fear and the notion that it is good to ask for help or advice is not part of the organizational culture. Staff are concerned that they will be criticized either for calling the MET or because of their management of the patient [42].

The MET is not "part of the team" for a department or service: Casamento and co-workers reported that an education program for ward nurses resulted in increased call rates [45]. Similarly, Buist and co-workers reported increased call rates associated with a sustained education program of new and existing ward medical and nursing staff [46].

Which Strategies Can Help to Reduce Delayed RRS Activation?

Delayed MET activation can be reduced through a number of mechanisms. An increase in the overall number of MET calls can result in a concurrent reduction of delayed activations [47]. This increase can be achieved by protocolling the recording of vital signs and their assessment with Early Warning Scores [26, 48]. Organizational learning over time might also mean that a more mature RRS might lead to shorter MET delays [19].

Automated systems can provide a second redundant feed for the activation of a MET. Published data in this area is still scarce [49, 50]. Bellomo [49] showed a reduction in the number of abnormal sets of vital signs prior to the call-out of an MET from three to four. Schmidt [50] demonstrated an association between the uptake electronic of vital sign

recording and the reduction in hospital mortality. Intelligent electronic alerts could improve timing in administration of disease-specific treatments in a study of septic patients [51]. An Utstein-style analysis of the impact of automated monitoring found however no evidence that this leads to a reduction in failure to rescue events [52]. It is unclear from this last paper whether only the recording of vital signs or also the notification of abnormalities was automated.

Proactive rounding of general wards has the potential to reduce events and might help to build inter-professional working relationships. Evidence for a reduction in adverse clinical events is however currently lacking [53].

We believe that it is important to regularly review MET activation rates, and instances where there has been partial or complete afferent limb failure. Such cases should be fed back to the appropriate medical or surgical units at peer review grand rounds or "mortality and morbidity" meetings. This should be performed in a non-confrontational and blame-free manner.

The studies outlined above suggest that the reasons for failed activation may vary between hospitals. Members of the RRT might need to be reminded that no member of staff should ever be criticized for calling the RRT, or for the management of the patient.

Finally, regular education and feedback should occur for all new and existing staff to reinforce or introduce the concept, background and principles of the RRS in identifying, reviewing and treating acutely unwell hospital ward patients.

References

1. Zajac JD. The public hospital of the future. Med J Aust. 2003;250–252
2. Andrews LB, Stocking C, Krizek T, Gottlieb L, Krizek C, Vargish T, et al. An alternative strategy for studying adverse events in medical care. Lancet. 1997;349(9048):309–313
3. Baker GR, Norton PG, Flintoft V, Blais R, Brown A, Cox J, et al. The Canadian adverse events study: the incidence of adverse events among hospital patients in Canada. CMAJ. 2004;170(11): 1678–1686
4. Davis P, Lay-Yee R, Briant R, Ali W, Scott A, Schug S. Adverse events in New Zealand public hospitals

I: occurrence and impact. N Z Med J. 2002; 115(1167):

5. Leape LL, Brennan TA, Laird N, Lawthers AG, Localio AR, Barnes BA, et al. The nature of adverse events in hospitalized patients. Results of the harvard medical practice study II. N Engl J Med. 1991; 324(6):377–384

6. Vincent C, Neale G, Woloshynowych M. Adverse events in British hospitals: preliminary retrospective record review. BMJ. 2001;322(7285):517–519

7. Wilson RM, Runciman WB, Gibberd RW, Harrison BT, Hamilton JD, Wilson DE, et al. The quality in Australian health care study. Med J Aust. 1995;163(12):754

8. Bell MB, Konrad D, Granath F, Ekbom A, Martling CR. Prevalence and sensitivity of MET-criteria in a Scandinavian University Hospital. Resuscitation. 2006;70(1):66–73

9. Buist MD, Jarmolowski E, Burton PR, Bernard SA, Waxman BP, Anderson J. Recognising clinical instability in hospital patients before cardiac arrest or unplanned admission to intensive care. A pilot study in a tertiary-care hospital. Med J Aust. 1999;171(1): 22–25

10. Hodgetts TJ, Kenward G, Vlachonikolis IG, Payne S, CastleN. The identification of risk factors for cardiac arrest and formulation of activation criteria to alert a medical emergency team. Resuscitation. 2002;54: 125–131

11. Hodgetts TJ, Kenward G, Vlackonikolis I, Payne S, CastleN, CrouchR, et al. Incidence, location and reasons for avoidable in-hospital cardiac arrest in a district general hospital. Resuscitation. 2002;54(2):115–123

12. Kause J, Smith G, Prytherch D, Parr M. A comparison of antecedents to cardiac arrests, deaths and emergency intensive care admissions in Australia and New Zealand, and the United Kingdom—the ACADEMIA study for the Intensive Care Society (UK) & Australian and New Zealand Intensive. Resuscitation. 2004;62:275–282

13. Blow O, Magliore L, Claridge JA, Butler K, Young JS. The golden hour and the silver day: detection and correction of occult hypoperfusion within 24 hours improves outcome from major trauma. J Trauma. 1999;47(5):964–969

14. Rivers E, Nguyen B, Havstad S, Ressler J, Muzzin A, Knoblich B, et al. Early goal-directed therapy in the treatment of severe sepsis and septic shock. N Engl J Med. 2001;345:1368–1377

15. Fresco C, Carinci F, Maggioni AP, Ciampi A, Nicolucci A, Santoro E, et al. Very early assessment of risk for in-hospital death among 11,483 patients with acute myocardial infarction. GISSI Investigators. Am Heart J. 1999;138(6 Pt 1):1058–1064

16. Troke STS, Roup STG. Tissue plasminogen activator for acute ischemic stroke. The National Institute of neurological disorders and stroke rt-PA stroke study group. N Engl J Med. 1995;333(24):1581–1587

17. England K, Bion JF. Introduction of medical emergency teams in Australia and New Zealand: a multi-centre study. Crit Care. 2008;12(3):151

18. Hillman K. Introduction of the medical emergency team (MET) system: a cluster-randomised controlled trial. Lancet. 2005;365(9477):2091–2097

19. Calzavacca P, Licari E, Tee A, Egi M, Downey A, Quach J, et al. The impact of rapid response system on delayed emergency team activation patient characteristics and outcomes—a follow-up study. Resuscitation. 2010 Jan [cited 2015 Jul 7];81(1):31–5.

20. Trinkle RM, Flabouris A. Documenting rapid response system afferent limb failure and associated patient outcomes. Resuscitation. 2011;82(7):810–814

21. Oglesby KJ, Durham L, Welch J, Subbe CP. "Score to door time", a benchmarking tool for rapid response systems: a pilot multi-centre service evaluation. Crit Care. 2011;R180

22. Benneyan JC, Lloyd RC, Plsek PE. Statistical process control as a tool for research and healthcare improvement. Qual Saf Health Care. 2003;12(6):458–464

23. Ma FT, Lee CE. Integrated control chart for vital signs early warning of long-term care patients. 2014 7th Int Conf Ubi-Media Comput Work. 2014;313–8.

24. Cretikos M, Chen J, Hillman K, Bellomo R, Finfer S, Flabouris A. The objective medical emergency team activation criteria: a case—control study. Resuscitation. 2007 Apr;73(1):62–72

25. Chen J, Bellomo R, Hillman K, Flabouris A, Finfer S. MERIT study investigators for the Simpson Centre and the ANZICS Clinical Trials Group. Triggers for emergency team activation: a multicenter assessment. J Crit Care. 2010;25(2):359.e1–7.

26. Ludikhuize J, Borgert M, Binnekade J, Subbe C, Dongelmans D, Goossens A. Standardized measurement of the modified early warning score results in enhanced implementation of a rapid response system: a quasi-experimental study. Resuscitation. 2014;85(5):676–682

27. Cretikos MA, Bellomo R, Hillman K, Chen J, Finfer S, Flabouris A. Respiratory rate: the neglected vital sign. Med J Aust. 2008;188(11):657–659

28. Khalid I, Qabajah MR, Hamad WJ, Khalid TJ, Digiovine B. Outcome of hypotensive ward patients who re-deteriorate after initial stabilization by the medical emergency team. J Crit Care. 2014;29(1):54–59

29. Buist MD, Moore GE, Bernard SA, Waxman BP, Anderson JN, Nguyen TV. Effects of a medical emergency team on reduction of incidence of and mortality from unexpected cardiac arrests in hospital: preliminary study. BMJ. 2002;324(7334):387–390

30. Jones D, Opdam H, Egi M, Goldsmith D, Bates S, Gutteridge G, et al. Long-term effect of a medical emergency team on mortality in a teaching hospital. Resuscitation. 2007;74(2):235–241

31. Jones DA, McIntyre T, Baldwin I, Mercer I, Kattula A, BellomoR. The medical emergency team and end-of-life care: a pilot study. Crit Care Resusc. 2007;9(2):151–156

32. Downey AW, QuachJL, Haase M, Haase-Fielitz A, JonesD, BellomoR. Characteristics and outcomes of patients receiving a medical emergency team review for acute change in conscious state or arrhythmias. Crit Care Med. 2008;36(2):477–481

33. Quach JL, Hons B, Downey AW, Hons B, Haase M, Bpharm AH, et al. Characteristics and outcomes of patients receiving a medical emergency team review for respiratory distress or hypotension. J Crit Care. 2008 Sep;23(3):325–331

34. Bucknall TK, Jones D, Bellomo R, Staples M. Responding to medical emergencies: system characteristics under examination (RESCUE). A prospective multi-site point prevalence study. Resuscitation. 2013;84(2):179–183

35. Robb G, Seddon M. A multi-faceted approach to the physiologically unstable patient. Qual Saf Health Care. 2010 Oct;19(5):e47

36. Boniatti MM, Azzolini N, Viana MV, Ribeiro BSP, Coelho RS, Castilho RK, et al. Delayed medical emergency team calls and associated outcomes. Crit Care Med. 2014;42(1):26–30

37. Mardini L, Lipes J, Jayaraman D. Adverse outcomes associated with delayed intensive care consultation in medical and surgical inpatients. J Crit Care. 2012;27(6):688–693

38. Galhotra S, DeVita MA, Simmons RL, Dew MA, Members of the Medical Emergency Response Improvement Team (MERIT) committee. Mature rapid response system and potentially avoidable cardiopulmonary arrests in hospital. Qual Saf Health Care. 2007 Aug;16(4):260–265

39. Guinane JL, Bucknall TK, Currey J, Jones DA. Missed medical emergency team activations: tracking decisions and outcomes in practice. Crit Care Resusc. 2013;15(4):266–272

40. Jones D, Bellomo R, Bates S, Warrillow S, Goldsmith D, Hart G, et al. Patient monitoring and the timing of cardiac arrests and medical emergency team calls in a teaching hospital. Intensive Care Med. 2006;32(9):1352–1356

41. McQuillan P, Pilkington S, Allan A, Taylor B, Short A, Morgan G, et al. Confidential inquiry into quality of care before admission to intensive care. BMJ. 1998;316(7148):1853–1858

42. Jones D, Baldwin I, McIntyre T, Story D, Mercer I, Miglic A, et al. Nurses' attitudes to a medical emergency team service in a teaching hospital. Qual Saf Health Care. 2006;15(6):427–432

43. Foraida MI, DeVita MA, Braithwaite RS, Stuart SA, BrooksMM, SimmonsRL. Improving the utilization of medical crisis teams (Condition C) at an urban tertiary care hospital. J Crit Care. 2003;18(2):87–94

44. Jones DA, Mitra B, Barbetti J, Choate K, Leong T, BellomoR. Increasing the use of an existing medical emergency team in a teaching hospital. Anaesth Intensive Care. 2006;731–735

45. Casamento AJ, Dunlop C, Jones DA, Duke G. Improving the documentation of medical emergency team reviews. Crit Care Resusc. 2008;10(1):29

46. Buist M, Harrison J, Abaloz E, Van Dyke S. Six year audit of cardiac arrests and medical emergency team calls in an Australian outer metropolitan teaching hospital. BMJ. 2007;335(7631):1210–1212

47. Moriarty JP, Schiebel NE, Johnson MG, Jensen JB, CaplesSM, MorlanBW, et al. Evaluating implementation of a rapid response team : considering alternative outcome measures. International J Qual Health Care. 2014;26(1):49–57

48. Mitchell IA, Mckay H, Van Leuvan C, BerryR, MccutcheonC, AvardB, et al. Clinical paper A prospective controlled trial of the effect of a multi-faceted intervention on early recognition and intervention in deteriorating hospital patients. Resuscitation. 2010;81(6):658–666

49. Bellomo R, Ackerman M, Bailey M, Beale R, Clancy G, Danesh V, et al. A controlled trial of electronic automated advisory vital signs monitoring in general hospital wards. Crit Care Med. 2012;40(8):2349–2361

50. Schmidt PE, Meredith P, Prytherch DR, Watson D, Watson V, Killen RM, et al. Impact of introducing an electronic physiological surveillance system on hospital mortality. BMJ Qual Saf. 2015;24(1):10–20

51. Umscheid CA, Betesh J, VanZandbergen C, Hanish A, Tait G, Mikkelsen ME, French B, Fuchs BD. Development,implementation, and impact of an automated early warning and response system for sepsis. J Hosp Med. 2015;10(1):26–31

52. Tirkkonen J, Ylä-Mattila J, Olkkola KT, Huhtala H, Tenhunen J, Hoppu S. Factors associated with delayed activation of medical emergency team and excess mortality: an Utstein-style analysis. Resuscitation. 2013;84(2):173–178

53. Butcher BW, Vittinghoff E, Maselli J, Auerbach AD. The impact of proactive rounding by a rapid response team on patient outcomes at an academic medical center. J Hosp Med. 2013;8(1):7–12

Kathy D. Duncan, Terri Wells, and Amy Pearson

Studies have shown and clinicians are keenly aware that subtle signs of deterioration can precede life-threatening events, and early identification and treatment of unstable patients may rescue them from progressing to serious instability or death [1, 2, 3]. Many healthcare systems are now implementing Rapid Response Systems (RRS) designed to provide for an immediate match between the needs of rapidly deteriorating patients with the knowledge, skills, and resources to meet those needs. Whereas the detection of instability and placing the call for help represents the afferent (crisis detection) arm of the RRS, the response to the call represents the efferent arm (crisis response), and can take a variety of forms. In many hospitals and healthcare facilities, the efferent response to recognized instability is to deploy a specially trained team of professionals to immediately respond to the needs of deteriorating patients. There are many names for such teams such as the Medical Emergency Team (MET) or Rapid Response Team (RRT), or Critical Response Team. For the purposes of this chapter, RRT and MET can be used interchangeably.

The differences between physician-led and nurse-led models will be described. The physician-led model describes a "high capability" team (both in terms of numbers of responders and treatment options). These capabilities include: (1) ability to prescribe therapy, (2) advanced airway management skills, (3) capability to establish central venous access, and (4) ability to begin an ICU level of care at the bedside. Nurse-led models provide "intermediate capability" or "ramp up" team with additional members such as a respiratory therapist. Nurse-led capabilities include: (1) rapid assessment of patient needs, (2) beginning basic care to stabilize the patient, (3) rapid triage of patients to a higher level of care if needed, and (4) ability to call in other resources to provide immediate ICU-level care on an expedited basis [4]. As healthcare facilities and systems embark upon developing, implementing, and evaluating their efferent crisis response structure, there are several key elements to consider:

- Engage senior leadership support.
- Determine the best structure for the Rapid Response Team.
- Establish criteria for activation of the Rapid Response Team.
- Establish a simple process for activating the Rapid Response Team.
- Provide education and training.
- Use standardized tools.

K.D. Duncan, RN (✉)
Institute for Healthcare Improvement,
Cambridge, MA, USA
e-mail: kduncan@ihi.org

T. Wells, RN, MSN, CCRN • A. Pearson, RN, BSN
Adult Medicine Service Line, Presbyterian Hospital,
Albuquerque, NM, USA

- Establish feedback mechanisms.
- Measure effectiveness [5].(IHI):

There are hypothesized advantages and disadvantages to each model. For example, it is proposed that physician-led advantages may be the application of definitive care as quickly as possible, and "one-stop shopping" for emergent services. Disadvantages may include the requirement of highly trained (and costly) first responders, and could be intimidating to nurses, leading to delayed call. There is evidence that delay in notification and intervention of deterioration can adversely impact patient outcomes by increasing lengths of stay and possibly increased mortality [6]. Studies find that successful response teams are contingent upon nurses feeling comfortable to active the team and feel supported [7]. Proposed advantages to the nurse-led model may be that it feels less intimidating to nurses resulting in earlier calls, focus on education and prevention of deterioration, and less costly resources to organizations. Therefore, examining patient needs as well as the hospital's available services and culture may be important when determining which response team model is chosen. For example, Children's Healthcare of Atlanta, a tertiary referral system with 474 staffed beds across three campuses, opted for the nurse-led model around findings from root cause analyses of patient deteriorations. In some instances, they had uncertainty of their own clinical assessment and wanted validation prior to calling. Their nurse-led team was created to provide staff with a "second look" and support when the staff might be hesitant to call a provider or escalate care. Thus, the RRT model seemed to be the best fit to address instability in their institution. In this chapter, we will describe characteristics and logistics of a nurse-led RRT.

Identification of Hospital Resources

As facilities design their rapid response system, a key component in making this decision is determining "who" is available and able to assist patients who are deteriorating in a timely matter.

For many hospitals, namely community and rural hospitals generally do not have the option of providing a response team led by a physician intensivist certified in critical care medicine. Indeed, many community hospitals may not have physician coverage—either intensivists or hospitalists—in the facility around the clock. Instead, they must look within their current facility resources. There is much data to support the effectiveness of both models of RRTs. Depending on each organization's needs and resources, prevention and detection of deterioration of patients should be the focus over mere survival. Nurse-led teams can make significant impacts in numerous ways when the key elements are established, results evaluated and revised as needed.

The development of RRT personnel makeup and roles depends on several factors:

1. Availability of RRT members: It is crucial that the staff of the hospital can call for a RRT whenever needed: 24 h per day, 365 days per year. Small community or rural hospitals may have difficulty identifying available resources; they must look at several areas of the hospital that *could* provide resources to the RRT but currently do not. When the RRT is called, the need is immediate, so the team members must be able to stop whatever they are doing and respond to the call. If the team members—especially the leader—have to prioritize tasks and make a snap decision, they may make incorrect choices. For example, they may choose to complete their current activity, and not make the priority the unseen patient who has begun to deteriorate. Thus, the goal of intervening early in the patients' downhill spiral is thwarted before the response even starts. RRT membership, in particular the designation of the team leader, must provide for immediate availability.

2. Accessibility to the RRT: Calling the RRT should be simple—1 number, 1 call. Staff members will not call for the "subtle changes" or when they are "worried" if it is difficult to make the call. For example, if there are different numbers to call on the day shift or the weekend, it becomes a chore to call. Also,

educating staff to request the RRT becomes more complex as the number of methods (phone numbers) to activate the crisis response increases. Simplicity and standardization are key. If the RRT is easy to reach, the staff is more likely to call at the first sign of instability [7].

3. Ability/Skills of RRT members: To form a treatment plan, each team member must be able to assess the patient quickly and critically, perform their specified duties, and be confident in their decision-making skills. The team leader must not only be clinically competent in diagnosis and treatment of patients in crisis, but must also possess and be confident in the skills needed to lead a small group in crisis. The team members must possess skills that match the tasks they are being asked to complete. For example, it would be neither prudent nor safe to delegate the role of airway manager to someone who is untrained, inexperienced, and unskilled. Nevertheless, non-physicians can perform advanced skills when appropriate training and credentialing is ensured. Often facilities choose to denote specially trained staff, especially nurses, as an "RRT nurse," "MET nurse," or "Outreach nurse." This notation indicates a nurse with rescue and resuscitation training as well as noted leadership within the RRT.

Nursing Leadership of RRTs

With these factors in mind, an experienced critical-care nurse frequently fulfills the RRT leadership role. Intensive care units, emergency departments, and post-anesthesia recovery rooms offer nurses opportunities to develop vital skills, such as:

- The ability to identify both overt and subtle signs of impending or present patient instability;
- The ability to accurately collect and recognize key laboratory data;
- The ability to quickly assess a variety of complex patients;
- The opportunity to implement evidenced-based protocols and observe immediate patient outcomes;
- The ability to quickly respond and effectively perform in critical patient situations;
- Confidence in ability and motivation by the urgency of the patient populations;
- The ability to work with physicians in consultation rather than at the bedside.

Nurse-led RRTs have been successful in various hospital settings, from the small community hospital to the very large tertiary referral centers. Success can be described in a multitude of ways: A decrease in mortality rate, decrease in the number of cardiac arrests, a decrease in the delay in transferring patients to a higher, more appropriate level of care, and arguably the most widespread of all staff satisfaction. After implementing their nurse-led team in 2004, Presbyterian Healthcare Services (PHS) in Albuquerque, New Mexico, a 500-bed, non-profit community hospital achieved the entire above list of successes. In addition, staff survey responses that included hospitalist physicians stated "best thing this hospital has ever done!" "I love the MET nurse!" "Great to have a resource to give a second look at my patients." New physicians were told by their colleagues "if you have any trouble, call the MET nurse!" This kind of rapport between staff nurses, physicians, and the MET RN is integral to ensuring the key elements of best structure, simple process and in the moment education occurs.

Support for the Nurse-Led Rapid Response Team

An effective nurse-led RRT must contain the following components:

- Specific Triggers and protocols
- Standardized Communication tools
- Chain of command process

Specific Triggers and Protocols

In order for any response team to be effective, there must be recognition and the decision to notify at the point of care. Organizations must determine specific indicators for staff to initiate the call for assessment. Most teams begin with what is defined as *single-parameter triggers*. If a patient meets any of the single triggers, the staff nurse should notify the MET.

Examples of single-parameter triggers may include:

- Chest pain or Acute Shortness of breath
- Systolic Blood pressure ≤ 90
- Change in heart rhythm or rate ≥ 120 or ≤50
- Oxygen saturation ≤ 90 OR increased oxygen requirements
- Respiratory rate < 8 or >28
- Acute Level of Consciousness (LOC) changes
- Suspect sepsis
- Unable to reach MD in timely manner
- Worried about your patient/resource for questions

These single triggers can be defined to meet the organization and patient population needs. Extensive staff education must accompany the new implementation of the response team with expectations set from senior leadership to notify per the policy.

As response teams formed and evaluated their results, evidence was developing that in addition to single-parameter triggers, vital signs could be combined to form an "early warning score" in pediatric and adult patients. Early Warning Scoring (EWS) tools have become a valuable addition to detecting patient deterioration early and implementing proper interventions in a more timely way [8–10]. Rather than looking at one aspect of the patient's vital signs (such as low blood pressure), the scoring tools look at *multiple parameters* that can signal deterioration in early phases. For this reason, many response teams are adding EWS in addition to single-parameter triggers as an indication to activate the response nurse.

This might appear as the above list of single-parameter triggers with the addition of:

- Call for EWS of 4–5 if not improved after intervention & f/u score
- Call for any EWS ≥ 6

Various EWS tools will be discussed later in this chapter.

Specific Protocols: When a response team is under the direction of an experienced nurse, protocols may offer resources for immediate action. Treatment protocols and algorithms that have support of the physician staff may be utilized by the team; these protocols may include early interventions such as stat lab work, ECGs, respiratory support, and emergency medications. There has been much attention to screening and initiating labs such as blood cultures, lactate, and IV fluids for SIRS/sepsis in an effort to impact sepsis survival among hospitalized inpatients. These initial order sets may be included when patients meet SIRS/sepsis screening criteria as part of response team protocols.

Protocols are facility specific and must be approved by the appropriate departments and medical staff committees. The protocol should be highly detailed: as specific as the approval to start an IV and/or move to a higher level of care [11]. It is important that the RRT protocols be written such that they match available skills, and exclude procedures or tasks that cannot be performed by the team members designated. Thus, the protocol development will guide the team development, and vice versa.

Communication Tools: A common barrier is the ability of the bedside nurse to communicate a concern to the patient's physician, especially by telephone. Frequently, the on-call physician may not be familiar with the patient, and the nurse will only relate the issue that is of concern. For example, the nurse may call and say "Mr. Smith's temperature is 101.4." The physician may ask for more information but without the entire picture of the patient, and this may result in an incorrect order of treatment, or in directing the nurse to "watch him and call if he gets worse." It is imperative that staff and response nurses have a standardized, concise method of communicating with physicians by phone. This tool should be brief and include several aspects that construct a complete picture of the patient for the physician who is not in the room. Perhaps a most beneficial addition to communication of patient status is using the standard language of the EWS score to illustrate patient status. Instead of the above "Mr. Smith's temperature is 101.4" the RN might state "Mr. Smith's EWS score has increased from 2 to a 5 in the past 8 h. He is requiring more oxygen and meets 3 sepsis screening criteria." Even a physician unfamiliar with Mr. Smith would be able to determine whether this patient is showing deterioration or simply spiking having a pattern of fevers. Another communication tool is the SBAR (Situation, Background, Assessment, and Recommendation) that allows the staff RN and response nurse to gather all the information and communicate all aspects to the physician when care decisions require escalation.

Chain of Command Process: In a community and/or rural hospital where a physician is not a member of the crisis response team, or when there are limited physician resources in the hospital during the off hours, there must be a clear, well-articulated chain of command process.

The response nurse should have the confidence to implement proper interventions per protocol without delay for patient safety, but must also keep the physician informed of all status changes and orders that have been implemented prior to physician assessment or arrival. If staff is unable to reach the patient's physician, the RRT must be well versed in the facility's physician chain of command. An important task for the nurse-led RRT and physician leadership is to develop and articulate a simple chain of command process for ready reference by RRT members. The RRT must be able to demonstrate the ability to use the established chain of command to obtain physician direction when needed. For example, intensivists, medical directors, or emergency department physicians may be prospectively

designated as resources for the RRT, along with a dedicated rapid contact mechanism so that consultation and escalation of care is not delayed.

While most organizations strive for interdisciplinary collaboration and professional rapport between caregivers, cultures vary widely regarding physician's acceptance of response nurses' autonomy for decisions regarding specific patient interventions. In addition to barriers between nurse-physician collaboration, a culture of hesitancy might exist related to physician to physician consults as well. In situations when the physician and response nurse are not in agreement regarding treatment or need for escalation to higher level of care, organizations must provide specific detailed steps of determining the safest decisions for patients. It is imperative to have the key element of senior leadership support when establishing and maintaining a response team. The goal must always be patient safety and evidence-based treatment.

An example of specific escalation steps when using an EWSS might be:

1. On initial assessment, RRT RN will request additional assessment and intervention by the attending physician.
2. At the 2 h reassessment, if the patient EWs score remains 6 or greater despite intervention, the RRT RN will again request additional assessment and intervention by the attending physician.
3. At the 4 h reassessment, if patient EWs score remains 6 or greater despite intervention, the RRT RN will notify the attending MD of the required Intensivist consult to request additional assessment and intervention.
4. Transfer patient to higher level of care if impending arrest (cardiac or respiratory) is indicated on RRT RN assessment.

Note there are a variety of EWS scoring tools in existence and the score or trigger must be specific to each organization's defined notification parameters.

Data Collection

Just as with other forms of response teams, data should be gathered from each RRT call. Data can then be analyzed to identify opportunities for improvement. The RRT data collection tool can include the following:

- *Situation* or Trigger for the call (why?) Who initiated: Nursing, Physician, or Family activation of MET?
- *Background* of the patient (Brief medical history and events leading up to the deterioration).
- *Assessment* of the patient (Patient clinical findings; vital sign assessment) Acuity status of patient when MET arrives.
- *Recommendations* and interventions.
- *Outcomes* (for example, transferred to a higher level of care, cardiac or respiratory arrest, and survival, observations from a follow-up visit, etc.) [5].

In addition to using these data to track the utilization and efficacy of the RRT, the information can also provide validation for bedside nurse that the RRT call was beneficial, thereby giving them confidence to respond to their instincts and ensure that this behavior will be repeated. By reinforcing the behavior of attempting to rescue the patient, it will encourage continued placement of calls and may provide confidence to make the call even earlier in the patient's deterioration.

Review of the data collected from the nurse-led RRT described above can also help to reveal trends of patient problems; staff knowledge gaps or neglect to notify team; or trends in certain nursing units that can be further evaluated and corrected in quality improvement initiatives such as:

1. *Failure to Communicate*: For example, a failure in the nurse-to-physician or nurse-to-nurse communication, communication between departments, or failure to reach the provider may need to be improved.
2. *Failure to Recognize*: These failures may include a failure to note a change in heart rate, blood pressure, respiratory status, behavior change, or change in level of consciousness and subsequently result in a failure to act.
3. *Failure to Plan:* These failures are often system failures that are multi-faceted. For example, an inability of critical care beds may allow critically ill patients to be placed in a lower level of care. Additional examples include extended time spent in ED while waiting on appropriate bed and the frequent use of narcotic reversals in a specific area (Outpatient department, GI lab).

Many of these discrepancies can be directly addressed with the goal of support and rapport between the response nurse and staff RN. The slogan of all successful response teams must be "There is no inappropriate call" [12]. In addition, senior leadership support must adhere to enforcement of the expectation to call for all triggers and staff should be coached when triggers to call were missed, delayed, or consciously ignored. Conversely, any response nurse who is determined to be found unapproachable or discouraging to staff should not be a member of the team.

Other trends that can be identified through data collection are number of code blues outside of critical care; number of transfers to higher level of care; common triggers for notification; time from admission to need to transfer to higher level of care which could signify various missed assessments from ED to inpatient arrival; time of day of most calls; and common "other questions or resources" being asked of the response RN. An example of "other questions" identified at PHS in Albuquerque was related to central venous access devices, dialysis catheters, accessing ports, and PICC line questions. The identification of this trend resulted in hospital-wide education surrounding the differences, assessment, and maintenance of the various devices.

Once such trends are identified, leadership can work to develop mechanisms to address these system-wide failures and improve processes. For example, failure to recognize a crisis might lead to the development of mnemonic tools like pocket cards or posters, electronic alerts, and the development of educational opportunities to foster better knowledge and performance. The use of data gleaned from RRT events and the institutional response to shortcomings can make the hospital environment safer for all patients [13, 14].

Response teams must continually evaluate their own goals and desired outcomes to ensure continued improvement and change strategies as evidence-based practice dictates. In Albuquerque, PHS was achieving the initial goals set for the team related to decreasing out of ICU code blues and having compliance with staff calling for single triggers. The team researched new ways to further impact patient outcomes and determined adding the EWS tool in addition to their single-parameter triggers might make an impact. PHS piloted several cycles of change to determine the best use and compliance in scoring and notification. The initial pilot was performed on a general medical unit with education, paper tools, response team and physician involvement, auditing, feedback, and coaching. Senior leadership determined EWS was beneficial in detecting patient deterioration in its earliest phase and took the tool further to automation and integration with the EMR. Organization-wide implementation of EWS to all hospital units has made an impact on decreasing code blues, mortality rates, lengths of stay, and transfers to higher level of care. The automation resulted vital sign devices at every bed head that calculate the EWS in the moment with the nurse assessing vitals and inputting the LOC for a final score. The score is displayed at the nurses' station and in the EMR in real time, allowing for improved detection, notification, and intervention. In addition, the automation allows for collection of data to analyze delay or failure to recognize or notify the response team. If response teams continually assess their own results and strive to implement evidence and technology, code blues resulting from predictable indicators can become a thing of the past. The original general medical pilot unit went 898 days without a code blue (*Oct 2014 data*).

Data collection can also assist organizations in determining the proper model and dedicated resource for their response team. For example, as discussed in smaller rural hospitals the role is often a combined nurse leader role such as house supervisor or a charge nurse. In order for a response nurse to be effective, there must be clear criteria and minimal conflicting duties that might inadvertently cause a delay to treat a patient. Data should be collected on the number of calls as well as time spent on each call to assess and treat patients. This could assist with determining if additional resources should be utilized to have a dedicated role, independent of other conflicting duties.

In Atlanta, the Rapid Response Team was rolled out simultaneously with education to all staff on recognition of shock, implementation of mock shock codes, and simulations with the PediaSims mannequins including calling the RRT as a part of simulation for these patient scenarios. Atlanta Children's has a database that notes the entire assessment form so that each element can be queried, for example, how many 2 years olds were found in shock with no IV access.

Benefits of a Nurse-Led RRT

Aside from data supporting decreased code blues, lengths of stay, and transfers to higher level of care, there are many unforeseen benefits of nurse-led response teams. One study determined having an RRT had profound effects for staff nurses who utilize the team [7]. Examples of these effects include statements that nurses would not work in an institution that did not have a team; improvement of overall work environment; a sense of relief knowing they have the extra set of hands, eyes, minds, and bodies to help meet a patient's immediate needs; facilitated timely transfers to higher level of care; and better physician response to the reports and recommendations of the RRT nurse [7]. Another study echoes these sentiments finding in an institution with an RRT that 93 % of nurses feel the RRT improved patient care, 84 % felt it improved the nurses' work environment, and 64 % would consider institutional RRTs as a factor ion seeking a new job [15]. Yet, another study indicates that nurse-led RRTs contribute to the educational needs of staff, patient assessment skills, assistance with patient care when acuity changes, timely transfers, transport assistance, and physician communication facilitation [12].

When considering the cost of nursing turnover, estimated to be $21,000–$64,000 per nurse this could be a powerful recruitment and retention tool.

In an acute care hospital environment, staff nurses are often overwhelmed with multiple complex patients. When a nurse-lead RRT is called to assess a patient, the interaction between the RRT leader and the bedside nurse is that of peer-to-peer, with a sense of collaboration for the good of the patient. The nurse leader—the right nurse leader—will keep the discussion and actions focused on what is best for the patient and refrain from judgment or criticisms. This attitude of mentoring also provides for the learning opportunities for the staff. The nurse-led response team has had great success in mentoring less experienced staff into understanding of the signs of deterioration, with the goal bedside nurse recognizing instability earlier and based upon more subtle findings when faced with their next case. As these positive interactions occur frequently, the staff RNs can begin to accumulate their own experiences to draw upon in similar situations, while sharing thoughts regarding patient assessments, expected interventions, and witness outcomes from these interactions in a safe manner with the mentor nurse. The nurse-led RRT can also help the staff by organizing their thoughts into a structured framework (SBAR) and calling the physician while the less experienced nurse listens and learns. Alternatively, the more experienced nurse can stay with them while they call in the event and assist them if the physician asks questions and they are uncertain how to answer [5].

The call to an RRT should not trigger feelings of judgment as to what did or did not happen before the call—that someone may have missed a crucial element in the assessment, or that the nurse does not know what he or she is doing. Teaching should occur at appropriate times in the moment or serious concerns regarding failure to recognize be addressed through unit leadership.

It is important that the RRT members not "take over" the care of the deteriorating patient. The role of the RRT is to bring critical care assessment skills and care to the bedside, ensuring deterioration is prevented or treated quickly. Staff nurses who have cared for this patient for a prolonged period of time will not learn from the event if they are pushed out of the way and the RRT takes over completely. Conversely, it is important that the assigned bedside nurse remains involved in all communications and interventions and does not assume the response nurse is now assuming total care. The bedside nurse must not simply place the call and then go about caring for her other assigned patients. Every call should be used as an experiential teaching moment and the bedside nurse must be ready to continue care in the event the response nurse is called to another priority. Many hospitals that may have demonstrated improvement in patient outcomes with the implementation of a nurse-led team have also observed a noticeable improvement in the relationship between ICU nursing staff and ward nursing staff. The team can rescue the patients from an acute event and often an ICU stay. Many activations of the response nurse result in treatment with an increase in monitoring while the patient remains at the same level of care. In fact, if the deterioration is truly detected in its earliest phase, this should be the normal course of action: detection, notification, intervention, monitoring, and improvement. In summary, the response nurses should be carefully selected for not only their advanced assessment skills, but also their ability to mentor and teach the less experienced nurse in a productive manner while ensuring the patients receive safe and appropriate care.

In another example, Children's Healthcare of Atlanta implemented its nurse-led team in December 2006, consisting of an ICU RN and Respiratory Therapist. Atlanta has seen their rate of preventable codes decrease as well as experienced a decrease in the number of patients being found in shock by the Rapid Response Team. Staff has verbalized great satisfaction with the program and the historical dissonance between the ICU staff and the General Care staff has also improved. In over 350 calls, the majority were for respiratory concerns, averaging 30 min for the call, with only 40 % of patients requiring ICU admission.

Nursing Leadership and Mentoring after the RRT Call

Several models of nurse-led RRTs provide a follow-up visit after the initial RRT call is completed. The follow-up visit is made by the nurse 2–12 h (as per protocol) after the initial visit and is an intentional redundancy that provides another safety net for the patient. During this visit, the nurse assesses the patient and reviews the events that have occurred since the RRT visit to ensure the interventions were effective and that the current level of care is still appropriate for the patient. This single follow-up can be a convincing argument to involve the response nurse when a patient meets established criteria and a physician is aware and present on the unit. Some physicians may question "why did you call the RRT?" The bedside nurse can simply explain this is an organizational patient safety protocol in place and the patient will then receive follow-up visits from the next shift RRT. The goal is always to ensure the patient is showing signs of improvement from any interventions and not allowed to deteriorate further. This visit also provides an opportunity for a debriefing with the staff currently assigned to the patient. The discussion and review of the patient during a less-urgent time provides a great opportunity for learning for staff members, and is a rare opportunity for collaboration of two professionals to discuss the care of their patient. This follow-up visit should be noted on the "call tool," which then can be used in data collection and given to the frontline management team of the area initiating the call for further learning.

A Review of Triggers/Early Warning Scoring Tools and Continuous Improvement

As mentioned previously, many response teams have integrated EWS tools in addition to single-parameter triggers. Additionally, technology and Electronic Medical Record (EMR) systems have provided even further real-time detection advantages for health care providers. The capability for remote surveillance of patients' vitals, EWS, and other parameters can further improve early detection. Common Early warning scoring tools are known as Pediatric Early Warning Score (PEWS), Modified Early Warning Score (MEWS), National Early Warning Score (NEWS), and VIEWS [16]. There have been numerous studies internationally attempting to validate a single tool. This has proven difficult as response teams have evolved and implemented systems specific to their own organizational needs, resources, and patient populations. Whichever tool an organization uses, there should be assessment and validation of the efficacy compared to their own previous results. If a response team triggers and EWS tool does not currently exist in an organization, sharing of best practices is strongly encouraged among like facilities to expedite improved recognition of patient deterioration, notification, response, and intervention.

Studies have confirmed that patients show signs of deterioration 6–8 h before an arrest or emergent transfer. Schien and colleagues [1] demonstrated 84 % of patients had identifiable deterioration long before they had their arrest. These included changes in breathing pattern, pulse rate, and LOC. Respiratory events are generally the initial cause of deterioration that ultimately leads to cardiac arrest [1]. Subbe and colleagues [10] found that in unstable patients, relative changes in respiratory rate were much greater than changes in heart rate or systolic blood pressure, and thus the respiratory rate was likely to be a more accurate predictor of at-risk patients. There has been a trend in technology to address respiratory rate as an earlier predictor of deterioration versus cardiac rhythm monitoring, heart rate, and blood pressure. In addition, recording of respiratory rates in hospitalized patients has often been inaccurate and viewed with little awareness of a marker of serious illness [9].

Rapid Response systems are increasingly integrating all aspects of critical intervention with teams responding to "Stroke Alert," "Code Sepsis," and "Code Blue." As evidence, technology and the ability to assign protocols and algorithms for standard response and care, patient outcomes should continue to improve. The tools and systems in place are only beneficial if properly implemented and utilized. The challenge to response teams remains to monitor our own team's effectiveness and continually evaluate ways to improve. Some suggested data measures for the team's effectiveness include:

- Trigger to RRT call time
- Trigger to treatment time
- Trigger to ICU arrival time
- Outcomes of RRT visit
- Time to admit to ICU

Summary Nurse-led RRTs

Effective nurse-led rapid response teams require several key elements to be successful. Support of senior leadership is essential. The structure must contain defined expectations for all staff accompanied by education for vitals signals assessment, interpretation, and recognition of signs of deterioration. The parameters to activate a call must be supported by a policy that allows for assessment and intervention in the interest of the patients.

Monitoring for deterioration may take many forms from single-parameter triggers, multi-parameter EWS, signs of sepsis or stroke. Utilization of technology such as remote surveillance of EMR, vital devices with automated scores, telemetry or respiratory monitoring devices, and automated sepsis screening alerts should be considered. Criteria should be included with increased monitoring for known patients at risk such as first 12 h of admission, high respiratory rates, higher EWS scores, or repeated triggers for activation of RRT. Assessment and action plans surrounding failures or delay in recognition and intervention should be part of internal assessment for optimal results. It is helpful to have standardized definitions of delay or failure to assist with data collection. The structure for staff

to call for assessment or assist should be simple and the responder should not be conflicted by dual roles. The responders should be carefully selected as both leaders and mentors with the overall goals to benefit both patient outcomes and staff work environment. The final structure should be standardized processes and contingencies for response to patient deterioration. Whether the responder is nurse-led or physician-led there could be varied factors that may influence the speed of intervention occurring at the bedside. Leadership must have chain of command and decision algorithms clearly spelled out to alleviate interference with patient treatment. Response teams should pro-actively monitor their own results and form action plans on identified opportunities for improvement at regular intervals. In addition, organizations should review best practices and new evidence to ensure their efforts are forward-moving in patients' best interest. Data collection should be regularly analyzed and updated per best practice recommendations and in collaboration with Quality Care specialists within the organization. Nurse-led response teams have shown to be an extremely successful model that has flexibility to bring a unique perspective to the leadership role in a Rapid Response Team process. Experience, instinct, determination, and a spirit of collaboration with the nurse at the bedside are attributes that can enhance and sustain the RRT process, improve patient outcomes, and over time improve the patient safety culture of the facility.

Conclusion

Nurse-lead RRTs may be the ideal mechanisms for crisis intervention, particularly when physician resources are scarce. RRTs frequently utilize a variety of tools and mechanisms to increase effectiveness and ensure patient safety such as communication pathways, treatment protocols, specialized training in crisis response skills, physician chain of command documentation, and post-event debriefing of involved staff to improve patient care.

References

1. Schein RM, Hazday N, Pena M, Ruben BH, Sprung CL. Clinical antecedents to in-hospital cardiopulmonary arrest. Chest. 1990;98(6):1388–92.
2. Franklin C, Mathew J. Developing strategies to prevent in hospital cardiac arrest: analyzing responses of physicians and nurses in the hours before the event. Crit Care Med. 1994;22(2):244–7.
3. Buist M, Bernard S, Nguyen TV, Moore G, Anderson J. Association between clinically abnormal observations and subsequent in-hospital mortality: a prospective study. Resuscitation. 2004;62(2):137–41.
4. DeVita MA, Bellomo R, Hillman K, et al. Findings of the first consensus conference on medical emergency teams. Crit Care Med. 2006;34:2463–78.
5. Institute for Healthcare Improvement (IHI). www.ihi.org
6. Paterson R, MacLeod DC, Thetford D, Beattie A, Graham C, Lam S, Bell D. Prediction of in-hospital mortality and length of stay using an early warning scoring system: clinical audit. Clin Med. 2006 May–Jun;6(3):281–4.
7. Shapiro S, Donaldson N, Scott M. Rapid response teams seen through te eyes of the nurse: how nurses who activate such teams feel about the experience and why it matters. Am J Nurs. 2010;110(6):28–33.
8. Gardner-Thorpe J, Love N, Wrightson J, Walsh S, Keeling N. The value of Modified Early Warning Score (MEWS) in surgical in-patients: a prospective observational study. Ann R Coll Surg Engl. 2006 Oct;88(6):571–5.
9. Goldhill DR, McNarry AF, Mandersloot G, McGinley A. A physiologically-based early warning score for ward patients: the association between score and outcome. Anaesthesia. 2005 Jun;60(6):547–53.
10. Subbe CP, Davies RG, Williams E, Rutherford P, Gemmell L. Effect of introducing the modified early warning score on clinical outcomes, cardio-pulmonary arrests and intensive care utilization in acute medical admissions. Anaesthesia. 2003;58(8):797–802.
11. Funk D, Sebat F, Kumar A. A systems approach to the early recognition and rapid administration of best practice therapy in sepsis and septic shock. Curr Opin Crit Care. 15:301–7.
12. Metcalf R, Scott S, Ridgway M, Gibson D. Rapid response team approach to staff satisfaction. Orthop Nurs. 2008;27(5):266–71.
13. Chan PS, Khalid A, Longmire LS, Berg RA, Kosiborod M, Spertus TA. Hospital wide code rates and mortality rates before and after implementation of a rapid response team. JAMA. 2008 Dec 3;21:2506–13.
14. DeVita MA, Smith GB. Rapid response systems: is it the team or the system that is working? Crit Care Med. 2007;35:2218–9.
15. Galhotra S, Schoole CC, Dew MA, Mininni NC, Clermont G, DeVita MA. Medical emergency teams: a strategy for improving patient care and nursing work environments. J Adv Nurs. 2006 Jul;55(2):180–7.
16. Prytherch DR, Smith GB, Schmidt PE, Featherstone PI. ViEWS—towards a national early warning score for detecting adult inpatient deterioration. Resuscitation. 2010 Aug;81(8):932–7.

MET: Physician-Led RRTs

Daryl A. Jones and Rinaldo Bellomo

Introduction

Patients admitted to acute care hospitals are complex and have increasing co-morbidity [1]. Several studies from multiple countries around the world reveal that patients suffer serious adverse events (SAEs) that prolong hospital length of stay, and may result in permanent disability and death [2–13]. Other studies have shown that these events may be preventable and avoidable [14, 15] and are often preceded by objective signs of deterioration that manifests as derangement in commonly measured vital signs [16–19].

Further studies have suggested that the response of ward doctors and nurses to these deteriorations may be suboptimal and not commensurate to degree of instability [14, 15, 20, 21]. Every hospital must develop strategies to deal with this problem. One such strategy is the Physician-led Medical Emergency Team (MET) [22].

Principles Underlying the Physician-Led MET

The principles underlying the physician-led MET are similar to those of all Rapid Response Teams (RRTs) (Table 18.1). Up to 17 % of patients admitted to hospital develop an SAE [2–13]. Accordingly, there needs to be a screening mechanism to detect and identify these deteriorations reliably and promptly. Several studies have shown that in up to 80 % of SAEs there are derangements of vital signs in period leading up to the event [16–19]. Such derangements form the basis for the calling criteria for METs (Fig. 18.1). The criteria are usually simple, and do not require the ward to staff to interpret, calculate, or formulate an "at-risk" score.

At least three studies have shown that if a patient develops these criteria they are more likely to die than patients who do not develop them [23–25]. Thus, the calling criteria are not only simple, but are predictive of a subsequent SAE. Other studies have shown that the evolution of the deterioration is often slow, occurring over hours, and thus there is time to intervene [16, 19, 26].

Examination of the actions of ward doctors and nurses during this period of clinical decline suggests that the response is frequently suboptimal, as they do not have sufficient skills to identify and treat such deteriorations [14, 15, 20, 21]. In contrast, intensive care staff are specifically

D.A. Jones (✉) • R. Bellomo
Department of Intensive Care, Austin Hospital, Studley Rd, Heidelberg, Melbourne, VIC 3084, Australia
e-mail: daryl.jones@austin.org.au; Rinaldo.bellomo@austin.org.au

© Springer International Publishing Switzerland 2017
M.A. DeVita et al. (eds.), *Textbook of Rapid Response Systems*, DOI 10.1007/978-3-319-39391-9_18

Table 18.1 Physiological rationale why the MET is a logical approach for preventing serious adverse events in hospitalized patients

- **Principle one:** *There is time for intervention*
  - The evolution of clinical and physiological deterioration is relatively slow
- **Principle two:** *there are warning sign.*
  - Clinical deterioration is preceded by physiological deterioration in commonly measured **vital signs**
  - These observations are easy to measure, are inexpensive, and are non-invasive (measuring them does not hurt the patient)
- **Principle three: there are** *effective treatments* if dangerous conditions are recognized
  - Examples include beta-blockers for myocardial ischaemia, fluid therapy for hypovolemia, non-invasive ventilation and oxygen for respiratory failure, and anticoagulation for thrombo-embolic disease
  - The majority of interventions of the MET are inexpensive, relatively simple, and non-invasive
- **Principle four:** *that early intervention improves outcome*
  - The assumption that early intervention saves lives has been shown for the treatment of trauma as well as septic shock
  - The hospital survival for cardiac arrest is at best 14 %
  - It is intuitive that sick people are easier to fix than dead people.
- **Principle five:** *the expertise exists and can be deployed*
  - Intensive care doctors and nurses are experts in the delivery of advanced resuscitation

trained in the advanced resuscitation of acutely unwell patients. Such expertise can be deployed from the ICU when patients develop one or more MET activation criteria.

One of the most important tenets underlying the MET concept is that early intervention in the course of deterioration improves outcome. This phenomenon has been seen in the early management of severe trauma [27], the early administration of antibiotics in patients with sepsis [28], and in association with early administration of thrombolytic therapy for acute myocardial infarction [29] and selected cases of ischemic stroke [30].

Importantly, the MET is a primarily reactive approach to the recognition and response to deteriorating patients. Thus, patients will have evidence of clinical deterioration before the system is activated, and patients are often moderately unwell when reviewed. This differs from critical care outreach teams which is primarily a pre-emptive and pro-active approach (Fig. 18.2).

What Is a Physician-Led MET?

The MET is an example of an RRT (see the chapter). The major difference between the MET and other RRTs is that the team leader of the MET is a physician (M = medical). The team should review the deteriorating patient promptly (less than 10 min). According to the statement of the first international conference on METs the MET should have core competencies that (1) ability to prescribe therapy; (2) advanced airway management skills; (3) capability to establish central vascular lines; and (4) ability to begin an ICU level of care at the bedside [31]. Studies conducted in the Netherlands and Australia reveal that there is considerable variability in the team leader of the RRT [32, 33]. In many instances, the assembled team would not be able to perform all of the tasks required of a highly proficient MET [32].

In Australia and New Zealand, the doctor is often a registrar (fellow) who is training to be a specialist in Intensive Care Medicine [32, 34]. Such trainees undertake rotations in internal medicine, anaesthesia, and at least 2 years training in a University-affiliated teaching hospital Intensive Care Unit. Accordingly, the MET team leader is usually credentialed to supervise or perform all aspects of advanced resuscitation, including endo-tracheal intubation and insertion of invasive vascular access.

Ideally, the team should be available 24 h per day and 7 days a week, as a number of studies have shown that many MET calls occur out of hours and on the weekend. In some cases, the MET supersedes cardiac arrest team and the MET is called for all medical emergencies [35]. In other cases runs in parallel with cardiac arrest team and the MET are summoned to review all emergencies other than arrests [36–38] (Fig. 18.1).

The key members of the MET typically include the ICU fellow, the internal medicine

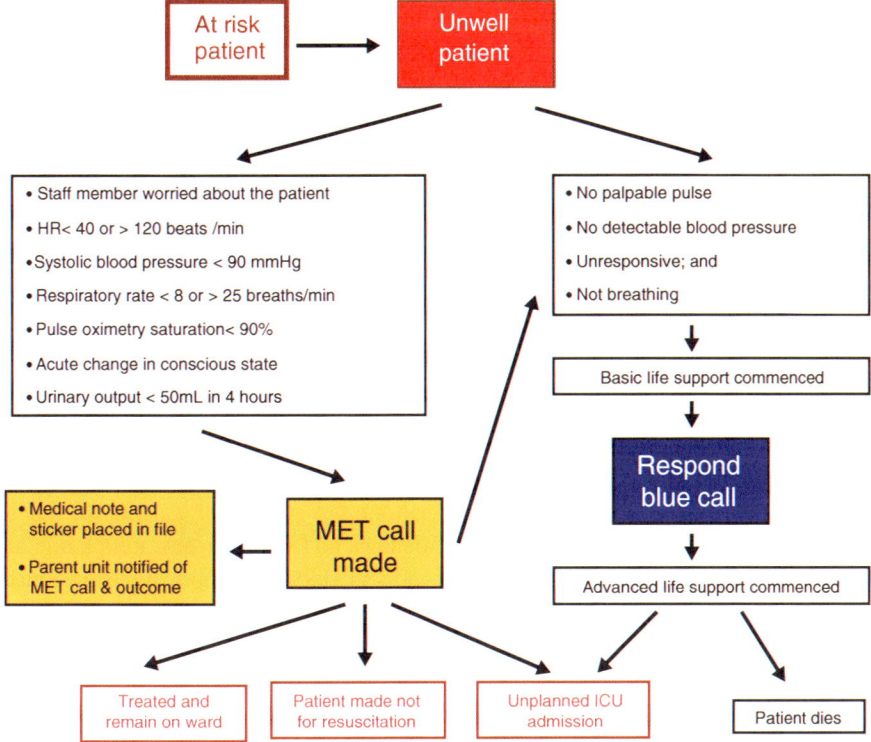

Fig. 18.1 Figure showing parallel processes of medical emergency team and cardiac arrest team for deteriorating patients

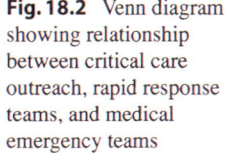
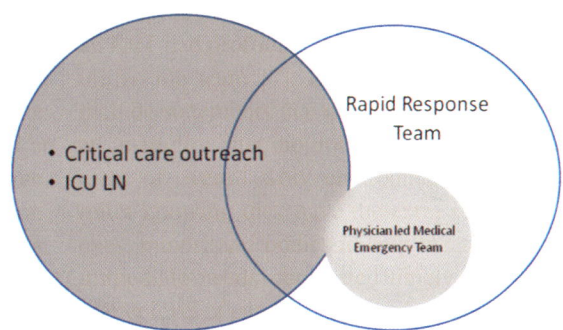

Fig. 18.2 Venn diagram showing relationship between critical care outreach, rapid response teams, and medical emergency teams

fellow, and an ICU nurse. Additional members include the ward nurse, and in the United States, a respiratory care practitioner (Table 18.2).

The major role of the MET is to act as a triage system in the early phases of clinical deterioration. As stated by England and Bion, the principle of the MET is to "take critical care expertise to the patient before, rather than after, multiple organ failure or cardiac arrest occurs" [39].

Why Do Patients Need MET Calls

There are relatively few studies examining the cause of MET calls. A study of 400 calls at our institution revealed that the triggers for the calls were hypoxia (41 %), hypotension (28 %), altered conscious state (23 %), tachycardia (19 %), increased respiratory rate (14 %), and oliguria

Table 18.2 Structure and roles of personal comprising the MET

Staff member	Role/responsibility
Intensive care fellow	• Thorough understanding of interplay between clinical medicine, mechanism of disease, and therapies for reversal of acute physiological derangement (advanced resuscitation techniques)
	• Skills in airway management and advanced cardiac life support
	• Facilitation of advanced treatment directives
	• Documentation of issues surrounding MET for ongoing audit and quality control
Intensive care nurse	• Advanced knowledge in the application of therapies required in advanced resuscitation
	• Provision of ongoing information and advice to ward nurses for patients remaining on the ward following MET call
	• Liaising with intensive care unit regarding potential for patient admission
Medical fellow	• Skills in diagnosis and management of underlying aetiology of medical condition
	• Follow-up and ongoing management of patients remaining on ward following MET call
Ward nurse	• Knowledge of patients nursing issues since admissions and leading up to MET call
Respiratory therapist (USA)	• Assistance with respiratory related therapies including endo-tracheal intubation

(8 %) [40]. Common causes of MET calls include pulmonary oedema, seizures, sepsis, and atrial fibrillation [41]. A single-centre observation study revealed that between 27.1 and 44.4 % of 358 MET calls had objective diagnostic criteria for sepsis [42].

Studies of the outcomes of patients subject to MET calls reveal that they are often critically unwell. Approximately one-fifth of patients reviewed by the MET will have more than one call during the same hospital admission [41]. Admission to critical care areas occurs in 10–25 % of patients following an MET call, and in approximately one third of patients, there are limitations of therapy and issues around end of life care. The in-hospital mortality of MET patients is approximately 20–25 % [41]. In patients without documented limitations of medical therapy, the in-hospital mortality is 15 %, and for those with documented limitations of medical therapy, this rises to 50 % [41].

What Does the Physician-Led MET Do

The MET provides prompt patient review, institutes acute resuscitation, and formulates a management plan [37]. In many cases subsequent management is delegated to ward staff who then follow up the patient and liaise with ICU staff as required. The patient may remain on the ward for full active therapy, or have a limitation of medical therapy or "Do Not Resuscitation" order instituted [43, 44]. Alternatively, if the acuity of the patient exceeds the care that can be provided on the ward, the patient may be urgently transferred to the ICU (Fig. 18.1). In this regard, the MET is providing a prompt second medical opinion for the acutely ill. It also provides a mechanism for expediting transfer of the critically ill patient to a higher level of care. A systematic review of interventions provided by the MET suggested that implementation of limitations of medical therapy is the most common intervention that the team performs [45].

In a study of 5389 calls in 3880 patients, NIV was delivered during 483 (9.0 %) calls to 426 patients (11 % of the total). The four most common MET diagnoses associated with NIV were acute pulmonary edema (156 calls, 32.3 %), pneumonia (84 calls, 17.4 %), acute respiratory failure of unclear origin (59 calls, 12.2 %), and exacerbation of chronic obstructive pulmonary disease (32 calls, 6.6 %) [46].

In a separate study of 5431 MET calls, 557 (10.3 %) calls in 458 patients were triggered by AF. The mean age for AF patients was 74.8 years, 230 (50.2 %) were female, and 271 (59.1 %) were in a surgical ward. Ninety-two (20.1 %) of the patients with MET calls due to AF died in hospital compared with 131 (28.6 %) in the control group [47].

We have previously proposed that there should be a minimum standard for the management of an

Table 18.3 An "A → G" approach to managing an MET call

Ask and Assess Ask the staff how you can help them Ask about the reason for the MET call Assess for the etiology of the deterioration
Begin basic investigations and resuscitation therapy
Call for help/call consultant if needed

Discuss, Decide, and Document
    Discuss MET with parent unit/consultant
    Discuss advanced care planning if appropriated
    Decide where the patient needs to be managed
    Document the MET and subsequent frequency of
    observations

Explain: the cause of the MET, the investigations   required, and subsequent management plan
Follow-up: which doctor to follow up the patient?   What are the criteria for doctor re-notification?
Graciously thank the staff at the MET

MET call [40] including: (1) determining the cause of the deterioration; (2) documenting the events surrounding the MET call; (3) prescribing a management plan and ensuring that appropriate medical follow-up occurs; (4) initiating a medical referral in cases where a surgical patient receives an MET call for a medical reason; (5) communicating the occurrence of the MET with the appropriate parent unit doctors; (6) liaising with the ICU consultant on call if the patient fulfils predefined criteria or remains unwell despite the initial resuscitation.

An approach to the management of an MET has also been proposed (Table 18.3). This AG approach can be adapted to the management of commonly encountered "MET syndromes" [40].

Like all RRTs the MET should be part of RRS. It should be linked to governance and quality arms and overseen by an administrative structure [31].

What Are the Advantages and Disadvantages of Physician-Led MET

The rationale behind, and method of activation of the MET are simple. The system allows a deteriorating ward patient to be reviewed promptly by a team of experienced and senior staff, where traditionally they would have been seen by a junior member of medical staff in isolation. The calling criteria are objective, simple and stress the importance of addressing deranged vital signs. There is no gradation of response which may reduce delays in intervention. The calling criteria are meaningful for the ward nurse, who is the typical caller of the MET. The MET is a hospital-endorsed mechanism of rapid patient review that may empower nurses to seek help for their deteriorating patients. Questionnaires of nursing staff reveal that the MET assisted them in managing sick ward patients, reduced their work load when managing such patients, and actually taught them how to better manage acutely ill patients [48, 49].

The MET may assist in establishing end of life care planning for patients in whom a switch to comfort care is most appropriate [43, 44]. Because the MET has a limited number of members, only a relatively small number of personnel need to be trained each year. In addition, doctor involvement in the team allows prescription of medications and the conduct of complex and invasive procedures [31]. These interventions may be delayed in the case of a nurse-led RRT.

The major advantage of the physician-led MET relates to improved patient outcome. Of all the comparative studies of the RRT that demonstrate improved patient outcome, relatively few involved a nurse-led RRT [50, 51]. Multiple studies in both adults and children demonstrate that a physician-led MET can result in reductions in cardiac arrests, unplanned ICU admissions, in-hospital deaths, and complications following major surgery.

There have been a number of stated disadvantages of the physician-led MET (Table 18.4). It has been argued that the MET is resource intensive and deskills ward doctors and nurses. However, it is arguably more labour intensive to train all ward doctors in the management of acutely ill ward patients. In addition, nurses at our institution state that the MET improves their skills in managing unwell ward patients [48]. The MET review process may create conflict and the MET staff may make errors because of lack of familiarity with the patient. Involvement of the parent unit doctors in the assessment and management plan is

Table 18.4 Aims and potential benefits of the medical emergency team (MET)

Aim	Potential benefit
• Assist ward doctors and nurses in the management of acutely unwell and complicated patients • Improve awareness and ability of doctors and nurses to identify and manage acutely unwell patients	• Reduction of cardiac arrests and unplanned ICU admissions • Reduction in morbidity and hospital length of stay • Increased use of hospital bed for management of primary surgical diagnosis rather than complications following surgery
• Provision of objective calling criteria for activation of the MET	• Empowering of nursing staff and doctors to seek help by a system which is supported by hospital policy
• Early identification and treatment of patients requiring ICU therapies	• Reduced ICU length of stay, disease-related morbidity, and mortality
• Assist in advanced treatment directive decision making	• Avoiding unnecessarily invasive therapies and cardio-pulmonary resuscitation in patients for whom CPR is futile and undignified

strongly encouraged to limit this problem. In at least one institution the composition and method of MET activation was modified because ward staff perceived it as excessive ramp up for a minor problem.

The MET may remove senior ICU staff from their primary role, impacting on the outcomes of those patients already in the ICU. It may also distract hospital administrations and clinicians from addressing other mechanisms of improving patient outcome such as staffing levels and training, and hospital-wide policies for end of life care planning. Finally, despite the simplicity of the approach, even in hospitals with a mature MET, there is frequently delayed activation of the MET, which has been associated with increased patient mortality (see Chap. 16).

Developing alternative strategies for providing prompt and competent medical review of deteriorating ward patients appears daunting. This would require repeated education of multiple junior medical staff on multiple occasions per year. Even with such an approach, it is unlikely that ward staff would attain the competency of an ICU fellow. In addition, there would need to be a mechanism for review of deteriorating surgical patients in the event that the surgical staff were in the operating room and unable to attend. Finally, a prompt and reliable mechanism of referral to the ICU would need to be ensured.

References

1. Zajac JD. The public hospital of the future. Med J Aust. 2003;179:250–2.
2. Andrews LB, Stocking C, Krizek T, et al. An alternative strategy for studying adverse events in medical care. Lancet. 1997;349:309–13.
3. Baker GR, Norton PG, Flintoft V, et al. The Canadian adverse events study: the incidence of adverse events among hospital patients in Canada. CMAJ. 2004;170:1678–86.
4. Bellomo R, Goldsmith D, Russell S, Uchino S. Postoperative serious adverse events in a teaching hospital: a prospective study. Med J Aust. 2002;176:216–8.
5. Brennan TA, Leape LL, Laird NM, Hebert L, et al. Incidence of adverse events and negligence in hospitalized patients. Results of the Harvard medical practice study I. N Engl J Med. 1991;324:370–6.
6. Brennan TA, Leape LL, Laird NM, et al. Identification of adverse events occurring during hospitalization. A cross-sectional study of litigation, quality assurance, and medical records at two teaching hospitals. Ann Intern Med. 1990;112:221–6.
7. Davis P, Lay-Yee R, Briant R, Ali W, Scott A, Schug S. Adverse events in New Zealand public hospitals I: occurrence and impact. N Z Med J. 2002;115:U271.
8. Davis P, Lay-Yee R, Briant R, Scott A. Adverse events in New Zealand public hospitals II: preventability and clinical context. N Z Med J. 2003;116:U624.
9. Leape LL, Brennan TA, Laird NM, et al. The nature of adverse events in hospitalized patients. Results of the Harvard medical practice study II. N Engl J Med. 1991;324:377–84.
10. Schimmel E. The hazards of hospitalization. Ann Intern Med. 1964;60:100–10.
11. Thomas EJ, Studdert DM, Burstin HR, et al. Incidence and types of adverse events and negligent care in Utah and Colorado. Med Care. 2000;38:261–71.
12. Vincent C, Neale G, Woloshynowych M. Adverse events in British hospitals: preliminary retrospective record review. BMJ. 2001;322:517–9.
13. Wilson RM, Runciman WB, Gibberd RW, et al. The quality in Australian health care study. Med J Aust. 1995;163:458–71.

14. Bedell SE, Deitz DC, Leeman D, Delbanco TL. Incidence and characteristics of preventable iatrogenic cardiac arrests. JAMA. 1991;265:2815–20.

15. Hodgetts TJ, Kenward G, Vlackonikolis I, et al. Incidence, location and reasons for avoidable in-hospital cardiac arrest in a district general hospital. Resuscitation. 2002;54:115–23.

16. Buist MD, Jarmaolowski E, Burton PR, et al. Recognising clinical instability in hospital patients before cardiac arrests or unplanned admissions to intensive care. Med J Aust. 1999;171:22–5.

17. Hodgetts TJ, Kenward G, Vlackonikolis I, et al. The identification of risk factors for cardiac arrest and formulation of activation criteria to alert a medical emergency team. Resuscitation. 2002;54:125–31.

18. Nurmi J, Harjola VP, Nolan J, et al. Observations and warning signs prior to cardiac arrest. Should a medical emergency team intervene earlier? Acta Anaesthesiol Scand. 2005;49:702–6.

19. Shein RMH, Hazday N, Pena M, et al. Clinical antecedents to in-hospital cardiopulmonary arrests. Chest. 1990;98:1388–92.

20. Hayward RA, Hofer TP. Estimating hospital deaths due to medical errors: preventability is in the eye of the reviewer. JAMA. 2001;286:415–20.

21. McQuillan P, Pilkington S, Allan A, et al. Confidential inquiry into quality of care before admission to intensive care. BMJ. 1998;316:1853–8.

22. Jones DA, DeVita M, Bellomo R. Current concepts: rapid-response teams. N Engl J Med. 2011; 365:139–46.

23. Bell MD, Konrad F, Granath A, et al. Prevalence and sensitivity of MET-criteria in a scandinavian university hospital. Resuscitation. 2006;70:66–73.

24. Buist M, Bernard S, Nguren TV, et al. Association between clinically abnormal observations and subsequent in-hospital mortality: a prospective study. Resuscitation. 2004;62:137–41.

25. Goldhill DR, McNarry AF. Physiological abnormalities in early warning scores are related to mortality in adult inpatients. Br J Anaesth. 2004;92:882–4.

26. Franklin C, Mathew J. Developing strategies to prevent in hospital cardiac arrest: analyzing responses of physicians and nurses in the hours before the event. Crit Care Med. 1994;22:244–7.

27. Blow O, Magliore L, Claridge JA, et al. The golden hour and the silver day: detection and correction of occult hypoperfusion within 24 hours improves outcome from major trauma. J Trauma. 1999;47:964–9.

28. Zubert S, Funk DJ, Kumar A. Antibiotics in sepsis and septic shock: like everything else in life, timing is everything. Crit Care Med. 2010;38:1211–2.

29. Fresco C, Carinci F, Maggioni AP, et al. Very early assessment of risk for in-hospital death among 11,483 patients with acute myocardial infarction. GISSI investigators. Am Heart J. 1999;138:1058–64.

30. The National Institute for Neurological Disorders and Stoke rt-PA Stroke Study Group. Tissue plasminogen activator for acute ischemic stroke. N Engl J Med. 1995;333:1581–7.

31. DeVita MA, Bellomo R, Hillman K, et al. Findings of the first consensus conference on medical emergency teams. Crit Care Med. 2006;34:2463–78.

32. The ANZICS CORE MET dose Investigators. Rapid response team composition, resourcing and calling criteria in Australia. Resuscitation. 2012;83:563–7.

33. Ludikhuize J, Hamming A, de Jonge E, Fikkers BG. Rapid response systems in the Netherlands. Jt Comm J Qual Patient Saf. 2011;37:138–44.

34. Jacques T, Harrison GA, McLaws ML. Attitudes towards and evaluation of medical emergency teams: a survey of trainees in intensive care medicine. Anaesth Intensive Care. 2008;36:90–5.

35. Lee A, Bishop G, Hillman KM, Daffurn K. The medical emergency team. Anaesth Intensive Care. 1995;23:183–6.

36. Jones D, Mitra B, Barbetti J, et al. Increasing the use of an existing medical emergency team in a teaching hospital. Anaesth Intensive Care. 2006;34:731–5.

37. Bellomo R, Goldsmith D, Uchino S, Buckmaster J, et al. Prospective controlled trial of effect of medical emergency team postoperative morbidity and mortality rates. Crit Care Med. 2004;32:916–21.

38. Bellomo R, Goldsmith D, Uchino S, et al. A prospective before-and-after trial of a medical emergency team. Med J Aust. 2003;179:283–7.

39. England K, Bion JF. Introduction of medical emergency teams in Australia and New Zealand: a multicentre study. Crit Care. 2008;12:151.

40. Jones D, Duke G, Green J, et al. Medical Emergency Team syndromes and an approach to their management. Crit Care. 2006;10:R30.

41. Jones D. The epidemiology of adult Rapid Response Team patients in Australia. Anaesth Intensive Care. 2014;42:213–9.

42. Cross G, Bilgrami I, Eastwood G, et al. The epidemiology of sepsis during rapid response team reviews in a teaching hospital. Anaesth Intensive Care. 2015;43:193–8.

43. Jones DA, Bagshaw SM, Barrett J, et al. The role of the Medical emergency team in end of life care: a multicenter, prospective, observational study. Crit Care Med. 2012;40:98–103.

44. Jones D, Moran J, Winters B, Welch J. The rapid response system and end-of-life care. Curr Opin Crit Care. 2013;19:616–23.

45. Tan LH, Delaney A. Medical emergency teams and end-of-life care: a systematic review. Crit Care Resusc. 2014;16:62–8.

46. Schneider A, Calzavacca P, Mercer I, et al. The epidemiology and outcome of medical emergency team call patient treated with non-invasive ventilation. Resuscitation. 2011;82:1218–23.

47. Schneider A, Calzavacca P, Jones D, Bellomo R. Epidemiology and patient outcome after medical emergency team calls triggered by atrial fibrillation. Resuscitation. 2011;82:410–4.

48. Jones DA, Baldwin I, McIntyre T, et al. Nurses' attitudes to a medical emergency team service in a teaching hospital. Qual Saf Health Care. 2006;15:427–32.

49. Bagshaw SM, Mondor EE, Scouten C, Capital Health Medical Emergency Team Investigators, et al. A survey of nurses' beliefs about the medical emergency team system in a Canadian tertiary hospital. Am J Crit Care. 2010;19:74–83.

50. Winters BD, Weaver SJ, PFoh ER, Yang T, Pham JC, Dy SM. Rapid response systems as a patient safety strategy. Ann Intern Med. 2013;158:417–25.

51. Chan PS, Jain R, Nallmothu BK, et al. Rapid response teams. A systematic review and meta-analysis. Arch Intern Med. 2010;170:18–26.

Pediatric RRSs

Christopher P. Bonafide, Patrick W. Brady,
James Tibballs, and Richard J. Brilli

Introduction

Cardiac arrest in hospitalized children is uncommon, but the outcome is often poor, despite expert resuscitation. For example, in two large series of outcomes, only 24% of 544 children [1] and 27% of 880 children [2] experiencing cardiac arrest survived to hospital discharge. In the latter study 34% of the survivors had severe neurological dysfunction. In smaller contemporaneous single hospital series, survival at 1 year was 34% [3], 19% [4], and 15% [5].

Revised for 2nd Edition by Bonafide and Brady.
Original author of 1st Edition are Tibballs and Brilli.

C.P. Bonafide, MD, MSCE (✉)
Perelman School of Medicine at the University of
Pennsylvania, The Children's Hospital of
Philadelphia, 3401 Civic Center Boulevard, Room
12NW80, Philadelphia, PA 19104, USA
e-mail: bonafide@email.chop.edu

P.W. Brady, MD, MSc
University of Cincinnati College of Medicine,
Cincinnati Children's Hospital Medical Center,
Cincinnati, OH, USA

J. Tibballs, MD, MBA, MEd
Royal Children's Hospital, Melbourne, VIC, Australia

R.J. Brilli, MD, FCCM, FAAP
Nationwide Children's Hospital, Columbus, OH, USA

Cardiac arrest and life-threatening critical illness in children, as in adults, are usually preceded by warning signs and symptoms [6]. Uncommonly cardiac arrest in children may be sudden and without warning; it is more often due to progressive respiratory failure, hypotension, or both, resulting from diverse illnesses. With earlier recognition of the severity of a deteriorating condition, it may be possible to intervene and prevent cardiopulmonary arrest and death.

Hospitals and healthcare systems throughout the world have adopted various strategies to recognize critical illness and to mobilize early assistance with the aim of preventing cardiopulmonary arrest. These interventions fit within systems approaches to reducing adverse events in hospitals. The principles described for adult patient systems elsewhere in this volume apply equally to systems for children.

This chapter describes the characteristics of pediatric rapid response systems (RRSs), recognition of critical illness on general inpatient units, and the outcomes following implementation of RRSs. Although various systems solutions have been adopted, all have the common themes of early recognition of acute illness outside the ICU and a triggered therapeutic response with follow-up.

Structure of Pediatric Rapid Response Systems

The general structure of pediatric RRSs is the same as in adults, consisting of four main components: two clinical components (the afferent and efferent limbs) and two organizational components (the process improvement and administrative limbs). In this chapter we will focus on the unique aspects within each of these components that distinguish pediatric from adult systems.

The Afferent Limb of Pediatric Rapid Response Systems

If children at risk for cardiopulmonary arrest can be identified, more resources and effort can be devoted to their care in order to prevent respiratory or cardiac arrest. The afferent limb of RRSs focuses on identifying patients at high risk of cardiopulmonary arrest or its immediate antecedents so that an appropriate response can be triggered. The vast majority of the research in this area has focused on detecting early indicators that deterioration is beginning to occur, often using vital signs, laboratory studies, and other observations that may change rapidly over time. The goal is to detect deterioration early in order to prevent life-threatening events.

A wide range of schema have been developed to alert the medical and nursing staff that a patient is deteriorating and may be at risk for cardiopulmonary arrest. Two general approaches have been developed. They are not mutually exclusive.

Single-Parameter Calling Criteria

One approach is to specify individual triggers or calling criteria to activate the RRS. In contrast to adult RRSs, pediatric systems are faced with the problem of adjusting the trigger or calling criteria according to different patient ages, which translate to vastly different normal, or expected values of vital signs [7, 8]. Many institutions have chosen age-based values for heart rate, blood pressure, and respiratory rate to reflect this variation

Table 19.1 Criteria for activation of medical emergency team from Royal Children's Hospital, Melbourne

Any one or more of:		
1. Nurse, doctor, or parent *worried* about clinical state		
2. Airway threat		
3. Hypoxemia	SpO$_2$ <90% in any amount of oxygen	
	SpO$_2$ <60% in any amount of oxygen (cyanotic heart disease)	
4. Severe respiratory distress, apnea, or cyanosis		
5. Tachypnea		
	Age	Respiratory rate/min
	Term 3 months	>60
	4–12 months	>50
	1–4 years	>40
	5–12 years	>30
	12 years+	>30
6. Tachycardia or bradycardia		
Age	Bradycardia beats/min	Tachycardia beats/min
Term 3 months	<100	>180
4–12 months	<100	>180
1–4 years	<90	>160
5–12 years	<80	>140
12 years+	<60	>130
7. Hypotension		
	Age	BP (systolic mmHg)
	Term 3 months	<50
	4–12 months	<60
	1–4 years	<70
	5–12 years	<80
	12 years+	<90
8. Acute change in neurological status or convulsion		
9. Cardiac or respiratory arrest		

(example in Table 19.1). Calling criteria also often include the option for a clinician to activate the team because they are worried, even if other calling criteria are not met. In addition, some hospitals have empowered parents to activate the team, a topic we will discuss later in this chapter.

To date, none of the pediatric triggers or calling criteria have been evaluated to determine their sensitivity and specificity for cardiac arrest due to the infrequency of events outside the ICU setting. Brilli and colleagues (2007) attempted to identify reliable activation triggers from over one thousand combinations of pre-arrest variables derived from previous codes but were unable to do so with sufficient sensitivity and specificity [9]. Instead, they chose criteria based on chart analysis and expert opinion. The evidence supporting single age-based vital sign parameters as activation criteria is very limited, and this is reflected in the differences in parameter cut points across studies [9–15].

Multiparameter Early Warning Scores

Development of pediatric early warning scores that use combinations of criteria to generate scores intended to detect clinical deterioration may help improve the system of identifying the child at risk of cardiopulmonary arrest. The scores are compilations of points attributed to various physiological abnormalities. Two scoring systems, the Paediatric Early Warning Score (PEWS) developed in the United Kingdom and the Bedside Paediatric Early Warning System Score (Bedside PEWS) developed in Canada, are the most commonly used and thoroughly evaluated to date.

The first PEWS was developed by Monaghan at Royal Alexandra Children's Hospital in Brighton (UK) [16]. The score was based on three types of variables: behavioral (e.g., playing, lethargic), cardiovascular (skin color, capillary refill, and heart rate), and respiratory parameters (chest wall retractions and relationship to normal respiratory rate). Additional scoring points are added according to treatment such as need for added oxygen and nebulizers. The summed score was associated with a color that indicated a suggested response by the team at the bedside. Depending on the score's indicated severity of illness, the nurse actions would be to inform the nurse in charge, increase the frequency of observations, call for a medical review, or call the critical care outreach team.

Since the original report by Monaghan, two studies have evaluated PEWS. In the first, Tucker and others (2008) [17] at Cincinnati Children's Hospital (US) evaluated an adapted version of Monaghan's PEWS among children admitted to a single medical unit over a 12-month period [17]. The outcome measure was the need to transfer a patient to the PICU as a substitute for cardiac arrest. Fifty-one patients needed admission to PICU, and there was a significant association between this outcome and the highest PEWS the patient had during hospitalization. The test characteristics were excellent. However, the study was limited because the score was calculated as part of clinical care and as such may have directly influenced decision-making to transfer the patient to the ICU, which would make the score's performance appear better than if the score had been assessed independent of the clinical care decisions.

A second study by Akre evaluated the PEWS in a case series of patients who required assistance from an MET or code blue team at Children's Hospitals and Clinics of Minnesota (US) [18]. At the score cut point they selected, the PEWS had a sensitivity of 86%. Neither the specificity nor any other test characteristics were reported, making the implications of this result for clinical care unclear.

The most rigorously evaluated pediatric early warning score is the Bedside PEWS, developed at the Hospital for Sick Children at Toronto, Canada. Originally published in 2006 [19], the score has been successively refined [20, 21]. The score was initially created using expert opinion and consensus methods. The most recent iteration of the score has seven items, including heart rate, systolic blood pressure, capillary refill time, respiratory rate, respiratory effort, oxygen therapy, and oxygen saturation (Table 19.2). Bedside PEWS has performed well in multiple retrospective studies, including a multicenter validation. [20, 21] At the score cut point they selected, the sensitivity was 64%, and the specificity was 91%. The positive predictive value was estimated at 9% assuming a baseline clinical deterioration rate of 10 per 1000 patient-days.

The Bedside PEWS is currently being evaluated in the Evaluating Processes of Care and the Outcomes of Children in Hospital (EPOCH) study [22]. EPOCH is measuring the impact of Bedside PEWS implementation on mortality, cardiac arrest rates, and processes of care among

Table 19.2 The Bedside PEWS tool. The total score is calculated as the sum of the sub-scores from each of the items (Reprinted from Parshuram CS, Duncan HP, Joffe AR, et al. Multi-centre validation of the Bedside Paediatric Early Warning System Score: a severity of illness score to detect evolving critical illness in hospitalized children. Crit Care. 2011;15(4):R184). This open access article was distributed under the terms of the Creative Commons Attribution License (http://creativecommons.org/licenses/by/2.0), which permits unrestricted use, distribution, and reproduction in any medium, provided the original work is properly cited

Item	Item sub-score				
	Age group	0	1	2	4
Heart rate	0–<3 months	>110 and<150	≥ 150 or ≤ 110	≥ 180 or ≤ 90	≥190 or ≤ 80
	3–<12 months	>100 and <150	≥150 or ≤ 100	≥ 170 or ≤ 80	≥180 or ≤ 70
	1–4 years	>90 and <120	≥120 or ≤ 90	≥150 or ≤ 70	≥170 or ≤ 60
	>4–12 years	>70 and <110	≥110 or ≤ 70	≥130 or ≤ 60	≥150 or ≤ 50
	>12 years	>60 and < 100	≥100 or ≤ 60	≥120 or ≤ 50	≥140 or ≤ 40
Systolic blood pressure	0–<3 months	> 60 and < 80	≥ 80 or ≤ 60	≥ 100 or ≤ 50	≥ 130 or ≤ 45
	3–<12 months	>80 and < 100	≥100 or ≤ 80	≥120 or ≤ 70	≥150 or ≤ 60
	1–4 years	>90 and < 110	≥110 or ≤ 90	≥125 or ≤ 75	≥160 or ≤ 65
	>4–12 years	>90 and < 120	≥120 or ≤ 90	≥140 or ≤ 80	≥170 or ≤ 70
	>12 years	>100 and <130	≥130 or ≤ 100	≥150 or ≤85	≥190 or ≤ 75
Capillary refill time		<3 s			≥3 s
Respiratory rate	0–<3 months	>29 and < 61	≥ 61 or ≤ 29	≥ 81 or ≤ 19	≥ 91 or ≤ 15
	3–<12 months	>24 or < 51	≥51 or ≤ 24	≥71 or ≤ 19	≥81 or ≤ 15
	1–4 years	>19 or < 41	≥41 or ≤ 19	≥ 61 or ≤ 15	≥71 or ≤ 12
	>4–12 years	>19 or < 31	≥31 or ≤ 19	≥41 or ≤ 14	≥51 or ≤ 10
	>12 years	>11 or < 17	≥ 17 or ≤ 11	≥ 23 or ≤ 10	≥30 or ≤ 9
Respiratory effort		Normal	Mild increase	Moderate increase	Severe increase/any apnea
Saturation %		>94	91–94	≤90	
Oxygen therapy		Room air		Any – <4 L/min or <50%	≥4 L/min or ≥ 50%

children hospitalized outside ICU settings in a prospective, cluster randomized trial. The results of this trial are of great interest to the pediatric RRS community because it will be by far the most thorough evaluation of any afferent tool for detecting pediatric deterioration.

Multiparameter early warning scores have the potential to identify early deterioration in children. More research in this area is needed, however, in order to determine the best mechanisms to trigger activation of the efferent arm.

Family Activation

In recent years hospitals and RRS leadership have developed an interest in engaging families in the afferent arm of RRSs, either by participating in the decision-making with the clinical team or by activating the medical emergency team directly. In pediatrics, much of this interest seems to have stemmed from the Josie King story. Josie was a toddler who was hospitalized in 2001 for burn injuries from climbing into a hot bath. During her hospitalization, just days before she was planned for discharge, she deteriorated and died. Her death was attributed in part to critical delays in escalation of Josie's care despite her family's persistently verbalized concern [23].

In the wake of Josie King's death, numerous hospitals initiated programs that enable families to directly activate multidisciplinary immediate response teams to their child's bedside when they detect concerning changes in their child [24–26] or adult relative's [27–31] condition. Since deterioration is so uncommon on regular inpatient units and the proportion of deterioration events when families activate is very small, it is difficult to determine if family activation is an effective intervention. Combining pediatric with adult data, we know that the calls that do occur are usually requests to address communication and coordination issues between patients and providers [24, 27, 30, 31] and perceived delays in care [28]. In 6.25 hospital-years described across seven published reports that provided call outcomes, 6 of 117 family activations (5%) required critical interventions and/or transfer to a higher level of care [24–28, 30, 31]. This is generally viewed as a success, although there are certainly opportunities to explore how to help families better identify deterioration and feel empowered to call for help if necessary. Implementation of family activation likely has other benefits; one study among adults found that, while families called rarely, rates of staff calling the MET increased fourfold, suggesting that the implementation may have indirectly improved safety by facilitating conversations about deterioration between staff and families [29].

One issue that has been raised is that simply enabling families to directly activate an MET may not be the best method for families to participate in the monitoring of their hospitalized children. In addition, there may be complex unintended consequences, including misuse of the MET, inappropriately asking parents to make assessments without clinical training, undermining therapeutic relationships, and burdening families [32]. Future research in this area should focus on finding new ways to improve shared decision-making between families and clinicians in the care of hospitalized children at risk of deterioration, capitalizing upon the strengths of families in recognizing changes from their child's baseline and the expertise of clinicians in identifying the need for intensive care.

The Efferent Limb of Pediatric Rapid Response Systems

Once patients experiencing deterioration have been identified, the next step is to bring the appropriate expertise to the bedside to rapidly assess, triage, and treat the patient in collaboration with the primary team. While conventional "code blue" teams that respond to patients with existing cardiac or respiratory arrest are technically included in the efferent limb, for the purposes of this textbook, we will focus on the teams that are available to respond to deteriorating patients who have not yet arrested. The aim of these teams is to rapidly intervene and prevent further deterioration, including cardiac or respiratory arrest.

Like adult-oriented systems, the efferent component of pediatric RRSs comes in a few different models, and each model has a classical definition that is not universally adhered to, but is worth mentioning. Medical emergency teams (METs) are composed typically of doctors and nurses. Rapid response teams (RRTs) are composed of either doctors and nurses or nurses alone. Critical care outreach teams (CCOTs) and patient-at-risk teams (PARTs) are usually composed of nurses alone but with rapid access to physician assistance. In this chapter, we will use "MET" to refer broadly to all of these efferent models.

Single-Tier vs. Two-Tiered Response Systems

Two different strategies have been adopted regarding the urgency of responding to a request for expert assistance. Some pediatric institutions consider a request for assistance as needing the same urgent response as the code blue team would provide for a cardiac or respiratory arrest. These are single tier systems. These teams are multidisciplinary including physicians, nurses, respiratory therapists, pharmacy personnel, security, social service, and sometimes surgeons. Other institutions have adopted a two-tiered system in which two response options are available depending on the urgency and severity of the patient's condition. The first tier is a small focused team that often serves in a consultative role and is not required to drop everything and run to the bedside immediately but must do so within a specified period, e.g., within 30 min [33].

The second tier is a larger multidisciplinary team that usually also functions as a code blue team and must respond immediately.

There are advantages and disadvantages to both single tier and two-tiered efferent systems. Advantages of the single-tier system include (1) quick provision of definitive care and (2) provision of all services, from administering a fluid bolus and supplemental oxygen all the way to cardiopulmonary resuscitation and defibrillation. Disadvantages of the single-tier system include (1) requiring a large group of highly skilled personnel, (2) intimidating barrier for staff to call the team for a consultation or evaluation, and (3) potential costs—financial as well as opportunity costs—that come from pulling expert staff away from the patients they are directly caring for in intensive care units and other areas. In contrast, the first tier of a two-tiered system may be less costly and less intimidating for clinical staff to activate when consultation and advice are sought. However, in the two-tiered system it is also possible that the initial smaller more focused team will be inappropriately called in a genuine life-threatening emergency which its members are under-skilled to handle. If clinicians on the wards will activate the less intimidating first tier for true life-threatening emergencies such as circulatory shock that merit an immediate response, a 30-min wait might allow a patient to continue deteriorating, introducing additional risk. Each institution must balance the advantages and disadvantages of the two systems because the personnel who respond and their other clinical commitments will be quite different.

Proactive Liaison or Rover Teams

Some institutions utilize liaison or "rover" teams whose tasks are to help colleagues proactively identify children with critical illness on wards before the need for an MET activation. At Duke University Children's Hospital and Health Center, the rover team is composed of the same team members as the hospital's MET: a pediatric critical care nurse practitioner or fellow, the PICU charge nurse, and a PICU respiratory therapist [34].

The team roves about the hospital in a systematic way, making scheduled stops at each of the intermediate care areas. They discuss any patients at risk of deterioration identified by each ward's charge nurse and on call senior resident. The team also evaluates all children who were discharged from the PICU in the preceding 12 h and all new admissions to the progressive care unit.

Safety Huddles

A second mechanism to more effectively and proactively identify at-risk patients is through scheduled safety huddles. Huddles are short, structured briefings that in this context are used to identify patients that may benefit from extra attention including the MET. At Cincinnati Children's Hospital Medical Center, three-times daily safety huddles were tested and implemented to improve situation awareness and reduce unrecognized clinical deterioration [35]. Charge nurses from each unit reported out on patients with elevated EWS or other safety concerns, and a senior nurse and pediatrician provided coaching on communication, developing treatment plans, and parameters that, when exceeded, would result in a MET call. Huddles were part of a complex intervention associated with reductions in unrecognized clinical deterioration and an increased sense of collaboration among attendees [35, 36].

Impacts of Pediatric Medical Emergency Team Implementation

METs have been the most widely researched aspect of pediatric RRSs. The most relevant studies describing the clinical impacts associated with implementation of METs or, in some cases, comprehensive RRSs with robust afferent components are summarized in Table 19.3. All have been quasi-experimental before-and-after studies, i.e., evaluating the incidence of outcomes like cardiac arrest and death before and after the introduction of a RRS, and the analytic rigor of the studies varies widely. Several have shown gratifying improvements in patient outcomes.

Table 19.3 Quasi-experimental studies of pediatric rapid response system implementation

Publication	Study period	Number of centers	Intervention	Number of response tiers	MET responders	Main findings
Brilli et al. 2007 [9]	2003–2006	1	MET + CC	2	• PICU fellow • Resident • PICU nurse • Respiratory therapist • Nursing supervisor	Significant reduction in combined respiratory and cardiac arrests outside ICU
Sharek et al. 2007 [13]	2001–2007	1	MET + CC	1	• PICU attending or fellow • PICU nurse • Respiratory therapist • Nursing supervisor	Significant reductions in combined respiratory and cardiac arrests outside ICU and hospital-wide mortality
Zenker et al. 2007 [15]	2004–2006	1	MET	2	• PICU nurse • Respiratory therapist	Nonsignificant reductions in combined rate of respiratory and cardiac arrests outside ICU
Hunt et al. 2008 [11]	2003–2005	1	MET + CC	1	• PICU fellow • Three residents • PICU nurse • Respiratory therapist • Nursing supervisor • Pharmacist	Significant reduction in respiratory arrests outside ICU
Tibballs et al. 2009 [14]	1999–2006	1	MET + CC	1	• PICU consultant or registrar • PICU nurse • Emergency department physician • Emergency department registrar	Significant reductions in hospital-wide mortality, hospital ward unexpected deaths, hospital ward preventable cardiac arrests, mortality from preventable hospital ward cardiac arrests
Hanson et al. 2010 [10]	2003–2007	1	MET + CC	1	• PICU fellow • Resident • PICU nurse • Respiratory therapist	Significant increase in the mean number of patient days between ward cardiac arrests, nonsignificant reductions in ward death, and cardiac arrest rates
Kotsakis et al. 2011 [12]	2004–2009	4	MET + CC	2	• PICU attending and/or fellow and/ or resident • PICU nurse • Respiratory therapist	Significant reduction in mortality rate among patients readmitted to PICU within 48 h of being discharged
Bonafide et al. 2014 [33]	2007–2012	1	MET + CC + EWS	2	• PICU fellow or nurse practitioner • PICU nurse • Respiratory therapist	Significant downward change in the preintervention trajectory of critical deterioration, 62% net decrease in critical deterioration relative to the preintervention trend, nonsignificant reductions in ward cardiac arrests, and deaths during ward emergencies

Abbreviations: *CC* calling criteria, *EWS* early warning score, *ICU* intensive care unit, *MET* medical emergency team

A meta-analysis published in 2010 showed an overall 38% reduction in cardiopulmonary arrest rates outside the ICU and a 21% reduction in hospital mortality rates associated with pediatric MET implementation [37]. However, the authors of the meta-analysis raised questions about the mechanistic plausibility of the MET intervention actually being responsible for the changes in all-hospital mortality (which presumably includes deaths in patients who were never eligible to be saved by an MET). A large cluster randomized trial remains highly desirable to sort out the effects of RRS implementation [38], but, given the diffusion of RRSs throughout the world, it is unlikely to be feasible.

Process Improvement

How to Best Measure the Impact?

Defining and measuring the success of an RRS implementation are more challenging than might be immediately apparent. Many of the outcomes we care about most are exceedingly rare in pediatrics, with cardiac and respiratory arrests averaging fewer than ten events per hospital per year in a large group of children's hospitals [39]. While no one would argue that these events should not still be measured, it is unlikely that these events will show statistically significant change over the short periods of time during which a single institution will seek to measure improvement.

To augment these important but rare outcome measures, two proximate outcome measures have emerged. These outcomes occur more frequently than arrests and deaths and thus can be used to measure improvement over shorter periods of time.

Critical deterioration events are defined as ICU transfers with noninvasive ventilation, intubation, or vasopressor infusion initiated in the 12 h following arrival in the ICU [40]. This measure was associated with a >13-fold risk of mortality and occurred more than eight times more commonly that arrests outside the ICU. It was also used as the primary outcome measure in a

recent quasi-experimental study of the impacts of RRS implementation [33]. The other proximate measure, UNrecognized Situation Awareness Failure Events (UNSAFE) transfers, is defined as ward to ICU transfers after which patients are intubated, placed on vasopressors, or receive three or more fluid boluses in the first one hour after transfer. An intervention designed to improve the afferent arm of the RRS has been associated with a significant and sustained reduction in UNSAFE transfers at one center [35].

Process of care measures are also useful for monitoring and improving the RRS. Commonly tracked process measures include the rate of MET calls per week or month and the percentage of METs that result in transfer to an ICU. The rate of MET calls, particularly when stratified by unit, is important both in assessing how well the afferent limb is functioning (e.g., a nursing ward with no MET calls for a several month period likely has a poor afferent limb or a culture that does not support MET calls) and in ensuring the MET is adequately staffed. A low "dose" of MET calls is associated with smaller reductions in cardiac arrests in adult MET studies [41]. The percentage of MET calls transferred to the ICU can also be useful in assessing if the RRS is functioning as intended. In our two tertiary care hospitals with mature RRSs, we have found that 50–60% of MET calls are transferred to the ICU (unpublished data). A much higher percentage than this may raise concern that the MET is being under-called, and a substantially lower percentage may serve as reason to examine if the MET is not being overcalled and/or not escalating care when appropriate.

Cost is an important but little studied balancing measure. The costs of a RRS include the financial cost of the team members' time and the opportunity cost of bringing critical care clinicians from the ICU to the floor. If team members also participate in direct care in the ICU, it is conceivable, although unproven, that the patients in the ICU would receive less attention. One study has examined the financial costs of a pediatric MET. A research team at the Children's Hospital of Philadelphia found that critical deterioration events cost almost $100,000 in each instance and that an MET comprised of a nurse, respiratory therapist, and ICU fellow with concurrent responsibilities would need to prevent only 3.5 critical deterioration events per year to recoup its cost [42].

Using Qualitative Methods to Better Understand Barriers to Optimal RRS Function

An important question to ask frequently is "What isn't working well and what could we do to optimize the system?" Two studies have reported barriers to recognizing deteriorating patients and delivering effective, appropriate care to those patients, with a focus on MET activation. Both studies used qualitative methods. In the first, researchers at Cincinnati Children's Hospital Medical Center explored facilitators and barriers to identifying, mitigating, and escalating the recognition of patient risk from the perspectives of nurses, respiratory therapists, and resident physicians [43]. Three themes and supporting subthemes emerged, highlighting key facilitators including (1) team-based care that empowered nurses and families and supported a culture of teamwork, accountability, and safety; (2) availability of standardized data including an EWS and tools for displaying and monitoring data and data trends; and (3) standardized processes and procedures at the organizational level including proper education and training on recognizing critical illness, a shared language around at-risk patients, and structure to proactively support risk identification, handoffs, and workload/staffing. Each focus group noted value in scheduled multidisciplinary huddles or briefings to identify at-risk patients and form treatment plans. In the second study, researchers at The Children's Hospital of Philadelphia interviewed nurses and physicians about barriers to calling for urgent assistance that existed despite the hospital having recently implemented a comprehensive RRS. The most important themes identified were that (1) self-efficacy, both in terms of (a) recognizing deterioration and (b) activating the MET, was a strong determinant of whether care would be

appropriately escalated for deteriorating children, (2) intraprofessional and interprofessional hierarchies could be challenging to navigate and lead to delays in care, and (3) expectations of adverse interpersonal or clinical outcomes from MET activations and ICU transfers could lead to a reluctance among physicians to transfer patients to the ICU for fear of inappropriate (or at least different) management.

The facilitators and barriers identified in these two studies provide useful data for institutions to consider when aiming to optimize their RRS.

Rapid Response System Administration

Meaningful adoption of an RRS is a cultural change which must overcome many of the barriers discussed above. Like any institutional change, it will not be successful without the full support of senior hospital management whose influence is particularly important in facilitating communication between disciplines and departments. An effective afferent limb requires empowered junior nurses and doctors. These clinicians, as well as parents of children, must be able to summon help without deferring to senior colleagues. Traditional medical hierarchy is a powerful barrier to change. Junior personnel are not accustomed to questioning senior physician staff or even nurses questioning physicians. Hospital leadership can help the RRS and its administrative team to succeed by endorsing that unexpected and preventable death can be reduced by the use of an RRS. In our experience the RRS leadership team can address culture concerns by messaging stories of successful RRS calls and noting that the system requires the skills of the activating and responding team. A multidisciplinary group of personnel (physicians, nurses, respiratory therapist, physiotherapists, managers) should oversee, regularly review, and provide feedback to hospital leadership and clinical staff regarding: (1) the effectiveness and usability of afferent tools such as early warning scores, (2) the response mechanisms and roles of the efferent response (usually an MET) and how they might evolve over time to meet the needs of patients and to align with institutional goals (e.g., sepsis reduction), and (3) the overall effectiveness of the RRS using quantitative patient outcome data and qualitative data from staff and families, including proactively identifying any unintended adverse consequences. Further improvements in outcomes may relate to better skills of frontline nurses and doctors in recognizing critical illness and overcoming RRS activation barriers. Team composition, active surveillance of patients, factors related to willingness to activate the system, and determination of preventability of adverse events are likely all factors that determine the success of RRSs, and research is needed to identify how best to configure these components to optimize hospital safety. An institutional culture wherein all staff members are comfortable calling for advice and help without fear of recrimination or embarrassment for being wrong in their assessment of the situation also likely contributes to the success of an RRS. Indeed, one may argue that irrespective of timely recognition of critical illness, the biggest challenge to RRS implementation and effectiveness is the reluctance to activate the system.

Availability of Rapid Response Systems in Hospitals that Care for Children

Although RRSs have been the subject of discussion and debate in adult hospitals for many years, the uptake of these systems in hospitals that care for children has only recently taken off. In North America, in 2005, all of the 181 hospitals with more than 50 acute pediatric beds had an immediate-response code blue team for patients with cardiac or respiratory arrest, but only 17% had an MET that responded to children with early signs of potential clinical deterioration [44]. These METs were also often only available during the daytime. In just 21% of the hospitals with METs, discrete calling criteria were used to determine when to activate the team. [44]. Similarly, in 2005 in the UK, only 22% of 144 hospitals caring for children had an early warning

system to identify patients at risk of physiological deterioration. [45]

Since 2005, dissemination of RRSs was rapid and extensive. A recent study of 130 US children's hospitals with pediatric ICUs in 2010 found that 79% had an MET, most of which had been implemented in the preceding 5 years [46]. Of those hospitals with an MET, 34% had predetermined activation triggers based on vital signs or overall clinical status. In 69%, families could activate the team. The most recent study on this subject, completed in 2012, surveyed 30 academic US pediatric hospitals and found that 100% had 24 h/day, 7 days/week MET availability [47]. Half of the hospitals used an early warning score to activate the team, and family activation was available in 77%.

Summary

Rapid response systems have now been implemented widely at pediatric hospitals throughout the world. While some controversy still occasionally emerges, the systems are now widely regarded to be effective and cost-efficient. Numerous research questions must be addressed, however, in order to determine how to optimize both the afferent mechanisms used to identify deteriorating patients and the efferent mechanisms used to rapidly triage and manage them.

References

1. Young KD, Seidel JS. Pediatric cardiopulmonary resuscitation: a collective review. Ann Emerg Med. 1999;33(2):195–205.
2. Nadkarni VM, Larkin GL, Peberdy MA, Carey SM, Kaye W, Mancini ME, et al. First documented rhythm and clinical outcome from in-hospital cardiac arrest among children and adults. JAMA. 2006;295:50–7.
3. Tibballs J, Kinney S. A prospective study of outcome of in-patient paediatric cardiopulmonary arrest. Resuscitation. 2006;71(3):310–8.
4. Suominen P, Olkkola KT, Voipio V, Korpela R, Palo R, Räsänen J. Utstein style reporting of in-hospital paediatric cardiopulmonary resuscitation. Resuscitation. 2000;45(1):17–25.
5. Reis AG, Nadkarni V, Perondi MB, Grisi S, Berg RA. A prospective investigation into the epidemiology of

in-hospital pediatric cardiopulmonary resuscitation using the international Utstein reporting style. Pediatrics. 2002;109(2):200–9.

6. McQuillan P, Pilkington S, Allan A, Taylor B, Short A, Morgan G, et al. Confidential inquiry into quality of care before admission to intensive care. BMJ. 1998;316:1853–8.

7. Fleming S, Thompson M, Stevens R, Heneghan C, Pluddemann A, Maconochie I, et al. Normal ranges of heart rate and respiratory rate in children from birth to 18 years of age: a systematic review of observational studies. Lancet. 2011;377(9770):1011–8.

8. Bonafide CP, Brady PW, Keren R, Conway PH, Marsolo K, Daymont C. Development of heart and respiratory rate percentile curves for hospitalized children. Pediatrics. 2013;131:e1150–7.

9. Brilli RJ, Gibson R, Luria JW, Wheeler TA, Shaw J, Linam M, et al. Implementation of a medical emergency team in a large pediatric teaching hospital prevents respiratory and cardiopulmonary arrests outside the intensive care unit. Pediatr Crit Care Med. 2007;8:236–46.

10. Hanson CC, Randolph GD, Erickson JA, Mayer CM, Bruckel JT, Harris BD, et al. A reduction in cardiac arrests and duration of clinical instability after implementation of a paediatric rapid response system. Postgrad Med J. 2010;86:314–8.

11. Hunt EA, Zimmer KP, Rinke ML, Shilkofski NA, Matlin C, Garger C, et al. Transition from a traditional code team to a medical emergency team and categorization of cardiopulmonary arrests in a children's center. Arch Pediatr Adolesc Med. 2008;162:117–22.

12. Kotsakis A, Lobos A-T, Parshuram C, Gilleland J, Gaiteiro R, Mohseni-Bod H, et al. Implementation of a multicenter rapid response system in pediatric academic hospitals is effective. Pediatrics. 2011;128:72–8.

13. Sharek PJ, Parast LM, Leong K, Coombs J, Earnest K, Sullivan J, et al. Effect of a rapid response team on hospital-wide mortality and code rates outside the ICU in a children's hospital. JAMA. 2007;298:2267–74.

14. Tibballs J, Kinney S. Reduction of hospital mortality and of preventable cardiac arrest and death on introduction of a pediatric medical emergency team. Pediatr Crit Care Med. 2009;10:306–12.

15. Zenker P, Schlesinger A, Hauck M, Spencer S, Hellmich T, Finkelstein M, et al. Implementation and impact of a rapid response team in a children's hospital. Jt Comm J Qual Patient Saf. 2007;33:418–25.

16. Monaghan A. Detecting and managing deterioration in children. Paediatr Nurs. 2005;17:32–5.

17. Tucker KM, Brewer TL, Baker RB, Demeritt B, Vossmeyer MT. Prospective evaluation of a pediatric inpatient early warning scoring system. J Spec Pediatr Nurs. 2009;14:79–85.

18. Akre M, Finkelstein M, Erickson M, Liu M, Vanderbilt L, Billman G. Sensitivity of the pediatric early warning score to identify patient deterioration. Pediatrics. 2010;125:e763–9.

19. Duncan H, Hutchison J, Parshuram CS. The Pediatric Early Warning System Score: a severity of illness score to predict urgent medical need in hospitalized children. J Crit Care. 2006;21:271–8.

20. Parshuram CS, Hutchison J, Middaugh K. Development and initial validation of the Bedside Paediatric Early Warning System score. Crit Care. 2009;13:R135.

21. Parshuram CS, Duncan HP, Joffe AR, Farrell CA, Lacroix JR, Middaugh KL, et al. Multi-centre validation of the Bedside Paediatric Early Warning System Score: a severity of illness score to detect evolving critical illness in hospitalized children. Crit Care. 2011;15:R184.

22. The Hospital for Sick Children. Evaluating Processes of Care & the Outcomes of Children in Hospital (EPOCH) [Internet]. Available from: http://clinicaltrials.gov/show/NCT01260831.

23. King S. Our story. Pediatr Radiol. 2006;36:284–6.

24. Dean BS, Decker MJ, Hupp D, Urbach AH, Lewis E, Benes-Stickle J. Condition HELP: a pediatric rapid response team triggered by patients and parents. J Healthc Qual. 2008;30:28–31.

25. Hueckel RM, Mericle JM, Frush K, Martin PL, Champagne MT. Implementation of Condition Help: family teaching and evaluation of family understanding. J Nurs Care Qual. 2012;27:176–81.

26. Ray EM, Smith R, Massie S, Erickson J, Hanson C, Harris B, et al. Family alert: implementing direct family activation of a pediatric rapid response team. Jt Comm J Qual Patient Saf. 2009;35:575–80.

27. Bogert S, Ferrell C, Rutledge DN. Experience with family activation of rapid response teams. Medsurg Nurs. 2010;19:215–23.

28. Dunning E, Brzozowicz K, Noel E, O'Keefe S, Ponischil R, Sherman S, et al. FAST track beyond RRTs. Nurs Manage. 2010;41:38–41.

29. Gerdik C, Vallish RO, Miles K, Godwin SA, Wludyka PS, Panni MK. Successful implementation of a family and patient activated rapid response team in an adult level 1 trauma center. Resuscitation. 2010;81:1676–81.

30. Greenhouse PK, Kuzminsky B, Martin SC, Merryman T. Calling a condition H(elp). Am J Nurs. 2006;106:63–6.

31. Odell M, Gerber K, Gager M. Call 4 Concern: patient and relative activated critical care outreach. Br J Nurs. 2011;19:1390–5.

32. Paciotti B, Roberts KE, Tibbetts KM, Paine CW, Keren R, Barg FK, et al. Physician attitudes toward family-activated medical emergency teams for hospitalized children. Jt Comm J Qual Patient Saf. 2014;40(4):187–92.

33. Bonafide CP, Localio AR, Roberts KE, Nadkarni VM, Weirich CM, Keren R. Impact of rapid response system implementation on critical deterioration events in children. JAMA Pediatr. 2014;168(1):25–33.

34. Hueckel RM, Turi JL, Cheifetz IM, Mericle J, Meliones JN, Mistry KP. Beyond rapid response teams: Instituting a "rover team" improves the

management of at-risk patients, facilitates proactive interventions, and improves outcomes. In: Henriksen K, Battles JB, Keyes MA, Grady ML, editors. Advances in patient safety: New directions and alternative approaches. Rockville, MD: Agency for Healthcare Research and Quality; 2008.

35. Brady PW, Muething S, Kotagal U, Ashby M, Gallagher R, Hall D, et al. Improving situation awareness to reduce unrecognized clinical deterioration and serious safety events. Pediatrics. 2013;131: e298–308.

36. Goldenhar LM, Brady PW, Sutcliffe KM, Muething SE. Huddling for high reliability and situation awareness. BMJ Qual Saf. 2013;22(11):899–906.

37. Chan PS, Jain R, Nallmothu BK, Berg RA, Sasson C. Rapid response teams: a systematic review and meta-analysis. Arch Intern Med. 2010;170:18–26.

38. Bonafide CP, Priestley MA, Nadkarni VM, Berg RA. Have we MET the answer for preventing in-hospital deaths or is it still elusive? Pediatr Crit Care Med. 2009;10:403–4.

39. Hayes LW, Dobyns EL, DiGiovine B, Brown A-M, Jacobson S, Randall KH, et al. A multicenter collaborative approach to reducing pediatric codes outside the ICU. Pediatrics. 2012;129:e785–91.

40. Bonafide CP, Roberts KE, Priestley MA, Tibbetts KM, Huang E, Nadkarni VM, et al. Development of a pragmatic measure for evaluating and optimizing rapid response systems. Pediatrics. 2012;129: e874–81.

41. Jones D, Bellomo R, DeVita M. Effectiveness of the medical emergency team: the importance of dose. Crit Care. 2009;13:313.

42. Bonafide CP, Localio AR, Song L, Roberts KE, Nadkarni VM, Priestley M, et al. Cost-benefit analysis of a medical emergency team in a children's hospital. Pediatrics. 2014;134(2):235–41.

43. Brady PW, Goldenhar LM. A qualitative study examining the influences on situation awareness and the identification, mitigation and escalation of recognised patient risk. BMJ Qual Saf. 2014;23(2):153–61.

44. VandenBerg SD, Hutchison JS, Parshuram CS. A cross-sectional survey of levels of care and response mechanisms for evolving critical illness in hospitalized children. Pediatrics. 2007;119:e940–6.

45. Duncan HP. Survey of early identification systems to identify inpatient children at risk of physiological deterioration. Arch Child. 2007;92:828.

46. Chen JG, Kemper AR, Odetola F, Cheifetz IM, Turner DA. Prevalence, characteristics, and opinions of pediatric rapid response teams in the United States. Hosp Pediatr. 2012;2:133–40.

47. Sen AI, Morgan RW, Morris MC. Variability in the implementation of rapid response teams at academic American pediatric hospitals. J Pediatr. 2013;163(6):1772–4.

Patrick Maluso and Babak Sarani

Introduction

Sepsis leading to multisystem organ failure is the leading cause of death in the ICU and the 11th leading cause of death in the USA [1–3]. The population-adjusted incidence of septic shock continues to increase worldwide and rose by 8.7% per year between 1979 and 2000 in the USA. Although figures are more readily available for developed nations, estimates of the worldwide burden of sepsis are on the order of 15–19 million cases per year [3, 4]. Despite the fact that the risk of death remains 20–50% in this population [2, 5, 6], the risk can be mitigated using an aggressive strategy of early, goal-directed interventions.

Beyond its direct impact on patients, sepsis imposes a dramatic burden on health care infrastructure and costs. Annually, it is responsible for 727,000 hospital admissions and accounts for $14.6 billion in health care spending in the USA alone [7]. The mean per-case cost for care of each septic patient is over $85,000—higher than the mean cost of any other single diagnosis in the USA [8]. Although cost varies significantly worldwide, a similar relationship between the cost for treatment of sepsis as opposed to other disorders has also been reported outside of the USA [9]. The majority of patients with severe sepsis receive treatment in a critical care setting which is also associated with greater use of hospital resources and a higher overall cost of care [1]. With the increased attention on the cost, efficiency, and effectiveness of therapies rendered, improvement of both expenditures and outcomes for septic patients represents an important goal in any modern health care system. Despite their mutual importance, the relationship between cost and quality of care is not a simple one; indeed, there appears to be no association between the cost of treating septic patients and improvements in outcomes [10].

Pathophysiology of Sepsis

The systemic inflammatory response syndrome (SIRS) is a broad diagnostic entity resulting from a generalized inflammatory response with systemic manifestations. The presence of two or more of any of the following signs is diagnostic of SIRS: respiratory rate over 20 breaths per minute, white blood cell count greater than $12,000/mm^3$ or less than $4000/mm^3$, heart rate greater than 90 beats per minute, or body temperature greater than

P. Maluso, MD (✉)
Department of Surgery, George Washington University, 2150 Pennsylvania Ave, NW. Suite 6B, Washington, DC 20037, USA
e-mail: pmaluso@email.gwu.edu

B. Sarani, MD, FACS, FCCM
Associate Professor of Surgery Director,
Center for Trauma and Critical Care Director,
George Washington Transfer Center,
George Washington University, Washington, DC, USA
e-mail: bsarani@mfa.gwu.edu

© Springer International Publishing Switzerland 2017
M.A. DeVita et al. (eds.), *Textbook of Rapid Response Systems*, DOI 10.1007/978-3-319-39391-9_20

38 °C or less than 35 °C. Sepsis refers to SIRS caused by infection and is further subcategorized into severe sepsis and septic shock based on the presence of clinical signs of organ hypoperfusion/ failure or hypotension, respectively. Septic shock exists when hypotension or organ dysfunction cannot be corrected with fluid resuscitation alone, thereby necessitating the use of vasopressors [11].

Systemic manifestations of SIRS are due to inappropriate elaboration of various inflammatory mediators including tumor necrosis factor alpha and various eicosanoids. In addition, there is suppression of compensatory anti-inflammatory response syndrome (CARS) pathways. This results in inappropriate dilation of arterioles and opening of vascular shunts between arterioles and venules, thereby bypassing the capillary bed. Such intravascular shunting results in both systemic hypotension, due to lack of resistance to flow at the capillary level, as well as an increase in the serum lactate level. The latter is due to cellular hypoperfusion due to decrease blood flow through the capillary bed [12] as well as inherent mitochondrial dysfunction [13], both of which result in anaerobic metabolism.

In addition to lactate, the mixed venous oxygenation saturation (MVO2) decreases in the under-resuscitated patient with septic shock due to a left shift in the oxyhemoglobin disassociation curve and hyperextraction of oxygen from hemoglobin. Somewhat paradoxically, in the appropriately resuscitated patient with septic shock, the MVO2 will be elevated due to shunting of oxygenated blood past the capillary bed and inability of the mitochondria to use what oxygen is delivered to the cell. Persistently elevated MVO2 and lactate are associated with multisystem organ failure and death due to ongoing cellular ischemia. Thus, serum lactate and MVO2 can be used to diagnose septic shock, assess the adequacy of resuscitation, and prognosticate survival in critically ill patients [14].

Early Intervention

Numerous studies over the last 20 years have shown that rapid initiation of appropriate therapy is a key factor for improving patient survival. Unfortunately, to date, no single intervention or medication has been shown to independently improve mortality. Thus, appropriate therapy for septic shock refers to the three independent but critical interventions: fluid and vasopressor based resuscitation to optimize perfusion, removal of the source of infection where possible, and the prompt initiation of appropriate antimicrobial therapy necessary to combat the infectious insult. The time to implementation of these therapies is directly related to risk of mortality.

In 2001, the early goal-directed therapy (EGDT) study by Rivers et al. effectively changed the paradigm for the management of the septic patient [15]. The trial showed dramatic improvement in mortality when resuscitative efforts were started immediately in the emergency department and specific endpoints where met. Although the specific endpoints chosen should be tailored to the individual patient, the study clearly shows that the most important determinant of patient survival was not the setting in which the care was delivered but was instead the speed with which interventions were begun. Fig. 20.1 depicts a modification of the EDGT algorithm.

Although EGDT pioneered the modern approach to rapid resuscitation of the septic patient, the necessity of the specific parameters involved in its strict protocol have come into question. The 2014 ProCESS trial sought to further refine management strategies for sepsis by assessing more modern critical care techniques within the framework of early intervention [16]. The study was a prospective randomized trial with three arms. The first arm replicated the EGDT. A second arm also utilized an algorithmic resuscitation strategy, however it differed from EGDT in that did not mandate central venous catheterization and that it had narrower threshold laboratory triggers for blood product transfusion (hemoglobin <7.5 g/dL instead of < 10 g/dL). Moreover, therapy in this cohort was titrated to systolic blood pressure and hypoperfusion as judged by the bedside physician rather than to specific, predetermined central venous oxygen saturation, blood pressure, and central venous pressure goals as in EGDT. Finally, the third arm allowed for usual, nonprotocolized care as deemed appropriate by the treating physician.

Fig. 20.1 Modified algorithm for goal directed resuscitation of the septic patient

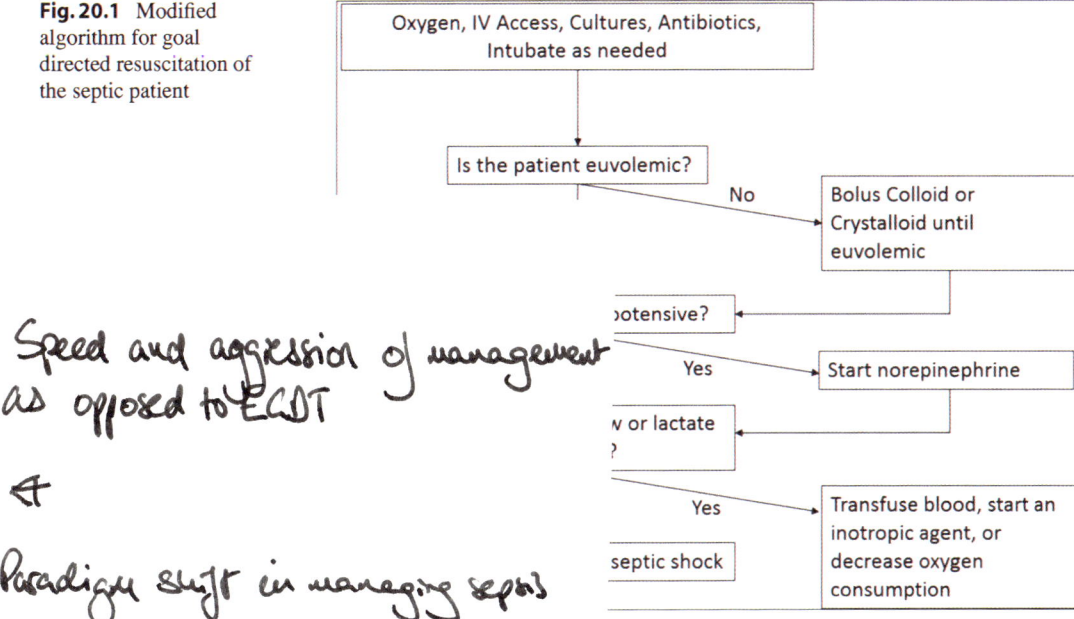

[Handwritten annotation:] Speed and aggression of management as opposed to EGDT

&

Paradigm shift in managing sepsis

between the arms in the amount and types of therapy received (i.e., use of vasopressors, volume of crystalloid or blood transfused) and in hemodynamic and laboratory markers during initial resuscitation, no statistically significant difference was observed in hospital length of stay or mortality (60-day, 90-day, or 1 year). The authors contend that Rivers EDGT trial resulted in a paradigm shift where early, aggressive resuscitation has now become standard practice such that all arms in the trial were appropriately resuscitated. ProCESS underscores the notion that early, aggressive therapy is a key determinant of patient survival in sepsis and that the specific methodology how of that care is delivered is of secondary importance.

In the same vein, rapid control and treatment of the underlying infectious cause of sepsis is of paramount importance in improving patient mortality. As illustrated in cases such as necrotizing soft tissue infections or catheter-related infections, control of the infectious source, when possible, is of utmost importance and should not be delayed for any reason [17]. Unfortunately, the majority of causes of septic shock, such as pneumonia and urinary tract infections, do not lend themselves to operative or catheter-based removal

e., drainage) of the source. Kumar et al. demonstrated a direct relationship between time to initiation of appropriate antimicrobial therapy and patient survival. In their study, every hour of delay from the onset of hypotension to the initiation of appropriate antimicrobial therapy conferred a 7.6% increase in mortality [18].

In a study designed to assess the effect of timely antimicrobial therapy in the setting of uniform EGDT, Gaieski et al. showed that administration of appropriate antibiotics within 1 h of qualification for EGDT yielded a 12% decrease in mortality. A similar mortality benefit was also seen when appropriate antibiotics were initiated within 1 h of triage [19]. Simply stated, the prompt and appropriate treatment of an underlying infectious process confers a further direct mortality benefit even in the setting of early, aggressive hemodynamic support.

Rapid Response Teams and Sepsis

Within the inpatient wards setting, early recognition and treatment of sepsis remains a diagnostic and logistical challenge and may contribute to increased morbidity and mortality in this patient [4, 20, 21]. Although Kumar, Rivers, and Gaieski focused primarily on the transition of care from the emergency department to a critical care setting, their broader findings regarding the importance of the timely initiation of appropriate multimodal therapy are broadly generalizable and should hold true regardless of the initial care setting. Clearly, any initiative designed to improve outcomes in sepsis should focus on removing the barriers to timely and appropriate medical care, irrespective of location. Multidisciplinary rapid response teams are meant to address this need.

As noted elsewhere in this book, there are still no universally accepted criteria for activation of the rapid response system (RRS) despite evidence showing that delay in doing so can result in failure to rescue and death. Objective measurements that have been frequently used to trigger RRS activation include the following: acute changes in respiratory rate (<8 or >25 breaths per minute), heart rate (<40 BPM, >120 BPM), systolic blood pressure (<90 mmHg), oxygen saturation despite supplemental oxygen therapy (<90%), urinary output (<50 ml over 4 h), and level of consciousness. Clearly, many of these criteria broadly overlap with SIRS and can be late manifestations of septic shock. In the past 5 years, increasing attention has been paid to creating scoring systems that may be more effective in identifying clinically occult septic shock, but such scoring systems still need to be prospectively validated in various patient populations [22].

Given the common criteria involved in both the definition of sepsis and in triggers for rapid response activation, it is not surprising that rapid response teams frequently are the first to identify and treat septic patients. Jäderling et al. found through a single institution retrospective study that ICU admissions from hospital wards which were initiated by rapid response team calls rather than by traditional transfer were three times more likely to have severe sepsis [23]. Other similar studies have found that sepsis is among the most common causes of RRS activation [24].

Following identification of septic shock, timeliness of intervention is directly associated with mortality. Unfortunately, inpatient hospital wards are complex and implementation of specific

therapy in a timely fashion using standard processes of care is frequently difficult, if not impossible. In a single-institution interventional study conducted at the University of Pennsylvania, Sarani et al. demonstrated significant improvement in the timely delivery of antibiotics using a streamlined medical emergency team (MET) response [25]. By including a clinical pharmacist on the MET and utilizing verbal orders in place of computerized order entry, they were able to decrease the median time to administration of therapy by almost 100 m.

It is clear, however, that rapid antibiotic administration is useless if the drugs themselves are ineffective. Frequently, practitioners order the same empiric antibiotics regardless of the patient's recent antibiotic use, local bacterial resistance patterns, and possible underlying cause of septic shock. By creating an algorithm tailored to institutional microbial resistance patterns and the speed with which each individual antibiotic can be administered, Miano et al. demonstrated a 32% improvement in adequate coverage of empiric antibiotic regimens during MET activations [26] (Fig. 20.2, Table 20.1). The algorithm called for administration of beta-lactam antibiotics first because these agents can be administered rapidly and administration of vancomycin last because this agent has to be infused slowly.

Combining the two interventions, a clinical pharmacist on the MET can rapidly determine a patient's recent antibiotic exposure and allergies, discuss the possible underlying cause of infection with the prescribing responder (e.g., physician or advanced practitioner), and verbally request the appropriate antibiotics from his/her partner in the central pharmacy. The nurse on the MET can then quickly administer the antibiotics when they are sent. Depending on a particular hospital's processes of care, some or all of the antibiotics in the algorithm can be placed on the wards for emergency release, thereby further decreasing time to administration of medication. Orders can be placed retroactively in the computer system for charting purposes, but, most importantly, the patient will have received appropriate, timely care.

Empiric Antimicrobial Selection[28]

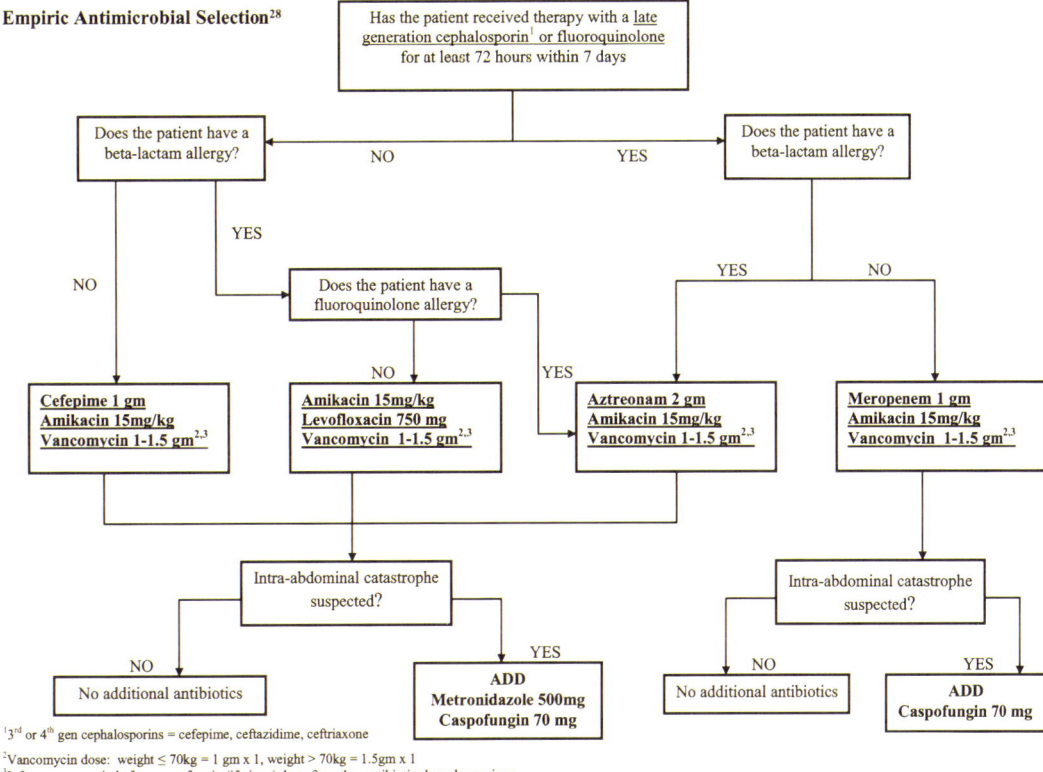

Fig. 20.2 Algorithm for emperic antibiotic prescription in patients with septic shock

Table 20.1 Antimicrobial dosage regimens

Drug	Dosage regimen	Infusion time
Amikacin	15 mg/kg × 1	30 min
Aztreonam[a]	2 gm IV q 8 h	15 min
Caspofungin[b]	70 mg × 1, then 50 mg IV q 24 h	60 min
Cefepime[a]	1 gm IV q 8 h	2–5 min
Levofloxacin[a]	750 mg IV q 24 h	60–90 min
Meropenem[a]	1 gm IV q 8 h	10–15 min
Metronidazole	500 mg IV q 12 h	30 min
Vancomycin	≤70 kg = 1 gm × 1, >70 kg = 1.5 gm × 1	60–90 min

[a]Dosage adjustment required with renal dysfunction
[b]Dosage adjustment required with hepatic dysfunction

Conclusion

Septic shock is exceedingly common in both the hospitalized and non-hospitalized patient population and is associated with mortality. Rescuing these patients requires early, aggressive, and appropriate fluid resuscitation, control of the source of infection, and antimicrobial therapy. Rapid response systems should be specifically tailored to this patient population.

References

1. Angus DC, Linde-Zwirble WT, Lidicker J, Clermont G, Carcillo J, Pinsky MR. Epidemiology of severe sepsis in the United States: analysis of incidence, outcome, and associated costs of care. Crit Care Med. 2001;29:1303–10.
2. Martin GS, Mannino DM, Eaton S, Moss M. The epidemiology of sepsis in the United States from 1979 through 2000. N Engl J Med. 2003;348:1546–54.
3. Adhikari NK, Fowler RA, Bhagwanjee S, Rubenfeld GD. Critical care and the global burden of critical illness in adults. Lancet. 2010;376:1339–46.
4. Sundararajan V, Macisaac CM, Presneill JJ, Cade JF, Visvanathan K. Epidemiology of sepsis in Victoria, Australia. Crit Care Med. 2005;33:71–80.

5. Annane D, Aegerter P, Jars-Guincestre MC, Guidet B. Current epidemiology of septic shock: the CUB-Rea network. Am J Respir Crit Care Med. 2003;168: 165–72.

6. Harrison DA, Welch CA, Eddleston JM. The epidemiology of severe sepsis in England, Wales and Northern Ireland, 1996 to 2004: secondary analysis of a high quality clinical database, the ICNARC Case Mix Programme Database. Crit Care. 2006;10:R42.

7. Hall MJ, Williams SN, DeFrances CJ, Golosinskiy A. Inpatient care for septicemia or sepsis: a challenge for patients and hospitals. NCHS Data Brief. 2011;1–8.

8. Bates DW, Yu DT, Black E, et al. Resource utilization among patients with sepsis syndrome. Infect Control Hosp Epidemiol. 2003;24:62–70.

9. Chalupka AN, Talmor D. The economics of sepsis. Crit Care Clin. 2012;28:57–76 .vi

10. Lagu T, Rothberg MB, Nathanson BH, Pekow PS, Steingrub JS, Lindenauer PK. The relationship between hospital spending and mortality in patients with sepsis. Arch Intern Med. 2011;171:292–9.

11. Bone RC, Balk RA, Cerra FB, et al. Definitions for sepsis and organ failure and guidelines for the use of innovative therapies in sepsis. The ACCP/SCCM Consensus Conference Committee. American College of chest physicians/society of critical care medicine. Chest. 1992;101:1644–55.

12. Trzeciak S, Dellinger RP, Parrillo JE, et al. Early microcirculatory perfusion derangements in patients with severe sepsis and septic shock: relationship to hemodynamics, oxygen transport, and survival. Ann Emerg Med. 2007;49:88–98 .e1-2

13. Brealey D, Brand M, Hargreaves I, et al. Association between mitochondrial dysfunction and severity and outcome of septic shock. Lancet. 2002;360:219–23.

14. Gutierrez G, Comignani P, Huespe L, et al. Central venous to mixed venous blood oxygen and lactate gradients are associated with outcome in critically ill patients. Intensive Care Med. 2008;34:1662–8.

15. Rivers E, Nguyen B, Havstad S, et al. Early goal-directed therapy in the treatment of severe sepsis and septic shock. N Engl J Med. 2001;345:1368–77.

16. Yealy DM, Kellum JA, Huang DT, et al. A randomized trial of protocol-based care for early septic shock. N Engl J Med. 2014;370:1683–93.

17. Marshall JC, Maier RV, Jimenez M, Dellinger EP. Source control in the management of severe sepsis and septic shock: an evidence-based review. Crit Care Med. 2004;32:S513–26.

18. Kumar A, Roberts D, Wood KE, et al. Duration of hypotension before initiation of effective antimicrobial therapy is the critical determinant of survival in human septic shock. Crit Care Med. 2006;34: 1589–96.

19. Gaieski DF, Mikkelsen ME, Band RA, et al. Impact of time to antibiotics on survival in patients with severe sepsis or septic shock in whom early goal-directed therapy was initiated in the emergency department. Crit Care Med. 2010;38:1045–53.

20. Esteban A, Frutos-Vivar F, Ferguson ND, et al. Sepsis incidence and outcome: contrasting the intensive care unit with the hospital ward. Crit Care Med. 2007; 35:1284–9.

21. Lundberg JS, Perl TM, Wiblin T, et al. Septic shock: an analysis of outcomes for patients with onset on hospital wards versus intensive care units. Crit Care Med. 1998;26:1020–4.

22. Smith GB, Prytherch DR, Meredith P, Schmidt PE, Featherstone PI. The ability of the National Early Warning Score (NEWS) to discriminate patients at risk of early cardiac arrest, unanticipated intensive care unit admission, and death. Resuscitation. 2013;84:465–70.

23. Jaderling G, Bell M, Martling CR, Ekbom A, Bottai M, Konrad D. ICU admittance by a rapid response team versus conventional admittance, characteristics, and outcome. Crit Care Med. 2013; 41:725–31.

24. Jones D, Duke G, Green J, et al. Medical emergency team syndromes and an approach to their management. Crit Care. 2006;10:R30.

25. Sarani B, Brenner SR, Gabel B, et al. Improving sepsis care through systems change: the impact of a medical emergency team. Jt Comm J Qual Patient Saf. 2008;34:179–82 .25

26. Miano TA, Powell E, Schweickert WD, Morgan S, Binkley S, Sarani B. Effect of an antibiotic algorithm on the adequacy of empiric antibiotic therapy given by a medical emergency team. J Crit Care. 2012; 27:45–50.

Other Efferent Limb Teams: Crises that Require Specialized Resources

21

Dan Shearn, Francesca Rubulotta, and Michael A. DeVita

Most of the world's literature on rapid response systems (RRS), rapid response teams (RRT), and medical emergency teams (MET) focuses on in-hospital crises for patients with sudden deterioration in vital signs or cognitive function. At UPMC Presbyterian Hospital, we found that certain low-frequency, high-risk events require specialized expertise not available on our "routine" MET. As a result, UPMC created a series of teams, all part of the rapid response system, which can address a variety of these critical events. The "system," then, is not just a system for responding to a specific physiological event, but rather a system for responding to all critical situations that require a speedy and effective

D. Shearn, RN, MSN (✉)
UPMC Presbyterian Hospital,
Fairfield Drive, Seneca, Pittsburgh, PA 15213, USA
e-mail: shearndp@upmc.edu

F. Rubulotta, MD, PhD, FRCA, FFICM, eMBA
Department of Surgery, Intensive Care Unit Charing Cross Hospital, Bariatric Anaesthesia St Mary's Hospital, Imperial College London,
NHS Trust London, London, UK
e-mail: francesca.rubulotta@imperial.nhs.uk

M.A. DeVita, MD, FCCM, FRCP
Department of Surgery, Critical Care,
Harlem Hospital Center, 506 Lenox Avenue,
New York, NY 10037, USA

Department of Internal Medicine, Critical Care,
Harlem Hospital Center, 506 Lenox Avenue,
New York, NY 10037, USA
e-mail: michael.devita@NYCHHC.ORG

organized response to prevent harm. The purpose of this chapter is to describe how and why UPMC expanded the medical emergency team and rapid response system to promote patient safety across a diverse range of critical events. We describe each team response, staffing, purpose, and outcomes.

The RRS in its "native" form is a system that includes a team response that will rescue patients from critical situations or emergent situations. The goal is to bring the critical care unit and resources to the bedside of the critical patient in need. *Specialized teams responding to specific needs are consistent with the concept of RRS being a quality improvement mechanism and a patient safety key tool. The use of these teams can improve the quality of care by facilitating appropriate allocation of important resources.*

At UPMC, after the RRS became part of the hospital culture, hospital leaders recognized that crisis events remained that did not fit neatly into one of the original existing calling criteria, and for which the response team was ill equipped because of either mismatched personnel or equipment. Because the team did not have the skills, or the crises are not medical in nature and not amenable to a clinical intervention team, a new type of response would be needed. These events could benefit from a new organized response to a clear triggering event. So as new crisis types were identified, new teams utilized an RRS approach to improve their management. In this chapter, we list some of the various teams that were developed. We describe teams developed in different organizational structures such as: stroke team, trauma team, blood administration team (BAT), chest pain team, condition L (for lost patient) team, condition M (for mental illness crisis—usually a belligerent or dangerous patient event), difficult airway team (DAT), pediatric response team, sepsis team, trach*eostomy* team, and end of life/*palliative care* team. While this list is not inclusive of all teams developed in the world, it does compromise a broader scope for the RRS than most have described. Additional examples of specialized teams are the "secondary victim" team and the obstetric crisis team described in chapters 28 and 22 respectively. We also do not discuss the cardiac arrest team because these have been well described elsewhere, and because we strongly believe the concept of responding "after cardiac arrest" is counterproductive to the premise that RRSs are created to prevent cardiac arrest [1]. The initial purpose of the entire RRS movement is to prevent in hospital severe adverse events including cardiac arrest. We therefore decided not to include any description of a cardiac arrest team considering that in a full implement RRS environment calls should be addressed either to prevent deterioration or to empower end of life care. No unplanned cardiac arrest should occur in the hospitals in the future. We acknowledge that there may be a generalizability issue for some of these teams especially in smaller hospitals. Our point in this chapter is to describe how the RRS model can be adapted to other crises, and show examples of this RRS structure.

Stroke Team

Why—The stroke team is created to improve the hospital's ability to manage efficiently and effectively patients brought to the emergency department (ED). These teams are very effective in speeding the process of intake, physical evaluation, diagnostic testing, and therapeutic intervention. The team usually supports ED physicians, but may also support hospital floor physicians when and if they need to make the complex decision of providing thrombolysis. The primary goal is to ensure the accurate completion of the task in a time sensitive manner. Initially the teams were intended for patients in the ED, but soon hospitals noticed that patients already in a hospital ward who developed stroke like symptoms did not have the same efficiency of care. As a result, centers have implemented a stroke team for both emergency department and hospitalized patients [2].

The inpatient stroke team is normally instituted to efficiently treat patients that have exhibited symptoms of a stroke. The aim is to get the experts in stroke therapy to the bedside of a patient with emergent neurological symptoms suggestive of an acute neurovascular event, and enable prompt therapeutic interventions like tPA, angioplasty, craniotomy, or even transfer if no adequate neuro-expertise is available in the hospital. With the goal being early treatment, be it medical treatment or surgical intervention, having the personnel that know how to get the job done was essential. Specialized neuro centers are not present in all hospitals. Nevertheless, a method for rapidly treating or triaging stroke patients is needed [3]. We believe a stroke team should be available in all hospital because the recognition and treatment of patients with acute neurological conditions is life saving. Quality of life after a neurological event is also very important and it is related to the time needed to recognize and treat the underling cause.

Who—This team consisted of a physician trained and expert in the treatment of strokes. Alberts and colleagues have reported that almost 100% of stroke teams, the leader is either a neurologist or neurosurgeon, and virtually all work 24 h/day, every day. At UPMC, the stroke team is activated only by the physician in charge of the basic MET, or the ED physician that is caring for the patient. This helps to ensure that calls would be activated that are legitimate, thus decreasing unnecessary calls, and also promotes use of the MET team: the "caller" has only to decide if there is a crisis, and not diagnose the crisis. However, in other hospitals physicians and nurses could activate the team.

How—Should a patient have neurologic symptoms, a MET response is triggered, bringing critical care resources to maintain respiration and circulation. The stroke team could be triggered directly if the diagnosis is made or the suspicious of a neurological acute condition is very high. Should the treating physician in the team response perceive an acute neurovascular event, then the stroke team must be always activated. In UPMC model, the MET remains to provide basic critical care support (circulation, respiration, etc.), and the stroke team leader performs an assessment and determines neurovascular care. In the absence of a MET or outreach team the ward registrar and the nurse in charge should provide support to the stroke team until the patient is stabilized or transfer to another unit. Other hospitals report that only a stroke team responds.

The Data—Data of outcomes is important in learning if the team is working. It is also helpful to continue to gain financial support for the team. Suggested stroke team outcome data can consist of monitoring time to treatment, number of calls activated or mortality of patients treated, and time lapse from onset of symptoms to initiation of treatment (e.g., tPA or surgery) if any. Post-stroke quality of life is key because cost related to major disabilities is elevated and can justify the implementation of an emergency stroke team in every hospital.

Trauma Team

Why—Trauma teams are useful in emergency departments among hospitals which are designated trauma centers [4]. The purpose, methodology, and success for these teams are now widely reported. Rarely, hospitalized patients, visitors, and staff may have an acute traumatic event. Examples include falls, suicide attempts, and assault. Should a severe traumatic event occur, often the resources brought by the MET or outreach nurses are not sufficient to manage the crisis. Therefore, some hospitals created the ability to call to an inpatient's bedside the responders usually delegated to respond to the emergency department for an out-of-hospital trauma. At UPMC, like the stroke team initiation, only the MET team leader can trigger the in-hospital trauma team call.

Who—Normally, there is not the need for the full trauma team to respond because the MET or other outreach team is already on site and has significant critical care resources. In this setting only a scaled down trauma team (usually the trauma resident and attending) is needed to respond and assist the MET response.

How—When a patient has a significant trauma, any staff member may trigger the rapid response system and the MET responds as usual. If the MET senior physician feels it appropriate, then a "trauma team" call is initiated as well. The MET is responsible for circulation and respiration, while the trauma team has responsibility for diagnosis, decision making regarding needed diagnostic or therapeutic interventions, and performing procedures. The UPMC experience shows that this team is usually called for sudden massive postoperative bleeding events, but may also be activated for those who have fallen down a flight of stairs.

The Data—Data outcomes are measured by the amount of non-ED Trauma team calls and the outcomes of individual patients. Patient safety events related to the Trauma team activation is reviewed. If needed, serious incidents forms must be filled according to local policy. The organization may learn from the event and implement measures to prevent similar events in future. The trauma team has the responsibility to complete the documentation including incident reports if required.

Blood Administration Team (BAT)

Why—A BAT may be developed to promote rapid and accurate delivery of blood products in the setting of acute large volume blood product resuscitation. Organizations may find that there are administrative, logistic, and clinical causes of delay in obtaining blood products, bringing them to the bedside, it would be given according to policy, performing required checks, and delivering the products rapidly using appropriate administration devices like warmers or rapid infusers.

The recognition of a need for this type of service may come about in review of cases of multiple unit transfusions wherein delays in obtaining blood were identified as well as failure to follow protocol for blood administration due to over-tasking of MET responders.

Who—At UPMC the BAT consists of an a ICU nurse and a nurse aide. The former's responsibility is to confirm orders as well as check, administer, and document delivery of the blood products. The nurse aide's responsibility is to obtain the blood products from the blood bank expeditiously. Organizations may choose other individuals for these tasks.

How—The BAT may activated by the primary MET, or by any ICU or ED nurse caring for a critically ill patient with a sudden large blood replacement need. At UPMC the triggering criteria is any case where at least two units of blood are to be administered immediately. One of the benefits of a BAT is the bedside nurses (or MET) have additional resources at the bedside of a patient who has sudden need for blood. The burden of all the steps for transfusion is lifted from the MET, ICU, or ED team so that they may focus on other concerns. The BAT is called for through the operator of the institution.

The Data—Data outcomes for this measure are number of BAT calls activated and number of patient safety events that have occurred since the initiation of the team. One might also survey the time from bleeding event to infusion of blood products.

Chest Pain/Coronary Syndrome Team

Why—This team was developed to treat acute myocardial infarctions in a timely manner. A goal is for ailing patients to get timely treatment and reduce infarct size. This type of team is commonly available to EDs, but the accuracy and efficiency of care may not be as good when the events occur on patients already in the hospital or outside a coronary care unit. The treatment may be to bring the patient to cardiac catheterization or provide a thrombolytic agent. In either case,

speed is essential for optimal outcome. The ED usually has built an efficient and effective system for ensuring that all patients with symptoms of an acute coronary syndrome receive diagnostics and interventions in under 90 min, with "door-to-needle" times being an important quality metric. In contrast, hospitalized patients have delays from symptom onset to treatment caused by the desire to consult a cardiologist who may not be on site, or delays in obtaining and interpreting the ECG. Inpatient units should have a means to mimic the ED's capabilities and create a similar if not identical response for the hospitalized patient. When implemented at UPMC, this intervention drove down the time from onset of symptoms to intervention.

Who—As the critical care resources are on site, the chest pain team consist of a Cardiology physician who can respond immediately. The capabilities of the physician on the chest pain team included ability to diagnose an acute coronary syndrome, order and perform an intervention, and mandate access to the cardiac catheterization laboratory as needed.

How—The MET treatment leader will determine the need to call for the chest pain team. This team is called for using the appropriate local resources. The level of cardiologist (fellow, cardiologist, interventional cardiologist) will be determined by the availability of the physician on call, but should always have the skill set described above. As with our other supplementary teams, the MET can remain with the patient to ensure circulatory and respiratory support.

The Data—Suggested data collection to point out outcomes are time of initial condition call to catheterization lab or delivery of tPA

(event onset to treatment initiation time; should be less than 90 min), number of chest pain team calls, and mortality data related to chest pain team calls.

Condition L (Lost Patient)

Why—This team may be created after recognition that a patient may leave her room and wander away—a not uncommon and potentially dangerous occurrence. In spite large responses which may take hours, and even extend to the neighboring community, patients not be found for some time, if at all. In some cases, patients may be found severely injured. When such events occur, a hospital performs a root cause analysis to understand how such a large-scale search could be unable to find the patient in a timelier manner. Indeed, the patient may be found in an area that had been searched repeated without success. It is recognized that a patient might wander in a way as to be unintentionally (or intentionally) avoiding searchers. Based on procedures learned from the US Forestry Service, a new strategy following national benchmarks for search and rescue teams creates an organized team response to simultaneously search all areas in the hospital and environs. This reduces the likelihood that a patient may elude searchers. When this system was set up and tested at UPMC, the time to locate the staff member simulating a "lost" patient was about 5 min on average.

Who—Condition L is an organized notification of all staff. It is an "all hands on deck" approach to notifying staff that a patient is "lost" and signals the initiation of a search for the lost patient. In essence, all staff have a search responsibility and the entire facility can be searched within a few minutes of the call. After an initial search, a huddle is completed to determine next steps in the search if the patient has not been found, or ceasing the Condition L if the search was successful. The Condition L can be called for by any staff member in the institution. This RRS will alert each staff member of a lost patient. The call also alerts security to become involved and look at exits in the institution, housekeeping to search the staircases in the building, and nursing staff to search each room and the staircase above and below their floor. An administrator on duty coordinates the response. In addition, an overhead announcement describing the lost patient enables visitors to help in the search should they see someone matching the description.

How—Condition L may be activated by any employee in the institution. The activation occurs through the hospital operator. The operator initiates the Condition L over the hospital page system. In addition, the operator calls on the overhead speaker system the condition L and may provide the first name of the patient, age of the patient and a general description of the patient that is missing.

The Data—Suggested data collection for condition L are the number of Condition L calls per month, time to find the patient, whether the appropriate assessments were completed prior to the condition L to prevent the patient from wandering away, and whether key process points were followed (e.g., was the patient assessed as a wanderer, did the post condition L huddle occur on the floor the patient was missing from, did the patient have a wanderer identification gown on). UPMC data show a remarkably short search time is now needed. In the first mock event, it took under 10 min to locate a "patient" trying to avoid discovery. Subsequent mock events have found the wanderer in under 5 min. In real "lost" patient event, the patient is typically found in the same time frame. The authors advocate this capability and system for all hospitals to prevent unintended harm.

Difficult Airway Team (DAT)

Why—The DAT's primary responsibility is to gain an artificial airway for a patient who needs an airway and the team already caring for the patient is unable to do so. Many RRS teams include a critical care medicine physician or anesthesiologist as part of the basic RRS response. However there is on occasion airway management issues that may be beyond that person's skills. Thus there is always a need for the availability of a planned response by experienced personnel and equipment to assist in managing the "difficult airway" scenario [5]. The hope is that a difficult airway does not become a "failed" airway, resulting in patient harm. The causes of a difficult airway requiring the DAT to respond vary. Some reasons are a large patient, abnormal anatomy, bleeding in the airway, or the need for surgical airway intervention.

Who—The DAT is activated by the rapid response airway manager who identifies the problem. The DAT should bring an anesthesiologist, an anesthesia technician, a surgeon, and a "difficult airway cart" which includes an intubating bronchoscope as well as other specialized airway equipment including a tracheostomy surgery tray.

How—When an airway is unsuccessfully instrumented more than twice, or if oxygenation cannot be maintained with noninvasive means, a difficult airway is considered to exist. In some cases, the DAT may be called prior to any attempt by the MET responders.

The Data—Suggested data outcomes are the amount of times the DAT is activated, the success of obtaining an airway, the need for surgical intervention at the bedside, and patient harm from delayed or failed airway management. DAT should be reviewed by an independent patient safety review panel.

Tracheostomy (Trachy) Team

Why—The tracheostomy team (Trachy team) is needed in centers with a high number of in hospital patients with tracheostomies. These include neuro and neurosurgical centers, burn and trauma centers, major ENT oncology centers, rehabilitation centers.

Who—The trachy team may be activated by the ward doctors or nurses in the event of occluded, dislodged or damaged tracheostomy that the primary nurse or physician cannot manage. The team should include a nurse and an anesthesiologist. In addition to this emergency response, the trachy team may review the condition of the tracheostomy in all hospitalized patients who have a tracheostomy tube. The trachy team can plan and perform timely changes of old devices to prevent untoward events. At a predetermined scheduled time after any tracheostomy procedure, the trachy team nurse will visit the patient and may change the original cuffed cannula with a new tube. The trachy team doctor does not necessary need to supervise tracheostomy changes unless the nurse requires it or specific concerns are present.

The Data—Suggested data are the amount of times the trachy team is activated, the number of

tracheostomy changes performed with no complications, those performed with minor or major complications, and the number patients discharged from the hospital without a tracheostomy. The trachy team should be reviewed by an independent patient safety review panel and can be variably related to the anesthetic team or ICU team in the hospital.

Pediatric Response Team

Why—Pediatric patients may require a response that is capable of diagnosing and treating sudden critical events. In an adult acute care facility, the expertise for caring for pediatric patients may be confined to a few staff. Even in a pediatric hospital, there may be few individuals with critical care experience needed to manage acute deterioration. Thus there is a need to define a specific trained pediatric response. Hospitals should develop the capability to maintain competency of individuals as well as efficiency of the team. The pediatric response team is activated when a pediatric patient (under 14 or under 40 kg.) meets age-specific critical condition triggering criteria. The goal of the team is to treat the patient acutely, rescue the patient from immediate danger, and if needed, escort them promptly to trained staff in the ER (if there are no pediatric critical care areas) or pediatric intensive care unit (PICU). The intention is to rapidly treat or triage the patients to a pediatric facility, or the appropriate unit able to deliver the needed level of care. Interestingly, at one large UPMC hospital, most pediatric MET calls are for children who are visiting relatives and suffer an event, or children who have an event in the vicinity of the hospital and parents brought their child into the front door of the hospital. The response material and emergency bag is different for the pediatric call. Nurses and doctors need to be familiar with the devices and emergency drugs in the pediatric emergency bag. Pediatric Rapid Response Systems improve outcome for pediatric patients who develop sudden critical illness outside an ICU [6]. In addition, Pediatric Medical Emergency Teams have been shown to improve patient outcome when they routinely visit patients 24 and 48 h after transfer from the PICU to the general ward [7].

Who—Pediatric team members consist of a (pediatric if possible) critical care physician, critical care nurse, a respiratory therapist and perhaps security and escort personnel. The optimal physician is trained in the general airway management. The team should be competent in the use of the Broselow pediatric resuscitation system. A pediatric crash cart should be available and brought to the scene.

How—Pediatric condition response occurs when staff recognize a patient who meets pediatric rapid response criteria.

The Data—Suggested data outcomes to be measured are number of pediatric response team calls, resultant outcomes of the calls. The event rate for pediatric cardiac arrests is exceedingly low, so cardiac arrest rate is not a good indicator of benefit. Bonafide and colleagues have recommended evaluating the "trajectory" of critical deterioration instead. Pediatric teams have been discussed in greater detail in chap. 19.

Condition M (Mental Illness Critical Event)

Why—Condition M is a crisis intervention that may be called for any patient or visitor who is experiencing a crisis that could pose a potential threat to themselves, patients, staff, or visitors. It is a "behavioral code." While most of the events occur with an unruly individual who is angry and has lost control, it also may include individuals under the influence of psychotropic medications or patients who are having an acute psychiatric episode. The condition M will provide resources trained in dealing with the behavioral situation that occurs, including the ability to stop physical altercations. In most cases, a security officer is not needed, but they are reassuring to have on site and can intervene if force is required to ensure safety.

Who—The condition M response team consists of a behavioral resource nurse, psychiatric physician at the trainee or attending level, other psychiatric responders, security staff, and may include an administrator on call. The purpose of providing these personnel is to bring the experts to the bedside that have the knowledge and interpersonal skills to deal with the problem (like the ability to de-escalate a crisis). Some responders should be able to authorize the use of force when needed (rarely), and have the knowledge of how to get other appropriate resources for the patient.

How—Condition M response is called for by the staff on the unit who feels an individual is in crisis. This crisis may be evidenced by patient's shouting, hitting objects or other people, or throwing objects. Other criteria may be pacing, verbal threats, reddening face, increased heart rate or blood pressure associated with threatening behavior.

The Data—Suggested data outcomes to consider are amount of condition M calls and the outcome of those calls. Analysis of each condition M is required to ensure that all appropriate personnel responded that all points of the policy were followed.

Sepsis Team

Why—Sepsis is a leading cause of death. Failure to treat effectively and with speed increases mortality risk. Outcome from patients admitted to the ICU from the ward is overall worse than that of patients admitted via the ED or the operating theater because of delays in recognition and treatment. Sepsis teams have been shown to provide early recognition and resuscitation of patients with severe sepsis and septic shock discovered outside the ICU [8]. In this study, the sepsis team was better than weekly education and feedback to staff. It seems that a dedicated team focused on this entity is preferable in terms of both process of care and outcome.

Who—The sepsis team consists of a senior nurse with the ability to prescribe the resuscitation and antibiotics according to protocol, or a physician trained in the care of the patient in severe sepsis and septic shock. They will require the support of pharmacy and clinical laboratories to obtain cultures and deliver antibiotics in a timely manner.

How—The sepsis team is called for by the staff on the unit who feels an individual is in crisis or is deteriorating and who meet severe sepsis or septic shock criteria.

The Data—Suggested data outcomes to consider are amount of sepsis calls and the outcome of those calls. Important is to track process measures such as time to delivery of 30 cc/kg initial resuscitation to patients (20 cc/kg to children), time to delivery of antibiotics, time to culture, time to evaluation of lactate level and time to admission to the ICU. Patient outcome measures like mortality, and length of stay in ICU and the hospital are important.

End of Life Team

Jones and colleagues and Hillman and colleagues have identified that a significant proportion of Rapid Response patients are actually dying, and may benefit more from appropriate implementa-

tion of palliative care resources than addition of critical care measures. This team is discussed in greater detail in chap. 27.

Summary

Low-frequency, high-risk events are most likely to cause harm to patients, visitors, and staff in hospitals. These events require special skills and equipment. While most of the early literature pertaining to rapid response systems relate to patients who have deterioration in heart rate, blood pressure, respirations or cognitive function, there are many other events which can be as dangerous. Because they are more rare, the need for a specific planned response including both personnel and equipment is heightened. This has led to the creation of other rapid response teams as part of a larger, more complex rapid response system (Tables 21.1 and 21.2). These creative and innovative teams allow rescue of patients by

Table 21.1 Rapid response team members and their responsibilities

Role	Personnel	Responsibility
1. Airway manager	MD	Assess, assist ventilation, intubate
2. Airway assistant	RT	Assist airway manager, oxygen and suction setup, suction as needed
3. Bedside assistant	Floor RN	Check pulse, obtain vital signs, assess patent IVs, push meds
4. Crash cart manager	ICU RN	Deploy equipment, prepare meds, run defibrillator
5. Treatment leader	MD or ICU RN till MD arrives	Assess team responsibilities, data, direct treatment, set priorities, triage patient.
6. Circulation	CPR certified personnel	Check pulse, place defib pads, perform chest compressions
7. Procedure MD	MD	Perform procedures, IVs, chest tubes, ABGs
8. Data manager (ICU RN)	ICU RN	Role tags, AMPLE, lab results, chart, record interventions

Table 21.2 Other rapid response teams and their responders

RRT or MET name	Reason developed or purpose	Responders
Stroke team	Instituted to treat inpatients with symptoms of a stroke.	Physician trained to treat strokes plus the basic condition response team
Trauma team	Needed to respond to the emergency department for an out of hospital trauma *as well as* inpatient trauma events	Trauma physician, and the equivalent of MET responders
Blood administration team (BAT)	Errors in transfusion of large volume blood products in haste may lead to patient harm. Special forms, procedures and equipment are needed	2 ICU nurses and a nurse aide.
Chest pain team	Developed to treat rapidly treat acute myocardial infarctions among hospitalized patients outside of critical care areas	Cardiologist plus the basic condition response team

(continued)

Table 21.2 (continued)

RRT or MET name	Reason developed or purpose	Responders
Condition L (lost) team	To find a patient that is unaccounted for or lost	Unit staff, security, escorts, housekeeping staff, patient's attending physician, administrator on duty
Difficult airway team (DAT)	The DAT's primary responsibility is to prevent a failed airway and death due to airway obstruction	Anesthesia personnel, surgeon, plus basic response team
Pediatric response team	Pediatric patients deteriorate and benefit from rapid care	Physician, ICU RNs, respiratory therapy
Condition M—behavioral crisis team	Need to de-escalate a crisis due to mental illness that is a potential threat to themselves, patients, staff, or visitors	Behavioral resource nurse, psychiatrist or other psychiatric responder, security staff, an administrator on call

enabling the delivery of appropriate resources to the bedside. The RRS is a safety improvement mechanism that is adaptable to all conditions and flexible to all hospitals.

References

1. Smith G, DeVita M, Jones D, Hillman K, Welch J. Education for cardiac arrest. Resuscitation. 2015;92:59–62. doi:10.1016/j.resuscitation.2015.04018.

2. Alberts MJ, Chaturvedi S, Graham G, Hughes RL, Jamieson DG, Krakowski R, Raps E, Scott P. Acute stroke teams. Results of a national survey. Stroke. 1998;29:2318–20.

3. Chapman SN, Mehndiratta P, Johansen MC, McMurry TL, Johnston KC, Southerland AM. Current perspectives on the use of intravenous recombinant tissue plasminogen activator (tPA) for treatment of acute ischemic stroke. Vasc Health Risk Manag. 2014;10: 75–87.

4. Deane SA, Gaudry PL, Pearson I, Misra S, McNeil RJ, Read C. The hospital trauma team: a model for trauma management. J Trauma. 1990;30:806–12.

5. Gonzalez MN, Weston B, Yuce TK, Carey AM, Barnette RE, Goldberg A, McNamara RM. One year experience with the institution of the critical airway team at an academic medical center. J Emerg Med. 2015;50:194–7. doi:10.1010/j.jemermed.2015.o9.011.

6. Bonafide CP, Localio AR, Roberts KE, Nadkarni VM, Weirich CM, Keren R. Impact of rapid response system implementation on critical deterioration events in children. JAMA Pediatr. 2014;168:25–33. doi:10.1001/jamapediatrics.2013.3266.

7. Lobos AT, Fernandes R, Williams K, Ramsay C, McNally JD. Routine medical emergency team assessments of patients discharged from the PICU: description of a medical emergency team follow-up program. Pediatr Crit Care Med. 2015;16:359–65. doi:10.1097/PCC.0000000000000354.

8. Schramm GE, Kashyap R, Mullon JJ, Gajic O, Afessa B. Septic shock: a multidisciplinary response team and weekly feedback to clinicians improve the process of care and mortality. Crit Care Med. 2011;39:252–8. doi:10.1097/CCM.0b013e3181ffde08.

Patricia Dalby, Gabriella G. Gosman, Karen Stein,
David Streitman, and Nancy Wise

Continuous Quality Improvement Inpatient obstetric care involves periodic maternal and or fetal crisis situations. During events such as fetal bradycardia, shoulder dystocia, anaphylaxis, and maternal hemorrhage, patient care needs greatly

P. Dalby, MD (✉)
Associate Professor, Department of Anesthesiology,
University of Pittsburgh School of Medicine,
Magee-Womens Hospital of UPMC, Room 3407,
300 Halket Street, Pittsburgh, PA 15213, USA
e-mail: dalbypl@anes.upmc.edu

G.G. Gosman, MD
Associate Professor, Department of Obstetrics,
Gynecology, and Reproductive Services, University
of Pittsburgh School of Medicine, Magee-Womens
Hospital of UPMC, Room 2314, 300 Halket Street,
Pittsburgh, PA 15213, USA
e-mail: ggosman@mail.magee.edu

K. Stein, RN, BSN, MSED
Department of Nursing Education, University of
Pittsburgh School of Nursing, Magee-Womens Hospital
of UPMC, 300 Halket Street, Pittsburgh, PA 15213, USA
e-mail: KStein@mail.magee.edu

D. Streitman, MD
Assistant Professor, Department of Maternal Fetal
Medicine, Saint Luke's Health System Kansas City,
Missouri USA, 4401 Wornall Rd, Peet Center 1,
Kansas City, MO 64111, USA
e-mail: dstreitman@gmail.com

N. Wise, RNC, BNS
Department of Woman Child Birthing Center of
Magee-Womens Hospital of UPMC, Labor and
Delivery Department, 300 Halket Ave, Pittsburth, PA
15213, USA
e-mail: Wisen@mail.magee.edu

exceed the resources allocated to routine care. Unfortunately these emergencies in the past half century have led to increases in maternal morbidity in the USA, especially in the case of maternal hemorrhage [1]. Many of these emergencies require rapid, coordinated intervention of a multidisciplinary team to optimize outcome. Increasingly, hospitals have incorporated obstetric teams into their rapid response system to address these recurring, but unpredictable maternal and/or fetal events. The American College of Obstetricians and Gynecologists (ACOG) Committee Opinion "Preparing for Clinical Emergencies in Obstetrics and Gynecology" emphasized the importance of crisis response teams for clinical emergencies relevant to obstetric patients [2]. The US Department of Health and Human Services along with the American Hospital Association and the Heath Research and Educational Trust which partners with the American Heart Association updated the Obstetrical Harm Care Change Package with a 2014 Update: Recognition and Prevention of Obstetrical Related Events and Harm [3]. Other groups such as the Institution for Health Care Improvement (IHI) have issued recommendations also.

Many institutions established obstetric-specific crisis teams as local quality improvement initiatives. In the past decade more reports on such teams appear in the published literature [4, 5, 6, 7]. This chapter describes the implementation, training and maintenance of an obstetric-specific crisis team at Magee-Womens Hospital of University of Pittsburgh Medical Center (UPMC) from 2005 thru 2014. A previous chapter described the early efforts (first 5 years) of this process in the first edition of this book. Included in this chapter is the subsequent year's information as the rapid response system for obstetrics evolved. This also includes descriptions of alternate obstetric team approaches chosen by other institutions. This information was solicited through query of several medical associations (Council of Women's and Infants' Specialty Hospitals, the Society for Obstetric Anesthesia and Perinatology, and the Society for Simulation in Healthcare), the Institute for Healthcare Improvement, and via personal communication by two of the authors (PD and GG).

Background and Justification

Magee-Womens Hospital of UPMC added and sustained an obstetric-specific team response to its rapid response system for multiple reasons.

1. The single call system was the most rapid way to bring multidisciplinary providers to the patient who needed care urgently. One call assembled the necessary personnel and expertise to provide optimal evaluation and intervention. After calling, the bedside provider could focus on immediate crisis care of his or her patient, rather than making multiple sequential phone calls.
2. The multidisciplinary response facilitated interdisciplinary communication, as team responders arrive and receive a briefing about the patient at nearly the same time. Poor communication was the number one root cause identified in the JCAHO Sentinel Event Alert *Preventing Infant Death and Injury During Delivery*" [8].
3. The UPMC health system had improved patient outcomes by introducing a crisis team response for inpatient pre-arrest medical emergencies (Condition C). After the institution of Condition C, inpatient cardiac arrests and deaths decreased [9].
4. Incorporation of obstetric crises into the health system's rapid response system held

promise to enhance data collection and quality efforts in obstetric care [10].
5. The team response provided a designated team member to do real time documentation of patient status and interventions during critical obstetrical events. This promised to improve documentation problems caused by multiple providers retrospectively recording their recall of critical events.
6. Crisis response teams provided a valuable resource for staff satisfaction and peace of mind. For a staff member who recognizes a patient in crisis, help is only a single call away [11].
7. Rapid-Response Teams have become a globally accepted mechanism for emergency response, driven by the belief that they make hospitals safer based on the rational that early intervention will improve patient outcomes [12].

Design and Introduction

Magee-Womens Hospital of UPMC is a full-service, academic urban hospital and a tertiary referral center. It is the largest maternity hospital in Western Pennsylvania, performing over 11, 000 deliveries in 2013. At the time Magee considered adding an obstetric team, the UPMC health system already had a well-established rapid response system for medical emergencies, in addition to a full cardiac arrest team (Condition A). The medical crisis team (Condition C) had been activated occasionally for obstetric patients. Event review of these calls suggested that the team composition was not ideal for obstetric patients. Key personnel not included on the Condition C team include obstetricians, obstetric nurses, newborn resuscitation team, and anesthesia providers. The obstetric-specific team response was called "Condition O." Table 22.1 compares personnel who respond to Condition O and Condition C. Some institutions have opted to use their medical crisis team to respond to obstetric patient events.

It took approximately 1 year to design and fully implement the team. The process began in early 2005, and requires constant reevaluation and revision. As the number of obstetrical patients taken care of at Magee-Womens Hospital has increased, so have the number of Condition O

Fig. 22.1 Crisis team calls on obstetric patients, rate per 10,000 obstetric discharges.

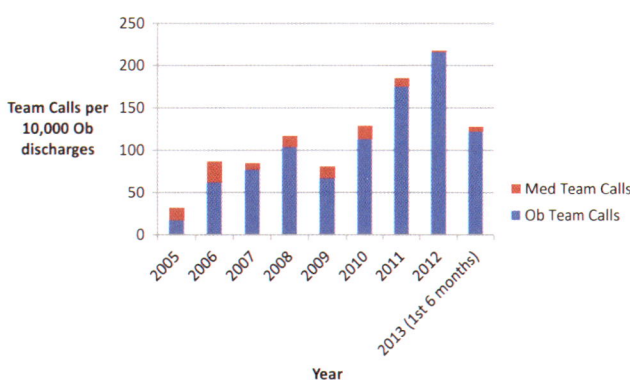

Table 22.1 Medical crisis vs. obstetric crisis team responders at Magee-Womens Hospital

Responder	Obstetric crisis (Condition O)	Medical crisis (Condition C)
In-house obstetrician	×	
Ob/Gyn resident (third and fourth year)	×	
Anesthesiology MD and/or nurse anesthetist	×	
Critical care medicine MD	×	×
Patient's nurse	×	×
Administrative clinician (nurse)	×	×
L&D charge nurse	×	
L&D clinician or manager (nurse)	×	
Newborn resuscitation team	×	
Respiratory		×
Emergency medicine MD		×
Resident on service		×
Emergency department nurse		×
Telemetry unit nurse		×
Safety/security officer	×	×

Ob/Gyn obstetrics and gynecology; *MD* physician; *L&D* labor and delivery

calls. Use of Condition O has also been associated with less Condition C calls in the labor and delivery suite.

Figure 22.1 in which is shown the growth of the obstetric rapid response utilization from 2005 thru the first 6 months of 2013.

Stakeholders in the following patient care areas: obstetrics, maternal–fetal medicine, obstetric nursing, critical care, neonatology, and anes-

thesiology convene to determine the appropriate team composition and size for the characteristics of our institution. Key considerations in team composition include provision of adequate nursing manpower, involvement of anesthesia providers, involvement of newborn resuscitation providers, and capability for real-time documentation. Activation criteria for Condition O include clinical events such as shoulder dystocia, seizure, or hemorrhage. Additionally, staff members are encouraged to call Condition O for acute situations in which the physician or nurse believes immediate evaluation/intervention is needed to avoid fetal/maternal harm. Activation criteria at other institutions with obstetric teams include "staff concern" with or without a list of clinical events such as those listed above. Additional clinical event triggers reported by other institutions include fetal distress, prolonged fetal bradycardia, and cord prolapse, absent fetal heart tones, vaginal bleeding, uterine rupture, emergent delivery, maternal respiratory distress, and maternal cardiac arrest. Some institutions have incorporated protocols that include recognition of events that can be considered "triggers" but not the actual onset of maternal/fetal emergencies. These include things such as agitation, pain, or changes in vital signs. Such an example is that of the Modified Early Obstetric Warning System (MEOWS) developed in Great Britain [13].

Table 22.1 shows the obstetric response team members at Magee-Womens Hospital. Table 22.2 shows the roles and duties that these responders fulfill during a crisis. Magee opted for a large team with full crisis care capabilities. Nursing contributes the highest number of responders.

Table 22.2 Obstetric crisis medical emergency team personnel and duties at Magee-Womens Hospital

Team member		Duties
Treatment leader *(obstetrician, occasionally anesthesiologist, as indicated)*		Obtain briefing from appropriate person, assess team organization/composition, assess data, direct treatment, set priorities, collaborate with anesthesia team on patient plan, triage patient
Bedside nurse *(usually patient's nurse)*	**Nursing team members select one of these roles as appropriate**	Stay by patient and communicate what is going on with the condition to the patient, attach monitoring, deliver briefing to responders, report IV size/location, adjust IV rate, draw up and administer medications
Runner *(L&D clinician or other personnel)*		Obtain medications and equipment, deliver to appropriate person
Senior obstetrical resident responder Nurse responder *(usually L&D charge nurse)* Safety and security personnel		Call for/dismiss personnel and family, call for/facilitate equipment acquisition, call for/facilitate patient transfer, get results
Documenter *(usually administrative clinician)*		Obtain record sheet, document (team leader, situation, vital signs and clinical data, treatments), brief personnel who come later
Procedure MD *(usually ob/gyn resident)*		Examine patient, inform team of maternal/fetal assessment, perform procedures
Anesthesia team *(attending anesthesiologist, anesthesia residents, nurse anesthetists and student nurse anesthetists, anesthesia technicians)*		Obtain briefing from obstetric team, assess analgesia, assess airway, perform anesthesia procedures, communicate anesthesia plan to team, arrange for cell salvage, collaborate with treatment leader on maternal issues
Newborn resuscitation team		Obtain briefing from obstetric team, assess newborn, resuscitate newborn

MD physician; *IV* intravenous; *L&D* labor and delivery; *ob/gyn* obstetrics and gynecology

This is because adequate nursing manpower is critical for implementing crisis interventions. Anesthesiology responds because they provide essential evaluation and intervention skills regarding anesthesia, analgesia, airway, and hemodynamic status. During the first 8 years of Condition O's at the hospital a critical care medicine (CCM) physician was designated to respond because almost one-quarter of crises at Magee are maternal. Currently the practice is to only call CCM by a "ramp up" mechanism if their services will be required, so as to decrease the very large number of responders. Similarly respiratory therapists initially came to all conditions but their services were rarely required. The neonatal resuscitation team was originally called only for gestations $\geq$ 24 weeks. However, a revised policy included them for every call on the labor and delivery suite. This change was motivated by the desire to eliminate an extra call, the need for timely arrival of the neonatal team, and gestational age uncertainty. Responders who are not needed for the crisis at hand are excused ("ramp down" strategy). This team composition suits Magee-Womens Hospital as a high volume, tertiary referral center with all of the described providers in the hospital 24/7.

Many other institutions with a high volume of obstetrics have obstetric-specific teams with similar personnel to the Condition O team. In general the obstetrical rapid response teams can be divided into four components necessary to optimize the response within the system. These components are the (1) activators of the response (generally the patients direct caregivers) (2) the responders to call, (3) quality improvement personnel who analyze the process, and (4) administrators who coordinate and perpetuate the effort. The following considerations help institutions who care for smaller volumes of inpatient obstetric patients to design an appropriate obstetric team. Skills needed by a full team include

Table 22.3 Core skills and potential personnel to include on an obstetric team

Skill	Possible provider type
Team leadership	Obstetrician Critical care physician Anesthesiologist Emergency physician Hospitalist physician
Adult medical crisis expertise (airway, breathing, circulation)	Critical care physician Emergency physician Anesthesiologist Hospitalist physician Respiratory therapy
Delivery and other obstetric management	Obstetrician Midwife Emergency physician Family medicine physician
Anesthesia for emergency procedures (or preparation for this)	Anesthesiologist Certified registered nurse anesthetist
Nursing task performance	Nurses from multiple units of the hospital (e.g., obstetric care, emergency department, medical-surgical unit, intensive care unit)
Coordination of additional resources (e.g., personnel, equipment, patient transfer, crowd control)	Nurse administrator Safety/security personnel
Acquisition of additional resources (e.g., medications, equipment)	Nurse Medical assistant/ Respiratory therapy Anesthesia technicians
Newborn resuscitation	Providers trained in newborn resuscitation (e.g., obstetrician, neonatal intensive care unit team, pediatric team, nurses)
Real-time documentation	Nurse Nurse administrator Physician

1) team leadership for data analysis and treatment decisions (this skillset may overlap with that of the team member serving in 2, 3, and 4 below), (2) adult medical crisis expertise, (3) delivery/obstetric management expertise, (4) provision of anesthesia for emergency operative procedures, (5) performance of nursing tasks, (6) coordination to acquire additional resources if needed, (7) acquire additional resources if needed, (8) newborn resuscitation, and (9) real-time documentation. Table 22.3 lists potential personnel who could participate. A single indi-

vidual may play multiple roles depending on the size of the team. As an alternate strategy, some institutions have opted for a "ramp up" approach with a small team (1–2 individuals). This smaller team responds, rapidly assesses, and has a process to summon additional personnel with the skills listed in Table 22.3 if indicated.

Staff Education:

Prior to initiating Condition O, the institution held education sessions for potential callers and potential responders. Sessions occurred during staff meetings for these caregivers. Written material about Condition O appeared in institutional newsletters and as postings on patient care units. Condition O was added to the list of emergency preparedness resources on the back of employee badges. New caregivers who are on-boarding are now fully educated on Condition O and how to implement it. Sustained implementation of the response is emphasized in monthly obstetrical crisis simulation training exercises.

Both callers and responders expressed initial resistance during these sessions and during the first 6 months of Condition O use. During the first few activations of the team, some physician responders criticized the caller (usually an obstetric nurse). Fear of this negative physician reaction resulted in few Condition O calls for about 6 months after implementation. To overcome this, further educational efforts included case-based discussions of teamwork during critical obstetric events, review of videotaped simulated crises with Condition O vs. usual sequential calling pattern, and an institutional multidisciplinary patient safety day. Facilitators of these sessions focused on two major points. (1) Responders must not criticize the caller for summoning the team to help a patient; and (2) Condition O greatly streamlines the crisis response process.

Response Team Training

Initial Condition O case review revealed opportunities for improvement in team organization, leadership, and crisis communication. In the beginning a multidisciplinary team from Magee-Womens Hospital initiated simulation-based team training at the Peter M. Winter Institute for Simulation, Education and Research to develop the Obstetric Crisis Team Training course (OCTT). The OCTT course trains both potential Condition O callers and responders, including obstetricians, anesthesiologists, and obstetric nurses. The course format involves online and in-person didactic presentations combined with filmed simulated emergencies and debriefing. The course curriculum was designed to meet the needs identified during the initial Condition O experience re: team performance and specific crises encountered. Course participants learn, practice, and debrief with a focus on the following key elements: crisis communication, team organization and leadership, and appropriate emergency care.

A streamlined version of the course is also utilized to facilitate learning during obstetric crisis drills done in situ on Magee's patient care units. Just like in the simulation center, these drills are filmed for video-based debriefing of team performance and participants practice methods of debriefing that can be used in actual crisis. Many other institutions with obstetric-specific teams use simulation-based crisis team training at simulation centers and/or in situ. Structured simulation-based team training for obstetric emergencies improves patient outcomes, including hypoxic-ischemic encephalopathy, 5-minute APGAR scores <7, and shoulder dystocia. [14, 15]

Data Collection, Review, and Process Improvement

The hospital developed a peer-review process of the obstetric crisis team calls which was similar to the review of cardiac arrests and medical crisis team calls. Obstetric crisis event records and patient medical record are reviewed by a designated physician to detect opportunities to improve patient management, team function, or systems issues that may have resulted in or influenced the crisis. Details of each team response are entered into the hospital's code response database. Multiple improvements have resulted from issues identified in obstetric crisis team events and crisis team drills. Additional major patient safety interventions that have resulted from this event review include interdisciplinary rounds every four hours on the labor and delivery unit and an increased number of attending obstetricians supervising care on the unit 24/7. In addition, a special group of hospitalist Obstetricians was also developed who expressly work in the Obstetrical Triage, and Labor and Delivery Suite.

Institutions initiating an obstetric-specific crisis response might consider collecting data on the following: (1) event rate; (2) event location; (3) reason for the call; (4) services provided by the team; (5) time (and duration) of initial call, team arrival, and end of resuscitation; (6) maternal and fetal clinical characteristics; (7) maternal and fetal/neonatal clinical outcomes; and (8) patient events for which the team should have been called but was not. Staff perception of the patient safety environment in obstetric care services may also give valuable feedback about the obstetric crisis team.

National Initiatives for Rapid Response Teams

As part of a national initiative led by the Institute for Healthcare Improvement there was a "How-to Guide" generated from data of five million incidents of medical harm between 2006 and 2008. This can serve as a basic guide to any group contemplating setting up such a response to obstetrical emergencies with in their maternal/fetal/neonatal care facility. [16]

Usage of Condition O at Magee-Womens Hospital and Discussion

Providers began using Condition O regularly beginning about 6 months after its introduction. Figure 22.1 shows crisis team call rates for obstetric patients since 2005. Providers called Condition O primarily for threats to fetal wellbeing (up to 90% in recent years). Use of the team for this indication suggests that the single call mechanism allows the caregivers (especially nursing) to focus

Table 22.4 Indications for obstetric crisis team activation, June 2005 through December 2013 listed in decreasing frequency of occurrence for each category

Indication		Number of Events
Fetal	Non reassuring fetal heart rate (Prolonged deceleration, heart rate lost, etc.)	Most frequent
	Shoulder dystocia	
	Cord prolapse	
	Imminent or precipitous delivery term	
	Imminent or precipitous delivery preterm	
	Imminent delivery of fetus with malpresentation (Footling breech, face, etc.)	
	Difficult delivery during cesarean section	
	Preterm labor	
	Rupture of membranes off of the obstetric unit	
	Contraction/abdominal/back pain off the obstetric unit	
	Head entrapment during breech delivery	Least frequent
Maternal	Postpartum hemorrhage	Most frequent
	Seizure	
	Syncope or lightheadedness	
	Patient unresponsive	
	Postpartum hypoglycemia	
	Respiratory distress	
	Chest pain/pressure	
	Possible intravenous injection of epidural medications	
	Upper gastrointestinal bleeding	Least frequent
Both	Abruption	Most frequent
	Antepartum vaginal bleeding	
	Hemorrhaging (placenta previa)	
	Home delivery preterm	Least frequent

Table 22.5 Indications for crisis team activation for obstetric patients, June 2005 through January 2013 (listed in decreasing order of events)

Indication
Most frequent
Syncope or lightheadedness
Seizure
Postpartum hemorrhage
Respiratory distress
Hemorrhage due to miscarriage
Patient unresponsive
Change in mental status
Trauma or fall
Anaphylaxis
Hypotension
Chest pain
Least frequent

on patient care interventions instead of summoning each member of the team individually. Emergencies that pose a direct risk to both mother and fetus have made up almost 10% of calls. Maternal crises constituted the remaining other percentage of events. Tables 22.4 and 22.5 describe the reasons for these calls and indicate their relative frequency. Obstetric caregivers are instructed to call Condition C purely for maternal indications, but many call Condition O anyway (perhaps because of familiarity with the call on the labor and delivery suite). In simulation training sessions it is taught that if an initial call later requires addition resources that it can always be escalated to another condition; for example an initial Condition O call can be followed by a Condition A in the case of a maternal arrest.

The majority of Condition O calls come for patients on labor and delivery and the obstetric triage unit. These units are adjacent to each other and staffed with multiple obstetricians, anesthesia personnel, and multitiered nursing providers. During the initial 6 months of Condition O, many nurses

Table 22.6 Obstetric crisis team activation locations, June 2010 through June 2013

Location	Number of events (Per Year)
Labor and delivery	>100
Triage unit	>40
Antepartum unit	>20
Emergency department	>20
Postpartum unit	>20
Ultrasound department	<10
Parking lot	<5
Cafeteria	<5
Staff meeting room	<5
Obstetric Antepartum Clinic	<5

Activation events for obstetric crisis (> is greater than, < is less than, yr is year)

Table 22.7 Patient and family satisfaction tool for obstetric emergency response

Questionnaire	Family	Patient
Cronbach's alpha	0.841	0.905
Test–retest Pearson's r	0.85	0.80
Subscale correlation	0.806	0.850

The questionnaire contains two different subscales—the first segment, which is composed of ten items, focuses on satisfaction with overall care and the second, which is composed of 2 Likert items and 3 comment free-writing sections, assesses satisfaction with regard to medical decision-making. All questions employ Likert-5 response scales

The patient and family satisfaction questionnaire in obstetric crisis has been found psychometrically sound with regard to measurement of satisfaction with care and medical decision-making of patients and families

For adaptation of actual tool to your institution please contact the primary author of this chapter

and physicians highlighted the ready availability of personnel on the unit. For this reason, they did not perceive that an obstetric crisis response team was needed. However, routine staffing on the unit is targeted to routine patient needs. Condition O use patterns demonstrate that providers' attitudes have shifted to recognize the periodic need for a rapid bolus of care resources. Table 22.6 indicates the patient location for Condition O calls on obstetric patients and their frequency.

Condition O patient events divert patient care resources from lower to higher acuity patients. This has raised the concern that the crisis response abandons lower acuity patients. However, Condition O's have thus far not resulted in staffing shortages for other obstetric patients at our hospital. The median duration of Condition O responses is less than 10 min. The majority of team members disband after a brief event review. Remaining members document the event for the medical record (physician team leader—several minutes) and for code response data collection (nurse administrator 5–30 min). Further review of the condition response occurs at the every 4 h patient safety interdisciplinary meetings, as well as later at formal conference time if deemed necessary.

Providers initially expressed concern that the Condition O response would scare patients and families. However, unsolicited patient comments at our institution indicate that patients and family are not frightened by the sudden influx of personnel

and flurry of activity during Condition O. This feedback suggests that patients and their families perceive the crisis team response as evidence of high quality emergency care. A quality improvement anonymous survey project at Magee-Womens Hospital of UPMC concerned patients and families whom had experienced a Condition O, queried their reactions to the event. The surveys found that both of the parties had appreciated the prompt and organized response to their emergency. Also it validated and proved reliable a patient and family satisfaction questionnaire that can be utilized for obstetrical emergency care situations [17, 18] See Table 22.7.

A need for patient and family education about what a Condition O response is and the possibility of a Condition O call during their hospitalization has been identified in our hospital. Some institutions, including ours have rapid response team information on their website; and separate literature and/or posters that they use to educate patients and families on the chance that they may experience such an event during their hospital stay.

Providers have used Condition O at a steady rate at our institution. An obstetric-specific crisis response team may be particularly important for institutions with lower volume and/or lower acuity obstetric units. Such units have fewer staff present 24/7 and fewer crises. For such institutions, a designated team may facilitate efficient training of team members and an improved response to obstetric crises.

The entire condition O response was reevaluated in 2014 at Magee-Womens Hospital of UPMC with the goal of optimization of the process from both the patient and provider perspectives. The most recent year's data of Condition O data was reviewed. Five areas of concern were identified and reviewed and the recommendations of the reviews follow.

Area of Concern 1. Definition of the optimal response team and the training of the team members.

It was found the overwhelming numbers of the Condition O's were called for perceived need for imminent delivery, for actual delivery problems, or immediate postpartum problems. On analysis the ICU team members and respiratory therapy providers (who until this time had been routinely responding to the calls) were found not to be routinely required for the response., NICU team members remained an integral part of calls from the labor and delivery areas but not for calls from the postpartum floors. The Condition O team members and response were reorganized and a new hospital based multidisciplinary simulation training course developed that emphasizes the new team composition and interactions.

Area of Concern 2. Determination of the leadership of the Condition O response and the delineation of the roles of various team responders.

The predominant leadership of the Condition O response was redesigned and designated to the Labor Suite Generalist who is a hospitalist obstetrician. One of the perceived problems with the Condition O response was the overwhelming number of responders to the call. It was determined that a senior obstetrical resident physician will take responsibility for the "ramp down" of too many Condition O responders since they have a very good knowledge of which responders are needed for the specific condition. This senior resident also coordinates with the labor and delivery nursing supervisor on duty the resources and locations utilized for the response. The patient's primary nurse remains with the patient to communicate the

response to the patient and continue direct patient care activities. Improvement in real time documentation of the response continues with a designated documenter and towards an electronic format with the help of the administrative clinicians.

Area of Concern 3. Further evaluation of the triggers for a Condition O call and elimination of barriers for the calling of a Condition O response.

Some recent criticism of called responses by some providers (primarily supervisory caregivers) had resulted in adverse psychological impact on the potential callers of the Condition O response (who were primarily the patient's direct care givers). This represented a "back-sliding" of the original intent of the Condition O call. Broad agreement reinforced the concept that nurses and any other obstetrical care provider could initiate the Condition O response and were not to be criticized for doing so. The culture that calling for help is to be congratulated for acting with patient safety concerns as a priority was reemphasized. The already established criteria for initiating a Condition O were validated and the concept that any clinical deterioration is grounds for making the call also required reinforcement.

Area of Concern 4. Establish an optimal debriefing process for Condition O responses and a schedule of Condition O Group meetings to assure continuous quality improvement.

Consensus was reached that all Condition O responses would be debriefed after the event at every 4 h group patient safety rounds. A mechanism for information to be fed forward to the Labor and Delivery Charge Nurse for presentation of the Condition O debriefing, if the providers themselves could not be present to discuss.

Area of Concern 5. Establishment of robust mechanisms for patient education prior to and after the occurrence of a Condition O

Patient education was enhanced about potential Condition O responses in the labor and delivery suite by adding additional information to the computerized electronic messages and consents available to patients on the hospital's website. New posters and direct signage in the patient rooms about the possibility of the response were introduced. All clinicians were strongly encouraged to debrief the patient and family after the event as soon as clinically appropriate.

These five areas of concern are issues that were identified as having become problematic with Magee-Womens-Hospital of UPMC initial Condition O response and so required restudy. It is very probable that the five areas of concern discussed above are similar to issues that have been found (or will be found) in other health care systems obstetrical emergency response. These areas of concerned may need to be reviewed to ensure the sustainability of an obstetrical specific rapid response team.

Part of the justification for introduction of Condition O was to apply the health system's successful experience with the rapid response system to a different clinical setting, widely recognized to be high risk and in need of periodic emergent multidisciplinary expert care. Condition O accomplished the goal of providing a reliable and effective resource that improves the patient care process. It is a resource that hospital staff members have used with consistent frequency since 2006. This provides evidence of both staff satisfaction with the process and a safety culture change.

Condition O has not had a detectable impact on the perinatal quality and safety data collected and reported by our institution. These parameters include The Joint Commission Obstetrical Pregnancy and Related Conditions Core Measures, the Agency for Healthcare Research and Quality Perinatal Patient Safety Indicators, the National Perinatal Information Service/Quality Analytic Services Obstetric Quality Indicators, and the Adverse Outcome Index. Specifically, these include event rates of vaginal birth after cesarean section, third or fourth degree laceration, obstetric trauma, postpartum readmissions, wound complications, anesthesia complications, neonatal mortality, birth trauma injury to neonates, and birth trauma linked to maternal shoulder dystocia. The Adverse Outcome Index includes maternal deaths, intrapartum neonatal death, uterine rupture, unplanned maternal intensive care admission, birth trauma, return to the operating room or labor and delivery, neonatal intensive care unit admission ≥37 weeks and ≥2500 g, maternal

blood transfusion, and third or fourth-degree laceration. Many of these measures are not directly related to the crisis team activities. Some of the potentially relevant outcomes such as maternal and neonatal death are such rare events that crisis team impact is difficult to assess. The institution also evaluated malpractice claims data for possible impact of Condition O on malpractice activity. However, not enough time has elapsed since 2005 to assess the impact on professional liability activity, given the long statute of limitations on obstetric cases.

The following patient outcome measures may help assess the impact of an obstetric crisis team. For events with emergency concerns about fetal wellbeing that result in cesarean section (prolonged bradycardia, cord prolapse, etc.) collect data on time from decision for cesarean section to incision ("decision to incision"), APGAR scores, cord blood gases, neonatal seizures, and unanticipated neonatal intensive care admission. For patients with obstetric hemorrhage, collect data on the number and type of blood products administered, estimated blood loss, use of the cell salvage equipment as well as rapid infusion devices, utilization of interventional radiology for urgent bleeding situations, and unanticipated hysterectomy. For shoulder dystocia events, collect data on the time from delivery of the newborn's head to delivery of the body ("head to body interval"), APGAR scores, cord blood gases, and neonatal fracture and nerve injuries.

Patient safety initiatives are commonly criticized because of the inability to detect and demonstrate a causal link between process change and outcome. Obstetric quality and patient safety indicators are in need of evaluation and revision to boost their ability to discriminate between high and low quality care. [1, 2, 18] This revision process is currently underway. Future measures may improve the ability to evaluate the impact of patient safety initiatives such as Condition O. However, in the modern patient safety environment, clinical areas often have multiple safety and quality improvement projects ongoing at any given time [19]. Thus it can be difficult to show a causal link between a specific initiative and a specific patient outcome measure.

Conclusion

An obstetric-specific crisis team allows institutions to optimize the care response for patients with emergent maternal and/or fetal needs. Characteristics of an optimal obstetric rapid response team are team member role designations, streamlined communication, prompt access to resources, and ongoing education, rehearsal, and training along with continual team quality analysis. The team response provides a key resource to reassure staff, physicians, and patients that prompt crisis care is only a single call away. Data on the obstetric-specific crisis response at Magee-Womens Hospital show that team activation is common, improves the care process, and has promise to improve outcomes directly and/or through event analysis and subsequent process improvement. Each individual obstetrical care situation should be encouraged to develop an emergency obstetrical response that fits its situation and multidisciplinary approach.

Acknowledgement No author has any conflicts of interest related to the content of this chapter.

References

1. Callaghan WM, Creanga AA, Kuklina EV. Severe maternal morbidity among delivery and postpartum hospitalizations in the United States. Obstet Gynecol. 2012;120:1029–36.
2. ACOG. ACOG Committee Opinion: Preparing for Clinical Emergencies in Obstetrics and Gynecology. Obstet Gynecol. 2014;123(3):722–5.
3. Obstetrical Harm Change Package 2014 Update; recognition and prevention of obstetrical related events and harm Available at: www.hret-hen.org/index.php.
4. Guise JM. Anticipating and responding to obstetric emergencies. Best Pract Res Clin Obstet Gynaecol. 2007;21(4):625–38.
5. Al Kadri HM. Obstetric medical emergency teams are a step forward in maternal safety! J Emerg Trauma Shock. 2010;3(4):331–415.
6. Clark ES, Fisher J, Arafeh J, Druzin M. Team training/simulation. Clin Obstet Gynecol. 2010;53(1):265–77.
7. Clements CJ, Flohr-Rincon S, Bombard AT, Catanzarite V. OB team stat: rapid response to obstetrical emergencies. Nurs Womens Health. 2007;11:194–9.
8. JCAHO. Preventing infant death and injury during delivery. Sentinel Event Alert. 2004;30:1–3.
9. DeVita MA, Braithwaite RS, Mahidhara R, Stuart S, Foraida M, Simmons RL. Use of medical emergency team responses to reduce hospital cardiopulmonary arrests. Qual Saf Health Care. 2004;13(4):251–4.
10. Braithwaite RS, DeVita MA, Mahidhara R, Simmons RL, Stuart S, Foraida M. Use of medical emergency team (MET) responses to detect medical errors. Qual Saf Health Care. 2004;13(4):255–9.
11. Galhotra S, Scholle CC, Dew MA, Mininni NC, Clermont G, DeVita MA. Medical emergency teams: a strategy for improving patient care and nursing work environments. J Adv Nurs. 2006;55(2):180–7.
12. Jones DA, DeVita MA, Bellomo R. Rapid response teams (current concepts). N Engl J Med. 2011;365(2):139–46.
13. Singh S, McGlennan A, England A, Simons R. A validation study of the CEMACH recommended modified early obstetric warning system (MEOWS). Anaesthesia. 2012;67:12–8.
14. Draycott T, Sibanda T, Owen L, Akande V, Winter C, Reading S, et al. Does training in obstetric emergencies improve neonatal outcome? BJOG. 2006;113(2):177–82.
15. Draycott TJ, Crofts JF, Ash JP, Wilson LV, Yard E, Sibanda T, et al. Improving neonatal outcome through practical shoulder dystocia training. Obstet Gynecol. 2008;112(1):14–20.
16. Million lives campaign. Getting started kit: rapid response teams. Cambridge, MA: Institure for Healthcare Improvement; 2008 (Available at www.ihi.org).
17. Wall RJ. Refinement, scoring, and validation of the family satisfaction in the intensive care unit (FS-ICU) survey. Crit Care Med. 2007;35(1):271–9.
18. Zhan Hanzi, Kwon Carolyn, Stein Karen, Gosman Gabriella, Slater Brian, Dalby Patricia. Patient and family satisfaction following emergency obstetric crisis: development of a valid and reliable questionnaire, Abstract: at society for obstetrical anesthesiology and perinatology 2014 Annual Meeting proceedings (unpublished).
19. Grobman WA. Patient safety in obstetrics and gynecology: the call to arms. Obstet Gynecol. 2006;108(5):1058–9.

Sonali Mantoo, Michael A. DeVita,
Andrew W. Murray, and John J. Schaefer III

Introduction

Care for patients who are in a medical crisis has historically entailed management by their physician and nursing staff in a way that was somewhat haphazard and reactive. The system's success was based largely on whether the established hierarchy (nurse to resident to attending; or nurse to generalist to specialist) was followed in an appropriate and timely manner, allowing the patient to receive the required attention rapidly enough to prevent further deterioration. Staff often learned how to respond to crises on the job: they were handed pagers and told to respond, but rarely received specific instruction regarding who else should respond, who had responsibility for what, and what was expected of them during a crisis event. It is no wonder that crisis responses have often been described as chaotic.

This chapter is an overview of the personnel and skills required to achieve a successful rapid-response system. Although the majority of the chapter discusses the response team and necessary skills of the responders, it is a misconception to think that only the responders need to be trained. The RRS is a facility wide endeavor requiring some form of education for all.

S. Mantoo, MD
Critical Care Medicine, Harlem Hospital,
New York, NY 10026, USA
e-mail: Mdevita06@gmail.com

M.A. DeVita, MD, FCCM, FACP (✉)
Department of Surgery, Critical Care,
Harlem Hospital Center, 506 Lenox Avenue,
New York, NY 10037, USA

Department of Internal Medicine, Critical Care,
Harlem Hospital Center, 506 Lenox Avenue,
New York, NY 10037, USA
e-mail: michael.devita@NYCHHC.ORG

A.W. Murray, MD
Department of Anesthesiology and Perioperative Medicine,
Mayo Clinic, Phoenix, AZ 85054, USA

J.J. Schaefer III, MD
Medical University of South Carolina,
96 Jonathan Lucas St, Charleston, SC 29425, USA

Impact of Hierarchy on Care

There is a hierarchy making the patient's individual attending physician the "captain of the ship." This is a great strategy for coordinating care in routine situations, but can become an obstruction to rapidly responding to changes in a patient's status especially if the attending does not have critical care skills or is not present at the patient's bedside. In a medical education model, a nurse assistant would first call the nurse, who would then call the intern, who would call the resident, who would then call the attending physician of record, with each call occurring when the individual perceived that he or she was incapable of managing the situation. A similar problem occurs in a community hospital: the nurse assistant notifies the nurse who calls the primary physician, who then calls one or more consultants. For a patient with sudden onset of respiratory distress, one can imagine that it could take 30 min or more just to contact the person best able to manage the problem. By then, the patient's condition could have significantly deteriorated, to the point where the patient could be *in extremis*. Further, when multiple parties are involved, who the "captain" is may become ambiguous.

Hierarchical considerations are found in many settings and create a social framework that in a crisis setting can interfere with optimal patient care [1]. For example, a nurse responsible for a patient experiencing a crisis may feel reluctant to offer suggestions or important information to a perceived higher authority because they feel that it is not their "place" in the social order [2]. The rapid response system (either using a medical emergency team (MET) or a rapid response team (RRT) as the responders) is an improved method of providing care for these patients, because it brings the necessary individuals to the bedside within minutes and establishes a "flat" hierarchy that prioritizes communication and cooperation. A number of studies have shown that there is an inverse relationship between the number of rapid response system (RRS) activations and the incidence of cardiac arrest and unexpected death [3–6].

Unfortunately, devising trigger and response strategies is insufficient by itself to create change. Behavioral changes need to occur as well, and that relies on culture change to call for help sooner. While this paradigm requires individual behaviors, to be effective it must reach the institutional level. Implementation of change in response to patient deterioration is difficult primarily because it requires institutional commitment of leadership and resources.

Health Care Education for Crisis: Focused Training and Experience to Achieve Expertise

One may assume that once physicians, nurses, and other health care professionals (HCP) have completed their training, they are adequately equipped to deal with any crisis that may arise.

The method of training has been based on an apprenticeship model, relying on individuals to learn by observing more experienced individuals, and then work under close supervision. There is an assumption that the more frequently one encounters a situation, the more expert one becomes. Some people do this very well, but others do not because of inattentive mentors, or nonequivalent exposure to events. Clinical learning is an inherently time-inefficient process. Expertise requires in addition to competence, a wealth of experience. There is a question as to whether all staff can be trained to a point where all have expertise in caring for suddenly deteriorating patients. If all staff could be trained to become expert, then in theory people will be able to deal effectively with crises. The problem is that people encountering few events lack the experience to become expert. This level of personnel training for the organization may be impossible. It is more efficient to train specialized teams to effectively and efficiently provide care and rely on them to provide the care throughout the organization. The support required to enable expert response will be less because fewer people have to be trained. This model does not absolve the rest of the hospital staff from being part of the RRS. They too play a part, and require training to be successful. The majority of the hospital workers need training to (1) recognize a crisis, (2) trigger a response, and (3) do an efficient handoff. Basic life support (BLS) and/or advanced cardiac life-support training remain important, but they are not sufficient for managing crises. Crisis care is rarely delivered well by one individual. Teamwork is required [7, 8].

Educational Targets for Crisis Response Personnel

Some basic skills for responders have been reported and include the ability to review the health care record, obtain a focused history, create a management plan, and explain thought processes to other staff, patients, and their loved ones. Technical tasks include examining circulation, respiration, and consciousness, ability to adjust oxygen, perform an EKG, administer fluids, and infuse medications [9].

Best care also requires a well-coordinated team. The knowledge set "teamwork" is distinct from other HCP education. Knowledge of the causes of respiratory distress and what treatments are indicated certainly facilitates care management of patients. Advanced education and training in a profession, specialty, or subspecialty are beneficial because they impart this knowledge. An additional form of training is necessary: teamwork training [7, 8]. Behaving as a team requires training to be a team. While each individual may be capable, groups cannot be expected to be as effective as a trained team. Without a role-specific action plan that coordinates the individuals and group practice they will not be a team. Uncoordinated ad hoc responses are risky for both the HCP and patient [5, 10].

When first exposed to a crisis scenario in a simulated setting, inexperienced anesthesiology residents may respond in the following ways:

1. Compulsion to do something
2. Loss of routine
3. Fixation on a task
4. Loss of effective communication

In a crisis, caregivers may feel compelled to do something to help the patient, even if they are not certain as to the best course of action, leading to unfocused activity.

There may be an emphasis by educational programs on some aspects of emergency care while not promoting actions that support accomplishing the necessary tasks. For example, advanced cardiac life support (ACLS) learners to perform the ABC's (airway–breathing–circulation) of resuscitation. The ABC's of course are important because successful completion of the ABC's result in improved outcome. However, focus on A-B-C does not consider team dynamics during a crisis response. As a result of the focus on "what-to" instead of "how-to," all responders may attempt to do the same interventions, or neglect some necessary aspects of care. The uncoordinated response is therefore danger-ous and can only be averted through interdisciplinary training. Other clinicians may undertake an action even though there is no benefit to the action or it is a low priority. An example is obtaining an arterial blood gas (ABG) when a patient is hypoxic. The most important step is not an ABG, it is supplementing oxygenation and ventilation.

The loss of the routine has the effect of putting "blinders" on the provider, as they may ignore data and thus be unable to respond [1]. The ability to maintain treatment and diagnostic priority as well as consider the social, personnel, and equipment characteristics of a crisis is termed "situational awareness" (SA). Effective team personnel maintain SA. Loss of SA may cause focus on one aspect of care and neglect of the situation as a whole. Communication during a crisis response may break down to the point that no data is shared, no leadership is apparent, and no decisions are made in a timely fashion. Team members may not know what happened to the patient, what has been done, or what still needs to be addressed. Planning and practice are needed to overcome both intrapersonal and interpersonal barriers to effective crisis management [10, 11].

How Organization Can Help in Crisis Response

Organizing the response to a crisis is an attempt to ensure that a team of different people can respond to an unexpected event and, once there, cooperate to perform a series of interrelated tasks and adapt to overcome barriers so as to benefit the patient [2, 5, 10]. This concept of adaptability is a highly useful team attribute considering the potential spectrum and complexity of medical crises. From an educational *design* perspective, this concept allows trainers to teach the trainees to focus on role-oriented goals and objectives and apply them to the collective team goals and objectives. The goal is not only to simply perform designated tasks but also to constantly monitor the situation and note how an individual's response has to change to coordinate with that of others. From a learner perspective, the role-specific tasks within the collective response allows them to focus on their own task set for treatment, monitoring, and communication. Through a focused understanding of how their actions influence, and are influenced by other team members' goals, the learner can become more able to achieve individual goals and contribute to other's performance. The institutional or system advantage of training individuals in teamwork is that while the personnel may change with each response, the individual and the team objectives are standardized. As long as the responders know what the roles are, what role they are taking on, and the role interactions among the group, then any combination of trained individuals can gather to solve the address the crisis [10].

The team's collective skill set and knowledge transcends that of the individual [2]. To put this to best advantage, teamwork skills should include social or professional behaviors and expectations centered on the primary goal of the patient's welfare. Hierarchal professional and social barriers can decrease a team's performance. Adherence to determine "what" to do rather than "how to get it done" can lead to inefficiency. Based on this premise, some team training courses promote "O-ABC" instead of "ABC," where O equals "organize." The few seconds it takes to organize responders according to roles enables more coordinated responses and more efficient and effective care [10]. ABC happens faster with an organized group response.

The process of training responders also provides an opportunity to uncover and correct latent errors. Simulation is a useful tool. Repetition of simulated events enables discovery of the types of errors that are made in a particular setting. A chaotic response may add risk (e.g., performing a treatment that includes a risk of complication or failure to perform an important task). In the simulation training environment, actions can be identified, corrected, and reevaluated. Errors can be allowed to "play out" so the team members can observe the consequences of their actions. For example, fixation on one task while the situation requires that several tasks be completed leads to poor outcome. Organizing crisis response enables triaging tasks to specific individuals as a routine

and avoid fixation errors. The division of labor should reduce each person's required workload. Planning enables prioritization of tasks and focuses effort on what needs to be completed first. With fewer tasks to accomplish (due to better division of labor) and improved speed of completion (due to rehearsal), the team members become positioned to either help with another team member's tasks or to perform their next required task. Thus "choreographing" tasks for the team beforehand can directly improve the efficiency of both the individuals' and the team's performance. In crisis situation, where speed and accuracy are most important, the planning and rehearsal lead to improved outcome for the patient.

When the position of leader is predetermined or accepted by all members of the team, it allows that person to observe the situation and make clear-minded, informed decisions regarding care. This role should be regarded more as a coordinating position than a hierarchical one. In the crisis team training approach, individuals know what his or her skill set and responsibility are before they arrive. This enables team members to self-assign. Because team leaders do not have to organize personnel resources or perform a specific therapy, they can instead focus on collection of data, data interpretation, treatment prioritization, reassessment, etc. Focus on organizing the team, diverts the leader's attention and may lead to error.

Organizing the Personnel

The thought processes involved in the management of a crisis need to be quick, reliable, and able to adapt easily to a changing situation. Effective performance requires that the team member be able to perform routine tasks and use sensorimotor input to make adjustments. Cognitively, this implies the efficient combination of pattern recognition and reflexive response. Until recently, health care educators have expected this development to occur through experience in an apprenticeship training process. However, the optimal routines may not be established through experience alone. This is especially important for the leader. This role requires the individual to be able to step back from the situation, observe, analyze, and intervene through the other responding personnel. The leader should ensure that tasks assigned are done, the right interventions are occurring, data is collected and reported, and treatment decisions are made. This can be difficult for the less experienced leader because functioning occurs on two levels. The first level includes the following: what is happening? what is--> the problem/diagnosis, what actions are needed? and are interventions effective? This is focus is patient centered. The second level is that of team performance oversight. The leader should supervise the amount of attention that team members are devoting to any given task. The better defined the roles and tasks are, the more likely that task completion occurs. The leader should create a mental priority list for the next point of care rather than focusing on who needs to be doing what. "Resource management" is included in this level of cognition. This skill focuses on using resources (human and otherwise) most effectively. This may occasionally entail changing the roles of the team members to ensure that the efficiency is maintained.

Structure

One of the keys to caring for suddenly critically ill patients better is being able to treat the patient early in the progression of the crisis. This entails equipping the nursing staff and junior physicians with the tools and training that they need to feel comfortable asking for help at the best possible time: earlier rather than later. This requires specific training for the persons who call the response (as opposed to the responder training). This afferent limb training should address what the crisis criteria are, how to communicate the need for help, and how to hand off care to the responder. Every person in the organization should be trained on these three objectives, making the entire organization responsible for crisis management.

One goal of crisis management is the personnel and equipment resources to be applied to the medical emergency situation once the call for help occurs. This is the efferent limb. A second aspect is the structure of team activation, from

the initial recognition of trouble, to the call for help, to the responder arrival: the afferent limb. Both limbs need to be reliable, consistent, and unambiguous. Both the responder and the caller actions need to be taught to the appropriate staff and monitored to ensure adherence. They require separate educational efforts. These two types of training (caller/crisis recognition, and responder/crisis response) are best accomplished with simulation training techniques.

Personnel

Whereas it would be very comforting to have a dedicated team that has no responsibility other than responding to crises, this may not be feasible in most hospitals because of the cost. To address the need for 24 h availability, the medical emergency team must have access to people with the necessary knowledge and skill set and who can be called together at a moment's notice. It is possible that they may have to come from different ends of the hospital, and they should be trained to be capable of focusing their collective capabilities to care for a single individual. The team needs to be large enough to be able to provide all the technical and knowledge resources that are required but not so big that it becomes cumbersome. In this section, we are promoting the skills the personnel must have to fulfill the various roles needed on the response team. We specifically are avoiding assignment to the team based upon profession. Skills are more important that educational degree. Focus on educational degree may limit people from filling gaps in the team response. For example, a nurse can be the airway assistant, airway manager, or treatment leader as long as the requisite skills are present.

Work at the University of Pittsburgh demonstrated that simulated patient survival is best if the team has a treatment leader and a record-keeper/data gatherer. The latter must collect a complete data set to enable good decisions, and the former must be positioned to analyze the data and maintain an understanding of the larger picture of the unfolding crisis. The remaining team members must assume identified roles and complete the essential tasks for each, reporting back to the leader (and each other). The roles need to be designed to ensure application of monitors, airway management, intravenous access, and performing a patient examination. The details of these roles and responsibilities are described below in terms of skills required to assume the task, and a separate chapter in this book focuses on team training in detail (*see* Chap. 32). A study done in New Zealand demonstrated that the providers were unclear of the roles and responsibilities of various team members especially crossing professional boundaries indicating the continuing need for this to be addressed in the training phase [12].

In addition to knowing the roles, team members should consist of people who are experienced with crisis situations. These personnel most commonly are staffed to the critical care areas of the hospital, but other HCPs are reported. Intensivist physicians (fellow and attending), an intensive care nurse, are optimal but may not be available at all times. Howell has promoted using the medicine residents on duty that day for the specific patient. Specialists in airway management and surgical management should be available, but are often not primary responders. An additional response team member is an administrator to facilitate the rapid transit of the patient to an ICU location when necessary. While most hospitals will not have this wealth of resources, the functions undertaken by this group need to be done by the responder team irrespective of the team size.

It is not clear who the optimal responders to fill each role should be. Howell and colleagues reported a rapid response system that relied on a patient's usual care providers, not an "imported" critical-care-trained rapid-response team [13]. Their model utilized the above noted team characteristics and relied on widely disseminated criteria for escalation (calling in a superior in a tightly regulated time framework to avoid delays). In essence, they transformed the usual team into a de facto rapid response team. In the intervention period, patients were monitored for predefined, acute vital sign abnormalities or nursing concern. If these criteria were met, a team consisting of the patient's existing care providers was emergently assembled. This primary-team-based implementation of a rapid response system was independently associated with reduced unexpected mortality similar to that reported in other RRSs. We may call this an "at-home rapid response team."

This staffing system may offer an alternative approach for personnel required for a rapid response system and may be particularly attractive to hospitals with limited intensivist availability but with around the clock physician presence for every patient. As all RRSs, it relies upon careful training and adherence to the protocol, to prevent "return to the usual." It is not clear whether additional resources are brought to the bedside to fulfill responsibilities for medication preparation and delivery, and airway management. This schema relies on delineating the rapid response event from the "usual" event like a fever. The sustainability of this methodology will rely on maintaining training, auditing compliance, and feeding back to staff their performance. These results may provide a less costly approach for hospitals to protect the particularly vulnerable population of decompensating patients.

Another RRS team model is the nurse led rapid response team, using a nurse-to-nurse consult approach, often assisted by a respiratory therapist [14]. As previously noted, the majority of in-hospital cardiac arrests are preceded by observable indicators of deterioration within hours of the event. Nurses triggered a response by the nurse led team who were often able to provide sufficient support to the primary nursing team to obviate a need to call a physician to the bedside. The primary reason for team activation was nurses' concern about the patient. The patient often was managed without direct physician intervention; however, it is important to note that in this study, a physician was always immediately available by phone and if necessary at the bedside. The response team helped with urgent questions about medications, or recognition of problems. They followed care algorithms or obtained physician input by phone. This model may spare physician-responders from having to attend each event, and may be equally effective in preventing patient demise. One year after the implementation of this type of rapid response system, the incidence of cardiac arrest events outside of the intensive care unit was reduced by 9 % and overall hospital mortality by 0.12 %. Nurses' responses indicated that they valued the consultant team as a method to both foster professional growth and improve patient outcomes. The nurse-led team is by far the most common RRS approach in the UK. There the system is termed critical care outreach (CCO), and like other models responds to alerts regarding patients who have sudden deterioration. This national model goes further: the CCO team also makes routine rounds on high risk patients like those transferred recently from the ICU to the ward to prevent an RRS event.

Activation of the RRS: The Need for a "Global Team"

A response cannot occur if there is no call to initiate it. Therefore it is important to develop a methodology for this. Smith has identified four steps to this process: Education, detection, recognition, and trigger [15]. Education includes the knowledge that the RRS exists, why it is important, and everyone's role in the system. For most people, the education should focus on "finding" the patient in distress (detection), understand that a crisis is occurring (recognition), and make the call for the team (trigger). The whole hospital should receive this information, which in effect, turns everyone into an important part of the rapid response system [15, 16]. They must act quickly. The amount of time that the responders take to respond affects the outcome, as illustrated in a study in Italy that showed that in cardiac arrest cases where the crisis response took longer than 6 min, no patient survived [7]. Several studies have shown a dramatic increase in mortality when a patient meets triggering criteria for longer than 30 min prior to the response team getting to the bedside [17–20]. While the optimal response time for an RRS event has not been established, 30 min from achieving criteria to either resolution of symptoms or arrival of the team to the bedside seems a reasonable benchmark.

The Ad Hoc Responder Team

Personnel who have other duties but who will respond to a call will become part of an ad hoc team (Table 23.1). Each person who responds will bring experience and a skill set that is specific and necessary. The various skills can be a source of strength or weakness. The strength is that enough people respond to be able to divide the workload and function as a collective unit. The weakness is that the ad hoc structure promotes a chaotic response. If the team is too large or uncoordinated, individuals may not perceive themselves as useful or that their opinion will not be regarded thoughtfully. Ideally, the people who arrive upon activation of the MET previously would have practiced working together. More often than not however, they may have only occasionally worked together and in some cases not at all. Careful education regarding the required roles for the team members, and the tasks assigned to the roles can help overcome the ad hoc nature of the team [8, 10]. Each institution must create its own structure in response to the perceived needs that they experience on a day-to-day basis. And education is required to ensure that all know the structure.

Table 23.1 Roles and goals for crisis team in the operating room

Responder roles skills/expertise
Team leader experience in managing acutely ill patients, preferably current
attending anesthesiologist/surgeon
Advanced cardiac life support training
Technician blood sampling (arterial blood gas, coagulants, thromboelastography)
Troubleshooting equipment
Supply equipment needs
Scribe keep accurate record of interventions and results
Airway management if needed in airway emergency
Medication delivery knowledge of allergies
Knowledge of ongoing medicinal therapy
Knowledge of pharmacology
Advanced cardiac life support training
Circulatory support provide cardiopulmonary resuscitation support if needed
Surgeon surgical intervention to correct or prevent problems

Creating Culture Change

Culture change requires behavior change. If one is successful in creating behavior change, people's expectations of what should occur will follow. The expectation of behavior and the behavior itself are a major part of "culture." Nevertheless, much of the difficulty in altering the way things are done exists in changing the minds of the people involved. The longer things are done a certain way, the stronger the culture becomes. During many physicians' and nurses' training, there was an expectation that a skilled physician and nurse should be able to deal with any crisis. Failure to do so may imply weakness, inadequate knowledge or training, lack of industry or determination, or fear. Thus calling for help has a negative connotation. The organized management of crises has only been addressed in the past decade or so. A study published in 2008 showed that ICU trainees felt that the training and time spent on medical emergency teams was beneficial for their training and the care of patients on the wards but sounded alarm about the potential for decreased care for patients in the ICU. An additional concern was that there was insufficient supervision during MET activations [11]. Medical trainees should be introduced to the concept of a team approach to crisis and should receive team training. This will allow for the development of respect for one's limitations, as well as for the contributions of other responders. The training should stress that the concept of being "all-capable" is a false ideal: the well-trained team performs better than individuals.

Rapid Response System training should focus on non-medical, non-technical aspects of team management of a medical crisis [8]. The emphasis is on the concept of being a member of a team and having a role to play with specific tasks to accomplish. Communication is a key skill for outstanding teamwork. Communication needs to be clear and organized. Speaking should be limited to what is absolutely necessary in order to minimize confusion and missed orders. Such communication should function as a closed loop, so that the individual who asks the question or gives the order is absolutely sure that they were heard, understood, and that the request is being carried out or is already completed. Resource management is also a concept that needs practice and training. The person functioning as the leader needs to be trained so that all their resources, human and otherwise, are managed effectively and brought to bear to resolve problems.

An important component of resource management is recognizing the crisis and reliably triggering the team to respond. The UPMC had a system in place for responding to crises for a decade, but it saw limited use while physicians were still being paged urgently and sequentially to the bedside to care for their patients. The culture had remained the same in spite of the creation of a new system. The institution then started reviewing the incidences of sequential stat pages and observing the consequences. The findings were related to nursing units and nurses were encouraged to use the team. Individuals responsible for delay in team activation were given feedback on their actions. However, this did not impact behavior significantly. The most effective interventions to create behavior change were [1]: the establishment of objective calling criteria, and [2] the dissemination of these criteria to the nursing units and other caregiver groups. The result was a significant positive change in MET use, with a corresponding drop in the number of sequential stat pages, which was the "old" way of assembling a group to deal with a deteriorating patient [16].

Because hospital resources differ, team compositions are different (Table 23.2), but the roles and tasks are constant. We have identified a number of different roles that must be filled: airway manager, airway assistant, circulatory support person, someone to deliver medications, someone to deploy medications and equipment from the crash cart, a person who makes therapeutic decisions after analyzing the data, and finally, someone to collect data and record the events [10]. The skills and knowledge needed for each position is different. The **airway manager** will be responsible for assessing the airway, positioning the head, choosing whether ventilation needs to be assisted, and if so, determine the methodology for that. The airway manager must know

Table 23.2 Roles and goals of MET responders, Pittsburgh methodology

Responder roles Skills/expertise
Treatment leader management of acutely ill patients in ER, OR, or ICU
Airway manager mask ventilation
Endotracheal intubation
Neurological assessment
Administer medications (sedative, neuromuscular blocking agents)
Airway assistance mask ventilation
Bedside assessment attain reliable intravenous access
Delivery of medications
Knowledge of allergies
Obtain vital signs
Equipment manager deploy medications and equipment (crash cart) run defibrillator
Circulatory support rapid assessment of the patient's physical examination
Mechanical circulatory support
Place defibrillator pads
Data manager keep accurate recording of the events of the crisis
Obtain key data from chart, caregivers
Deliver data to treatment leader
Procedure physician check pulse, adequacy of chest compressions
Perform procedures

how to mask-ventilate the patient, suction the airway, and intubate the trachea if necessary. In addition, because of the location relative to the patient, the airway manager should be able to assess the patient's level of consciousness, check pupils, and feel carotid pulses. Finally, the airway manager must have the capability to order medications for sedation, anesthesia, or neuromuscular blockade to facilitate intubation when necessary. Because of the complexity of these skills for set of duties, the airway manager role can be filled by only a few types of professionals. Usually anesthesia, critical care, and emergency medicine physicians, as well as nurse anesthetists have this capability, and so they are usually responsible for this role. It is important to note that the defining characteristic for a person taking on a particular role is the skill and knowledge set and not the title, specialty, or profession. Respiratory care personnel have the training and

experience to noninvasively manage the airway, and therefore they may make excellent airway managers. At some hospitals, they also have the skills to perform endotracheal intubation using standardized physician order sets for sedation. With appropriate training, so may some nursing staff.

The point is training and skill, and not profession, determines what roles a person is qualified to fill. Trainees for the team must learn their own skill sets so they can understand their "menu of capabilities" for taking on various roles on the team. They should exclude themselves from roles they do not have the skills for, and position themselves for those that they can do.

Other roles in the team include the **airway assistant** to deploy and assemble a bag-mask unit for use, connect the oxygen source to the airway devices, set up suction, assist intubation, prepare the endotracheal tube and laryngoscope prior to insertion, testing carbon dioxide in exhaled air, and connect the patient to a ventilator if necessary.

A **crash cart manager** is needed to staff the crash cart because it contains a large variety of medications and equipment needed for a crisis response. The medications must be located swiftly and mixed expertly, and then delivered via the appropriate route. Pharmacists or nurses usually take on this role, although physicians may also possess the skills.

Most teams have a person responsible for recording what happens during the crisis, usually focusing on the vital signs and treatments delivered. Because one of the more common mistakes in a crisis response team is a failure to collect data and deliver it to the person who needs that information to make decisions, we advocate the "recorder" also be a "data gatherer." This role is titled "**data manager**." The personnel taking on this role is responsible for collecting a database that includes recent laboratory results, electrocardiogram and chest x-ray results, and physical findings by the team.

A "**bedside assistant**" is needed to deliver the medications and to obtain vital signs. There is strong reasoning for the patient's bedside nurse to assume this role because she or he usually is aware of the prior state of the patient, and is aware of allergies and recent medication administrations. This knowledge can prevent error or lead to a diagnosis of the etiology of the crisis.

The role and responsibilities of the **treatment leader** have been discussed earlier in this chapter. The two final roles are **circulation manager** and **procedures**. The tasks of the former are to continuously assess adequacy of circulation and ensure provision of circulatory support (often in the form of chest compressions) if needed. The latter is responsible for performing any necessary procedure, including obtaining blood for laboratory analysis and inserting tubes or catheters. If no procedure is needed, the procedure person should also assess adequacy of circulation and assist the circulation manager in providing chest compressions when needed.

Some hospitals will have sufficient personnel to have one person assume each of the eight roles. Other institutions may not have as many responders, and so one person may need to assume more than one role. In designing a crisis team response, the directors should attend to these roles, and make sure that responders with adequate skills and knowledge are assigned to them. Redundancy can be built in when establishing the teams by cross-training responders.

Operating Room Crisis Teams

Crisis teams may be needed for other purposes than a crisis on a hospital ward or lobby area. As noted in the chapter "Other Crisis Teams," there are critical events that require an RRS approach, but require skills beyond that of the usual RRT. One example is anesthesia or operating room (OR) crisis teams [1]. OR crisis teams respond to anesthetic emergencies, such as a difficult airway with failure to ventilate, malignant hyperthermia, OR fires, massive hemorrhage, and obstetrical emergencies as well as surgical emergencies. In contrast to the floor crisis response teams described previously, OR personnel that could be used in a MET are often largely already present on-site or immediately available (with other duties) when the crisis emerges

(Table 23.1). A surgical team is constructed, organized, and focused on a collective task such as a surgical procedure. It includes an anesthesiologist and/or anesthetist, a surgeon, a scrub nurse, and a circulating nurse. The hierarchal structure is quite variable, with ranges of perceptions: the surgeon, anesthesiologist, or nurse anesthetist may each believe him or herself to be "captain of the ship." The hierarchy should change with the introduction of a crisis, where the assumed team leader during a regular surgical procedure—usually the surgeon—switches to the anesthesiologist for management of the crisis (unless the crisis is a surgical one like massive hemorrhage). Additional resources are dictated by the type or severity of a crisis and may include equipment like a defibrillator, a bronchoscope, a "difficult airway cart," central line placement kit, blood products, blood administration devices including rapid infusers, and emergency medications that may require preparation (like dantrolene). The number and composition of additional personnel required, as well as specialized equipment, depends on the type and severity of the specific crisis. For purposes of discussion, an OR crisis can be viewed as any adverse event that requires additional personnel or equipment beyond that normally anticipated for the specific surgical procedure. OR crises can either present as a sudden, obvious event that requires significant immediate resources, or can arise as a slowly escalating continuum that requires a matching escalation of resources to manage appropriately. Crisis management and personnel decisions need to take this into account, as they draw resources from the same pool or from resources earmarked for other cases. Administrative control and communication channels of these resources are necessary and each organization will have its own structure. Like the team training noted above, design and training OR crisis management must include significant leadership training for the anesthesia team to be able to rapidly recruit and organize resources. A hospital's OR RRS should systematically address: 1) the composition of an RRS for the OR; 2) the method to activate this team, 3) effective cross-coverage for the responding members' responsibilities, so that they can focus on the crisis, and 4) an administrative process for capturing the information for quality improvement. Training objectives include learning the operational, administrative, and hierarchical operating room environment. This crisis training program focuses on training the anesthesia care team, and includes [1]: generic patient safety principles and concepts [2], how to rapidly tap into existing resources to organize an appropriate team response in the setting of an ongoing surgical procedure, and [3] methods for effectively treating all types of crisis through simulated experiential methods. This is an interdisciplinary approach including all members of the care team.

Conclusion

For crisis teams to be effective and efficient, they must have more than appropriate personnel, and they must be well designed. There is no consensus on the "best" personnel for the team response. All teams need delineated roles optimal functioning. How each institution fills these roles depends on local factors. The administrative limb of the RRS needs to ensure that sufficient people with knowledge and skills respond, and that appropriate equipment and resources are available. Crises by their nature require more than one person to respond effectively; cooperation and coordination of a group is necessary. Like any group effort, knowledge of what to do is insufficient. Group practice is needed to maximize potential. We believe that full-scale simulation is the best tool at this time to enable the responders to perform the skills needed to save lives.

References

1. Gaba DM, Fish KJ, Howard SK. Crisis management in anesthesiology. New York: Churchill Livingston; 1994.
2. Weick KE, Roberts K. Collective mind in organizations: heedful interrelating on flight decks. Adm Sci Q. 1993;38:325–50.
3. Chen J, Bellomo R. Flabouris A etal. The relationship between early emergency team calls and serious adverse events. Crit Care Med. 2009;37:148–53.
4. Buist MD, Moore GE, Bernard SA, et al. Effects of a medical emergency team on reduction of incidence of and mortality from unexpected cardiac arrests in hospital: preliminary study. BMJ. 2002;324(7334): 387–90.
5. Jones D, Bellomo R, Bates S, et al. Long term effect of a medical emergency team on cardiac arrests in a teaching hospital. Crit Care. 2005;9(6):R808–15.
6. Dacey MJ, Mirza ER, Wilcox V, et al. The effect of a rapid response team on major clinical outcome measures in a community hospital. Crit Care Med. 2007;35(9):2076–82.
7. Sandroni C, Ferro G, Santang elo S, Tortora F, Mistura L, Cavallaro F, Caricato A, Antonelli M. In-hospital cardiac arrest: survival depends mainly on the effectiveness of the emergency response. Resuscitation. Sep 2004;62:291–7.
8. Lightall GK, Barr J, Howard SK, et al. Use of a fully simulated intensive care unit environment for critical event management training for internal medicine residents. Crit Care Med. 2003;31:2437–43.
9. Topple M, Ryan B, Baldwin I, McKay R, Blythe D, Rogan J, Radford S, Jones DA. Tasks completed by nursing members of a teaching hospital medical emergency team. Intensive Crit Care Nurs. 2016;32:12–9 . doi:10.1016/j.iccn.2015.08.008.Epub October 22, 2015
10. DeVita MA, Schaefer J, Lutz J, Wang H, Dongilli T. Improving medical emergency team (MET) performance using a novel curriculm and a computerized human patient simulator. Qual Saf Health Care. 2005;14:326–31.
11. Jacques T, Harrison GA, McLaws ML. Attitudes towards and evaluation of medical emergency teams: a survey of trainees in intensive care medicine. Anaesth Intensive Care. 2008;36(1):90–5.
12. Weller JM, Janssen AL, Merry AF, Robinson B. Interdisciplinary team interactions: a qualitative study of perceptions of team functions in simulated anaesthesia crises. Med Educ. 2008;42(4):382–8.
13. Howell MD, Ngo L, et al. Sustained effectiveness of a primary-team–based rapid response system. Crit Care Med. 2012;40:2562–8.
14. Bertaut Y, Campbell A, Goodlett D. Implementing a rapid-response team using a nurse-to-nurse consult approach. J Vasc Nurs. 2008;26:37–42.
15. Smith GB. In-hospital cardiac arrest: 'is it time for an in-hospital chain of prevention'? Resuscitation. 2010;81:1209–11.
16. Foraida MI, DeVita MA, Braithwaite RS, Stuart SA, Brooks MM, Simmons RL. Improving the utilization of medical crisis teams (Condition C) at an urban tertiary care hospital. J Crit Care. 2003;18:87–94.
17. Jones DA, DeVita MA, Bellomo R. Rapid response teams. N Engl J Med. 2011;365:139–46.

18. Chen J, Bellomo R, Flabouris A, Hillman K, Finfer S. The relationship between early medical emergency team calls and serious adverse events. Crit Care Med. 2009;37:148–53.

19. Quach JL, Downey AW, Haase M, Haase-Fielitz A, Jones DA, Bellomo R. Characteristics and outcomes of patient receiving a medical emergency team review for respiratory distress or hypotension. J Crit Care. 2008;23:325–31.

20. Boniatti MM, Azzolini N, Viana MV, Ribeiro BS, Coelho RS, Castilho RK, Guimaraes MR, Zorzi L, Schulz LF, Filho EM. Delayed medical emergency team calls and associated outcomes. Crit Care Med. 2014;42:26–30.

Equipment, Medications, and Supplies for a Rapid Response Team

Edgar Delgado, Rinaldo Bellomo, and Daryl A. Jones

Introduction

Once a hospitalized patient suffers clinical deterioration, it is essential to deliver safe, accurate, and timely emergency care. Patient survival depends on the efficiency of the response [1]. This response must include not only the appropriate personnel but also the supplies, equipment, and medications that are needed. This chapter describes a methodology for providing an organized equipment and medication supply response.

Institutional Oversight of Equipment

To obtain a quality rapid response team (RRT), education of responding personnel is critical. All staff members in contact with direct patient care are required to have basic life support education, and critical care staff is also educated in advanced life support. However, depending upon the acuity of the patient's condition and observations, one

may not have experience in a crisis until it actually happens, and some medical staff may not feel adequately prepared to participate the management of clinically important patient deterioration. To help staff understand the importance of correct procedures, everyone should be educated during hospital and/or unit-based orientations regarding their specific role in an RRT or cardiac arrest call. Annual competency evaluations are another method of training for crisis event management; to reinforce and test the knowledge base, we use "mock code" scenarios. The mock code can also determine system and personnel deficiencies, and promote processes to decrease or eliminate them. By using programmable, computer-based, full-scale human simulation, events can be repeated and data obtained regarding specific personnel tasks. For example, one may determine the range of how long it takes for a crash cart to get to the scene of a crisis, or how long it takes personnel to defibrillate a patient in ventricular fibrillation. This data can determine equipment needs and personnel education. By retesting, frontline staff can gain the comfort level and knowledge necessary to improve patient outcomes in any crisis situation, and hospital leaders gain confidence in the adequacy of their crisis response program.

The RRT training programs are charged with ensuring that personnel and equipment are prepared for crisis events. RRT-dedicated nursing staff members are responsible for restocking the carts after the event. At times, because of nor-

E. Delgado
Respiratory Care Department UPMC Presbyterian Shadyside, UPMC Presbyterian Campus, Pittsburgh, PA, USA, 15213

R. Bellomo • D.A. Jones (✉)
Department of Intensive Care, Austin Hospital, Studley Rd, Heidelberg, Melbourne, VIC 3084, Australia
e-mail: daryl.jones@austin.org.au;
Rinaldo.bellomo@austin.org.au

© Springer International Publishing Switzerland 2017
M.A. DeVita et al. (eds.), *Textbook of Rapid Response Systems*, DOI 10.1007/978-3-319-39391-9_24

mal patient care activities, this task is delayed, thus a second cart should be available and ready at all times. When all the carts/trolleys are prepared, it is possible to employ a systematic method for stocking: some use a sectional medical tray system that can quickly be changed out, thus limiting the time it takes to restock the cart. The medication and equipment contents of the cart are determined by critical care nurses and physicians who respond to the events. Pharmacy's role is to ensure sufficient supply of medications for each event (how many vials of each medication), and create a convenient location for each item. The pharmacist should also provide guidance about appropriate storage and shelf life of items. Central supply had a similar role for all other equipment. The possible contents of the MET trolleys/carts are presented in Tables 24.1–24.7.

To improve patient safety, the intubation equipment can be removed from all non-intensive

Table 24.1 Emergency airway bag contents

Intubation kit	Other accessories
1. Surgi-lube	1. CO_2 detector
2. Tongue blade	2. Mask with filter setup
3. Gum bougie	3. Mask (child)
4. #3 Mac laryngoscope blade	4. Mask (small adult)
5. #4 Mac laryngoscope blade	5. Mask (large)
6. Laryngoscope handle with batteries	6. Exam gloves
7. #3 Miller laryngoscope blade	7. Suction catheter kit
8. Adult Magill forceps	8. Salem sump 16 Fr.
9. Green oral airway 80 mm	9. Tape
10. Yellow oral airway 90 mm	10. Nasal airway 28 Fr.
11. Red oral airway 100 mm	11. Nasal airway 30 Fr.
12. Intubation stylet	12. Nasal airway 32 Fr.
13. Yankauer suction	13. Syringe 30 cc Luer lock
14. #9 Endotracheal tube	14. Syringe 10 cc Luer lock
15. #8 Endotracheal tube	15. Biohazard specimen bag
16. #7 Endotracheal tube	16. Splash mask with shield
17. #7 Endotracheal tube	17. Endotracheal tube holder
	18. 20 gauge $1.5 \leq$ needles
	19. Jet ventilation kit

care units and can be placed in the cart/trolley or in a portable airway bag. This bag can be stocked in central supply to ensure reliable, functioning equipment. After every intubation, the old bag is exchanged for a new one. The bag can be kept only by the on-call anesthesia and critical care personnel. If the MET is manned by critical care clinicians, such intubation material can be provided as part of the MET trolley/cart (*see* Figs. 24.1–24.4).

Personnel Response

Efficiency in personnel response during an RRT call is also desirable. There is evidence that teamwork during crisis events may be deficient, and consequently errors may be made. Personnel response and teamwork therefore should be improved. Two models for teamwork improvement have been advanced: the first depends on the training for the crisis team leaders, and the second emphasizes a flat hierarchy wherein each team member has a specified role and responsibilities. The personnel designated to respond, the rationale for choosing those responders, and team training are discussed elsewhere in this book.

Nursing Responder Equipment

Airway Equipment

Success during a crisis response requires adequate ventilation and oxygenation as a first priority, and establishing a secure airway as part of that goal. Therefore, personnel, equipment, and medications must all be brought to the scene within about a minute of the onset of the event.

Over the years, when attempting to establish an airway, clinicians have been frustrated by unfamiliarity with the equipment, lack of available equipment, or lack of process standardization. This presents a significant challenge in an institution where residents, or fellows are required to learn and perform airway management. To facilitate and improve this skill set, a system can be set up which uses a portable emergency airway bag,

Table 24.2 Standard crash "code" cart/trolley supply contents

UNIT: _____
CART NUMBER _____

P.U.H.   COST CENTER: _____
STANDARD CRASH "CODE" CART   ISSUE # _____
SUPPLY CONTENTS

Item	Description	Qty.	Issue unit	Filled	Expir. date	Item	Description	Qty.	Issue unit	Filled	Expir. date
	Top of cart						Drawer 3				
8740	Electrodes	2	each/box	NO CHG		8962	Interlink luer lok	5	each		
8838	Gloves, non sterile exam	1	box			E056600	Vac holder (no charge)	1	each	NO CGE	
9289	Wipes, Alcohol	10	each/box	NO CHG		100235	Vac needle (no charge)	3	each	NO CGE	
8254	Swabs, Betadine	5	each/box	NO CHG		109730	Blood gas kit	5	each		
8030	Tape, Adhesive 1-inch	1	roll/box	NO CHG		8911	Lever lock	5	each		
8040	Tape, Adhesive 3-inch	1	roll/box	NO CHG		8913	Threaded lock	3	each		
8041	Tape, Transpore 2-inch	1	roll/box	NO CHG		6222	NaCl 0.9% 30 mL	3	each		
E051100	Tape, Mircopore 1-inch	1	roll			103557	Chloraprep swabs	3	each	NO CGE	
8046	Tape, Micropore 2-inch	1	roll/box	NO CHG		8251	Benzoin Solution	1	each		
100078	Needle Box w/Lid	1	each			8806	Tourniquet	2	each		
	Please secure lid onto top of needle box					6000	I.V D5 w/H$_2$O 100 mL	2	each		
						122877	Needle, Spinal 18 ga × 3–1/2	1	each	NO CGE	
8801	Resuscitator Bag "AMBU"	1	each			122851	Needle, filter 19 ga × 1–1/2	4	each	NO CGE	
8075	Airway 90 mm yellow	1	each			8740	Electrodes	2	each/box	NO CGE	
8076	Airway 100 mm red	1	each			19923	1 Ultrasonic gel	1	each		
	**** Resuscitator bag must be assembled and					109772	1 Vacutainer. Breen too	2	each	NO CGE	
	Placed in the draw string bag provided					70075	Vacu, purple top no charge	2	each	NO CGE	
	The red and yellow airways must be placed into the bag also					109763	Vacutainer, red top	2	each	NO CGE	
	The bag must then be hung in plain sight on					109751	Vacutainer, red top serum	2	each	NO CGE	
	The outside of the cart					109760	Vacutainer, grey top	2	each	NO CGE	
						122854	Syringe, 10 cc slip-tip	5	each	NO CGE	
						9780	Syringe, 30 cc luer-lock	1	each		
						122847	Syringe, 10 cc luer-lock	5	each	NO CGE	
	Drawers 1 and 2 are for pharmacy use. please do not place					8505	Cath. IV 14 ga protective	2	each		
	Any items in these two drawers					8506	Cath. IV 16 ga protective	2	each		

(continued)

Table 24.2 (continued)

UNIT: _____
CART NUMBER _____

P.U.H.   COST CENTER:
STANDARD CRASH "CODE" CART   ISSUE #
SUPPLY CONTENTS

Item	Description	Qty.	Issue unit	Filled	Expir. date	Item	Description	Qty.	Issue unit	Filled	Expir. date
	Top of cart										
	Drawer 3						Drawer 3				
B37370	5 CC Blunt Cannula	5	each	NO CGE		8507	Cath. IV 18 ga protective	2	each		
B37375	3 CC Blunt Cannula	5	each	NO CGE		9038	Gauze, pad 4 × 4 (2/pack)	6	pack/box		
B37385	10 CC Blunt Cannula	5	each	NO CGE		122823	Blunt Cannula	4	each	NO CGE	
116539	10 CC Syr Flushers	8	each	NO CGE		122865	Needle Safety 21 GA × 1 1/2	4	each	NO CGE	
						122875	Needle Safety 25 GA × 5/8	4	each	NO CGE	
						122841	3 cc syringe (lok)	4	each	NO CGE	

Table 24.3 Possible syringe drawer contents list, expiration dates, and billing

Medication	How supplied	Quantity Stocked	Expiration Date	# to bill	Mnemonic
Albuterol inhalation	5 mg/mL 20 mL vial	1			ALBT20L
Atropine syringe	1 mg/10 mL	3			ATRP1S
Topex spray (Benzocaine 20%)	54 g	1			
Dextrose 50% syringe	50 mL	2			D5050S
Dopamine premix	800 mg/250 mL	1			DPMN800I
Epinephrine syringe	1 mg/10 mL (1:10,000)	8			EPNP10S
Lidocaine jelly	2% 5 mL	1			
Lidocaine premix	2 g/250 mL	1			LDCN8I
Lidocaine syringe	100 mg/5 mL	4			LDCN25S
Esmolol premixed bag	2.5 g/250 mL or 10 mg/mL 2 50 mL	1			
Magnesium sulfate premixed bag	80 mg/mL 50 mL or 4 g/50 mL	1			MGS80
Racemic epinephrine inhalation	2.25% 0.5 mL	1			RCPN225
Sodium bicarbonate syringe	50 mEq/50 mL	6			SDBC50S
Colloid solution (place in Drawer #5 on cart)	500 mL	2			

Table 24.4 Possible vial tray contents, emergency cart medication list, expiration dates, and billing

Medication	How supplied	Quantity Stocked	Expiration Date	# to bill	Mnemonic
Adenosine	3 mg/1 mL 2 mL	5			ADNS6I
Amiodarone	150 mg/vial 3 mL	3			AMDR3
Aspirin, chewable	81 mg	2			
Calcium chloride	1 g/10 mL	2			CACH10I
Diphenhydramine	50 mg/1 mL 1 mL	2			DPHNI
Dobutamine	12.5 mg/mL 20 mL	2			DBT250
Epinephrine	1 mg/1 mL 30 mL (1:1000)	2			EPNPI
Syringe labels		10	N/A	N/A	N/A
Flumazenil	0.1 mg/mL 10 mL	1			FLMZ1I
Furosemide	10 mg/1 mL 10 mL	2			FRSM10S
Heparin	1000 units/mL 10 mL	2			HPRN10I
Lidocaine	2% 20 mL	1			LD20I
Methylprednisolone	125 mg	2			MTHL125I
Metoprolol	1 mg/mL 5 mL	4			MTPR1I
Midazolam	1 mg/mL 2 mL	5			MDZL2I
Naloxone with 10 cc sodium chloride	0.4 mg/mL 1 mL	4			NLXN4I
Nitroglycerine	0.4 mg tablets SL #25	1			NTRG4
Norepinephrine	1 mg/mL 4 mL	4			NRPNI
Phenobarbital	130 mg/mL 1 mL	4			PHNB130I
Phenylephrine	10 mg/mL 1 mL	4			PHNY10I
Phenytoin	50 mg/1 mL 5 mL	4			PHNY250
Procainamide	100 mg/mL 10 mL	3			PRCN10I
Vasopressin	20 units/mL 1 mL	3			
Vecuronium	10 mg	2			VCRN10I
Verapamil	2.5 mg/mL 2 mL	4			VRPM2I
Bacteriostatic water	30 mL	1			WTR30I
0.9% sodium chloride	10 mL	5			SDCL10

Table 24.5 Possible emergency cart replacement process

Medication cart exchange process:
Emergency cart is opened by nurse caring for patient:
• At completion of crisis care, nurse calls pharmacy department to exchange the cart
• Pharmacy technician brings new cart and a black plastic lock marked "do not use" (this denotes the cart as "used" and prevents unintentional redeployment) to central supply
• Central supply department technician brings new cart and black seal to unit. New cart is left on unit and black seal is placed on used cart
• Used cart is taken to pharmacy and two medication drawers/trays are removed
• Used cart is taken to central supply for cleaning and to replenish supplies and equipment. A form is placed on top of the cart stating the first expiration date of the supplies
• Newly stocked cart is taken to pharmacy
• Pharmacy replaces the two medication drawers/trays
• An inventory-tracking sticker is applied. The stick notes the date the cart was filled and checked, the supervising pharmacist's signature, and date and name of the first medication to expire
• The cart is secured with red plastic lock (denotes new cart that is ready to go)

Table 24.6 Possible syringe drawer or bag layout

Drawer 1 Layout: 1 Dopamine 800 mg/250 mL premixed bag will be placed on the top of the Bicarb		
Atropine 1 mg/10 mL Syringe 3	Dextrose 50% 50 mL Syringe 2	Sodium icarbonate 50 meq/50 mL Syringe 6
Epinephrine 1:10,000 1 mg/10 mL Syringe 8	Lidocaine 2 g/250 mL premix bag 1	Magnesium sulfate Premix 80 mg/mL 50 mL 1
	Lidocaine Jelly 2% 5 mL 1	Esmolol Premix 1 2.5 g/250 mL
Lidocaine 100 mg/5 mL syringe 4	Albuterol Inhalation 5 mg/mL 20 mL vial 1 Topex SPRAY 57 g 1	Racemic epinephrine inhalation 2.25% 0.5 mL 1

Table 24.7 Possible vial drawer layout

Drawer 2 vial layout						
Procainamide	Procainamide	Vasopressin	Vecuronium	Vecuronium	Verapamil	Verapamil
100 mg/mL	100 mg/mL	20 units/mL	1 mg/mL	1 mg/mL	2.5 mg/mL	2.5 mg/mL
10 mL	10 mL	1 mL	10 mL	10 mL	2 mL	2 mL
1	1	3	1	1	2	2
Naloxone	Naloxone	Naloxone	Nitroglycerine	Norepinephrine	Norepinephrine	Norepinephrine
0.4 mg/1 mL	0.4 mg/1 mL	0.4 mg/1 mL	0.4 mg	1 mg/mL	1 mg/mL	1 mg/mL
with 10 cc	with 10 cc	with 10 cc	SL	4 mL	4 mL	4 mL
NSS	NSS	NSS	#25			
			Tab bottle			
1	1	1	1	1	1	1
Flumazenil	Furosemide	Furosemide	Heparin	Heparin	Lidocaine	Methylpred
0.1 mg/mL	10 mg/mL	10 mg/mL	1000 units/mL	1000 units/mL	20 mg/mL	125 mg
10 mL	10 mL	10 mL	10 mL	10 mL	2%	
					20 mL	
1	1	1	1	1	1	1
Adenosine	Adenosine	Amiodarone	Amiodarone	Aspirin	Calcium	Calcium
3 mg/mL	3 mg/mL	150 mg	150 mg	81 mg	chloride	chloride
2 mL	2 mL	3 mL	3 mL	Chewable	1 g/10 mL	1 g/10 mL
3	2	2	1	2	1	1
Bacteriostatic	0.9% Sodium	0.9% Sodium	0.9% Sodium	0.9% Sodium	0.9% Sodium	

(continued)

Table 24.7 (continued)

Drawer 2 vial layout						
water	chloride	chloride	chloride	chloride	chloride	
30 mL	10 mL	10 mL	10 mL	10 mL	10 mL	
1	1	1	1	1	1	
Norepinephrine	Phenobarbital	Phenylephrine	Phenytoin	Phenytoin	Procainamide	
1 mg/mL	130 mg/mL	10 mg/1 mL	50 mg/mL	50 mg/mL	100 mg/mL	
4 mL	1 mL	1 mL	5 mL	5 mL	10 mL	
1	4	4	2	2	1	
Methylpred	Metoprolol	Metoprolol	Midazolam	Midazolam	Naloxone	
125 mg	1 mg/mL	1 mg/mL	1 mg/mL	1 mg/mL	0.4 mg/1 mL	
	5 mL	5 mL	2 mL	2 mL	with 10 cc NSS	
1	2	2	3	2	1	
Diphenhydramine	Dobutamine	Dobutamine	Epinephrine	Epinephrine	Syringe	
50 mg/mL	12.5 mg/mL	12.5 mg/mL	1:1000 (1 mg/mL)	1:1000 (1 mg/mL)	Labels	
1 mL	20 mL	20 mL	30 mL	30 mL		
			Injection	Injection		
2	1	1	1	1	10	

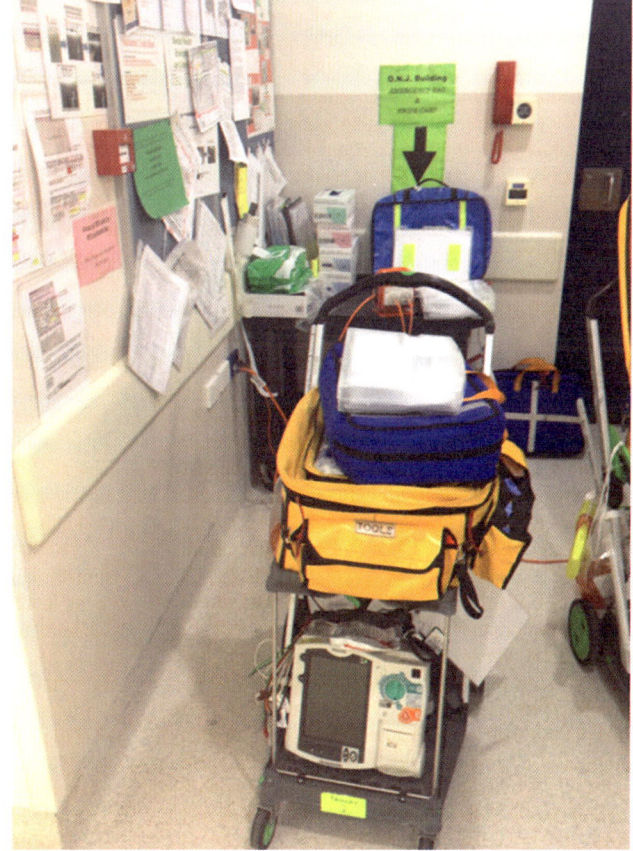

Fig. 24.1 Picture of a medical emergency team cart/trolley at the Austin Hospital. The cart has monitor/defibrillator and bags with medications and tools

Fig. 24.2 Picture of a second emergency cart/trolley with tools bag in the open position

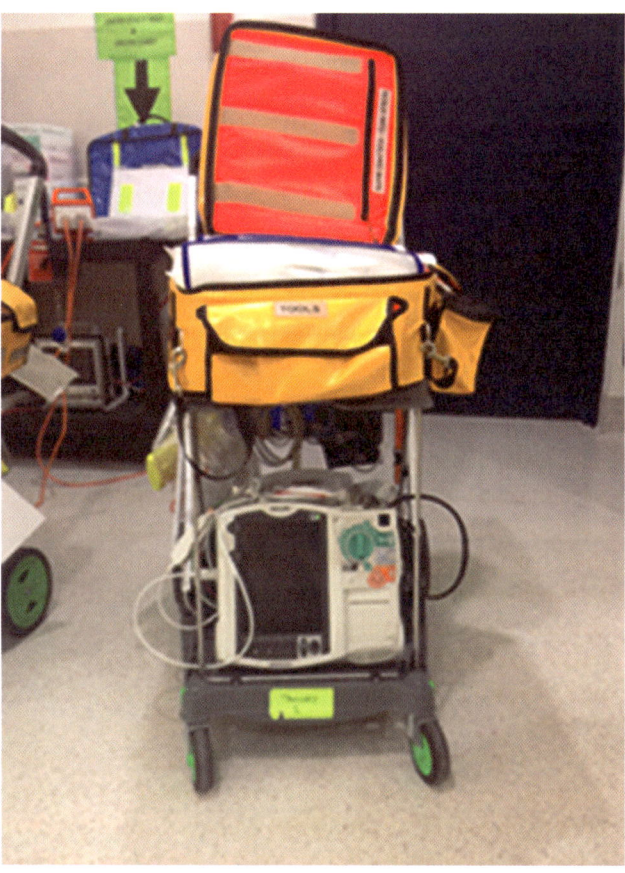

which contains the necessary equipment to allow a clinician to always quickly ensure adequate oxygenation and ventilation. In institutions where such activities are performed by intensive care clinicians and intensive care nurses, such equipment is contained within the MET cart.

The airway management contents are standardized, so that any member of the RRT will know where to find any needed item. The airway bag can be divided into two compartments: a "quick intubation kit" and "other accessories or adjuncts." The division improves organization and facilitates rapid intubation, since the equipment for most intubations is placed in one location. Possible bag contents are presented in Table 24.1. They include: an intubation kit with laryngoscopes and blades, and a variety of endotracheal tube sizes, a mask with a bacterial filter for mouth-to-mask ventilation, gloves, nasal and oral airways, a CO_2 detector, syringes, tape, an endotracheal tube fixation device, Magill forceps, suction equipment, and a hand-jet insufflator in case of an emergency

cricothyrotomy. A secured compartment contains medications to facilitate intubation, including: midazolam, fentanyl, morphine, rocuronium, suxamethonium, succinylcholine, propofol, benzocaine topical metered dose spray, oxymetazoline nasal spray, and lidocaine jelly are included. Regulations for storage of Opioid and benzodiazepines may vary according to jurisdiction, and their availability may need to be adjusted accordingly. The critical care medicine fellow or RRT nurse must ensure the integrity of the bag at each exchange between fellows or each shift. Once the crisis event is over, the airway bag is resupplied appropriately.

MET Cart/Trolley Standardization

To organize MET carts/trolleys, it is essential to thoroughly review all emergency carts in hospital departments and patient units, including the operating rooms and post-anesthesia care units.

Fig. 24.3 Tool bag in the open position and displaying endotracheal tubes and laryngoscopes

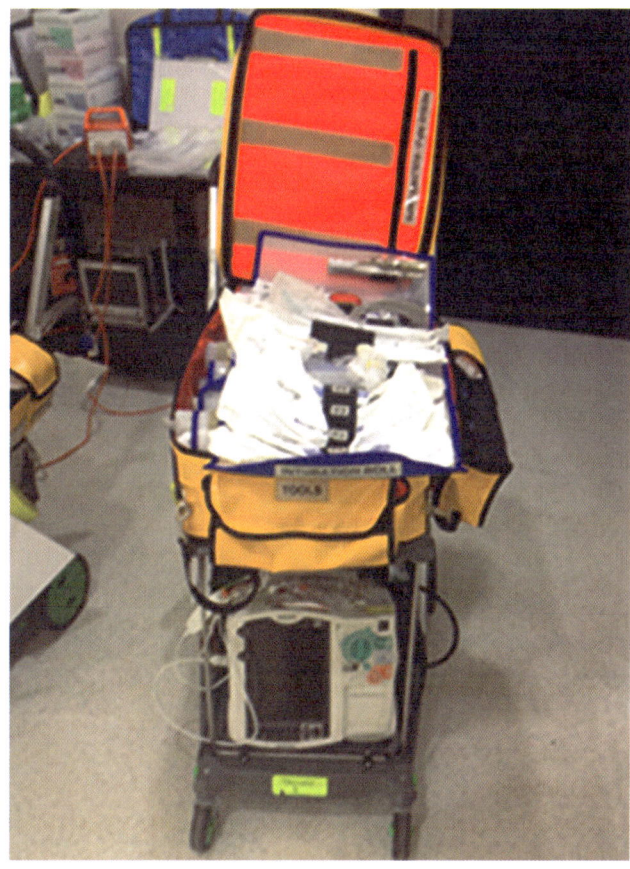

Fig. 24.4 Open drugs bag showing commonly used emergency drugs as presented to the user

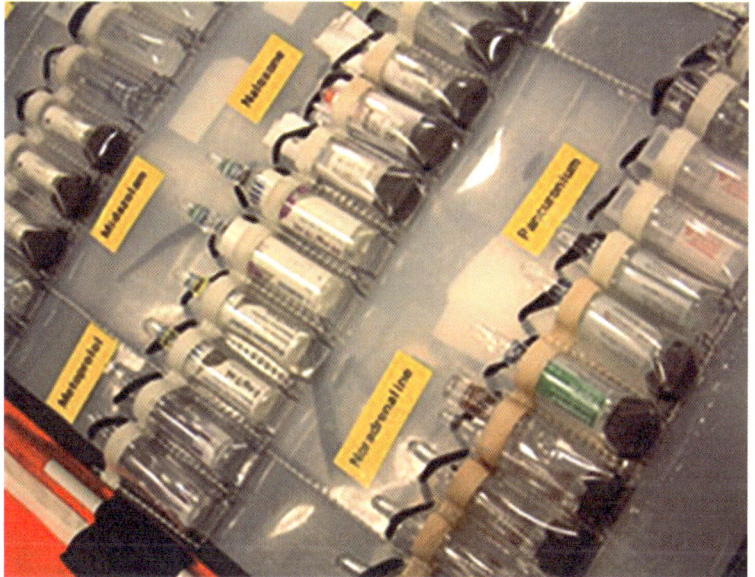

Emergency carts may differ in both organization and contents (disposable supplies, durable equipment, medications, and documentation). Standardization is important and includes medications, supplies, equipment, and layout for all general patient units, intensive care units, hospital departments, emergency department, post-anesthesia care units, operating room, and hospital-based outpatient clinics. On the outside of the cart/trolley, crisis algorithms and dosing charts can be securely attached for use by the emergency response team.

This strategy facilitates the actions of the RRT, reduces practice variation, ensures familiarity with equipment layout, and reduces the potential for error. Another potential mistake is a misreading error. If magnesium is stocked on one cart, but morphine is placed in the same spot on another cart, it is more likely there will be a morphine-for-magnesium mix-up. In addition, the committee must decide whether certain medications that are needed in only a few sites are worth putting on the standardized cart. The cost goes up as additional medications are included, and the probability of a medication being used goes down as medications are excluded. Stocking of cart contents is thus a collaborative and ongoing process. We continuously review and revise, and implement changes once a year. This facilitates and organizes the process for change and education.

Selecting an Emergency Cart/Trolley

The emergency cart/trolley can take on different characteristics (Figs. 24.1–24.3).

The cart/trolley needs to be durable, mobile, and secure; it should have sufficient capacity for the equipment and medications, and accommodate a workspace. A number of suppliers make carts/trolleys that meet these specifications.

The drawers/bags hold trays (medication cassettes) that can be pre-stocked and sealed in clear plastic by the pharmacy for easy replacement. The medications contained within the cassettes can be arranged alphabetically by generic drug name, so that they can be found and viewed easily through the plastic (Table 24.2).

Because the cart/trolley has a locking/sealing mechanism that can be secured with numbered, plastic, break-way seals, reviewers can determine whether the cart is "ready for use." This facilitates central supply restocking and storage.

Need for Specialty Carts/Trolleys

Pediatric crash carts present difficult logistic problems because a wide array of equipment and medications is required to meet the needs of the large range of ages and sizes of the patients. While our institution is not a pediatric facility, we have nevertheless prepared for the pediatric RRT call. Although we rarely have a pediatric inpatient, children visitors are common, and they may have a medical crisis while visiting. The most common events are seizures, syncope, and asthma exacerbation. Obviously, for any child less than 40 kilograms, the medications and equipment used to care for adults are inappropriate. The Joint Commission's Medication Management standards emphasize that it is important that emergency medications are available in unit-dose, age-specific, and ready-to-administer forms [3]. There are two techniques for pediatric crash carts that we briefly discuss. The first is a cart that is organized according to equipment type: for example, all airway equipment is stored together in a single drawer, and all medications in another. The second is the so-called Broselow cart. In this cart, each drawer is color-coded according with Broselow tape, which delineates medication dosing based on the child's weight and size. Each drawer contains the equipment and medications for a certain size child. These carts, like the adult carts, are standardized.

Medication Selection

Every hospital must decide which emergency medications and supplies will be readily available in patient care areas. One can reference the medications and supply requirements from the advanced cardiac life support (ACLS) algorithms and clinical experience. Because 90% of the events we respond to are not cardiopulmonary arrests, the cart/trolley is modified to accommodate relevant needs. Although the goal is to provide the necessary medications and equipment, another goal is to limit medication choices to one drug from each class where possible. The three reasons for this are: fewer medications reduces opportunity for error, practice standardization also reduces error, and fewer medications means lower costs. When medications are commercially available in a premixed dosage form, one can choose that formulation to reduce the chance for errors in admixing. A final goal is to create an emergency cart/trolley that requires minimum maintenance (except for the required daily checks by nursing staff to ensure that the cart is intact, up-to-date, and ready to go).

The cart/trolley is organized to improve efficiency and limit errors. Medications on the emergency cart/trolley are arranged in alphabetical order by the generic (not trade) drug name. The individual drug vials are placed in the vial trays/bags and are clearly labeled with the generic name (Fig. 24.4), the drug concentration, and the stock quantity. A drawer/bag can holds boxes of needle-less emergency medication syringes, premixed medication intravenous solutions, and odd-sized medications (i.e., topical gels or sprays that do not fit into the drawer 2 cassette). Table 24.3 displays a possible plan for such a drawer/bag 1. The second drawer/bag can be used to hold all of the medication vials and ampules in a vial display racks (Fig. 24.4) as shown in the plan in Table 24.4. When medications are stocked in the cart/trolley, they must have a minimum of at least 6 months until their expiration date. This reduces medication waste due to outdated items and reduces the frequency that carts/trolley need to be exchanged due to expiration.

The medications in the emergency cart are reviewed annually by the RRT committee members or by the intensive care team and can be based on the American Heart Association *Guidelines for Cardiopulmonary Resuscitation and Emergency Cardiovascular Care* [2]. Changes to the medications and other emergency cart stock are permitted only once per year, due to the workload involved in updating each of the emergency carts in the hospital.

The RRT committee members, in particular a pharmacist, ICU nurse, and a critical care medicine physician, can review requests to add or remove medications on the emergency cart. Medication requests that can be particularly troublesome include controlled substances (such as morphine), lorazepam (because of it activity against seizures), and insulin. Controlled substances can be difficult to add to the emergency cart because the federal requirements for double locking, daily audits, and concern for diversion create too much work. Medications that require refrigeration, such as fosphenytoin, lorazepam, and insulin, and have a reduced stability when not refrigerated (i.e., 30 days) should not be stocked in the crash cart/trolley. Again, the additional workload of maintaining and tracking short expiration medications on emergency carts is prohibitive. In addition, some medications (insulin) have a high propensity for error, and yet may not be required in virtually any emergency situation. While insulin may often be helpful (as in hyperkalemia), there may be other medicines that can be used with fewer risks and logistic difficulties. In addition, insulin may be obtained readily from most ward areas in hospitals.

Some medications in the cart/trolley require additional warning labels or information to ensure safety in preparation and administration. Examples are warning labels on phenytoin to note that the drug must be mixed in 0.9% sodium chloride solution, and specific dilution and administration instructions for use of naloxone injection to reverse opioid overdose or appropriate use of flumazenil to reverse benzodiazepine overdose.

Pharmacy Emergency Cart/Trolley Exchange Process

Regulatory agencies like The Joint Commission [3] have outlined standards for the managing emergency medications. Staff involved with the supervision of the RRT should be familiar with regulatory requirements in their own jurisdictions.

These include: restocking, maintaining appropriate inventory, ensuring that emergency medications and their associated supplies are readily accessible, and verifying that the carts themselves are secure in their location within the hospital [3]. After opening and using medications and equipment from the emergency cart/trolley, the supplies must be replaced as soon as possible in order to be prepared for the next event. We have an exchange process to meet performance standards developed with all of the involved disciplines and departments—nursing, respiratory therapy, central supply, pharmacy, risk management/patient safety, and critical care medicine physicians. Hospitals can utilize the transport tracking system run by the central supply department to assist in timely tracking and exchanging of crash carts after they have been used. They system tracks the number of requests for carts, time from dispatch of pharmacy technician to completion of the job.

Restocking Medications in the Emergency Cart/Trolley

As discussed previously, medications placed on the cart/trolley must have at minimum a 6-month expiration time. The outside of the cart/trolley contains the name and expiration dating of the first medication to expire in the cart. During the monthly pharmacy inspections of the patient units and hospital departments, the pharmacy checks for outdated carts and to ensure that nursing staff is performing the daily required emergency cart/trolley checks and documentation. Table 24.5 shows a possible cart/trolley replacement process. We offer it as an example; many different processes are possible, and the one chosen at a specific hospital depends on that institution's resources.

The pharmacy can keeps a sufficient supply of backup emergency carts/trolleys and backup medication trays on hand for immediate exchange with units that have used their carts or such work can be conducted by nurses within the ICU department. In addition, the pharmacy or ICU department maintains complete and sealed medication backup trays, so that the exchange process within the stocking area can be performed quickly on all shifts.

Additional Methods for Supplying Emergency Medications

In addition to the emergency cart/trolley process, other methods have been developed to provide emergency medication before or during an RRT response. We have created transport emergency boxes and airway management bags (Fig. 24.4). Both contain a small assortment of medications, and the airway bag also contains intubation equipment and supplies. Transport boxes are for units that care for patients on monitors and must be transported for a test or similar transport. The box contains the three most highly used medications for emergencies: atropine injection, epinephrine injection, and lidocaine injection. The emergency airway bag contains a sedating agent for intubation (fentanyl), local anesthetic (benzocaine aerosol and lidocaine jelly), and a neuromuscular blocking agent (succinylcholine). Other bag contents are described earlier in this chapter.

Barriers to Implementation

The potential barriers to implementation of the emergency medications, equipment, and supply exchange systems include cost, ability to standardize contents (resolving the variation), dynamic administrative backing and leadership, education and training needs, knowledge deficits, time involved, and the staff needed to maintain the processes. To break through these barriers, the focus must be on a common goal—patient safety. Our approach to standardizing the emergency carts/trolleys is to define a core group who shares the need to simplify the cart/trolley restocking procedure, and improve the reliability of the equipment. Consensus regarding content can be achieved, and the hospital administration can provide the funds to purchase the carts/trolleys and their content.

There is a cost associated with standardization. In many hospitals, purchases are part of a nursing unit's budget, and the individual unit must prioritize purchasing a new cart above other expense items. Most units see use of the emergency carts as exceptions to the rule, and many may therefore consider it a low priority. The administration was essential in creating funds for the purchases and creating the imperative for units to make the appropriate purchase. While there are costs, there are also savings. First, standardizing the carts reduces the number of medications, and provides a mechanism for systematically reviewing and choosing medications and supplies with global costs in mind. Second, it reduces nursing work for restocking and checking the medications. Third, less waste of outdated medications occurs. Fourth, staff became very familiar with their contents.

Cardiac arrests events may be low-frequency, high-stress occurrences. Therefore training is important, and performance is unreliable unless practiced frequently. Training nurses, respiratory therapists, and physicians to perform well during crisis situations is an essential component to crisis response preparedness. Standardizing the medication and equipment response dramatically facilitates training. However, if the hospital's educators are not involved in the process, there are two potential problems. First, they may not train people according to the hospital's process design. Second, the design team may make decisions that seem sensible from one perspective, but may create huge training issues. Overcoming this barrier is relatively simple if the education staff is included.

Supply Standardization in the Emergency Carts/Trolleys

The normal supply stock for the cart/trolley needs to be uniform for the same reasons as outlined above. To achieve this goal, central supply staff can be enlisted to develop consistency in all carts/trolleys. The methodology is similar: review of the current carts' contents, determine relevance and necessity, and consider which items could

reasonably be provided from floor stock. The emergency cart drawers/bags are standardized, which helps prevent restocking errors, limits the time crisis response staff needs to find items, and decreases the probability of error (either through misuse, or a mistaken impression that the equipment is not present). Tables 24.6 and 24.7 show a possible equipment drawer configuration and contents.

All emergency carts/trolleys in the institution are mandated to hold a defibrillator (with monitoring, pacing, defibrillation and synchronous cardioversion capabilities); however, they must be standardized. If cables, pads, paddles, and defibrillators are not standardized, mismatches result and the equipment cannot be used. Further, if the responding staff is not familiar with a particular model, an inability to use the equipment or serious errors could result. Both problems might appear to be "equipment failure" although the equipment might be in perfect working order.

Standardization facilitates and reduces the burden of education. Unfamiliarity may contribute to hesitation on the part of less experienced staff to perform defibrillation without an expert clinician. To address this, one can purchase "hands-free" and "auto-analyze" defibrillators. Because pads and not paddles are used, the staff is more willing to perform a "quick look" maneuver with the defibrillator. In addition, the hands-free pads free up a staff member, and are safer to use for staff and patients, because there is less chance of electrical "arcing" or short circuit (particularly if the patient or the person delivering the shock is wet). The auto-analyze function tells the staff whether a shock is indicated; when a shock is recommended, the staff needs only to assess consciousness, and, if absent, defibrillate.

Summary

To mount an effective emergency response, medication and equipment resources must be available, reliable, and organized in a way to make them easily usable. Staff must be trained adequately so that they know what their resources are and how to manage them. Standardizing the equipment and medications contributes to a safe system by improving a number of logistic issues, including staff training, performance, error reduction, equipment maintenance and replacement after a crisis, and finally the institution's ability to revise medication and equipment resources for crises. We believe that improving efficiency and reliability can reduce delays and errors, and contribute to the primary goal of improving patient outcomes following a crisis event.

References

1. Abella BS, Alvarado JP, Myklebust H, et al. Quality of cardiopulmonary resuscitation during in-hospital cardiac arrest. JAMA. 2005;293:305–10.
2. Cummings RO, Hazinski F. Guidelines for cardiopulmonary resuscitation and emergency cardiovascular care. Currents. AHA, Fall; 2000.
3. Joint Commission on Accreditation of Healthcare Organizations (TJC). Comprehensive Accreditation Manual for Hospitals: The Official Handbook (CAMH). Oakbrook Terrace, Illinois: Joint Commission Resources; 2009. p. 2009.

Governance of the Rapid Response System

25

Melodie Heland and Daryl A. Jones

Previous chapters have detailed the rationale behind the rapid response system (RRS), the various methods of activation, and the composition of the Rapid Response Team (RRT). In this chapter, we discuss the role of the administrative and governance limb of the RRS. Specifically, we outline why an administrative and governance limb is needed, what its goals should be, its various components, and finally, the importance of senior hospital medical, nursing, allied health and administrative staff contribution in ensuring successful RRS implementation and maintenance. The need to link audit activities of the RRT to research projects, quality improvement and clinical governance is also emphasized. The structure, members and roles of the administrative and governance arm at our hospital are used as an example.

M. Heland, RN, CritCareCert, GDip.
Surgical Clinical Services Unit, Austin Health, Studley Rd, Heidelberg, VIC 3084, Australia

D.A. Jones (✉)
Department of Intensive Care, Austin Hospital, Studley Road, Heidelberg, Melbourne, VIC 3084, Australia
e-mail: daryl.jones@austin.org.au

Why Is an Administrative Arm Needed?

The RRS is an example of a complex intervention as it "developed from a number of components that may act both independently and interdependently" [1]. All RRSs are composed of an afferent limb (including activations criteria and the trigger mechanism) as well as an efferent limb RRT [1]. To be successful in identifying and treating a deteriorating ward patient, there must be a timely progression of a complex chain of events. This includes measuring the vital signs, recognizing that there is an abnormality, making the decision to activate the system, actually activating the system, timely review by the RRT, ward staff conveying an accurate handover to the arriving RRT, accurate patient assessment and initiation of appropriate therapy, and finally, appropriate patient disposition and follow-up after the RRT review has occurred (Fig. 25.1).

The RRS is a resource intensive system involving staff that in many hospitals regularly rotate or turnover. It has been suggested that institutionalization of system change may fail because of turnover of key employees [2]. It is essential that all RRSs should have an administrative arm to ensure that the RRS is successfully implemented, efficiently run, and effective in achieving its stated goals. As stated by Berwick, "the effectiveness of these systems is sensitive to

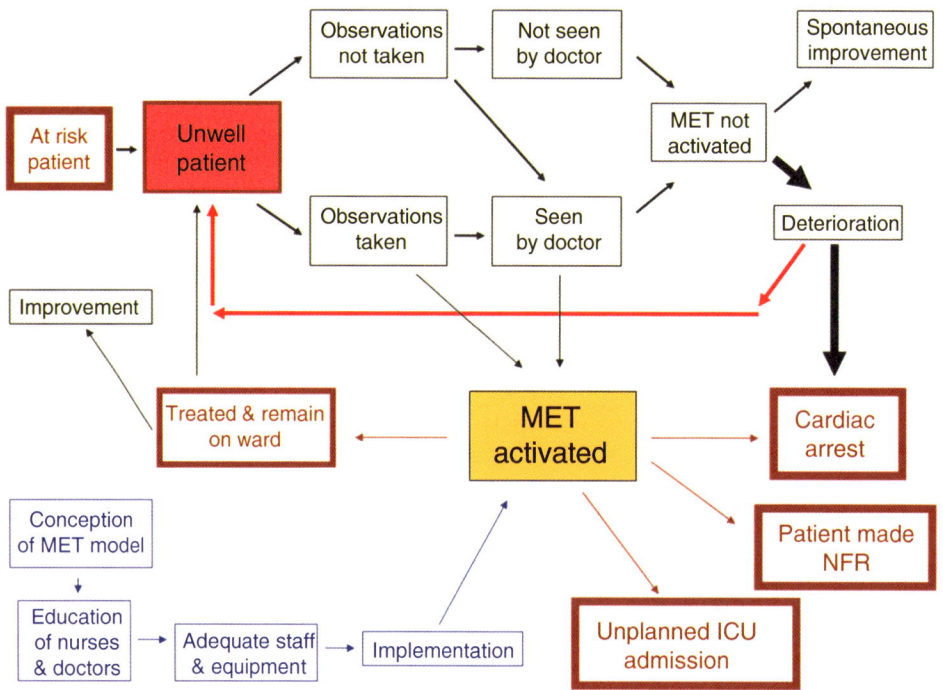

Fig. 25.1 Chain of events for identification, review, and treatment of acutely deterioration ward patient. MET—medical emergency team. ICU—intensive care unit. NFR—not for resuscitation

an array of influences: leadership, changing environments, details of implementation, organizational history, and much more" [3]. The RRS cannot exist in isolation. It must be part of an overarching strategic plan to make the hospital safer by developing strategies that identify at-risk and deteriorating patients as early as possible in the course of clinical decline and provide a standardized response about which all staff members are educated. In addition, many countries now have national policies regarding deteriorating hospital patients that are linked to hospital accreditation. The governance and administrative limb of the RRS must ensure that the hospital complies with such policies. In Australia the national policy standardizing expectations regarding management of deteriorating patients was established by the Australian Commission for Safety and Quality in Health Care [4]. All hospitals are expected to meet the standards as part of the process to gain accreditation.

In our hospital the governance of the RRS is overseen by a "Deteriorating patient commit-

tee" (DPC). The DPC is the central organizing body, consisting of clinicians from different craft groups and sites of the hospital, quality and safety experts, senior management staff and the Executive. It provides leadership and coordination to improve detection, recognition, and escalation of care for patients who deteriorate anywhere in our hospital. The administration of the RRT and the interaction of the RRT with the remainder of the hospital is overseen by a "MET-panel," all of whom are senior ICU clinicians.

The Deteriorating Patient Committee (DPC)

This section will review the role of the DPC and provide detail as to some specific strategies undertaken by the committee.

The RRS has multiple objectives including the detection of patient deterioration, reliable activation to the RRT, ensuring that the RRT responds

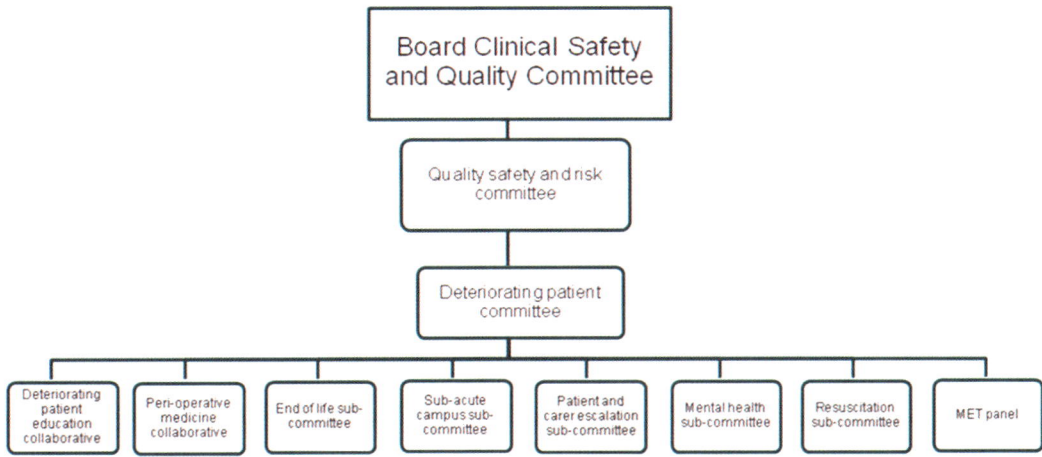

Fig. 25.2 Schematic diagram showing interaction of DP steering committee with other working committees and medical emergency team (MET) panel

promptly and provides effective treatment [1]. The large number of steps involved in recognizing and responding to clinical deterioration introduces the risk of practice variation. Deming argued that "uncontrolled variation is the enemy of quality" [5]. Accordingly, behind the clinical processes there must be a framework of organizationally established policies, procedures, and education programs which focus on standardizing the recognition and response system. The DPC is the vehicle to establish and monitor consistency, in addition to being an important forum for full and frank discussion on all principle matters surrounding patient deterioration. As the committee has grown and evolved, its governance responsibilities have been facilitated by numerous sub-committees to provide expertise and drive the work within various key areas. These are overseen by a formal governance structure (Fig. 25.2).

DPC Sub-Committees

The sub-committees of the DPC are essential for managing the large breadth and depth of work in the key clinical challenge of recognizing and responding to patient deterioration. Each sub-committee has terms of reference and a chair and provides an annual action plan to DPC. The chair of each sub-committee is also a member of DPC

and provides regular progress reports on the activities of each sub-committee. The members of each sub-committee are derived from experts in the field, quality and clinical staff who have an interest in improving current patient care processes. For example, the End-of-life care sub-committee has developed a detailed process based on providing a "good death" for patients who are going to die. They have developed a detailed model addressing matters at ward, hospital and government/community level. The chair of this sub-committee is the director of palliative care.

Similarly, the resuscitation committee examines data and incidents related to cardiac arrest. It also provides advice to DPC regarding changes to policy, equipment, and processes. When new national or international guidelines are released, the Resuscitation sub-committee reviews these and makes recommendations regarding implementation, impact, and resource requirements.

A third example of a sub-committee is the deteriorating patient education collaborative (DPEC). There are very few actions undertaken by DPC that do not require some form of implementation by the education team. This sub-committee ensures standardized practice by coordinating the education courses for all staff. Courses include basic, intermittent, and advanced life support; early recognition of the deteriorating patient and critical care education and skills series (termed COMPASS [6] and ACCESS programs in our hospital). DPEC has members who are at the forefront of new methods of training and education research, particularly in relation to simulation. This sub-committee ensures that the overall hospital educational approach to the deteriorating patient is consistent, well packaged and targeted and delivered to the right staff in an efficient, professional manner.

The Deteriorating Patient Coordinator

An essential element to the impact and momentum of the DPC's activities is the existence of a part-time coordinator. The objectives of the role are;

- Promote best practice in early detection, resuscitation, and escalation of medical emergency response to the deteriorating patient at Austin Health.
- Guide and support Austin Health to meet the requirements of Standard 9 under the NS&QHSS—"Recognising and responding to clinical deterioration in acute health care"[4].
- Implement and coordinate standardized interdisciplinary deterioration and resuscitation education programs, with particular emphasis on developing team training and a team approach to emergency medical situations.
- Facilitate deterioration and resuscitation training outcome data and quality improvement activities.

The role is located within the clinical education unit of our hospital. The coordinator works closely with the DPC chair and education unit manager to implement the strategies of the DPC, particularly in relation to education and projects to test and introduce change. For example, DPC introduced a new documentation chart to record the interventions when the medical emergency team was called (MET record) [7]. While several people were involved in the design of the chart, it was the coordinator who organized a trial on several wards, provided inservice education to staff, collated feedback and suggested changes,

presented recommendations back to DPC, facilitated the chart through the hospital forms committee for approval, and arranged printing and distribution of the new chart when it was complete. This example demonstrates the attention to detail required to successfully implement just one aspect of the system.

The deteriorating patient coordinator plays an important role in receiving and disseminating information from any source however is particularly important as a responsive focal point for queries, ideas, complaints and feedback from all staff within the hospital.

The Importance of an Organizational Approach

Our organization has three separate campuses and provides the full range of acute, sub-acute, rehabilitative services. While most services are directed towards adult physical and mental healthcare, there are also a significant range of pediatric services. DPC has therefore always taken an enterprise approach to its role, considering all policies and processes as needing to be implemented and/or adapted according to site, patient and resource profile. The committee ensures that policies are integrated with other functions that exist within such a complex organization. The following are some examples of activities that the committee has administered to facilitate the end aim of improving the recognition and response to patient deterioration.

- Developed real time, easily accessible data on medical emergency calls. The data can be accessed and formatted in various ways for a specific medical unit to understand the medical emergency calls occurring within its patient group. Data are transparent to the whole hospital and have been widely promoted for units to access as part of their morbidity and mortality audits. This has enabled recent findings such as the need for earlier end of life discussions in oncology and aged care patients, and the increased risk to patients who are "boarding" on a ward that is not the usual home location for the unit.

- Specified the responding team members and the areas to which they respond—each of the three campuses are very large, with clinical emergencies occurring internally and externally. We established separate teams with skills for external or "field" type responses and another directed at the inpatient group. These teams are resourced and trained accordingly. There are maps and lists by building and floor on our intranet as to the responsibilities of each team.
- Standardized the role of the switchboard staff—two incidents identified that switchboard staff were sometimes being provided with confusing information when a caller rang with an emergency response. This issue was addressed by three actions: establishing an agreed method of "caller control" by the switchboard operator; standardizing the wording used to confirm the location and type of call; and developing a training program for the switchboard staff to ensure a consistent approach continued. There have been no further incidents of delayed or incorrect response since this implementation.
- Liaison with external organizations—Due to the occasional need to transport unwell patients between sites, DPC has liaised with the ambulance service to establish the most efficient and safest way to achieve this. This has often required delicate negotiation to engage the ambulance service with our challenge of having multiple sites while having an emergency department, 24-hour theater, and intensive care on only one site.
- Linking all aspects of DPC work with the quality, safety and risk unit—this unit has a broad range of expertise and assists the committee to ensure compliance with regulatory requirements and other standards (e.g., coroner's findings), utilize current thinking around process improvement and promulgate the work of the committee via quality coordinators, which are distributed through the clinical service units of the hospital.

In summary, whether an organization is large or small, it is essential to have an organizing body with the authority of the executive to ensure the administration and governance of systems which promote early, standardized, and efficient recognition and response when a patient deteriorates. This central body needs to be clear on its aims, well connected to other key bodies, resourced to drive change, have a broad membership and a long term view to improving clinical management of the unwell patient.

Administration of the RRT is Performed by a MET Panel

Roles and Responsibilities of the MET Panel

The MET panel comprises four senior ICU nurses, the medical director of critical care outreach, and the nurse unit manager of the ICU. The objectives of the MET panel are to oversee the day to day running of the RRT (Table 25.1). In addition, members of the MET panel also sit on the deteriorating patient committee to participate in broader aspects of coordination of initiatives for deteriorating patients and the RRS. The MET panel meets regularly to revise and discuss issues around the RRT and members also attend the regular deteriorating patient committee meetings. The medical director of the MET panel is a

Table 25.1 Summary of role and responsibilities of the administrative MET panel

1. Induction of new and rotating medical and nursing staff about the RRT
2. Training of RRT staff in relation to response and team interaction
3. Ensuring data on all calls in entered into the electronic database
4. Following up critical RRT incidence involving clinical issues and/or undesirable behavior of RRT staff.
5. Participation and attendance in deteriorating patient committee
6. Design and conduct of research and audit related to the RRT

Table 25.2 Members and roles of intensive care MET panel and other administrative staff

Group member	Roles
Medical director of critical care outreach	• Educates new hospital medical staff about RRT • Educates ICU fellows about managing an RRT call • Reviews performance of RRT fellow • Provides mentorship to RRT fellows • Assists with complex RRT calls as needed • Together with RRT fellows identifies system problems uncovered by RRT which require "political"/"administrative" intervention. • Ensures all RRT calls data are entered in computerized database • Generates regular reports of RRT activity • Designs and executes RRT related research
ICU nurse educators	• Trains ICU nurses to be part of RRT • Teaches advanced resuscitation skills • Develops nursing research projects in relation to RRT • Conducts nursing research
Ward clerk	• Ensures all RRT calls data are entered in computerized database • Ensures completeness against ICU NUM shift report • Uses monthly report of all emergency activity (code blue calls and RRT calls) to identify areas of concern
RRT research fellows	• Identifies all aspects of RRT system which require research • Designs research project with RRT medical supervisor • Obtains ethics approval • Conducts research work with RRT administrative team • Develops manuscripts with RRT supervisor
MET panel	• Meets to review issues related to RRT • Develops strategic plan to resolve them • Develops plans for future developments • Identifies hospital-wide issues that require involvement of governance limb • Communicates with ward NUMs through open forum

ICU intensive care unit. *NUM* nurse unit manager. *MET* medical emergency team. *RRT* rapid response team.

member of the DPC and reports on updates related to the RRT.

The MET panel provides induction of new nursing staff and rotating medical staff about aspects of the RRT. Induction entails explanation of the history of the RRS, RRT calling criteria and method of activation, common causes of RRT calls, and the roles and expected behaviors of the various RRT members. RRT members are also taught a previously published "A G approach" for the management of an RRT call [8], the layout and contents of the RRT trolley and the method of data entry into the electronic RRT database (Table 25.2).

Training of the RRT Nurse Members

The four senior nurses of the MET panel oversee training of the nursing members of the RRT. To be accredited to work as a nurse on the

RRT, ICU nurses must undergo a 6 month training programme under the supervision of a mentor and the four senior nurses. A course handbook outlines a series of competencies including checking of the RRT trolley, assisting with endotracheal intubation, commencement of noninvasive ventilation and high flow oxygen. Evaluation involves a series of examinations and two oral presentations regarding assessment and initial management of two common RRT scenarios.

Reviewing Critical Incidences Related to the RRT

The MET panel also follow up critical incidences related to the RRT. These may include root cause analysis of critical incidence of clinical deterioration resulting in patient harm. Alternatively, they may involve review and feedback about undesirable behavior of members of the RRT, particularly perceptions of criticism of ward staff during the conduct of the call.

Finally, the MET panel are involved in the design and implementation of research and audit related to the RRS and deteriorating patients more broadly. Findings of audit and research are presented to the deteriorating patient committee to guide refinement of hospital policy.

References

1. Delaney A, Angus DC, Bellomo R, Cameron P, Cooper DJ, Finfer S, Harrison DA, Huang DT, Myburgh JA, Peake SL, et al. Bench-to-bedside review: the evaluation of complex interventions in critical care. Crit Care. 2008;12:210.
2. Jones D, Bates S, Warrillow S, Goldsmith D, Hart G, Opdam H, Goldsmith D. Long term effect of a medical emergency team on cardiac arrests in a teaching hospital. Crit Care. 2005;9:R808–15.
3. Berwick DM. The science of improvement. JAMA. 2008;299:1182–4.
4. Australian Commission on Safety and Quality in Health Care. National consensus statement: essential elements for recognising and responding to clinical deterioration. Sydney: ACSQHC; 2010. http://www.safetyandquality. gov.au/internet/safety/publishing. nsf/Content/F329E60CC4149933CA2577740009229 C/$File/national_consensus_statement.pdf. Accessed March 2015).
5. Chang WK, Paul HK. Basic statistical tools for improving quality. John Wiley and Sons, Inc.; 2012.
6. COMPASS. ACT Health, 2007. (Accessed March 2015, at http://www.health.act.gov.au/c/health?a= da&did=11025490.
7. Mardegan K, Heland M, Whitelock T, Millar R, Jones DA. developing a medical emergency team running sheet to improve clinical handoff and documentation. Jt Comm J Qual Patient Saf. 2013;39:570–5.
8. Jones D, Duke G, Green J, Briedis J, Bellomo R, Casamento A, Kattula A, Way M. Medical emergency team syndromes and an approach to their management. Crit Care. 2006;10:R30.

Part III

Monitoring of Efficacy and New Challenges

Magnolia Cardona-Morrell, Eyal Zimlichman,
and Andreas Taenzer

Introduction

Background and History

The practice of intermittent, incomplete, and inaccurate vital signs monitoring at long intervals in hospitalized patients is over 100 years old [1–4]. The relevance of episodic routine monitoring is still being questioned as undetected adverse events still occur, even with the average 2-hourly monitoring of postsurgical patients [5]. There is no agreement on the most optimal vital sign monitoring frequency associated with patient safety [6], and the heterogeneity of studies on intermittent observations makes the evidence for routine spot-checks inconclusive [7]. A major deficiency of episodic monitoring without attention to trends is the lack of effective and timely recognition of instability of individual patients in general care units (GCUs). This has often been cited as a key reason for "unexpected" patient deterioration and adverse events [8, 9].

Efforts to enhance intermittent physiological surveillance have included the use of palm-held assistants for wireless transmission of manually entered vital signs and automated alerts for escalation [10, 11], with development of software to improve the accuracy of collection and charting of vital signs along with calculation of early warning scores for adequate clinical response [12, 13]. A large multicenter before-and-after controlled trial in ten hospitals in US, Europe, and Australia examined the effect of electronic technology on frequency, type, and treatment of rapid response team calls and incidence of adverse events [14]. A bedside monitor electronically captured four vital signs intermittently when vital signs are measured as part of routine care and also accepted manual input of another three parameters for automated calculation of early warning scores and generation of clinical decision support prompts. This intervention shortened the acquisition of vital signs, and increased the demand for medical emergency teams to respond to unstable respiratory rates, but found a nonsignificant trend for decreased length of hospital stay. The above methods still rely on nurses manually entering episodic observations, albeit more frequently. With the extensive use of electronic medical records (EMR) today, it is possible to automate capture and produce a graphic profile of deteriorating patients for predictive modeling and triggering of a rapid [15]. Yet, as long as the frequency of vital sign monitoring is not near continuous, timely identification of the interval deterioration risk seems unlikely.

M. Cardona-Morrell, MBBS, MPH, PhD (✉)
E. Zimlichman • A. Taenzer
The Simpson Centre for Health Services Research,
South Western Sydney Clinical School and Ingham
Institute for Applied Medical Research, The
University of New South Wales, P.O. Box 6087,
UNSW Library Walk, Sydney, NSW 1466, Australia
e-mail: m.cardonamorrell@unsw.edu.au

© Springer International Publishing Switzerland 2017
M.A. DeVita et al. (eds.), *Textbook of Rapid Response Systems*, DOI 10.1007/978-3-319-39391-9_26

Unlike the intermittent vigilance of general wards, the practice of continuous monitoring of vital signs in semi-intensive and intensive care units (ICUs) has been widespread since the 1980s. ECG monitoring for early diagnosis of ischemia and therapeutic response [16] and continuous pulse oximetry for the detection of episodic desaturation to decrease risk of mortality [17] are now commonplace. In the past decade or so, a range of advanced technologies for monitoring additional single or multiple parameters have become a part of routine care in ICUs and in some noncritical areas [14, 18–20]. The introduction of these technologies has provided staff with a safety net to assist their assessments in busy hospitals, as clinicians can use live data to determine the status of their patients at any time during the day, whether during a face-to-face physical examination or when remotely supervising less senior staff. In contrast to ICUs, there is widespread variation of monitoring practices in GCUs. This variation ranges from intermittent spot checks of vital signs over selective monitoring of "patients-at-risk" to routine monitoring of all that requires the signing of waivers to opt out.

This chapter reviews some of the common suggestions for adoption of higher monitoring frequency in CGUs; characteristics of recent continuous monitoring technology and systems; their potential advantages and disadvantages; emerging evidence for effectiveness and cost benefit; and likely impact on patient safety.

Importance of Continuous Monitoring

New treatments and technological advances, along with general improvements in population health, have led to increased life expectancy and to a change in the profile of hospitals, with more elderly and complex cases increasingly being admitted to general care floors [21]. Given the high prevalence of frailty [22] and comorbidities in older age, these patients are more likely to deteriorate on general wards, require transfer to a high-dependency unit, have a prolonged length of stay or die during the admission [22, 23]. In ICUs, expert staff can continually observe patients directly or remotely and provide advice to clinicians to ensure better outcomes [24]. However, this remote consulting approach could be expensive if implemented on general wards where neither videoconferencing technology nor ongoing availability of experts is feasible or sustainable [24]. The establishment and standardization of rapid response systems [25] has attempted to address this gap and has shown varying degrees of improved patient outcomes after deterioration is identified. EMR-based capture and monitoring of manually entered vital signs with electronic automatic triggers for rapid response alerts when parameters meet the calling criteria have been integrated into ward care [26]. Results are mixed as reductions in intensive care transfers are not coupled with mortality reductions, with the latter only observed among elderly with multiple comorbidities.

The question remains as to whether continuous monitoring could bring about further gains [27]. Intuitively, introduction of continuous monitoring in noncritical areas where resources are low [28, 29], and patient acuity is increasingly high due to health system pressures [30], might increase the chances of identifying high-risk events earlier and prevent incidents during the long periods when mandatory observations are not taken. In semi-intensive stroke units, for instance bedside continuous monitoring of blood pressure, oxygen saturation, respiratory frequency, ECG, body temperature, and electro-encephalography has shown improvement in discharge outcomes for patients with ischemic stroke due to earlier intervention before complications become symptomatic [31]. New information is required, however, on the benefits that continuous monitoring may provide over and above existing practice on CGUs.

Attributes and Potential Advantages of the Ideal Continuous Monitoring System

Before we address the effectiveness of continuous monitoring technology, let us consider a wish list of the technical and contextual attributes of such systems if they were to become part of routine general ward care.

The fundamental requirement, and advantage, of continuous monitoring is the preservation of data integrity when transmitted to nurses' stations or to the hospital server. Infrastructure to store large amounts of data points, for example wave forms with date-time stamps, is paramount for correlation of alarms with clinical events. Accuracy of the vital signs information would also need to be equivalent to the "gold standard" of existing ward equipment [32]. Linkages to EMR or wireless transmission to the data repository can potentially reduce the time spent entering vital signs data [14] and error rates of manual documentation [33]. The ability to retrospectively rapidly review vital signs data from an electronic source enables rapid quality control and reflective learning for clinicians. Integration of continuous vital sign data with other clinical data in the EMR such as laboratory test results, medication, and diagnosis can further increase risk-scoring capabilities through big-data analysis and allow for more accurate alerts and decision support tools [34]. Providing multi-source clinical data along with the continuous monitoring data would allow improving alert accuracy and decreasing alert fatigue.

A continuous monitoring system for GCUs needs to be as unintrusive as possible to provide limited interruptions to patient's rest at night [35], minimize the "wake up" effect on vital signs [32], and avoid family concern and activations of rapid response systems [36] from repeat alerts. Visual or audible alarms when instability occurs are essential, but the need to minimize alarm burden to tolerable and actionable alarms is well established as it also minimizes ward staff ignoring or inactivating them [37]. Setting clinically meaningful delays in parameter abnormalities before alarms are triggered is also important for individualized response [38]. Alarm delays have shown good correlation with cardiorespiratory instability [20]. Thus, a balance needs to be achieved in setting the individual or multiparameter thresholds. An added desirable feature would be the ability to readjust alarm thresholds according to patient groups or individual patient need, after sound statistical validation [38]. For instance, raising the calling criteria for systolic

blood pressure in patients with traumatic brain injury from <90 mmHg to <120 mmHg [39]. Automation of early warning scores or average parameter values for predetermined time periods would assist evaluation of trends and risk prediction [18, 40]. Associating these risk profiles with automated clinical support prompts [14] has also been found to improve rapid response attendance for unstable patients [10]. Ideally, the system should provide an ability to adjust or turn these features off depending on user's experience.

From a research standpoint, continuously monitoring and storing physiological variables not only allows the review of adverse events, but to create a virtual patient environment [41]. These big data environments allow the development of deterioration detection algorithms and alarm modeling in adverse event and control groups before these alerting systems go "live." Hence, positive and negative predictive values as well as alarm burden can be estimated before exposing patients and healthcare professionals to the implementation.

Importantly, the system needs to be affordable in public hospitals to enable use on patients at all levels of risk, not only high-risk patients. After all, the driver for the introduction of rapid response systems in the early 1990s was the unexpected deterioration and death of younger people without comorbidities [42] along with patient safety incidents among people of all ages due to incomplete checking and oversight, inappropriate management of deterioration, failure of prevention, and equipment-related mistakes are still prevalent in hospitals today [43]. The cost-effectiveness and opportunity cost of continuous monitoring will need to be investigated. A study has found that in stroke patients, even if continuous monitoring could be used only for a limited time (e.g., the first 2–3 days of hospital admission), improved outcomes and prevention of complications could still be achieved [31].

An environment where ward staff can access real-time displays of a patient's condition, automated risk prediction, and clinical decision support at all times and notifications of parameter threshold violations [38] provides a safety net for patients. Theoretically, staff would have more time for face-to-face patient contact and other disease management activities such as medication administration and general care.

Potential Disadvantages

A system that may potentially capture instability outside scheduled manual observation times would require sufficient resources to identify abnormalities when displayed on monitors [19], and to undertake verification. Until the system is smart enough and automated with interpretive prompts, staff training may be required to enable pattern recognition and subtle vital signs deviations from the norm [44]. For instance, one study of the introduction of five-channel physiological monitoring in a UK hospital showed no difference in outcomes compared to standard care. The authors attributed the result to the absence of adequately trained staff to initiate appropriate response despite obvious instability [19]. At the other end of the spectrum, over-reliance on noninvasive technology, under the assumption of superiority to traditional assessment, may provide a false sense of security to nursing staff if they are unaware of the accuracy limitations of some parameters such as oxygen saturation through pulse oximetry [45]. While continuous monitoring can represent an improvement over 8- or 6-hourly observations, over-reliance on clinical decision-prompts based on automated early warning scores may detract from a comprehensive assessment of other patient risk factors such as demographic characteristics, other medical history [38], of simply how the patient appears. Less face-to-face assessment of patients may result if nurses are able to substitute patient contact for checking their vital-signs status from a remote screen.

As mentioned before, a major concern with continuous monitoring on GCUs is the potential for alarm fatigue due to an increase in number of alarms coupled with low positive predictive value (false alarms) [46]. Monitors that rely on contact with the patient, such as pulse oximeters, chest leads for ECG, etc., may alert due to detachment of sensors that, of course, would constitute a false alarm and prompt alarm fatigue among staff.

In addition to patient or caregiver anxiety about the number of alarms, whether false or true, other patient factors such as skin irritation or pressure ulcers may also become an issue due to longer duration of contact with devices if gels or straps are not bio-compatible [47].

Moving from a traditional manually operated to paper-free vital signs monitoring would require staff to embrace new technology, accept the tradeoff of incurring higher costs to reduce the risk of undetected adverse events, and take up the challenge of implementing practice change [1]. This would extend to alleviating hospital management's fear of loss of control or for the privacy of clinical data [1]. Gaps in transmission, for instance when battery life expires or when devices need to be replaced or swapped in the course of routine care, would undermine the purpose of this technology. Transfer errors with subsequent discrepancies in clinical interpretation or gaps in the clinical data cannot be ruled out, although previous small-scale studies suggest that these errors can be reduced [33]. Revolutionizing ward care with paperless electronic continuous monitoring may be compromised by the inability to conduct quality control in the absence of original paper-based manual measurements for comparison. In low-resource settings, the system might be unusable during down-time periods of power failures, data overload, or computer software or hardware malfunction, aside from a technically proficient team to routinely and regularly maintain the technology.

Arguably, the cost of installing some of these technologies can be reduced by using or enhancing existing IT and telecommunications infrastructure [48], but in acute public health systems with hundreds of beds using traditional manual technology the cost might be prohibitive if attempted globally instead of gradually. Certainly, the sheer volume of vital signs data will be a challenge to existing IT infrastructure.

Current Technology and Emerging Evidence on Effectiveness

The variety of continuous monitoring technologies available now include bedside [14, 20], patient-worn [48], wired [37], wireless [47], contact-less [49], single or multi-parameter monitoring devices [14, 20, 48], and can be stand-alone or linked to the electronic medical record [40]. Some are fitted with automated early warning scores [14], automated probabilistic risk estimations [20], can trigger audible or visual alarms [20, 48] and various degrees of severity alerts [37]; others feature graphical trend outputs, allow alert modifications, provide on-screen clinical decision support on the screen or issue alerts with the ability to reach a remote clinician by pager [15], telephone, hospital intranet, or other wireless mobile devices [40]. While many systems are released onto the market after small efficacy trials, only some have published results of their effectiveness testing in real-life situations and none have quantified the level of acceptability by staff. Below are some recent examples.

Work on continuous monitoring of patients in GCUs has been ongoing at some centers for over a decade. Using the experience of human factor and signal processing engineers in military field triage, a team of engineers, physicians, and nurses at Dartmouth (US) implemented a continuous surveillance system based on pulse oximetry that monitors all patients all the time. Data is sampled in one-second intervals and nurses are notified via a pager system when static alarm thresholds are crossed. Alarms are controlled by notification delay and a tiered alarm trigger implementation. The key premises of implementation consisted of controlling alarm burden and workload to nurses as well as improving outcomes of patients while controlling cost (no additional personnel and cost savings through avoidance of adverse events that would match or exceed maintenance cost of the system). Using a before/after study design with concurrent controls, the authors showed a reduction of ICU transfers by 50% and reduction of RRT activations by 65% as a result of continuous monitoring [50]. The avoidance of unanticipated ICU transfers saved the institution

approximately 150 ICU admissions in 1 year from one 32-bed unit alone. Based on the dramatic impact on outcomes patient surveillance was expanded to all patients in GCUs. Surveillance monitoring has been an institutional standard since 2009, individual physicians cannot "overrule" the institutional policy to monitor all at all times and patients are asked to sign waivers if they elect not to be monitored. The original 32-bed orthopedic study unit has not had a death or severe adverse event from respiratory cause since 2007. While respiratory events have not been entirely eliminated, RRT data shows that alerts of respiratory origin have been at about 5% for the last 5 years.

A recent systematic review of electrocardiograph monitoring concluded that studies had demonstrated little value in continuous monitoring of low-risk patients [34]. Further, it suggested that this redundant cardiac telemetry represented a financial burden to hospitals and could paradoxically lead to higher rates of missed cardiac events among higher-risk patients due to equipment shortages and demands on staff. This is due to the overuse of cardiac telemetry on GCUs for non-cardiac patients and has prompted investigators to look for more appropriate monitoring technologies that would better fit early detection of deterioration [38].

A before-and-after study of a continuous monitoring system that automatically combined five single parameters into a predictive index was phased in at a single noncritical unit in USA [20]. The technology was introduced initially without alerts or staff training and gradually the complete intervention in a relatively small number of patients to assess the correlation between alerts and patient instability. Analysis indicated that the number and duration of serious instability episodes was significantly reduced after the technology was in full use. As no information was collected on staff interventions before the alarms were triggered, the association between alerts and outcomes is not conclusive.

A pilot study of a device for contactless continuous monitoring for heart rate, respiratory rate, and bed motion was conducted among patients at high risk of respiratory failure in two medical wards in Israel. Alarms were disabled to retrospectively estimate the ability of the vital signs behavior within 24 h of an adverse event to predict cardiac arrest, need for intubation or ventilation, or transfer to intensive care [18]. The device was reported to accurately predict major deterioration, and trend algorithms rather than single-parameter alerts were found to provide the optimal cutoffs to identify deterioration with minimal false alerts. However, these thresholds were not validated for correlation with less severe clinical events, and the effect of clinical responses to earlier deterioration was not documented or incorporated in the prediction. The same device was assessed 2 years later in an interventional pre-post and concurrent control design at a medical-surgical unit at a community hospital in Los Angeles. Following a 9 month intervention period the results indicated no impact on the numbers of transfers to intensive care, but a significant reduction in the total length of stay in intensive care among transferred patients, and significant reduction incidence of code blue events [49]. The authors concluded that the continuous monitoring allowed for earlier transfer to the ICU of lower acuity patients who required shorter stays in the ICU.

Another single-center study of machine learning used data from the electronic medical records to compute an algorithm predicting risk of deterioration. Electronic data included manually entered vital signs from point assessment (rather than continuous monitoring) as well as medical data, pharmacy data, and laboratory data. Real-time automated alerts were then sent to the nurse's pager on the four non-ICU intervention wards, so physicians or a rapid response team could be contacted [40]. Comparisons with four control wards where alerts were stored in the database but not sent to the nurses' pager showed that impending deterioration was equally predicted in both groups but the pager alerts yielded no difference in the proportion of patients who were transferred to ICU or those who died. The absence of clinical support prompts for patient-directed intervention on the system was thought to be the reason for the lack of impact of the predictive algorithm on patient outcomes.

The concordance between manually charted vital signs and values from bedside continuous pulse oximetry technology was recently assessed in a single-center controlled study. Analysis of data from patients with prolonged oxygen desaturations of $\leq 90\%$ showed that the nurse's visit for manual observations was associated with a statistically significant arousal effect when compared to noninvasive monitoring recorded in the 5 min prior to the nurse's observations visit [32]. As manual saturation recordings were considered inaccurate and inflated, the authors concluded that spot checking of oximetry was insufficient for timely detection of deterioration and the difference in values was sufficient to have triggered a rapid response team attendance.

The introduction of intermittent electronic surveillance to improve collection, accuracy, and clinical use of vital signs recording appears to be a logical transition stage between intermittent manual charting and full-on continuous monitoring. This intervention consists of software to enter and view multiple vital signs on wireless PC tablets and desktop PCs for identification of deterioration. While this monitoring has shown to prevent adverse events during anesthesia, its mandatory use outside critical care without training in trend interpretation or changing clinical response did not appear to have an effect on adverse events (with ~50% requiring change in treatment) or mortality (17% in intervention and control group) [19]. However, its impact on mortality reductions in a more recent study of two UK hospitals from 56 selected causes was apparent within 2 years of deployment of the software and persisted after 6 years (relative risk of death 0.83 and 0.82) [12]. The difference in outcomes could have been attributed to the associated training on trend interpretation, and inclusion of clinical decision support prompts such as early warning scores, indication on when the next set of vital signs was due, and whether care should be escalated to senior staff.

Other Implications for Practice

Improper implementation of close monitoring may come at the cost of increased staff workloads related to non-actionable alarms such as self-correcting episodes of apnea or tachycardia or nuisance alarms from motion artifacts. This can lead to staff desensitization or alarm inactivation with the paradoxical effect of compromising patient safety [37]. While perfect alarm balance is unrealistic, strategies to minimize alarm fatigue to prevent staff from abandoning technology can also have unintended consequences on patient safety. This is due to the individual patient variations observed in clinical practice. For example, respiratory rate reductions are used as indicators of opioid-induced ventilatory depression. But there is evidence that hypoventilation from benzodiazepines can be associated with variable breathing patterns including increased respiratory rate in some patients [51]. In fact, data of 5000 patient-days of continuous monitoring of respiration indicates that respiratory rate remained normal in almost all cases of desaturation [49]. Thus, setting strict and generic thresholds for particular parameters may not be appropriate in isolation of patient profiles. Individualizing patient alarm thresholds and selective customization of audibility to ensure critical alarms are not ignored has shown to reduce alarms to a manageable 43%. Technology that is flexible to enable personalized modifications to parameters after careful clinical assessment is worth considering as an option for alarm management [37].

Potential shortcomings of continuous monitoring that could deter its adoption are the high cost of capital infrastructure, new equipment and consumables, and in some cases staff dissatisfaction and decreased retention [52]. These disadvantages have to be weighed against the potential benefits of earlier detection of instability with unpredictable crises resulting from episodic monitoring that misses trends and warning signs and generates transfers to higher-level care and deaths [25].

The challenge of staff engagement and training remains. Continuous monitoring for low-risk patients is still far from being routine as well as being a part of nurses' curriculum in nursing schools or more advanced training programs. Effective implementation will require change management and strong leadership support and direct involvement. New technologies and processes will need to be integrated into the current nursing and physicians work-flows in a way that would allow for maximum benefits while improving efficiency. This would require further research that would compare different implementation strategies and their effect on effectiveness, costs, and staff satisfaction and attitudes.

Finally, while it is technically feasible to address these issues and obtain value for money from the use of continuous monitoring, these can never replace physical examination, critical thinking, or clinical judgment. They should always be used as an adjunct to existing patient contact and rapid response systems, not a substitute.

Cost Considerations of Continuous Monitoring

Evidence of cost-effectiveness in the use of continuous monitoring technology as compared with standard care (manual or electronic) is still sparse [53]. A return on investment (ROI) model developed for the single-center community hospital in Los Angeles trial [44] has shown a ROI with a breakeven of 0.5–1.5 years. For this evaluation true implementation costs were used and cost savings based on favorable attributable outcomes such as reduction of ICU utilization, shorter hospital stays, and prevention of pressure ulcers were factored in. Robust sensitivity analysis allowed accounting for most uncertain factors that would affect the ROI, thus providing a model that might be generalized to most U.S. hospitals.

While cost-effectiveness considerations are rarely applied for code or rapid response teams, the principal ethical question for a technology that serves the purpose to save lives is no different.

Despite that, the demand for analyzing the cost of technology is greater than that of human labor as a resource. In a cost-effectiveness analysis using the reduction in length of stay and ICU transfers for cost calculation, it was estimated the cost equality between the investment cost of surveillance technology and improved outcomes to be reached if care escalations would be reduced by 9% [54]. Cost estimations are often difficult to quantify in the settings of quality improvement. The dramatic reduction of RRT alerts seen [50] are hard to assign with cost savings. Given that the highest cost in most production environments (including hospitals) is human labor, it is a logical step to replace the intermittent and inaccurate sampling of vital signs with technology. Indeed, as sensor technology has improved and become more common, cost per patient has decreased. From 2011 to 2014 the cost to monitor a single patient at one of the authors' institutions has decreased from $85 to $22 per hospital stay [54]. For now on, information on outcomes such as reduction of code blue events, total time spent in hospital, and duration of ICU stay for those transferred [49] indicates possible translation into cost-savings for hospitals. Automated sampling of vital signs and associated alerting may be of even greater value in small, non-academic, or resource-constrained hospitals that do not have the volume or personnel to afford a rapid response team.

Other Areas for Future Research

The effectiveness of rapid response systems is still debatable [55, 56] and likely this is due to the use of single parameters as calling criteria and to the low frequency of observations precluding a timely or early response before serious instability occurs. It would be interesting to see if outcomes of the RRS point toward definitive effectiveness after wider introduction of continuous monitoring.

One of the major areas of future research of continuous monitoring systems is the automation of support algorithms to understand and optimize permutations of vital signs to more accurately identify the patients at risk of clinical deterioration

and in need of additional intervention before serious deterioration events [30].

Research in the area of continuous monitoring is in its infancy and much work remains to be done. Only recently, "normality"—the underlying distribution of continuously sampled vital signs like heart rate and oxygen saturation had never been described [54]. The distribution of many other physiologic variables such as respiratory rate, blood pressure, temperature, ECG changes, or laboratory values and their respective changes over time are largely unknown; yet they are essential for the understanding of interpretation of continuous vital sign sampling. Furthermore, which of these parameters should be monitored and how frequent is entirely unknown, as is whether and how they should be weighted in algorithms.

The number of accuracy studies outside laboratory settings is also scarce [57], and it would be reassuring for clinicians to make informed decisions about introducing new systems based on validations comparing the performance of new technology with that of equipment currently used on wards if trials with "gold standards" are not feasible.

Overall Effect of Continuous Monitoring on Patient Safety

Continuous monitoring has the potential to improve patient safety not only through early detection of deterioration and through that prevention of avoidable in-hospital mortality, but also through possibly preventing other forms of patient harm. Detection of falls or predicting falls has been explored using continuous monitoring with technology such as wearable sensors, cameras, motion sensors, microphones, and floor sensors. Most smart beds today include a motion sensor that can alert when a patient has left the bed. Yet, a recent systematic review has found that very little real-world evidence exists that would show the effectiveness of such solutions in preventing patient falls in an in-patient setting [58].

Similarly, another avoidable in-hospital complication, pressure ulcers, can potentially be prevented using continuous monitoring technologies. Continuously monitoring patients' risk for developing pressure ulcers was demonstrated using technologies such as pressure sensors under the mattress [59] or wearable accelerometers [60]. Assessing risk continuously can provide a clear advantage for timely identification of quick changes in risks, such as can be seen in patients on a rapid deterioration phase. Although preliminary evidence is emerging that these monitoring technologies might be effective in preventing pressure ulcers [59, 61], much more research and development is needed before evidence of effectiveness is sufficient for widespread adoption of these and other technologies [62].

Summary

While the 1990s were the decade of the executive arm of RRTs, the realization that RRS are only as good as their notification system became obvious in the first decade of this century. Early approaches implemented continuous monitoring as part of RRS. With further developments of patient surveillance expanding from GCU in academic centers to community centers and patient home monitoring, it has become clear that surveillance monitoring is the overarching umbrella and system under which RRS have their place. As total knee replacement surgery in the elderly becomes an outpatient procedure in patients with multiple comorbidities who recover at home, surveillance monitoring in- and outside of health care organizations becomes increasingly important; often in settings that go beyond the scope of RRT as we know them.

Failure to rescue patients from inadvertent deterioration on general care units has long been associated with a combination of incomplete or infrequent patient vital signs monitoring, lack of recognition or inadequate interpretation of physiological derailment, and untimely clinical response. Fortunately, the last decade has seen impressive developments in the area of continuous monitoring to reduce these adverse events and ultimately avoidable hospital mortality. Initial cost-effectiveness studies of some technologies show promise. Currently, we still rely on clinical skill training, device testing, and RRT responses; much progress has been made but further research is needed to find the point where the benefits outweigh the cost. The future of patient safety is envisaged as a paperless continuous charting of vital signs integrated with laboratory profiles in the EMR, greatly assisted by smart automated interpretation and decision support tools. New, innovative technologies will allow for monitors designed and intended toward the specific attributes of patients in GCUs, either wearables or contactless, allowing for accurate readings of vital signs. These continuous readings, together with other clinical data, will offer a chance to improve healthcare outcomes without replacing human intervention. The quest continues today for a suitable algorithm to maximize accuracy of early detection, and minimize transmission errors and alert fatigue so that ward-based clinical care can deliver optimal survival without serious unexpected complications and reduced need for rapid response system calls, transfers to higher levels of care, other hospital resources, and ultimately preventable mortality.

References

1. Ahrens T. The most important vital signs are not being measured. Aust Crit Care. 2008;21(1):3–5.
2. Villegas I, Arias IC, Botero A, Escobar A. Evaluation of the technique used by health-care workers for taking blood pressure. Hypertension. 1995;26:1204–6.
3. Sneed NV, Hollerbach AD. Accuracy of heart rate assessment in atrial fibrillation. Heart Lung. 1992;21: 427–33.
4. Hooker EA, O'Brien DJ, Danzl DF, Barefoot JA, Brown JE. Respiratory rates in emergency department patients. J Emerg Med. 1989;7:129–32.
5. Abenstein JP, Narr BJ. An ounce of prevention may equate to a pound of cure: can early detection and intervention prevent adverse events? Anesthesiology. 2010;112(2):272–3.
6. Evans D, Hodgkinson B, Berry J. Vital signs in hospital patients: a systematic review. Int J Nurs Stud. 2001;38(6):643–50.
7. Storm-Versloot MN, Verweij L, Lucas C, Ludikhuize J, Goslings JC, Legemate DA, et al. Clinical relevance of routinely measured vital signs in hospitalized

patients: a systematic review. J Nurs Scholarsh. 2014;46(1):39–49.

8. Van Leuvan CH, Mitchell I. Missed opportunities? An observational study of vital sign measurements. Crit Care Resusc. 2008;10(2):111–5.

9. Chua WL, Mackey S, Ng EK, Liaw SY. Front line nurses' experiences with deteriorating ward patients: a qualitative study. Int Nurs Rev. 2013;60(4):501–9.

10. Jones S, Mullally M, Ingleby S, Buist M, Bailey M, Eddleston JM. Bedside electronic capture of clinical observations and automated clinical alerts to improve compliance with an early warning score protocol. Crit Care Resusc. 2011;13(2):83–8.

11. Smith GB, Prytherch DR, Schmidt P, Featherstone PI, Knight D, Clements G, et al. Hospital-wide physiological surveillance–a new approach to the early identification and management of the sick patient. Resuscitation. 2006;71(1):19–28.

12. Schmidt PE, Meredith P, Prytherch DR, Watson D, Watson V, Killen RM, et al. Impact of introducing an electronic physiological surveillance system on hospital mortality. BMJ Qual Saf. 2015 Jan;24(1):10–20.

13. Mitchell IA, McKay H, Van Leuvan C, Berry R, McCutcheon C, Avard B, et al. A prospective controlled trial of the effect of a multi-faceted intervention on early recognition and intervention in deteriorating hospital patients. Resuscitation. 2010; 81(6):658–66.

14. Bellomo R, Ackerman M, Bailey M, Beale R, Clancy G, Danesh V, et al. A controlled trial of electronic automated advisory vital signs monitoring in general hospital wards. Crit Care Med. 2012;40(8):2349–61.

15. Evans RS, Kuttler KG, Simpson KJ, Howe S, Crossno PF, Johnson KV, et al. Automated detection of physiologic deterioration in hospitalized patients. J Am Med Inform Assoc. 2015 Mar;22(2):350–60.

16. Goldstein B. Intensive Care Unit ECG Monitoring. Card Electrophysiol Rev. 1997;1(3):308–10.

17. Jubran A. Pulse oximetry. Crit Care. 1999;3(2):R11–7. (London, England).

18. Zimlichman E, Szyper-Kravitz M, Shinar Z, Klap T, Levkovich S, Unterman A, et al. Early recognition of acutely deteriorating patients in non-intensive care units: assessment of an innovative monitoring technology. J Hosp Med. 2012;7(8):628–33.

19. Watkinson PJ, Barber VS, Price JD, Hann A, Tarassenko L, Young JD. A randomised controlled trial of the effect of continuous electronic physiological monitoring on the adverse event rate in high risk medical and surgical patients. Anaesthesia. 2006; 61(11):1031–9.

20. Hravnak M, Devita MA, Clontz A, Edwards L, Valenta C, Pinsky MR. Cardiorespiratory instability before and after implementing an integrated monitoring system. Crit Care Med. 2011;39(1):65–72.

21. Hillman K. The changing role of acute-care hospitals. Med J Aust. 1999;170(7):325–8.

22. Le Maguet P, Roquilly A, Lasocki S, Asehnoune K, Carise E, Martin M, et al. Prevalence and impact of frailty on mortality in elderly ICU patients: a prospective, multicenter, observational study. Intensive Care Med. 2014 May;40(5):674–82.

23. Stelfox HT, Bagshaw SM, Gao S. Characteristics and outcomes for hospitalized patients with recurrent clinical deterioration and repeat medical emergency team activation. Crit Care Med. 2014;42(7):1601–9.

24. Breslow MJ, Rosenfeld BA, Doerfler M, Burke G, Yates G, Stone DJ, et al. Effect of a multiple-site intensive care unit telemedicine program on clinical and economic outcomes: an alternative paradigm for intensivist staffing. Crit Care Med. 2004;32(1):31–8.

25. DeVita MA, Smith GB, Adam SK, Adams-Pizarro I, Buist M, Bellomo R, et al. "Identifying the hospitalised patient in crisis"—A consensus conference on the afferent limb of rapid response systems. Resuscitation. 2010;81(4):375–82.

26. Huh JW, Lim CM, Koh Y, Lee J, Jung YK, Seo HS, et al. Activation of a medical emergency team using an electronic medical recording-based screening system*. Crit Care Med. 2014;42(4):801–8.

27. Galhotra S, DeVita MA, Simmons RL, Dew MA, Members of the Medical Emergency Response Improvement Team (MERIT) Committee. Mature rapid response system and potentially avoidable cardiopulmonary arrests in hospital. Qual Saf Health Care. 2007;16:260–5.

28. Twigg D, Duffield C, Bremner A, Rapley P, Finn J. The impact of the nursing hours per patient day (NHPPD) staffing method on patient outcomes: a retrospective analysis of patient and staffing data. Int J Nurs Stud. 2011;48(5):540–8.

29. Shekelle PG. Effect of nurse-to-patient staffing ratios on patient morbidity and mortality (Chapter 34). In: AQHR , editor. Making health care safer II: an updated critical analysis of the evidence for patient safety practices. Rockville: AHRQ Publication. Evidence Report/Technology Assessment No 211 AHRQ Publication No 13-E001-EF2013.

30. Dombrowski W. Acutely ill patients will likely benefit from more monitoring, not less. JAMA Intern Med. 2014;174(3):475.

31. Ciccone A, Celani MG, Chiaramonte R, Rossi C, Righetti E. Continuous versus intermittent physiological monitoring for acute stroke. Cochrane Database Syst Rev. 2013;5.

32. Taenzer AH, Pyke J, Herrick MD, Dodds TM, McGrath SP. A comparison of oxygen saturation data in inpatients with low oxygen saturation using automated continuous monitoring and intermittent manual data charting. Anesth Analg. 2014;118(2):326–31.

33. Smith LB, Banner L, Lozano D, Olney CM, Friedman B. Connected care: reducing errors through automated vital signs data upload. Comput Inform Nurs. 2009;27(5):318–23.

34. Bates D, Zimlichman E. Finding patients before they crash: the next major opportunity to improve patient safety. BMJ Qual Saf. 2015;24:1–3. doi:10.1136/bmjqs-2014-003499.

35. Yoder JC, Yuen TC, Churpek MM, Arora VM, Edelson DP. A prospective study of nighttime vital

sign monitoring frequency and risk of clinical deterioration. JAMA Intern Med. 2013;173(16):1554–5.

36. Winters BD, Weaver SJ, Pfoh ER, Yang T, Pham JC, Dy SM. Rapid-response systems as a patient safety strategy. A systematic review. Ann Intern Med. 2013;158(5_Part_2):417–25.

37. Graham KC, Cvach M. Monitor alarm fatigue: standardizing use of physiological monitors and decreasing nuisance alarms. Am J Crit Care. 2010;19(1): 28–34.

38. Taenzer AH, Pyke JB, McGrath SP. A review of current and emerging approaches to address failure-to-rescue. Anesthesiology. 2011;115(2):421–31.

39. Brenner M, Stein DM, Hu PF, Aarabi B, Sheth K, Scalea TM. Traditional systolic blood pressure targets underestimate hypotension-induced secondary brain injury. J Trauma Acute Care Surg. 2012;72(5): 1135–9.

40. Bailey TC, Chen Y, Mao Y, Lu C, Hackmann G, Micek STHK, et al. A trial of a real-time alert for clinical deterioration in patients hospitalized on general medical wards. J Hosp Med. 2013;00(00):1–7.

41. Pyke J, Taenzer AH, Renaud CE, McGrath SP. Developing a continuous monitoring infrastructure for detection of inpatient deterioration. Jt Comm J Qual Patient Saf. 2012;38(9):428–31.

42. Fourihan F, Bishop G, Hillman KM, Daffurn K, Lee A. The medical emergency team: a new strategy to identify and intervene in high-risk patients. Clin Intensive Care. 1995;6:269–72.

43. Donaldson LJ, Panesar SS, Darzi A. Patient-safety-related hospital deaths in England: thematic analysis of incidents reported to a national database, 2010-2012. PLoS Med. 2014;11(6):e1001667.

44. Odell M. Are early warning scores the only way to rapidly detect and manage deterioration? Nurs Times. 2010;106(8):24–6.

45. Puri N, Puri V, Dellinger RP. History of technology in the intensive care unit. Crit Care Clin. 2009;1: 185–200.

46. Mitka M. Joint commission warns of alarm fatigue: multitude of alarms from monitoring devices problematic. JAMA. 2013;309(22):2315–6.

47. Yilmaz T, Foster R, Hao Y. Detecting vital signs with wearable wireless sensors. Sensors (Basel). 2010; 10(12):10837–62.

48. Welch J, Moon J, McCombie S. Early detection of the deteriorating patient: the case for a multi-parameter patient-worn monitor. Biomed Instrum Technol. 2012;Fall(Suppl):57–64.

49. Brown H, Terrence J, Vasquez P, Bates DW, Zimlichman E. Continuous monitoring in an inpatient medical-surgical unit: a controlled clinical trial. Am J Med. 2014;127(3):226–32.

50. Taenzer AH, Pyke JB, McGrath SP, Blike GT. Impact of pulse oximetry surveillance on rescue events and intensive care unit transfers: a before-and-after concurrence study. Anesthesiology. 2010;112(2):282–7.

51. Curry JP, Jungquist CR. A critical assessment of monitoring practices, patient deterioration, and alarm fatigue on inpatient wards: a review. Patient Saf Surg. 2014;8:29.

52. DeVita MA. Should all hospitalized patients be continuously monitored?: Critical Care Canada presentation; 2011 [cited 2014 September 12]. Available from: http://www.criticalcarecanada.com/presentations/ 2011/all_hospitalized_patients_should_be_monitored.pdf.

53. Slight SP, Franz C, Olugbile M, Brown HV, Bates DW, Zimlichman E. The return on investment of implementing a continuous monitoring system in general medical-surgical units*. Crit Care Med 2014; 42(8):1862–1868. PubMed

54. Taenzer AH, Blike GT. Postoperative monitoring— The Darmouth experience. APSF Newsletter [Internet]. 2012 [cited 2014 November]; Spring-Summer. Available from: http://www.apsf.org/newsletters/html/2012/spring/01_postop.htm.

55. Chan PS, Jain R, Nallmothu BK, Berg RA, Sasson C. Rapid response teams: a systematic review and meta-analysis. Arch Intern Med. 2010;170(1):18–26.

56. Winters BD, Pham JC, Hunt EA, Guallar E, Berenholtz S, Pronovost PJ. Rapid-response systems: a systematic review. Crit Care Med. 2007;35(5): 1238–43.

57. Ben-Ari J, Zimlichman E, Adi N, Sorkine P. Contactless respiratory and heart rate monitoring: validation of an innovative tool. J Med Eng Technol. 2010;34(7–8):393–8.

58. Chaudhuri S, Thompson H, Demiris G. Fall detection devices and their use with older adults: a systematic review. J Geriatr Phys Ther. 2014;37(4):178–96.

59. Zimlichman E, Shinar Z, Rozenblum R, Levkovich S, Skiano S, Szyper-Kravitz M, et al. Using continuous motion monitoring technology to determine patient's risk for development of pressure ulcers. J Patient Saf. 2011;7(4):181–4.

60. Dhillon MS, McCombie SA, McCombie DB, editors. Towards the prevention of pressure ulcers with a wearable patient posture monitor based on adaptive accelerometer alignment. Conference proceedings: annual international conference of the IEEE engineering in medicine and biology society IEEE engineering in medicine and biology society annual conference; 2012.

61. Zimlichman E, Shinar Z, Rozenblum R, Levkovich S, Skiano S, Szyper-Kravitz M, et al. Using continuous motion sensing technology as a nursing monitoring and alerting tool to prevent in-hospital development of pressure ulcers. International society for quality in health care annual meeting; Hong Kong, China. 2011.

62. Cardona-Morrell M, Prgomet M, Turner RM, Nicholson M, Hillman K. Effectiveness of continuous or intermittent vital signs monitoring in preventing adverse events on general wards: a systematic review and meta-analysis. International journal of clinical practice. 2016;70:806–24.

Dying Safely

Magnolia Cardona-Morrell and Ken Hillman

Introduction

The burden of deaths due to noncommunicable disease, particularly in the elderly, is projected to rise from 59% in 2002 to 69% in 2030 [1]. The ageing population has increased the use of medical technology and life support systems for the support of elderly complex cases [2–4]—the so-called "sick elderly." Public expectations believe modern medicine and its associated miracles can prolong life almost indefinitely [5]. Sophisticated technology and the way media portrays the latest miracles generates unrealistic expectations by relatives and often causes potential conflict at the end of life (EoL) [6]. The medicalization of death

The original version of this chapter was revised. An erratum to this chapter can be found at DOI 10.1007/978-3-319-39391-9_37

M. Cardona-Morrell, MBBS, MPH, PhD (✉)
The Simpson Centre for Health Services Research, South Western Sydney Clinical School and Ingham Institute for Applied Medical Research, The University of New South Wales, P.O. Box 6087, Sydney, NSW 1466, Australia e-mail: m.cardonamorrell@unsw.edu.au

K. Hillman, MBBS, FRCA, FCICM, FRCP, MD
The Simpson Centre for Health Services Research, South Western Sydney Clinical School, UNSW Sydney, the Ingham Institute for Applied Medical Research and Intensive Care, Liverpool Hospital, Locked Bag 7103, Liverpool BC, NSW 1871, Australia e-mail: k.hillman@unsw.edu.au

and dying, despite its inevitability has contributed to the disappearance of the concept of a dignified natural death [7]. Dying and death are seen as the ultimate challenge for successful ageing [8] or as a failure of medicine if doctors cannot offer hope of recovery [9]. Unfortunately, in many terminal cases, efforts are made to prolong life under pressure from families as well as the culture of acute hospitals and their concentration on "curing." Clinicians are often reluctant to recommend limitations of treatment and instead, often administer inappropriate treatment in the face of futility.

This chapter is not about assisted dying, euthanasia, nor about the "right to die." It is about recognition of dying by clinicians; acceptance of death as a natural part of the cycle of life; understanding what constitutes a "good death"; considering the ethical aspects of futile interventions; and reviewing best practice in providing quality of EoL. We discuss the role of doctors, nurses, and the health system in supporting patients and family through the transition.

Recognizing and Managing the Dying Patient

Elderly and chronically ill complex patients constitute a large proportion of acute hospital patients today and many of these die in these institutions [10]. Nursing homes often are forced to transfer these patients to acute facilities when clinical deterioration occurs. Different providers have different levels of expertise in dealing with dying patients and often conflicting opinions about what constitutes best care. Despite the uncertainty of predicting imminent death, many clinicians are often not aware of indicative signs or symptoms associated with patients at the EoL. Features in the last weeks of life are frailty, severe fatigue, severe pain, anorexia, and cachexia [11–13]. Some of these are present in up to 50% of dying patients [14]. More obvious indicators in the last 2 days or hours of life are drowsiness, irregular breathing, cyanosis, respirations with mandibular movements, dehydration, confusion, delirium, and loss of consciousness.

Even when symptoms are recognized, busy acute hospitals are often not able to provide high quality EoL care as skills in communication [15], pain management [16], palliation and emotional care are often not readily available [14]. Instead, there is evidence since the mid-1990s of the increasing use of aggressive interventions near death, such as increased emergency department visits, hospitalizations, and repeated intensive care admissions [17, 18]. Markers of aggressive and/or futile interventions administered to dying patients include a chemotherapy in the last 2 weeks of life, oxygen therapy to treat chronic lung disease; physical restraint for agitation; invasive procedures such as ventilatory support; intubation/tracheostomy; parenteral nutrition; hemodialysis; blood transfusion; and CPR [14, 17, 19, 20]. In an ideal world, those reaching the end of their journey benefit from care by health professionals equipped to provide a *good death*.

What Is a "Good Death"?

In-hospital death after terminal illness can be an intrusive, painful, and long-drawn out experience where futile, life-sustaining treatments are administered sometimes, even against the patient's wishes to withhold aggressive care or resuscitation [19]. Well-meaning clinicians whose training is focused on "curing" often use inappropriate interventions to prolong life. On the other hand, death could be a planned event where patients are involved in recognizing the inevitable, express-

ing their preferences on active management or place of death, participating in advance care directives as well as decision-making on pain and other supportive management [20, 21].

High quality of dying is as important as good quality of life. The concept of *dying safely* denotes the values and choices of patients, families, and healthcare practitioners in achieving a less traumatic EoL experience. This involves delivery of clinical and psychosocial services to prepare patients for death; reducing the patient's suffering, including pain and symptom management; alleviating concerns about undertreatment and increasing caregiver's knowledge of and participation in the decision-making process [20]. This is facilitated by honest communication of information with families in a way they can digest and which encourages natural grieving [22]. Importantly, dying safely emphasizes the withholding or discontinuation of potentially harmful, burdensome or futile interventions such as inappropriate admissions to intensive care [2] and unnecessary procedures or administration of aggressive palliative treatments [23]. All of this can be achieved if the diagnosis of dying is recognized, the patient needs are anticipate, where there is improved patient–physician communication [24], and where there is cooperation among clinicians from various health services [25]. The failure to prevent or relieve unnecessary suffering and using scarce health funds for acute hospital treatments to prolong the process of dying can sometimes be considered futile, unethical [26] and even exaggerating inequity in healthcare [27, 28].

What Dying Patients Want and How to Help Them Die Safely

The majority of patients with an advanced illness wish to die at home [29, 30] and their next preference is for a hospice or nursing home death [31]. However, only about half of all terminally ill patients actually achieve it [30, 32]. This occurs despite the fact that a clinical *turning point* marking EoL could be identifiable within several months of death and could prompt modification

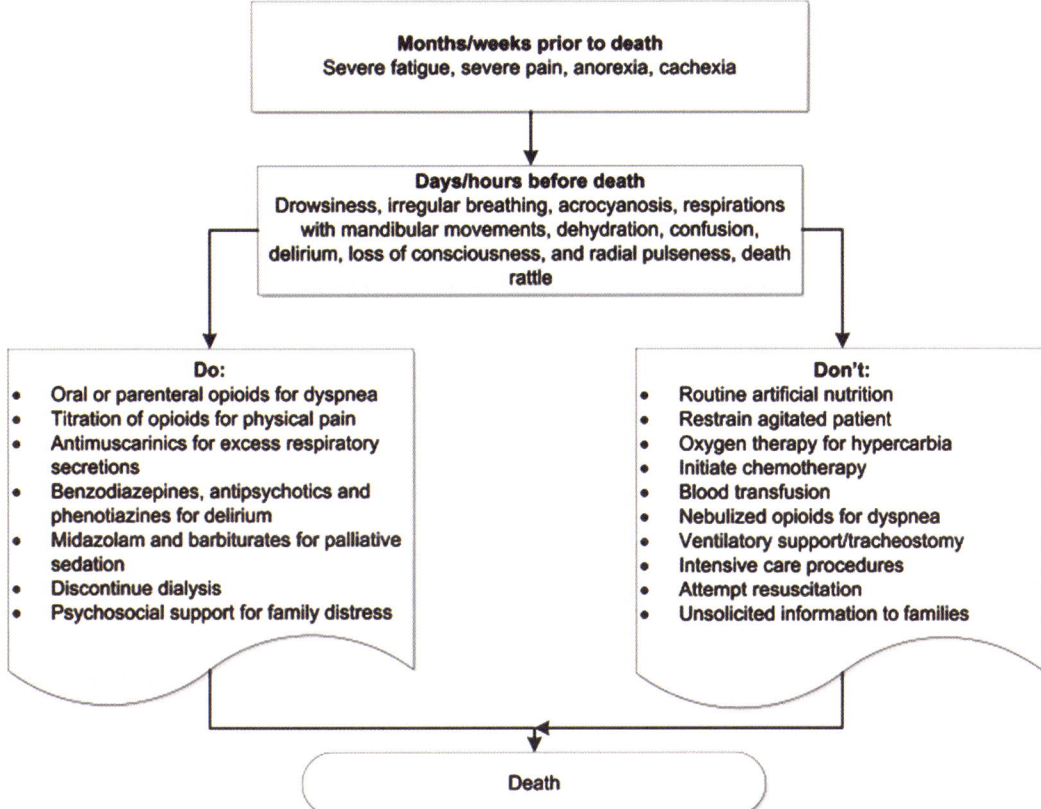

Months/weeks prior to death
Severe fatigue, severe pain, anorexia, cachexia

Days/hours before death
Drowsiness, irregular breathing, acrocyanosis, respirations with mandibular movements, dehydration, confusion, delirium, loss of consciousness, and radial pulseness, death rattle

Do:
- Oral or parenteral opioids for dyspnea
- Titration of opioids for physical pain
- Antimuscarinics for excess respiratory secretions
- Benzodiazepines, antipsychotics and phenotiazines for delirium
- Midazolam and barbiturates for palliative sedation
- Discontinue dialysis
- Psychosocial support for family distress

Don't:
- Routine artificial nutrition
- Restrain agitated patient
- Oxygen therapy for hypercarbia
- Initiate chemotherapy
- Blood transfusion
- Nebulized opioids for dyspnea
- Ventilatory support/tracheostomy
- Intensive care procedures
- Attempt resuscitation
- Unsolicited information to families

Death

Fig. 27.1 To treat or not to treat: journey from signs and symptoms to safe death

of treatment approaches from life-extending to palliative care [33]. However, decisions about limiting or changing the type of treatment are often delayed until the last day or week of life.

While often not employed by treating clinicians there are comprehensive guidelines for the control of symptoms in terminally ill patients [14]. Figure 27.1 summarizes approaches to symptom control.

The following measures are based on patient priorities and are recommended to prevent or alleviate suffering: oral or parenteral opioids are first-line therapy for terminal dyspnea; and titration of opioids for treatment of terminal physical pain. Routine artificial nutrition is not recommended for terminal care. More limited patient-oriented evidence from cohort studies or validated clinical decision rules suggests some benefit from hospice enrolment and palliative care programs. Other measures include antimuscarinics to manage excess respiratory secretions; benzodiazepines, antipsychotics, and phenothiazines

for management of terminal delirium; propofol, midazolam, and barbiturates for effective palliative sedation; and psychosocial support to improve caregiver distress and bereavement outcomes [14].

The amount of information about prognosis and dying requested by patients varies [33]. However, that is not a decision that the clinician should make. There is general agreement that prognosis should be discussed as soon as it becomes evident that the disease process is probably untreatable and will eventually become terminal even if the projected life span may be more than 1 year [34]. Included in any discussions should be the possibility of parallel active management and palliative care, especially in the face of uncertainty. Honest and transparent discussions with the patient could include the possibility of active treatment being appropriate but at the same time including information about the likelihood of success and plans to also ensure that the patient can have issues such as pain and suffering addressed. The patient should also be included in further discussions about the course of the illness and response, or lack of, to active management in order to change the balance of active and supportive treatment as appropriate.

The definition of *quality EoL care* has been generally accepted as a combination of domains, including: use of appropriate life-sustaining treatment; provision of desired symptom relief [14]; treatment of the dying with respect; supported shared decision-making as far as active management should be employed [23]; coordinated care; and the provision of information and emotional support for families [21]. A multidisciplinary team and open communication between members is essential. This is easier said than done and several aspects still need addressing in the current climate of restricted health budgets, lack of alternative care facilities, and increasing demand by complex patients.

Potential Models of Care to Improve Outcomes for Dying Patients

How do we know what works and what does not? Evidence of effectiveness or the best pathways in terminal care is not usually derived from randomized controlled trials due to the difficulty in enrolling dying patients [14]. Moreover, because of the inevitably high mortality rates of participants, follow-up sample sizes are too small and outcome measurements other than death, incomplete [35]. However, this should not deter us from attempting to determine the effects of interventions using lower level evidence (level III) such as cross-sectional surveys, retrospective studies, observational cohorts, or qualitative before and after studies. Even expert opinions (level IV), extrapolating practice from other stages of life could be used to inform strategies which might be useful to improve outcomes for the dying patient. The examples below illustrate this.

Home Care

Many patients prefer to have the dying process managed in their own home. Relatives or lay carers may be able to provide basic assistance with activities of daily living, supported by palliative or rehabilitation services. Unplanned visits to emergency department and respite care can be part of the package. Many health systems are increasingly offering EoL care in the home, although preferences vary by sex, age, and socioeconomic status [36]. By contrast, a recent decline in preference for home death has been reported in Japan, Italy, and the UK. The latter trend seems associated with poor coordination of services and cultural factors rather than availability of palliative care options. A systematic review of 22 studies of home-based EoL care a decade ago [31] reported substantial variation in the models of care provided. They included independent basic nurse or palliative care nurse specialists; individual doctors; or multidisciplinary teams. Most studies came from the US or the UK. Outcomes such as pain and symptom control and satisfaction with the service appeared to be better for models where staff had some level of palliative care training and there was an advantage of multidisciplinary over unidisciplinary models. More recently, another systematic review of four EoL home-based palliative care programs [35] found that patient satisfaction within the first month of home care was significantly higher than that of hospitalized patients. The likelihood of ending life at the preferred place of death was an important factor. However, there was no evidence of any difference in psychological well-being for patients or satisfaction with care for lay carers or families [35]. This could have been due to the variation in the occurrence of precipitous hospital admission while receiving home care, unmeasured quality of life for carers or other social/emotional circumstances not explored in these studies. While home-based care is attractive to patients, carers need to be aware of the enormous burden and change in lifestyle that it may impose on them [35].

Inpatient Hospice Care

Hospices offer EoL care focused on symptom management and emotional support in the last 6 months of life, so it is offered to people who have an understanding of the prognosis and have agreed to reorient care from cure to palliation [37]. It is expected that during that time, patients and their families will have an opportunity to express preferences and concerns, share the care and decision-making process, and accomplish goals of care and effective grieving [38]. The availability of hospices is associated with more relevant and less aggressive treatment near the EoL [17]. Also, the concept of hospice varies from one health system to another [39]. For example, some institutions only care for HIV or cancer patients, and there are racial and ethnic disparities in utilization [40], indicating the option may not be available to the chronically ill with other life-limiting conditions. Poor availability of hospice care can influence the appropriateness and quality of care terminal patients receive [18]. For instance, rural residence of patients [41] or low socioeconomic status [40] has been associated with continuing chemotherapy for longer than it otherwise would have been administered. Hospices in the USA are increasingly admitting patients that would otherwise seek acute hospital admission, yet referrals are often made too late in the last weeks or days of life. This is an indicator of poor quality EoL care [18]. Length of stay, however, varies and is generally a median of 20 days due to delayed medical referrals [17], family's lack of mental readiness for hospice care [37], or choice of late admission by patients [38].

As in home-based care, studies of inpatient hospice care suggest variation in the level of expertise of staff delivering it [31]. Despite this, studies consistently report higher carer satisfaction, better physical symptom control and lessened anxiety compared with conventional hospital or home care but no difference in the patient's quality of EoL. There is little data on outpatient hospice care for the EoL.

The main factors that predict high satisfaction with hospice services are related to being kept regularly informed about their loved one's condition, obtaining accurate information about the patient's medical treatment, receiving the right amount of emotional support to families and being able to identify one nurse as being in charge of their loved one's care [42].

Nursing Home Care

Nursing homes can potentially provide physical, social and behavioral services to terminally ill patients and their families. Comfort care is widely used and encompasses symptom management, emotional support, education, and spiritual care. They can use a variety of staff roles and various models of person-centered care, all complementing one another [43]. However, many nursing homes are not equipped or capable of offering this level of support and, as such, when the patient deteriorates, they are transferred to acute hospitals.

Given the nature of advanced age and multiple comorbidities of nursing home residents, and the low uptake of advance care directives in many countries, documentation of physician orders for life-sustaining treatment (POLST) can be a suitable proxy from the time of admission. This is essentially a form completed and signed by the treating medical officer in consultation with the patient which translates the patient's preference for aggressive medical interventions or comfort measures only into a medical order. The form becomes effective if the patient becomes seriously ill during their hospital admission or on return to the nursing home. It is usually valid for the following one year and can be modified if circumstances vary or if the patients change their mind [16]. A study of its effectiveness at eight nursing homes over a 1-year period revealed that nursing home residents who had POLST in place received significantly lower rates of aggressive life-extending interventions and high levels of comfort care aligned with their expressed wishes [44].

Hospital Palliative Care

This service is delivered by specialist palliative care doctors, anesthetists and/or nurses with emphasis on pain control and other symptom management and again, models of care vary across settings from individuals to multidisciplinary teams according to resources and levels of expertise. A systematic review of 12 studies concluded that the effectiveness could not be evaluated due to a combination of study quality and non-independent outcomes. Results were equivocal. There was reported improvement in some symptoms but not in others and this was associated with deterioration in the patient's quality of life over time [31]. There were no differences in other outcomes, such as satisfaction for patients or carers when compared with other services.

Dilemmas and Barriers to Improve the Care of the Dying

As illness progresses, a paradox of patient and caregiver information can occur. Caregivers can request more and patients may want less information. Both seek a trusted, empathic, and honest health professional that encourages questions, and offers customized explanations to their level of understanding. These conversations should take place as early as possible in the course of the illness [33]. A question prompt list can be used to assist terminally ill cancer patients and their caregivers in asking questions about prognosis and EoL issues. This seems to have promoted better communication without creating patient anxiety or impairing satisfaction [45].

The traditional definition of terminal care is confined to the last weeks of life [14]. However, this can be too late for many patients as it is too close to death for the patient to communicate effectively and to deal with many of the implications of a shortened life span. Despite some patient's request for access to all life-saving measures, there is pressure on treating doctors to be honest about the likelihood of continued active and aggressive measures being successful [23].

Continuing futile treatment also has important implications for the unsustainable cost of healthcare [27, 46].

The use of rapid response teams (RRT) as de-facto decision makers on limitations of care and *do-not-attempt-resuscitation* (DNAR) orders is not uncommon and suggests failure of the ward staff to either recognize the dying patient [47] or to act upon that identification. Over one-third (35.5%) of patients generating rapid response call are older people with a terminal illness who have a prior limitation of treatment order [48]. Ward staff seem to need these expert teams as support for these joint decisions at the EoL and hence valuable ICU staff resources and time are invested in those ward attendances [48]. Skill building at identifying and communicating the news [34] for decision-making would lead to better use of the RRS team and better management for patients.

Generally there are legal protections for the withdrawal of life-sustaining measures in terminal cases, but legal implications can arise when patients have an advance care directive and it is not followed by the treating or RRT. In fact surrogate consent is sometimes needed to withhold a resuscitation attempt [49]. Likewise, treating patients against their will might be considered a form of assault.

Fragmentation of care, as a result of the involvement of many specialist teams, can contribute to poor care of the dying [2]. While specialist teams bring individual expertise, it is based on seeing the illness through only one organ or from a similarly focused approach. This can sometimes lead to poor communication, confusion for families, and inadequate consensus on when to refer the patient to palliative care or when to introduce or cease aggressive treatment [50].

Clinicians are sometimes not proactive at initiating appropriate conversations with patients about EoL issues. This may be related to the uncertainty involved in prognosis; the sociocultural barriers; doubts about whether the patient or family desire to hear the truth; lack of knowledge of how families will manage the distressing news; and the patient's past experiences with terminal services [37, 51]. However, one of the consistent factors in the inability to communicate effectively about dying may be related to inadequate training [23, 51] and the concentration of medicine on "cures" and prevention rather than the inevitability of death and dying.

Advance care directives can be used to protect the rights and wishes of patients, encourage reflection on goals of care and guide treatment preferences [52]. Families of terminally ill patients who have made their wishes known, experienced significantly less stress, anxiety, and depression [52]. While the uptake is low in some countries [52], in some parts of the US up to 70.8% of people who died in a nursing home, hospital, or home had an advance care directive according to relatives surveyed by telephone [21]. Whether the difference in prevalence of advance care directives is driven by lack of awareness, spiritual or cultural beliefs, financial concerns or litigation, the promotion of written wishes on preferred care prior to entering the dying phase is important to assist treating clinicians and take much of the burden off carers.

Cost–Benefit of Services to Die Safely

One of the arguments for out-of-hospital EoL care is that health expenditure could be minimized if futile and aggressive interventions were reduced. The hospital costs of care for elderly patients over the age of 70 escalate with increasing limitations of daily living and with institutionalization in nursing homes [53]. The cost of care for patients receiving home palliative care has generally been reported as significantly lower than hospital or hospice-based care [31, 54]. However, not all health systems offer a safe, non-acute environment for the dying and some are more comprehensive than others. Aggressive treatments are still inflicted on those patients dying in acute hospitals, due to a combination of family pressure to prolong life [55], clinician's fear of litigation [26], or worse, the failure to recognize signs of impending death [14].

The shift to alternative EoL care has led to a promising decrease in in-hospital deaths but, unfortunately, it has not concurrently translated in reduced per capita utilization of expensive inpatient services in the last year of life [27].

While actual costing of alternatives to acute care for the dying are not readily available, a modelling study in the UK used scenarios for terminally ill patients receiving care in different settings (acute hospital, community, and hospice). The authors concluded that reducing reliance on acute care and increasing use of community services, hospices and home palliative care could release resources [4]. The study estimated cost-savings from the health system perspective but did not consider the burden of cost transfer to patient and families. The public may be better informed about the benefits of alternative care and may be more likely to use it for longer periods if it was offered several months before death rather than at crisis point [37]. Obviously this is more feasible when there is prognostic certainty for timely referral. The decision to administer costly treatments needs to weighed against the benefits of briefly extending low quality of life against the probability of relieving suffering through high quality of dying.

Managing EoL in non-hospital settings may represent cost-savings or are at least cost-neutral [4]. However, just as importantly, they provide terminal patients with the opportunity to die at the place of their choice.

Implications for Practice

Many patients may have individual insight into their own poor prognosis and many of those would want to be involved with the important decisions that, as a result, have to be made. For example, most patients would want to have a say about whether they would want to be subjected to complex interventions in an intensive care unit; and to be given the opportunity to prepare for the EoL, resolve conflicts, and say their goodbyes [56].

Understanding the reasons for the *mismatch between the dominant culture of recovery-focused medicine and the needs of an aging population* [10] is a first step in moves to advocate for policy and practice changes to minimize harm to dying patients; increase chances of meeting people's preferences; avoid behavioral and compassion fatigue among clinicians [55]; and to reduce the financial stress on the health system [4]. A joint medical-family decision to reduce active management is considered ethical and justifiable if there is evidence that the treatment is futile [23, 55].

To receive better quality and affordable care at the EoL, a culture change may be needed to prevent conflict between providers and recipients of care [50]. Health service reform may be needed to standardize policies in some places while others have already come a long way in implementing alternative services and taking up advance care planning. Integrating the skills for dying safely as part of routine health service delivery has many potential benefits. It can help plan EoL; enhance satisfaction and respect; reduce discomfort and stress for patients; enrich the debate for dying with dignity; provide families with a better starting point for bereavement; and minimize inequalities of resource allocation for other patients likely to survive.

Advance care planning is known to improve EoL care and patient and family satisfaction as it reduces stress, anxiety, and depression in surviving relatives [52]. But not all cultures or health systems are embracing of a simple patient directive and the emotional and legal concerns and burden may be responsible for the low uptake in some settings. Doctors and frontline nurses have a role in familiarizing with local legislation and promoting the benefits of advance care planning with their patients nearing death. In practice, healthcare providers can assist patients by giving information about the consequences of withdrawing treatment and mentally preparing for authorizing others to make decisions on their behalf.

An issue that is not often considered is the adverse effect on staff morale when the dying process is handled poorly [23, 55]. Distress can occur as a result of being obliged to deliver "care" that is not in the patient's best interest [23] and which violates the clinician's ethical values [55]. Open dialogue with nurses and allied health staff on the rationale for administering or withholding treatments and training and supporting clinical staff in communicating decisions to families has been recommended. Thus, nurses may have more opportunities for contact with families and are well placed to recognize and sensitively initiate discussions that doctors sometimes may avoid [50].

Conclusions and Recommendations

Dying safely involves complex dynamics between a clinician's knowledge of prognosis and the possible futility of treatment and the needs of the patient and their carers. The process can be significantly enhanced by a health system with appropriate policies and funding to provide facilities and trained staff to provide comfort care that facilitates a safe dying process.

There is still ambiguity and debate about the effectiveness of some of the life-sustaining interventions, but the often blurred line between active management, in the face of futility, and more appropriate care can become clearer when the definition of dying safely is better understood. It is possible to start resolving the puzzle of whether to treat or not to treat if we start shifting the paradigm from a *culture of cure to one that does not see every death as a failure* [5]. Recognition of the signs and symptoms of dying facilitates decisions on reorientation of care with a focus on relief of suffering to provide a "good death" [57]. Rationing the use of procedures and treatments near the time of death [27] becomes an end in itself as patients and families accept the inevitable.

As part of communication of a terminal prognosis and consultation on EoL care preferences, physicians need communication skills to deal with the associated EoL [15, 34]. They can facilitate an early hospice referral rather than wait for an end-stage crisis which distresses the family and burdens the health system [37]. Importantly, they need to address the ethical issues associated with misconceptions by some patient groups. Reassuring the elderly and terminal patients that the motivation is not to achieve cost-savings or hasten death due to old age or incurable disability but to improve palliation, decrease aggressive, harmful, and futile treatments [10].

There is still uncertainty about which sites are the more appropriate for EoL care. Much of the uncertainty could be clarified by informing our society more about aging and dying and including them in discussions about their own choices of care in these circumstances. Future research on the effectiveness of alternative EoL care could include indicators that matter to patients and families, such as level of comfort; outcomes of symptom relief; management of anxiety and pain; lay carer's quality of life; satisfaction with emotional support; and cost of home-based care from the societal perspective.

Governments and the private sector have a role in deploying health policies and infrastructure funding for expansion of non-acute care of the dying [46] to support patient and family choices and facilitate death in dignity and comfort.

The public needs information on the benefits of, and encouragement to, take up advanced directives and talk to their families about each other's wishes. Widespread discussion needs to continue so decision-making is not relegated to uninformed staff or proxies in the final moments of intense emotional pressure.

Finally, clinicians have a duty of care that extends to respecting life and allowing patients to die with dignity. The "first do no harm" principle also applies to EoL [58] care and it embraces both the provision and withdrawal of appropriate measures. Incorporating care for the dying patient in undergraduate, graduate, and continuing education activities [26, 50] may assist to reconsider the medicalization of death and dying. This may help society be aware of more real expectations about what modern medicine can offer and more importantly what it cannot.

References

1. Mathers CD, Loncar D. Projections of global mortality and burden of disease from 2002 to 2030. PLoS Med. 2006;3(11):e442.
2. Hillman K. Dying safely. International J Qual Health Care. 2010;22(5):339–40.
3. Hillman K. The changing role of acute-care hospitals. Med J Aust. 1999;170(7):325–8.
4. McBride T, Morton A, Nichols A, van Stolk C. Comparing the costs of alternative models of end-of-life care. J Palliat Care. 2011;27(2):126–33.
5. McConnell T, O'Halloran P, Porter S, Donnelly M. Systematic realist review of key factors affecting the successful implementation and sustainability of the Liverpool care pathway for the dying patient. Worldviews Evid Based Nurs. 2013;10(4):218–37.
6. Hillman K, Chen J. Conflict resolution in end of life treatment decisions: an evidence check rapid review brokered by the Sax Institute for the Centre for Epidemiology and Research. Sydney, NSW: The Sax Institute; 2008.
7. Soper RH. An unmerciful end. BMJ. 2001;323:217.
8. Patrick DL, Curtis JR, Engelberg RA, Nielsen E, McCown E. Measuring and improving the quality of dying and death. Ann Intern Med. 2003;139(5 Part 2):410–5.
9. Bowron C. Our unrealistic views of death, through a doctor's eyes. Opinion: Washington Post. 2012. http://www.washingtonpost.com/opinions/our-unrealistic-views-of-death-through-a-doctors-eyes/2012/01/31/gIQAeaHpJR_story.html. Accessed Oct 2014.
10. Tilden VP, Thompson S. Policy issues in end-of-life care. J Prof Nurs. 2009;25(6):363–8.
11. Fried LP, Tangen CM, Walston J, Newman AB, Hirsch C, Gottdiener J, et al. Frailty in older adults: evidence for a phenotype. J Gerontol A Biol Sci Med Sci. 2001;56(3):M146–57.
12. Jones D, Mitchell I, Hillman K, Story D. Defining clinical deterioration. Resuscitation. 2013;84(8):1029–34. PubMed.
13. Le Maguet P, Roquilly A, Lasocki S, Asehnoune K, Carise E, Martin M, et al. Prevalence and impact of frailty on mortality in elderly ICU patients: a prospective, multicenter, observational study. Intensive Care Med. 2014;2014:1–9.
14. Plonk Jr WM, Arnold RM. Terminal care: the last weeks of life. J Palliat Med. 2005;8(5):1042–54.
15. Goodman NW. Decisions not to resuscitate must not be left to junior doctors [Letter]. BMJ. 2001;323:1131.
16. Tilden VP, Nelson CA, Dunn PM, Donius M, Tolle SW. Nursing's perspective on improving communication about nursing home residents' preferences for medical treatments at end of life. Nurs Outlook. 2000;48(3):109–15.
17. Earle CC, Neville BA, Landrum MB, Ayanian JZ, Block SD, Weeks JC. Trends in the aggressiveness of cancer care near the end of life. J Clin Oncol. 2004;22(2):315–21.
18. Earle CC, Landrum MB, Souza JM, Neville BA, Weeks JC, Ayanian JZ. Aggressiveness of cancer care near the end of life: is it a quality-of-care issue? J Clin Oncol. 2008;26(23):3860–6.
19. Somogyi-Zalud E, Zhong Z, Hamel MB, Lynn J. The use of life-sustaining treatments in hospitalized persons aged 80 and older. J Am Geriatr Soc. 2002;50(5):930–4.
20. Teno JM. Measuring end-of-life care outcomes retrospectively. J Palliat Med. 2005;8(Suppl 1):S42–9.

21. Teno JM, Gruneir A, Schwartz Z, Nanda A, Wetle T. Association between advance directives and quality of end-of-life care: a national study. J Am Geriatr Soc. 2007;55(2):189–94.
22. Steinhauser KE, Clipp EC, McNeilly M, Christakis NA, McIntyre LM, Tulsky JA. In search of a good death: observations of patients, families, and providers. Ann Intern Med. 2000;132(10):825–32.
23. Willmott L, White B, Smith MK, Wilkinson DJ. Withholding and withdrawing life-sustaining treatment in a patient's best interests: Australian judicial deliberations. Med J Aust 2014;201(9):545–547. PubMed Epub 2014/11/02. eng.
24. The SUPPORT Principal Investigators. A controlled trial to improve care for seriously ill hospitalized patients. The study to understand prognoses and preferences for outcomes and risks of treatments (SUPPORT). JAMA. 1995;274(20):1591–8.
25. Patrick DL, Engelberg RA, Curtis JR. Evaluating the quality of dying and death. J Pain Symptom Manage. 2001;22(3):717–26.
26. Institute of Medicine. Approaching death: improving care at the end of life—a report of the Institute of Medicine. Health Serv Res. 1998;33(1):1–3.
27. Barnato AE, McClellan MB, Kagay CR, Garber AM. Trends in inpatient treatment intensity among Medicare beneficiaries at the end of life. Health Serv Res. 2004;39(2):363–75.
28. Gill B, Griffin B, Hesketh B. Changing expectations concerning life-extending treatment: the relevance of opportunity cost. Soc Sci Med. 2013;85:66–73.
29. Brazil K, Howell D, Bedard M, Krueger P, Heidebrecht C. Preferences for place of care and place of death among informal caregivers of the terminally ill. Palliat Med. 2005;19(6):492–9.
30. Higginson IJ, Sen-Gupta GJ. Place of care in advanced cancer: a qualitative systematic literature review of patient preferences. J Palliat Med. 2000 Fall;3(3):287–300.
31. Finlay IG, Higginson IJ, Goodwin DM, Cook AM, Edwards AG, Hood K, et al. Palliative care in hospital, hospice, at home: results from a systematic review. Ann Oncol. 2002;13(Suppl 4):257–64.
32. Beccaro M, Costantini M, Giorgi Rossi P, Miccinesi G, Grimaldi M, Bruzzi P. Actual and preferred place of death of cancer patients. Results from the Italian survey of the dying of cancer (ISDOC). J Epidemiol Community Health. 2006;60(5):412–6.
33. Parker SM, Clayton JM, Hancock K, Walder S, Butow PN, Carrick S, et al. A systematic review of prognostic/end-of-life communication with adults in the advanced stages of a life-limiting illness: patient/caregiver preferences for the content, style, and timing of information. J Pain Symptom Manage. 2007;34(1):81–93.
34. Clayton JM, Butow PN, Tattersall MHN. When and how to initiate discussion about prognosis and end-of-life issues with terminally ill patients. J Pain Symptom Manage. 2005;30(2):132–44.
35. Shepperd S, Wee B, Straus SE. Hospital at home: home-based end of life care. Cochrane Database Syst Rev. 2011;7:CD009231.
36. Decker SL, Higginson IJ. A tale of two cities: factors affecting place of cancer death in London and New York. Eur J Public Health. 2007;17(3):285–90.
37. Waldrop DP, Rinfrette ES. Making the transition to hospice: exploring hospice professionals' perspectives. Death Stud. 2009;33(6):557–80.
38. Teno JM, Shu JE, Casarett D, Spence C, Rhodes R, Connor S. Timing of referral to hospice and quality of care: length of stay and bereaved family members' perceptions of the timing of hospice referral. J Pain Symptom Manage. 2007;34(2):120–5.
39. Higginson IJ. End-of-life care: lessons from other nations. J Palliat Med. 2005;8(Suppl 1):S161–73.
40. Keating NL, Herrinton LJ, Zaslavsky AM, Liu L, Ayanian JZ. Variations in hospice use among cancer patients. J Natl Cancer Inst. 2006;98(15):1053–9.
41. Virnig BA, Ma H, Hartman LK, Moscovice I, Carlin B. Access to home-based hospice care for rural populations: Identification of areas lacking service. J Palliat Med. 2006;9(6):1292–9.
42. Rhodes RL, Mitchell SL, Miller SC, Connor SR, Teno JM. Bereaved family members' evaluation of hospice care: what factors influence overall satisfaction with services? J Pain Symptom Manage. 2008;35(4):365–71.
43. Waldrop DP, Kirkendall AM. Comfort measures: a qualitative study of nursing home-based end-of-life care. J Palliat Med. 2009;12(8):719–24.
44. Tolle SW, Tilden VP, Nelson CA, Dunn PM. A prospective study of the efficacy of the physician order form for life-sustaining treatment. J Am Geriatr Soc. 1998;46(9):1097–102.
45. Clayton JM, Butow PN, Tattersall MH, Devine RJ, Simpson JM, Aggarwal G, et al. Randomized controlled trial of a prompt list to help advanced cancer patients and their caregivers to ask questions about prognosis and end-of-life care. J Clin Oncol. 2007;25(6):715–23.
46. Angus DC, Barnato AE, Linde-Zwirble WT, Weissfeld LA, Watson RS, Rickert T, et al. Use of intensive care at the end of life in the United States: an epidemiologic study. Crit Care Med. 2004;32(3):638–43.
47. Hillman KM. Failure to recognise patients at the end of life in acute hospitals [Editorial]. Acta Anaesthesiol Scand. 2014;58(1):1–2.
48. Jaderling G, Bell M, Martling CR, Ekbom A, Konrad D. Limitations of medical treatment among patients attended by the rapid response team. Acta Anaesthesiol Scand. 2013;57(10):1268–74.
49. Weissman D. Policy forum. Policy proposal: do not resuscitate orders: a call for reform. Virtual Mentor. 2003;5(1):5.
50. CRELS Working Project Group. Conflict resolution on end of life settings (CRELS). Sydney, NSW: New South Wales Department of Health; 2010. p. 56.

51. Amati R, Hannawa AF. Relational dialectics theory: disentangling physician-perceived tensions of end-of-life communication. Health Commun. 2014;29(10): 962–73.

52. Detering KM, Hancock AD, Reade MC, Silvester W. The impact of advance care planning on end of life care in elderly patients: randomised controlled trial. BMJ. 2010;340:1345.

53. Lubitz J, Cai L, Kramarow E, Lentzner H. Health, life expectancy, and health care spending among the elderly. N Engl J Med. 2003;349(11):1048–55.

54. Brumley R, Enguidanos S, Jamison P, Seitz R, Morgenstern N, Saito S, et al. Increased satisfaction with care and lower costs: results of a randomized trial of in-home palliative care. J Am Geriatr Soc. 2007;55(7):993–1000.

55. Kompanje EJ, Piers RD, Benoit DD. Causes and consequences of disproportionate care in intensive care medicine. Curr Opin Crit Care. 2013;19(6):630–5.

56. Heyland DK, Dodek P, Rocker G, Groll D, Gafni A, Pichora D, et al. What matters most in end-of-life care: perceptions of seriously ill patients and their family members. Can Med Assoc J. 2006;174(5):627–33.

57. Jakobsson E, Bergh I, Gaston-Johansson F, Stolt CM, Ohlen J. The turning point: clinical identification of dying and reorientation of care. J Palliat Med. 2006;9(6):1348–58.

58. Queensland Health. Implementation guidelines. end-of-life care: decision-making for withholding and withdrawing life-sustaining measures from adult patients. Part 2. Ethical and special considerations. Brisbane: Queensland Health; 2010.

The Second Victim

28

Susan D. Scott, Laura E. Hirschinger, Myra McCoig,
Karen Cox, Kristin Hahn-Cover, and Leslie W. Hall

The longer we dwell on our misfortunes, the greater is their power to harm us.

Voltair

Gary Donnell MD, is a 2-year resident in Medicine caring for Mr. Pauley, a 64-year-old with a history of diabetes and chronic renal insufficiency. Mr. Pauley's nurse is Katie, a new graduate. Mr. Pauley was admitted for sudden-onset left side-weakness. A CT scan of his brain on admission showed no evidence of hemorrhage/mass. Katie paged Dr. Donnell 4 h later, when she found the patient to have a distinct change in his speech patterns from her initial admission assessment. Busy with several ER patients, Dr. Donnell did not evaluate Mr. Pauley, but ordered a STAT repeat head CT scan based on Katie's findings. Radiology assured Dr. Donnell that Mr. Pauley's CT would be completed within the hour. Dr. Donnell instructed Katie to perform hourly neurologic exams, and to page him with any changes.

Shortly before Katie was next due to perform a neurologic exam, Mrs. Pauley noticed her husband could not carry on a conversation. She found Katie in the hallway and asked for her help. Katie hurried to assess Mr. Pauley, and found him unresponsive. She immediately activated the rapid response team to help assess and stabilize her patient. A text page notification was also sent to Dr. Donnell informing him of the team's activation. Upon Dr. Donnell's and the rapid response team's arrival, Mr. Pauley was unarousable. His heart rate was 138, blood pressure 164/92, and he was afebrile. Dr. Donnell arranged immediate transfer to the neurological intensive care unit for progression of presumed stroke.

The morning after the transfer, intensivist Erin Boyd, MD, paged Dr. Donnell with an update. Mr. Pauley's blood glucose had been 20 when he arrived at the ICU. He was treated with a $D_{50}W$ bolus and a D_5-1/2 NS drip. Repeat head CT

S.D. Scott, PhD, RN, CPPS, FAAN (✉)
Office of Clinical Effectiveness, University of Missouri Health System, Columbia, MO, USA

University of Missouri Health, One Hospital Drive, DC 103.40, Columbia, MO 65212, USA
e-mail: scotts@health.missouri.edu

L.E. Hirschinger, RN, MSN, AHN-BC, CPPS
Clinic Administration DC121.00, University of Missouri Health System, One Hospital Drive, RM 1N04, Columbia, MO 65212, USA

M. McCoig, CPHRM
Corp Risk Management, University of Missouri Health Care, DC 103.40, Columbia, MO, USA
e-mail: McCoigM@missouri.edu

K. Cox, PhD, RN • K. Hahn-Cover, MD, FACP
University of Missouri Health, One Hospital Drive, DC 103.40, Columbia, MO 65212, USA
e-mail: CoxK@health.missouri.edu;
hahncoverk@health.missouri.edu

L.W. Hall, MD
University of South Carolina, Palmetto Health, 15 Medical Park, Suite 300, 3555 Harden Street Extension Columbia, Columbia, SC 29203, USA
e-mail: Les.hall@uscmed.sc.edu

showed no evidence of bleeding or ischemia. Mr. Pauley's blood glucose has now normalized, but he remains unresponsive. The team is concerned about brain injury due to profound hypoglycemia.

Identifying Emotional Vulnerability and Recognizing Second Victims

Dr. Donnell could not believe it. How could he have missed a hypoglycemic event? What must Dr. Boyd and the ICU team think of him? He would have to tell his attending and intern. How would he ever regain his credibility? Would he ever be trusted again?

Questioning one's abilities to meet the intense demands required of health care professionals in the aftermath of an unexpected clinical event can be the beginning of a long emotional road of silent suffering. Dr. Donnell encountered an inner turmoil that he had never experienced before in his training or career. He had a sickening realization that he was responsible for not recognizing sooner the hypoglycemic event that may have caused serious harm to his patient. Dr. Donnell could only think about this case, repeating each action and thought, step by step, over and over. One perplexing question remained on his mind: If he missed this simple problem, was he good enough to be a doctor?

Unexpected clinical events occur every day in hospitals; some involve mistakes, while others result from complications of the patient's condition. We are just now learning more about the vast emotional suffering experienced by many health care workers, irrespective of level of experience, gender or professional type. The intense work of health care often exposes clinicians to emotionally laden situations. Resilient members of the health care professions can typically review case events and make sense of what has unfolded under their watch. Occasionally, specific patient experiences trouble even the most confident clinician, resulting in a vulnerable period in which the clinician faces haunting reenactments of the event.

The personal impact of emotionally devastating clinical events has been described in health care literature as the "second victim" experience [1]. Second victims often experience a variety of physical and/or psychosocial symptoms in the aftermath of the event [2]. Many clinicians are perplexed about whom they can safely turn to for support and guidance. As a result, it is common for them to suffer in silence. Clinicians, like Dr. Donnell, often question their clinical decision making and ultimately their professional abilities. These events can result in heavy personal toll and potential career-altering changes.

In the 1980s, first-person stories began to appear in the literature, chronicling intense feelings of incompetence, inadequacy, or guilt following a medical error [3–6]. Additional renditions of the traumatic impact of unexpected clinical events continued in the 1990s when unique needs of second victims were described and hypothesized support strategies for clinicians were offered [7–13]. As patient safety and risk management professionals dealing with patient safety events, we witnessed emotional suffering first-hand, yet the literature lacked a clear roadmap of actions we could or should take when providing emotional support interventions during post-event investigations.

Since 2006, the multidisciplinary team charged with overseeing safety event reporting and risk management at University of Missouri Health System has been systematically studying this phenomenon in order to improve patient safety while also mitigating the impact of emotional trauma on clinicians. A steering team, consisting of interprofessional clinicians and individuals who provide crisis support as part of their job, was convened. Our team defined second victims as "*healthcare providers who are involved in an unanticipated adverse patient event, in a medical error and/or a patient-related injury, and become victimized in the sense that the provider is traumatized by the event. Frequently, these individuals feel personally responsible for the patient's outcome. Many feel as though they have failed the patient, second-guessing their clinical skills and knowledge base* [14]."

Using this definition, interviews were conducted with 31 clinicians known to have been personally affected by events in the workplace, to inquire about the experience and what institutional sup-

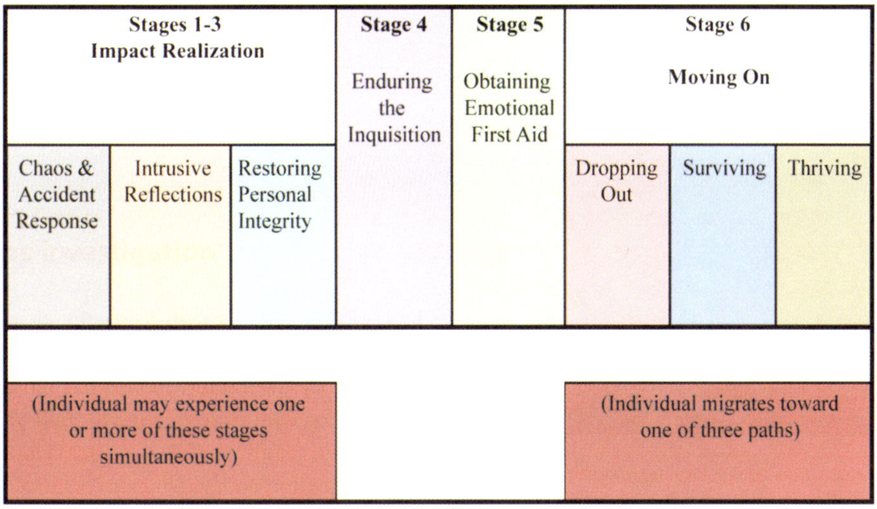

Stages 1-3 Impact Realization			Stage 4 Enduring the Inquisition	Stage 5 Obtaining Emotional First Aid	Stage 6 Moving On		
Chaos & Accident Response	Intrusive Reflections	Restoring Personal Integrity			Dropping Out	Surviving	Thriving
(Individual may experience one or more of these stages simultaneously)					(Individual migrates toward one of three paths)		

Fig. 28.1 The second victim recovery trajectory

ports might have mitigated the suffering. Most accounts clearly described specific career-jolting experiences, in meticulous detail, revealing the damaging impact of emotionally charged incidents. Unexpectedly, these narratives, once analyzed in the aggregate, revealed a largely predictable trajectory towards emotional recovery. These post-event stages include (1) chaos and accident response; (2) intrusive reflections; (3) restoring personal integrity; (4) enduring the inquisition; (5) obtaining emotional first aid; and (6) moving on (Fig. 28.1 [14]). Institutional support strategies were also described that match with the stages of emotional recovery. Interventions to help the second victim cope were desired from peers and supervisors immediately after the event as well as periodic support by valued colleagues long after the event.

Immediate Support During the Crisis

At the time of event identification and during the initial aftermath, enormous confusion is likely. "Impact realization" encompasses the first three stages of the recovery trajectory, where the second victim may experience a variety of emotional and physical reactions. These responses are normal human reactions to abnormal or unusual traumatic stressful situations or events [15].

Upon event discovery, patient stabilization is the first priority. However, the second victim is frequently distracted from immediate patient care demands by becoming engrossed in self-reflection replaying the activities preceding the event. Some providers may be unwilling or unable to discuss the event, compounding their anxiety and ability to work through the case events [16]. Once the patient's condition stabilizes, clinicians begin to worry about how the case might impact their careers. Specifically, physicians described apprehension about medical-legal proceedings, while nurses expressed fear of losing their jobs and/or licenses. Over days, the second victim tends to self-isolate in an attempt to concentrate and focus on precisely what transpired (Fig. 28.2). Over time, clinicians move from these worries to an intense fear that they will no longer be viewed as trusted colleagues. Ultimately, second victims desperately want to know post-event details so they can make a positive difference in future outcomes.

During these three stages of impact realization, peers serve an important role in emotional "first aid." In a study of physicians who experienced the second victim phenomenon, four specific needs were identified (1) the need to talk to someone; (2) the need for validation of decisions made during patient's care; (3) the need for professional reaffirmation of competence; and (4) the need for reassurance of self-worth [9]. Not addressing the specific unique needs of the second victim could leave an enduring emotional scar on the clinician that can be imprinted in their memories forever [17, 18]. Support by peers that is timely and effective can provide much-needed reassurance. Some clinicians benefit from immediate relief of patient care duties to allow them time to collect their thoughts prior to resuming patient care. After this respite from clinical care,

a "safe zone" can be offered to allow second victims to openly express their feelings and concerns regarding the event in a confidential and nonjudgmental environment. Given an opportunity to unload their emotional response with a trusted peer is likely to result in less emotional suffering and improved feelings of self-worth. This interaction requires a peer who can facilitate a dialogue with someone in crisis, someone trained in active listening skills that maximally allow event reflection, and scripted responses to reassure the victim that he is not alone. Peer supporters should reinforce their confidence in the second victim.

Astute supervisors can offset much emotional trauma. Supervisors should be aware of common high-risk situations likely to evoke a second victim response so that clinicians at the epicenter of such events can be deliberately identified, monitored, and supported in a timely manner. Figure 28.3 identifies events from our interviews that are likely to evoke emotional turmoil. It is important to touch base with potential victims more than once, as there may be cases in which an emotional impact is delayed or cases in which the victim is unable to talk about the emotional trauma immediately after the event.

Second victims articulated the need for specific key messages from their supervisor after a traumatic clinical event. For example, second victims desperately need to hear that their supervisor continues to have confidence in their clinical skills, that they were still trusted, and that the victim remains a valued member of their clinical team. Supervisors should also introduce the victim to formal investigative steps following safety events. It is important for the supervisor to be readily

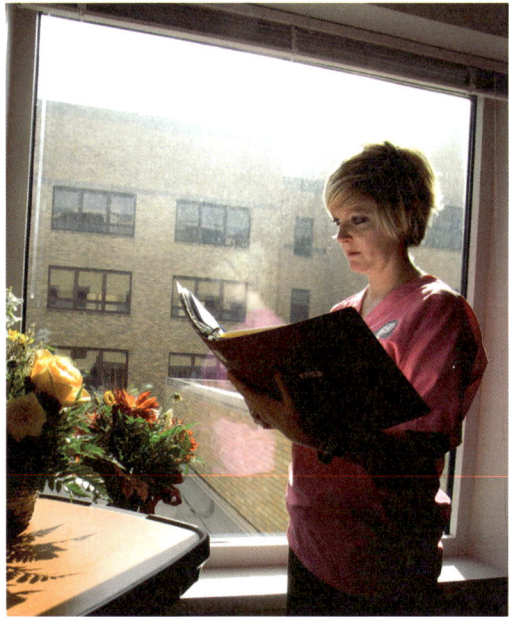

Fig. 28.2 Immediately following an adverse event, clinicians frequently reflect on the case to enhance their understanding of what has transpired

- Failure to identify patient deterioration and/or failure to rescue
- Medical error or preventable harm to patient
- Any patient which 'connects' a staff member to his/her own family (share mother's name, age of children, same appearance, red curly hair of grandchild, etc.)
- Cases involving children
- First death under their watch
- Unexpected patient demise
- Multiple patients with same poor outcomes within a short period of time within one clinical area

Fig. 28.3 High-risk clinical events for evoking second victim response

accessible during event investigations to explain steps in the process, make introductions with key safety and risk management personnel, and provide reassurance/support.

Support Long After the investigation

Well after the chaos of the event has settled and after the second victim has had time to personally process what happened, interviewees expressed the feeling that, given a choice, they would welcome conversations about their emotional response with a trusted peer or colleague. The ideal peer or colleague is someone familiar with the victim's specific professional role and setting, so that insights could be shared concerning common reactions and responses to similar case or event types. Through peer collaboration and reflection, the second victim senses a colleague who cares about him as an individual and as a professional. It is important for this person to practice active listening skills that will allow the second victim to share responses and feelings about the clinical event. Peers, especially those who have experienced this phenomenon, can offer powerful healing words and special support based on their personal experience. If the colleague has experience as a second victim, sharing personal stories can be powerful. Even without personal experience, the colleague can still be supportive while anticipating common second victim needs, free from judgment and blame. These brief conversations may take place spontaneously (Fig. 28.4). Ultimately, ongoing reassurance that the clinician remains a respected and trusted member of the clinical team is essential. However, some conversations may extend far beyond a few minutes and the second victim may rapidly lose composure, requiring the arrangement of a follow-up, by way of a more structured meeting. Some second victims—we estimate 10%—may benefit from support and counseling by professional experts. In these cases, the colleague must have the skills to recognize when additional assistance is warranted and be prepared

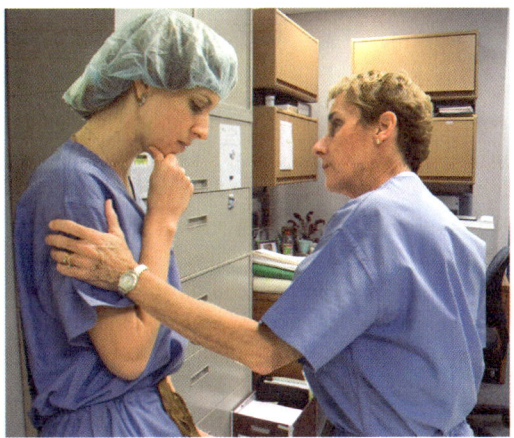

Fig. 28.4 Professional colleagues and peers can offer powerful healing words for their distressed coworker

to propose a professional referral, with contact information about available resources.

Healing for the second victim may take months or even years. We believe that professionals who are not supported after emotional trauma and who are allowed to suffer alone are at risk for premature career departure. On the other hand, future professional direction may be significantly influenced by support and guidance received within those institutions that prepare for and manage a formal second victim response team.

Emotional First Aid When Entire Teams Are Suffering

Occasionally, an entire health care team can be impacted by a clinical event, such as a rapid response team activation for a hospitalized coworker who ultimately dies, or trauma team activation for a maternal trauma that results in the deaths of both mother and baby. Dramatic events such as these may bring about long-lasting impact on team function and morale. In these situations, a team debriefing may be an effective and efficient approach for beginning the healing process as team members reflect on components of the event. Specifically, the team debriefing should focus primarily on the emotional impact, not individual team members' performances during the crisis.

Fig. 28.5 Team debriefings are opportunities for participants to discuss their unique perspectives regarding the event as well as their feelings/ reactions to it

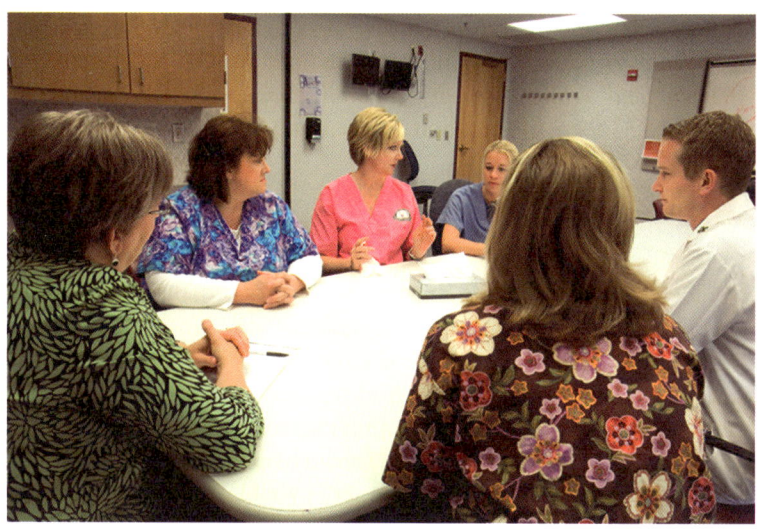

Also referred to as team defusings, team debriefings should be planned within 8–12 h of the event [19]. All team members closely involved, including licensed and non-licensed personnel, students or volunteers, should be individually contacted and invited to a 45–60 min team debriefing. Participation should be on a voluntary basis and no team member should be forced to speak up. A meeting location should be selected for the debriefing, which promotes an environment free of interruptions and other clinical distractions (Fig. 28.5). During these emotionally charged discussions, a facilitator skilled in group dynamics and critical incident stress management (CISM) should coordinate and lead the team discussion. CISM has been used effectively for years in the emergency medical community and was developed to help prevent potentially disabling stress responses among emergency responders to traumatic community disasters such as the Columbine shootings, the Oklahoma City bombing, and the 9/11 World Trade Center attack [20].

How to Formalize a Support Network

Clinicians should not have to seek support on their own. Key principles should serve as a guide for the institution's formalizing a peer support infrastructure, keeping in mind that affected staff should always be treated with respect, compassion, and administrative support immediately following adverse clinical events [21]. Denham proposes basic rights of second victims that should be guaranteed by one's workplace and summarizes these rights using the acronym "TRUST" (*T*reatment that is just, *R*espect, *U*nderstanding and compassion, *S*upportive care, and *T*ransparency) and the opportunity to contribute to learning [22] (p.107).

To support a rapid response for second victims at all times, formal peer support teams should be designed to complement existing support infrastructures within the facility. Appropriate resources can be allocated to ensure peer availability and support for members of the clinical team as well as the necessary team framework of polices and prcocedures [23]. Successful peer-to-peer support programs can be found in community emergency response systems and could serve as useful examples for designing a hospital-based support network. The Medically Induced Trauma Support Services Team (MITSS) provides support for patients/families as well as health care clinicians following an unexpected clinical event [24]. The University of Missouri Health System's support structure, the forYOU team, was designed in 2006 to increase awareness of the second victim phenomenon and to provide consistent "in-time" support for second victims [25].

Putting It All Together

Based upon emotional injury and recovery information acquired from second victims, institutions should formalize a second victim support network across every worksite to ensure that every health care clinician, student, or volunteer is monitored for second victim reactions. Institutions should design a structured response plan that results in ongoing surveillance for potential second victims and acts to mitigate emotional suffering immediately upon second victim identification. Using a peer-to-peer support model with specially trained individuals embedded in high-risk clinical environments (rapid response teams, ICU, ER, OR, helicopter/ambulance services, etc.) provides opportunities for continual surveillance as well as the capability for immediate basic emotional first aid.

Health care institutions more than likely have internal resources available that could provide the support structure needed by caregivers. Developing an infrastructure of support requires leadership and coordination by skilled personnel representing patient safety, risk management, employee assistance programs (EAP), chaplaincy, social work, and other holistic or mental health clinicians. These experts normally work with individuals during emotionally devastating times and have the passion to support these types of programs. These individuals, once organized, can serve as mentors for colleagues and on-unit peers who are interested in providing emotional first aid to identified second victims. An understanding of the second victim phenomenon, together with peer and supervisory surveillance in the aftermath of high-risk clinical events, provides a unique opportunity to enable second victims to return to full, rewarding professional roles.

> To have someone call me out of the blue, just to offer support, was a wonderful thing. It was like a burden was lifted off me, knowing I didn't have to get through it alone.
> Physician in response to peer support team activation
> I don't think I've met a doctor over the age of 30 that hasn't experienced at least two memorable adverse patient events. By the time folks get to my point in their careers they will probably have

experienced at least 4–6 such events. Even many years after these have occurred, I find myself thinking about them at least 2–3 times per year, rehearsing once again if there is anything else I could have done to avoid the negative outcome.
> Physician with more than 25 years' experience

References

1. Wolf ZR, Serembus JF, Smetzer J, Cohen H, Cohen M. Responses and concerns of healthcare providers to medication errors. Clin Nurse Spec. 2000;14(6):278-287
2. Scott SD, Hirschinger LE, Cox KR. Sharing the load: rescuing the healer after trauma. RN. 2008;71(12):38-43
3. Levinson W, Dunn PM. A piece of my mind. Coping with fallibility. JAMA. 1989;261(15):2252
4. Hilfiker D. Facing our mistakes. N Engl J Med. 1984;310(2):118-122
5. Hilfiker D. Healing the wounds: a physician looks at his work. New York, NY: Pantheon2009.
6. ElizabethR. The mistake I'll never forget. Nursing. 1990;20(9):50-51
7. Christensen JF, Levinson W, Dunn PM. The heart of darkness: the impact of perceived mistakes on physicians. J Gen Intern Med. 1992;7(4):424-431
8. Engel KG, Rosenthal M, Sutcliffe KM. Residents' responses to medical error: coping, learning, and change. Acad Med. 2006;81(1):86-93
9. NewmanMC. The emotional impact of mistakes on family physicians. Arch Fam Med. 1996;5(2):71-75
10. West CP, Huschka MM, Novotny PJ, et al. Association of perceived medical errors with resident distress and empathy: a prospective longitudinal study. JAMA. 2006;296(9):1071-1078
11. Wu AW, Folkman S, McPhee SJ, Lo B. Do house officers learn from their mistakes? JAMA. 1991;265(16):2089-2094
12. Wu AW, Folkman S, McPhee SJ, Lo B. How house officers cope with their mistakes. West J Med. 1993;159(5):565-569
13. Wolf ZR, Serembus JF, Smetzer J, Cohen H, CohenM. Responses and concerns of healthcare providers to medication errors. Clin Nurse Spec. 2000;14(6):278-287
14. Scott SD, Hirschinger LE, Cox KR, McCoig M, Brandt J, Hall LW. The natural history of recovery for the healthcare provider "second victim" after adverse patient events. Qual Saf Health Care. 2009;18(5):325-330
15. Mitchell JT, Everly GS. Critical incident stress debriefing: an operations manual for cisd, defusing and other group crisis intervention services. 3rd edition. Ellicott City, MD: Chevron Publishing; 1997.
16. Delbanco T, Bell SK. Guilty, afraid, and alone—struggling with medical error. N Engl J Med. 2007;357(17):1682-1683

17. Schwappach DL, Boluarte TA. The emotional impact of medical error involvement on physicians: a call for leadership and organisational account-ability. Swiss Med Wkly. 2009;139(1–2): 9-15

18. Serembus JF, Wolf ZR, Youngblood N. Consequences of fatal medication errors for health care providers: a secondary analysis study. Medsurg Nurs. 2001;10(4):193-201

19. Mitchell J. Critical incident stress management(CISM): group crisis intervention. 4th ed. Ellicott City, MD: International Critical Incident Stress Foundation; 2006.

20. Mitchell JT. Advanced group crisis intervention: strategies and tactics for complex situations. Participant manual. 3rd ed. Ellicott City, MD: International Critical Incident Stress Foundation; 2006.

21. Conway JB, Weingart SN. Leadership: assuring respect and compassion to clinicians involved in medical error. Swiss Med Wkly. 2009;139(1–2):3

22. Denham C. Trust: the 5 rights of the second victim. J Patient Saf. 2007;3(2):107-119

23. Robinson R, Murdoch P. Establishing and maintaining peer support programs in the workplace. 3rd ed. Ellicott City, MD: Chevron Publishing; 2003.

24. Medically Induced Trauma Support Services (MITSS). Organization located in Boston, Massachusetts, USA. http://www.mitss.org/. Accessed 6 Oct 2010.

25. for YOU team. Columbia, MO. www.muhealth.org/secondvictim; Accessed 6 Oct 2010.

Max Bell and David Konrad

Introduction

Although institutions for caring for the sick are known to have been around much earlier in history, the first teaching hospital was reportedly the Academy of Gundishapur in the Persian Empire during the Sassanid era. In addition to systemizing medical treatment and knowledge, the scholars of the Gundishapur academy also transformed medical education; students were authorized to methodically practice on patients under the supervision of physicians as part of their education. And rather than apprenticing with just one physician, medical students were required to work in the hospital under the supervision of the whole medical faculty. There is even evidence that graduates had to pass exams in order to practice as accredited Gundishapur physicians. This early teaching hospital is seen to have been the most important medical center of the ancient world (defined as Europe, the Mediterranean, and the Near East) during the sixth and seventh centuries [1].

Some things have changed since then, but not everything. Most teaching hospitals pursue three related enterprises:

- **Teaching**: training nurses, medical students, and resident physicians
- **Research**: conducting both basic science and clinical investigation
- **Patient care**: delivering healthcare services through a network that may include one or more hospitals, satellite clinics, and physician office practices.

This is sought to result in a health system that encourages the highest standards of quality and provides access to the most up-to-date treatments. It also meant to foster an environment where the staff is always thinking about the patient's condition, leading to more thorough patient care.

From one point of view, a teaching hospital is a high-risk environment. Usually these hospitals are large, with many beds, and complex medical conditions in patients with serious comorbidities are treated there. This is coupled with high numbers of trainees indicating a malignant combination. There have indeed been studies reporting adverse events in teaching hospitals [2–4]. To complicate matters, teaching hospitals have a

M. Bell, MD, PhD (✉) • D. Konrad, MD, PhD
Perioperative Medicine and Intensive Care,
Karolinska University Hospital,
171 76 Stockholm, Sweden
e-mail: max.bell@karolinska.se;
david.konrad@karolinska.se

high turnover in their ward staff; both junior doctors and nurses in training migrate to new positions as part of their education. The local know-how in a single ward is thus changed—and drained—on a regular basis. Junior doctors and nurses must also be considered by default to be inferior when it comes to medical judgment, practical skills, or knowledge of treatment protocols.

The system of medical management in teaching hospitals may then per se represent a milieu where the signs and symptoms of deterioration in patients at risk could be overlooked. Yet another system deficiency is how junior staff trains to deal with the critical ill patient. Nobody would expect a junior doctor to handle a brain hemorrhage by herself or himself. A neurosurgeon would immediately be alerted if a patient undergoing a CT scan was found to have a cerebral bleeding. Yet, even though critical care physicians undergo a subspecialty training equally long to that of a neurosurgeon, the deteriorating patient in the general ward is expected to (at least initially) be treated by the physicians that happen to work in that environment.

Another point of view is this: teaching hospitals are the perfect place to implement new systems of care, like the rapid response team (RRS). One could argue that the environment, by its very nature, is susceptible to change. Teaching hospitals are expected to frequently and critically review the way patients are treated. Pharmacological innovations, new treatment techniques, and systemic changes in how to manage patients represent changes in practice. The doctors and nurses in teaching hospitals may be eager to learn new things and are used to the constant struggle of lifelong learning. Another benefit of teaching hospitals is the fact that research and research projects are present in the day-to-day care. This is helpful, as the introduction of an RRS always should be preceded by the recording of baseline patient characteristics and outcome. Moreover, after the RRS is in place, it is recommended to continue the data collection to ensure that the RRS works and to make feedback possible.

In reality, however, teaching hospitals—just like any other hospital organization—do not implement new systems of care without a fight.

There will always be a reluctance to move from a familiar system to something novel, especially if this new system invites a whole new look on the responsibilities of the physicians, the nurses, and other ward personnel.

An introduction of a rapid response system represents a massive system change. In teaching hospitals—and in all hospitals—it is paramount to win the hearts and minds of key persons! The joke that eminence-based medicine is more important than evidence-based medicine works here too. Naturally, it is equally important to convince the nursing staff that this change will help them to help their patients. An insight from the Karolinska University Hospital, recently shared by Jones and coworkers, is that even after an implementation of an RRS, there is a perpetual need for continuous educational efforts. It may in fact take years before a rapid response system is up and running on all cylinders [5].

Implementing RRS in Teaching Hospitals

Due to its complexity, heterogeneity, and size, the process of change in teaching hospitals can be both time- and energy consuming but at the same time very rewarding. The key issue is to change the culture of an entire institution and not merely to add another process. Wide acceptance of a new course of action is crucial and depends largely upon educational efforts. There is a need to explain the expected effects of RRS implementation to a very diverse audience: physicians, nurses, department leaders, and hospital management, all of whom will have different viewpoints and reasons to accept or reject your proposals. Arguments need to be titrated in order to make all stakeholders embrace the common goal: to enhance your hospital's level of patient safety. Implementing an RRS is a major step in that direction.

The Afferent Limb

In order to have an efficient RRT, there need to be clear and readily available triggers. The ward caregivers, including physicians, should be well informed of these and encouraged to use them. Well-displayed posters and pocket-size stickers with the calling criteria and page-procedure will facilitate RRT activation. In a teaching hospital, there are a wide variety of wards and a high degree of specialization. Nonetheless, the triggers used should be the same all over your institution. Failing physiology constitutes a medical emergency regardless of cause and location. In teaching facilities, as mentioned above, there tends to be a high turnover of staff and change of working places. Also, in such settings, many students will rotate between wards. Having identical triggers regardless of different hospital locations will increase clarity, minimize confusion, and reduce the risk of delay in calling the RRT. Continuous feedback to the wards will also encourage the use of the RRT. At our institution, we use contact persons to ease communication between wards and the RRT, creating a channel for bilateral feedback.

The Efferent Limb

The responding arm of the RRT, the efferent limb, should be multidisciplinary. The most common setup is to use an ICU-based team consisting of an ICU physician and/or an ICU nurse that will meet up with the nursing and medical staff of the ward at the patient's location. This will ensure ample competence as well as staff familiar with the patient, thus facilitating assessment and treatment. Including the medical staff of the ward at the scene will also decrease the risk of the RRT being considered as intruders and will aid in planning the remainder of the patient's stay, possible referrals, and DNR status. It is prudent that the RRT behaves in a professional and inclusive manner to facilitate further collaboration. It is highly important that whoever triggered the RRT is encouraged rather than criticized. We have found it fruitful to think of every RRT call as an educational opportunity regarding management of the critically ill.

The introduction of the RRT is likely to cause an increased workload for the ICU staff. On the other hand it will also provide insight into working conditions and patient population at the general wards. In our experience ICU nurses consider RRT work as a privilege.

Hospital Culture and Management

In trying to change hospital culture and to implement the RRS, the value of information and education cannot be overemphasized. There will certainly be opposition since the implementation of an RRS affects current practices, possibly financial aspects, and may be seen as an intrusion. In our experience, a productive approach is to run a pilot study or otherwise assess your institution's baseline in order to highlight problems regarding patient safety. Patient safety—and changes in patient safety—can be measured in many ways, such as adverse events, cardiac arrest rate, length of stay, standardized mortality ratios, or other aspects, that may benefit from RRS implementation. The focus should always be on improving a faulty *system*, moving away from a culture of individual blame. Correct and timely feedback will also encourage hospital governance in facilitating the RRS process. The potential for cost savings may also be relevant.

Experiences with the RRS

Most of the current literature regarding RRS comes from single-center, before-and-after studies conducted at teaching hospitals. Many of these studies report beneficial effects on unexpected deaths, cardiac arrest rate, ICU length of stay, and some even on reduced hospital mortality. A more thorough review of the evidence is found in Chap. 6.

Clinical deterioration and abnormal vital signs are associated with increased risk of cardiac arrest and death [6–8]. Also, there seems to be a correlation between meeting one or more RRS trigger criteria and longer-term mortality. At the Karolinska, meeting such criteria once is associated with an increased risk of death up to 6 months [9] (Fig. 29.1). When acting upon such triggers, several authors have reported significant reductions in cardiac arrest rate [10–12]. Hospital mortality has been shown to decrease significantly [11] as well as morbidity and mortality for patients undergoing major surgery [13]. Interestingly, a dose-response relationship appears to exist: the more frequent your RRS is activated, the greater

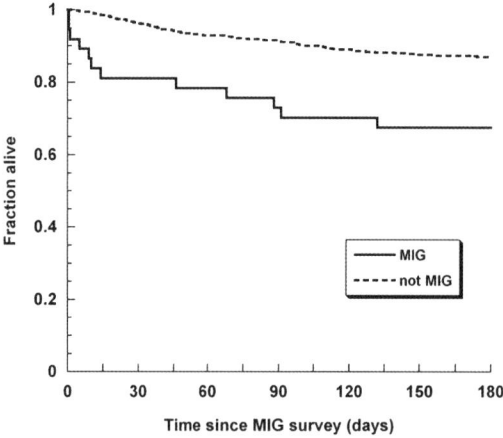

Fig. 29.1 Kaplan-Meier graph of survival for patients meeting any MET criteria. MIG = MET criteria fulfilled, not MIG = no MET criteria fulfilled. Modified from reference [9]. MIG (mobile intensive care group) is the Swedish acronym for MET

the reduction in cardiac arrest rate [14, 15]. A notable effect of implementing the RRS is the increase in NFR orders and the role of the RRS in end-of-life care [16]. This area is addressed in detail in Chap. 34.

The vast majority of these studies come from centers in Australia or North America, although the Karolinska University Hospital has shown the introduction of an RRS to be associated with a significant improvement in both cardiac arrest rate and overall adjusted hospital mortality [17]. Recently, a study of deranged physiological parameters and their association with mortality was tested in a low-income setting [18]. This collaboration between Swedish physicians and staff in Tanzania deserves further attention. However, reproducibility of results like these in other centers in other parts of the world is probable but not certain [19]. For this reason it is imperative to continue to pursue evidence regarding the efficacy of RRS. There is a need to understand by which mechanisms RRS functions, and in order to do so, attention should be paid to the RRS process itself.

The RRS, once implemented, is generally well accepted and often with great enthusiasm. For the nursing staff at the wards, the RRS constitutes a safety net which they can use either directly or when not getting the appropriate attention from their medical staff. It is therefore imperative that all the healthcare providers can rely on that activation of the RRT will lead to proper and swift action. The junior medical staff can find support in the RRT when faced with problems beyond their current level of competence, and using the RRT may also enhance their education. In our experience the ICU nurses are looked upon as experts by their peers at the ward, contributing to their work satisfaction. At our ICU it is seen as a privilege to be part of the RRT, and it is only available to those nurses with at least 1 year of ICU experience. Their skills and competence set an example for the ward staff and may also facilitate recruitment of ICU nurses in the future. For ICU residents and fellows, the RRT is a very good way of facing numerous patients with failing physiology, contributing to their training.

Conclusions

Adverse events and ward patient crises still pose a great challenge in modern teaching hospitals. Unlike the ancient academic institutions, such as the Academy of Gundishapur in the sixth century, inexperienced healthcare providers during their training are frequently either not supervised or backed up adequately. Also, experienced staff in the wards may not be sufficiently trained in the subspecialty of managing critically ill patients. The RRS has a great potential to intervene to reduce potential harm to our patients. In many single-center studies, early recognition and timely treatment have shown to decrease cardiac arrest rates, morbidity, and mortality. Apart from providing state-of-the-art healthcare, the teaching hospitals have a significant educational task where the RRS may serve two purposes: to facilitate the process of learning by a generous attitude in sharing knowledge of physiology and to avert the consequences of inexperienced staff. The success of rapid response systems depends largely on wide hospital acceptance, reliability, and feedback. To achieve this, a continuous educational effort is of utmost importance.

References

1. Frye R. The Cambridge history of Iran. Vol 4, The period from the Arab invasion to the Saljuqs. Cambridge: Cambridge University Press1975.
2. Brennan TA, LeapeLL, LairdNM, et al. Incidence of adverse events and negligence in hospitalized patients: results of the Harvard Medical Practice Study I. 1991. Qual Saf Health Care. 2004;13(2):145-151 Discussion 151–142
3. Wilson RM, Runciman WB, Gibberd RW, Harrison BT, NewbyL, HamiltonJD. The quality in Australian health care study. Med J Aust. 1995 Nov 6;163(9): 458-471
4. James K, Bellomo R, Poustie S, Story DA, McNicol PL. The epidemiology of major early adverse physiological events after surgery. Crit Care Resusc. 2000 Jun;2(2):108-113
5. Jones D, Bates S, Warrillow S, et al. Effect of an education programme on the utilization of a medical emergency team in a teaching hospital. Intern Med J. 2006 Apr;36(4):231-236
6. Schein RM, Hazday N, Pena M, Ruben BH, Sprung CL. Clinical antecedents to in-hospital cardiopulmonary arrest. Chest. 1990 Dec;98(6):1388-1392
7. Hillman KM, Bristow PJ, Chey T, et al. Antecedents to hospital deaths. Intern Med J. 2001 Aug;31(6): 343-348
8. Kause J, Smith G, Prytherch D, Parr M, Flabouris A, HillmanK. A comparison of antecedents to cardiac arrests, deaths and emergency intensive care admissions in Australia and New Zealand, and the United Kingdom--the ACADEMIA study. Resuscitation. 2004 Sep;62(3):275-282
9. Bell MB, Konrad D, Granath F, Ekbom A, Martling CR. Prevalence and sensitivity of MET-criteria in a Scandinavian University Hospital. Resuscitation. 2006 Jul;70(1):66-73
10. Buist MD, Moore GE, BernardS A, Waxman BP, Anderson JN, Nguyen TV. Effects of a medical emergency team on reduction of incidence of and mortality from unexpected cardiac arrests in hospital: preliminary study. BMJ. 2002 Feb 16;324(7334):387-390
11. BellomoR, GoldsmithD, UchinoS, et al. A prospective before-and-after trial of a medical emergency team. Med J Aust. 2003 Sep 15;179(6):283-287
12. DeVita MA, Braithwaite RS, Mahidhara R, Stuart S, ForaidaM, Simmons RL. Use of medical emergency team responses to reduce hospital cardiopulmonary arrests. Qual Saf Health Care. 2004 Aug;13(4):251-254
13. Bellomo R, Goldsmith D, Uchino S, et al. Prospective controlled trial of effect of medical emergency team on postoperative morbidity and mortality rates. Crit Care Med. 2004 Apr;32(4):916-921
14. Jones D, Bellomo R, Bates S, et al. Long term effect of a medical emergency team on cardiac arrests in a teaching hospital. Crit Care. 2005;9(6):R808-R815
15. ChenJ, BellomoR, FlabourisA, HillmanK, FinferS. The relationship between early emergency team calls and serious adverse events. Crit Care Med. 2009 Jan;37(1):148-153
16. Jaderling G, Bell M, Martling CR, Ekbom A, Konrad D. Limitations of medical treatment among patients attended by the rapid response team. Acta Anaesthesiol Scand. 2013 Nov;57(10):1268-1274
17. Konrad D, Jaderling G, Bell M, Granath F, Ekbom A, Martling CR. Reducing in-hospital cardiac arrests and hospital mortality by introducing a medical emergency team. Intensive Care Med. 2010 Jan;36(1):100-106
18. Baker T, Blixt J, Lugazia E, et al. Single deranged physiologic parameters are associated with mortality in a low-income country. Crit Care Med. 2015 Oct;43(10):2171-2179
19. Jaderling G, Calzavacca P, Bell M, et al. The deteriorating ward patient: a Swedish-Australian comparison. Intensive Care Med. 2011 Jun;37(6):1000-1005

The Nurse's View of RRS

Mandy Odell, Nicolette Mininni,
and Donna Goldsmith

Introduction

Nurses, like all other healthcare professionals, focus on patient safety and strive to deliver the right care at the right time. One example of this cultural focus of patient safety is the implementation of rapid response systems (RRSs) that include medical emergency teams (METs), rapid response teams (RRTs) and critical care outreach teams (CCOTs) [1]. Although there are different models of RRSs, all systems include an afferent phase where vital sign thresholds act as a trigger to activate a specialist team and an efferent phase where the expert team assesses and manages the deteriorating patient [1]. Therefore the bedside nurse plays a vital role in the initial activation and subsequent success of the RRS process. In order to properly utilise the RRS, we need to understand how the bedside nurses view RRSs, their role in the RRS process and what factors inhibit or enhance their engagement in the process.

M. Odell, RN, MA, PGDip, PhD (✉)
Royal Berkshire NHS Foundation Trust,
London Rd, Reading, Berks RG1 5AN, UK
e-mail: mandy.odell@royalberkshire.nhs.uk

N. Mininni, BSN, RN, MEd, CCRN
Nursing Education & Research, UPMC Shadyside,
Pittsburgh, PA, USA
e-mail: mininninc@upmc.edu

D. Goldsmith, RN, PGCert & Dip, MN, PhD
Austin Hospital,
Studley Road, Heidelberg, VIC 3084, Australia
e-mail: donna.goldsmith@austin.org.au

The Nurses' View

There is evidence supporting the notion that nurses and doctors consider the RRS valuable [2–5]. Both published and non-published results of nursing surveys document how much nurses value the response teams, whether they are physician led or nurse led. Nurses recognise that the RRS improves patient outcomes. In a small (n = 248) study conducted at the University of Pittsburgh Medical Center in 2005, 93 % of the responding nurses reported that the medical emergency teams (MET) improved patient care, and 84 % felt that they improved the nursing work environment. Nurses who had called the MET on more than one occasion were more likely to value their ability to call a team (P = 0.002) [3]. In addition, 84 % of nurses felt that it improved their work environment, and 65 % of nurses took the availability of an RRS into consideration when seeking future employment.

Similar positive attitudes towards the MET were found in a major teaching hospital in Australia. A simple survey of 351 ward nurses (51 % of the nursing population at the hospital) was carried out 4 years after the introduction of the MET. The survey determined that 91 % felt that the MET prevented cardiac arrests, and 97 % felt that the team helped manage unwell patients. Only 2 % of the surveyed nurses felt that they would restrict the number of MET calls for fear of being criticised [6]. The key to the success of this team project is thought to be the 1-year preparatory education programme that was undertaken prior to the commencement of the service to ensure that a major 'no-blame' culture change was adopted by all medical, nursing and allied health staff.

In contrast, surveys conducted on the general nursing staff from all 12 of the MERIT study intervention hospitals after both the 4-month implementation period and after the 6-month study period did not show that same unwavering support of the RRS. Importantly, these surveys also showed that there was a significant relationship between this lack of positive attitude and general awareness and understanding of the existence of the MET and the utilisation of the system [7].

The Nurses' Role in RRSs

The key factors required to recognise and manage the deteriorating and critically ill patient involve the bedside nurse recognising the deteriorating patient through vital sign recording and physical assessment, reviewing the patient's progress and reporting when further expert help is needed [8]. This process can be complex with problems occurring at any of the stages. Studies have been undertaken to establish why RRSs are not meeting the expectation to save lives. One phenomenon is identified as failure to rescue, not recognising that a patient is clinically deteriorating and appropriately responding to care for the patient [9]. Historically a number of studies have reported that recognition of the deteriorating patient can be hampered by excessive workloads [10], insufficient education [9], lack of expertise [11] and poor vital sign recording [9–15], as well as failure to report abnormalities to the appropriate healthcare provider or RRS and delayed response [9].

Recognising Deterioration

Observing the patient and recording vital signs have long been an established function of the bedside nurse. As the nurses' role has developed into more complex and medicalised areas, undertaking the patients' observations has become viewed as one of the more mundane tasks of the nurse [16]. The routinisation and 'basic' nature of vital sign recording mean that this key role can sometimes be delegated to the unregistered healthcare assistant or student nurse [10, 15].

As well as recording and interpreting vital signs, physical assessment of the patient is an important factor in identifying the deteriorating patient. The assessment process is regarded by nurses as being more complex [11], consisting of subjective and objective data obtained through the techniques of look, listen, feel and sense [17]. The nurses' role in the assessment process is unclear, and there is a lack of training for nurses beyond vital sign observations [18].

Problems with vital sign recording and failure to recognise the deteriorating patient have helped to drive the implementation of RRSs which, coupled with an increased emphasis on patient safety, has improved vital sign recording at the bedside [19]. However, while it has been difficult to provide empirical evidence that RRSs improve patient outcome [20], later studies have shown that the problem may lie with poor utilisation of the RRT [2, 21–23].

Activation of the RRT

While there has been a marked improvement in vital sign recording and evidence suggesting that nurses value RRSs, there still remains a problem with the activation of the RRT when vital sign thresholds are breached [24]. There is a growing interest in studying the afferent phase of the RRS and exploring the factors that contribute to 'failure to rescue'. Activating an RRT is a highly complex judgement call. Marshall et al. [25] developed a theoretical framework to describe the multitude of factors that may contribute to RRTs not being activated. This includes cognitive aspects: perception, comprehension and projection and sociocultural aspects – personal, professional and contextual [25].

Earlier research has identified that lack of knowledge and skill may have contributed to poor compliance with RRS protocols. Ward nurses who have had sufficient education in RRSs [5], more experience and expertise are more likely to effectively utilise RRSs [26]. One descriptive quantitative design study utilised a 13-multiple-choice questionnaire derived from the European Resuscitation Council Guidelines for Resuscitation 2005 [27]. The questionnaire was distributed to 150 randomly selected nurses working on a general medical or surgical unit. The results of the study identified that nurses who graduated from a 4-year education programme identified clinical situations and RRS activation at a significantly higher rate than nurses with a 2-year education. This study examines one facet of why and when RRS activation may occur. In contrast, Astroth et al. [28] found that senior nurses may believe that an RRT is more beneficial for inexperienced nurses and senior nurses are reluctant to activate an RRT, failing to model the desired behaviour that supports safe patient care [28]. However studies are now reporting that more complex sociocultural effects are influencing the effectiveness of RRSs.

Unit cultures and RRTs that support teamwork and willingness to care for each other's patients increase staff confidence in activating a RRT. Nurses that have experienced positive interactions with RRT activation have reported that the ICU nurse responders validated their concerns for the patient and offered their expertise and mentoring. Unit leadership, senior nurse modelling and RRT responder behaviour impact the utilisation of RRTs [27]. These findings are supported by Jones et al. [26] literature review that found responses and behaviours of the responding team can have a damaging or beneficial effect on the staff calling the team. Belittling comments, criticism and poor communication by the expert team can all negatively affect the nurses' future engagement with the RRS process [26].

Clinical staff do not necessarily follow protocols but can act on local sociocultural factors and

be influenced by professional hierarchies [21]. One of the main reasons for not activating the RRT was that the ward teams felt that they could manage the patient themselves or that activation was delayed while further tests and reviews were being carried out [21]. In addition nurses are concerned about an increase in their workload when they activate the RRT and are more likely to adhere to traditional medical cultural influences and call the patients' treating physician before the RRT [23].

Improving the Nurses' View of RRSs

Overcoming traditional hierarchical models of care can take considerably more time than we currently expect; as the vast majority of RRT activation is made by nurses, we must continue to change hospital culture in order to properly utilise and embed RRT programmes in support of a robust patient safety culture. For a successful RRS, hospital environments need to support frontline staff to call, call early and that no call is a bad call. It is not as simple as more education, better communication and policy development, but in exploring the cultural barriers to activating an RRT.

Physicians can potentially help or hinder implementation of the system, and nursing staff need to be supported in their decisions to activate the RRS within a safe reporting structure. Collaborative practice relationships need to be developed between the RRT and ward teams.

Communication is an essential component of a successful RRS. Staff nurses interact with physicians every day. During a crisis, communication patterns may change in a way that can render it ineffective. Communication and hierarchy may be challenged and result in poor transmission of important facts to key personnel who are making the decisions. The five 'Es' of successful RRSs have been described as education, empowerment, efficiency, equipment and evaluation [29]. Maintaining and sustaining activation of the RRS require ongoing communication to maintain awareness, and other in-patient units such as radiology and physical therapy will have special education needs.

The use of early warning scores or electronic warning systems may be an answer to early activation of RRS. Early warning scores have been standardised across the United Kingdom [30], and many other institutions have made changes to RRT activation criteria based on early warning scores. Early warning scores raise healthcare providers' attention to subtle changes in condition, serve as a common language surrounding a patient assessment and support staff making the decision to activate the RRT [31, 32].

Summary

Recognising patient deterioration and activating the RRT is a highly complex process. It involves communication, empowerment, education and knowledge within a culture that challenges traditional hospital hierarchies and cultures with a commitment to patient safety. We need to learn more about the afferent process of the RRS and build on what we are starting to learn about the factors that inhibit and encourage implementation and engagement with the rapid response concept. The efferent limb of the RRS cannot be successful unless bedside nurses are supported and empowered to take on this new responsibility.

References

1. Devita MA, Bellomo R, Hillman K, Kellum J, Rotondi A, Teres D, Auerbach A, Chen WJ, Duncan K, Kenward G, Bell M, Buist M, Chen J, Bion J, Kirby A, Lighthall G, Ovreveit J, Braithwaite RS, Gosbee J, Milbrandt E, Peberdy M, Savitz L, Young L, Galhotra S. Findings of the first consensus conference on medical emergency teams. Crit Care Med. 2006;34(9):2463–78.
2. Andrews T, Waterman H. Packaging: a grounded theory of how to report physiological deterioration effectively. J Adv Nurs. 2005;52(5):473–81.
3. Jones D, Baldwin I, McIntyre T, Story D, Mercer I, Miglic A, Goldsmith D, Bellomo R. Nurses attitudes to a medical emergency team service in a teaching hospital. Qual Saf Health Care. 2006;15(6):427–32.
4. Sarani B, Sonnad S, Bergey MR, Phillips J, Fitzpatrick MK, Chalian AA, Myers JS. Resident and RN perceptions of the impact of a medical emergency team on education and patient safety in an academic medical center. Crit Care Med. 2009;37(12):3091–6.
5. Radeschi G, Urso F, Campagna S, Berchialla P, Borga S, Mina A, Penso R, di Pietrantonj C, Sandroni C. Factors affecting attitudes and barriers to a medical emergency team among nurses and medical doctors: a multi-centre survey. Resuscitation. 2015;88:92–8.
6. Cretikos MA, Chen J, Hillman KM, Bellomo R, Finfar SR, Flabouris A. The effectiveness of implementation of the medical emergency team (MET) system and factors associated with use during the MERIT study. Crit Care Resusc. 2007;9(2):206–12.
7. Scott SA, Elliott S. Implementation of a rapid response team: a success story. Crit Care Nurse. 2009;29(3):66–76.
8. Odell M, Victor C, Oliver D. Nurses' role in detecting deteriorating ward patients: systematic literature review. J Adv Nurs. 2009;65(10):1992–2006.
9. Subbe CP, Welch JR. Failure to rescue: using rapid response systems to improve care of the deteriorating patient in hospital. Clin Risk. 2013;19:6–11. doi:10.1177/1356262213486451.
10. Hogan J. Respiratory assessment: why don't nurses monitor the respiratory rates of patients? Br J Nurs. 2006;15(9):489–92.
11. Cox H, James J, Hunt J. The experiences of trained nurses caring for critically ill patients within a general ward setting. Intensive Crit Care Nurs. 2006;22(5):283–93.
12. Chellel A, Fraser J, Fender V, et al. Nursing observations on ward patients at risk of critical illness. Nurs Times. 2002;98(46):36–9.
13. McBride J, Knight D, Pipe J, Smith GB. Long-term effect of introducing an early warning score on respiratory rate charting on general wards. Resuscitation. 2005;65:41–4.
14. Nurmi J, Harjola VP, Nolan J, Castren M. Observations and warning signs prior to cardiac arrest. Should a medical emergency team intervene earlier? Acta Anaesthesiol Scand. 2005;49:702–6.
15. Wheatley I. The nursing practice of taking level 1 patient observations. Intensive Crit Care Nurs. 2006;22(2):115–21.
16. Kenward G, Hodgetts T, Castle N. Time to put the R back in TPR. Nurs Times. 2001;97(4):32–3.
17. Cioffi J. Recognition of patients who require emergency assistance: a descriptive study. Heart Lung. 2000;29(4):262–8.
18. Cutler LR. From ward based critical care to educational curriculum 2: a focussed ethnographic case study. Intensive Crit Care Nurs. 2002;18(5):280–91.
19. Odell M, Rechner IJ, Kapila A, Even T, Oliver D, Davies CWH, Milsom L, Forster A, Rudman K. The effect of a critical care outreach service and early warning scoring system on respiratory rate recording on the general wards. Resuscitation. 2007;74:470–5.
20. Hillman KM, Chen J, Cretikos M, Bellomo R, Brown R, Doig G, Finfar S, Flabouris A. Introduction of the medical emergency team (MET) system: a cluster randomised controlled trial. Lancet. 2005;365(9477):2091–7.

21. Shearer B, Marshall S, Buist MD, Finnigan M, Kitto S, Hore T, Sturgess T, Wilson S, Ramsay W. What stops hospital clinical staff from following protocols? An analysis of the incidence and factors behind the failure of bedside clinical staff to activate the rapid response system in a multi-campus Australian metropolitan healthcare service. BMJ Qual Saf. 2012;21(7): 569–74.

22. National Patient Safety Agency. Recognising and responding appropriately to early signs of deterioration in hospital patients. London: NPSA; 2007.

23. Donohue LA, Endacott R. Track, trigger and teamwork: communication of deterioration in acute medical and surgical wards. *Intensive Crit Care Nurs*. 2010;26:10–7.

24. Hands C, Reid E, Meredith P, Smith GB, Prytherch DR, Schmidt PE, Featherstone PI. Patterns in the recording of vital signs and early warning scores: compliance with a clinical escalation protocol. BMJ Qual Saf. 2013;22:719–26.

25. Marshall SD, Kitto S, Shearer W, Wilson SJ, Finnigan MA, Sturgess T, Hore T, Buist MD. Why don't hospital staff activate the rapid response system (RRS)? How frequently is it needed and can process be improved? Implement Sci. 2011;6(39). http://www.implemntationscience.com/conyent/6/1/39.

26. Jones L, King L, Wilson C. A literature review: factors that impact on nurses' effective use of the Medical Emergency Team (MET). J Clin Nurs. 2009;18: 3379–90.

27. Pantazopoulos I, Tsoni A, Kouskouni E, Papadimitriou LO, Johnson E, Xanthos T. Factors influencing nurses' decisions to activate medical emergency teams. J Clin Nurs. 2012;21:2668–78.

28. Astroth KS, Woith WM, Stapleton SJ, Kegitz RJ, Jenkins SH. Qualitative exploration of nurses' decisions to activate rapid response teams. J Clin Nurs. 2013;22:2876–82.

29. Scholle CC, Mininni NC. Best-practice interventions: how a rapid response team saves lives. Nursing. 2006;36(1):36–40.

30. Royal College of Physicians. National Early Warning Score (NEWS): standardising the assessment of acute-illness severity in the NHS. Report of a working party. London: Royal College of Physicians; 2012.

31. Race T. Improving patient safety with a modified early warning scoring system. *American Nurse Today*. 2015;10(11). DA, DeVita MA, Bellomo MD. Rapid-Response Teams. N Engl J Med. 2011;365(2): 139–146.

32. Duncan KD, McMullan C, Mills BM. Early warning systems. Nursing. 2012;42(2):38–44.

Geoffrey K. Lighthall

Introduction

An increased focus on patient safety on the part of regulatory and accreditation agencies has led to a host of reforms aimed at improving patient welfare. Rapid response systems (RRS) have emerged at the same time as resident work hour restrictions have come into effect, public awareness of medical error has increased, and new models of residency program accreditation have been instituted [1, 2]. Initially, rapid response teams were perceived as a threat to the time-honored traditions of learning through experience and to the consummate professional who participates in all aspects of patient care. In the past ten years, however, work hour limitations have created huge disruptions in typical patient care workflow and have created a greater reliance on shift work and patient handoffs—a class of events believed to be associated with risks of their own [3, 4]. In this context of greater fragmentation of care, the demand for the safety net provided by rapid response systems has helped solidify their niche in the care of hospitalized patients. One can also imagine some conceptual synergy between the missions of general RRS

G.K. Lighthall, PhD, MD (✉)
Department of Anesthesia, Stanford University
School of Medicine, Palo Alto, CA 94305, USA
e-mail: geoffL@stanford.edu

teams and specialized teams for sepsis, pulmonary embolism, myocardial infarction, and so forth. While numerous other challenges abound for those involved in resident education, the question to be dealt with here is whether the implementation of rapid response systems—a classically patient centered-intervention—interferes with medical education or whether there are ways in which medical education can be enhanced through the existence of such a system.

Origins of Rapid Response Systems: A Solution to a Real Problem

Studies of antecedents to cardiac arrest demonstrated that between 75 and 85 % of the affected patients had some form of deterioration in the hours prior to the arrest [5, 6]. Nearly a third of such abnormalities persisted for greater than 24 h prior to arrest, with a population mean of 6.5 h [5]. In one series, the vast majority (76 %) of the disease processes eventually progressing to cardiac arrest were not considered to be intrinsically rapidly fatal. [6] In another series over half of the arrests presented with ample warning signs of decompensation; the majority had uncorrected hypotension, and half of these had systolic blood pressures less than 80 mm Hg for more than 24 h [7]. Other patients in this series had severe, but correctable, abnormalities such as hypokalemia, hypoglycemia, and hypoxemia. Problems with establishing proper care were found to exist at multiple levels: nurses were not calling physicians for patients with abnormal vital signs or changes in sensorium; physicians did not fully evaluate abnormalities when they were contacted; ICU consultants were not called in routinely, and even senior level or consulting ICU caregivers did not obtain routine laboratory studies that would have defined the patient's problem. In cases when laboratory studies were done, they were not always interpreted correctly, and when they were, therapy was not always initiated [8].

Studies evaluating patterns of ward care prior to ICU admission show a similar lack of time urgency in evaluating and treating patients with abnormal vital signs and other forms of deterioration [5, 9, 10]. Patients initially admitted to hospital wards (as opposed to ICU) had up to a fourfold increase risk of mortality, suggesting that the nature of the care was a more significant determinant of ultimate clinical trajectory than the admitting diagnosis [10]. Areas considered problematic were delays in admission and improper attention to oxygen therapy, airway, breathing, circulation, and monitoring. Reasons underlying suboptimal care were "failure of organization, lack of knowledge, failure to appreciate clinical urgency, lack of experience, supervision, and failure to seek advice." Our own experience in examining dynamic decision-making of house staff in a fully simulated ICU revealed similar classes of deficiencies, including nonadherence to established protocols [11].

All of the aforementioned studies were conducted in academic centers where junior team members are traditionally called to evaluate a patient and then there is a graded engagement of more senior staff members. Loss of valuable time in patient evaluation and stabilization may have been further compounded by attending staff that lack knowledge of seriously ill patients and their problems and who lacked the skills to direct an appropriate resuscitation [12, 13]. As noted previously, teaching hospitals have increased their reliance on cross coverage schemes, which too have been associated with an increased incidence of potentially preventable adverse events [4].

Goals of RRS Care

Therapeutic efficacy in many disease processes such as myocardial infarction, sepsis, traumatic injury, and pulmonary embolism is time critical. The goal of a rapid responses system is to promptly identify clinical deterioration in applicable patients and institute corrective action as rapidly as possible. Likewise, identification of patients for whom comfort care is most appropriate and providing this care is a typically unmet need that can be facilitated by an RRS [14]. Implicit in the creation of an RRS is that it can deliver important care in a manner that improves outcomes—either hard outcomes such as saving of lives and costs or surrogates for quality of care such as more timely institution of therapy. While the goals of rapid response systems seem to answer the majority of concerns related to suboptimal patient care, the efficacy is greatest in single-center interventions and less encouraging when targeted to multiple centers [15, 16]. A number of team compositions and leadership models have been utilized, and none has emerged as the definitive design [17–19], [20]. Thus, the MET is not like penicillin or balloon angioplasty or other interventions whose benefits are so robust that they can be reproduced in nearly any environment. Rather the benefits are tied to the interest and passions of those involved and their ability to effect change throughout complex organizations. I believe the latter needs to be kept in mind when considering the impacts of an RRS on medical education. Some benefits may be derived through passive diffusion, but the highest yield will come from situations where educational goals are intentionally designed into care delivery and other elements of the system [21]. Below I will list a number of patient care issues that have been highlighted through the development of rapid response systems. The topics include some that represent a general knowledge base and that can built into reading lists and case conferences and others that can be incorporated into patient care and research activities.

Educational Goals Related to Rapid Response Systems

Recognizing the Deteriorating Patient

For over five or more years, the majority of residents will have begun training in hospitals with an RRS already in place. However, understanding the origins of the RRS remains a valuable area of knowledge, as it is likely to promot e a deeper understanding of the epidem iology of patient deterioration and the development of critical illness. The ability to describe the normal course of therapy and to detect deviations from this course is a crucial area of discussion between physicians and nurses and one that can be informed by formal readings and discussions of the medical literature and of individual cases. Junior residents in particular can be a bit myopic in their care of patients, so having some sense of how an individual's vital sign changes signify higher risks is of great value. The predictive nature of individual vital signs and composite warning scores is an area of active research whose intellectual background is tied to development and optimization of rapid response systems [22, 23]. Results from prior and ongoing studies deserve attention as tools that potentially improve clinical decision-making.

Related to this topic is the question of why rapid response systems fail to work. A number of studies have demonstrated the impact of late MET calls or persistence of MET criteria for 24 h prior to critical events (afferent limb failure) [24–29]. Understanding that there are differences in outcomes depending on the interval between objective signs of instability and action should be part of the discussion as to how to derive the greatest benefit from the system and should help create support for greater time accountability of first responders [17]. A study in the emergency medicine literature suggested that MET calls within 24 h of ward admission may serve as a marker for mis-triage and should be investigated as part of quality improvement efforts in the field [30]. Accountability for transfer decisions within a hospital is an equally important area of feedback.

Care of the Deteriorating Patient

There is plenty of flexibility in RRS design, with some, but not all, containing junior trainees. In a few institutions, the primary team acts as the RRT; first the intern is summoned, and if the patient fails to stabilize within 30 min, the rules call for summoning the senior resident and then the attending [17]. Other more common varieties of RRTs include nurse-led RN + RT teams and full-blown ICU outreach teams led by either fellows or attendings. Some teams include the ICU resident, and others have used a senior ward resident. There is no evidence suggesting the superiority of one design over another in terms of clinical outcomes; however, the educational benefit for members is likely to be greatest in situations where more senior members of the same profession (RN or MD) are involved. If adequately staffed with attending- or fellow-level staff, there should be plenty of room for resident involvement. I am of the belief that junior-level trainees should be challenged with synthesizing the available information and committing to decisions, regardless of whether they are in charge of a team and ultimately responsible. This way, analytic and decision-making processes are still actively engaged, and these judgments are still evaluated and critiqued, but they are not allowed to harm patients if not correct. Thus active participation can exist without allowing the "learning from mistakes."

Additionally, the common denominator of nearly all rapid response systems in academic centers is a concurrent summons of the primary ward team [31–33]. From a training perspective, having the primary team work with the RRS not only maintains their exposure to interesting cases and their proper management but also respects the fact that the best solutions to patient problems involve sharing of information and establishing consensus regarding appropriate goals of care. Cross discipline training is also achieved when trainees from one discipline (medicine, anesthesiology) are called for care for patients admitted to other disciplines.

Despite a great deal of resistance during the initial phase of MET operation, resident acceptance

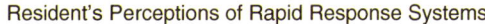

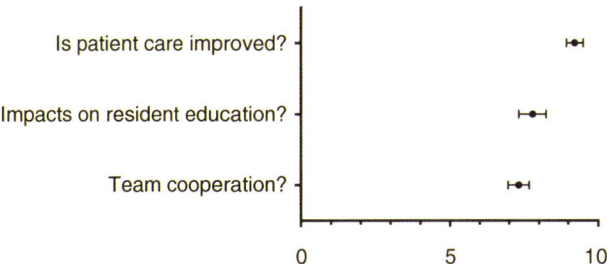

Fig. 31.1 Residents' perceptions of the impact of rapid response systems. Mean responses ± SE are shown for a confidential web-based survey of internal medicine residents. Residents were asked a series of questions including (1) whether they thought RRSs improved patient care, (2) whether the RRS had an adverse or positive impact on their education, and (3) to estimate the level of coopera-tion between the MET and the primary team. Survey questions were anchored to a 1–10 scale where 1 represented the lowest or most negative response, 5 was listed as neutral, and 10 was the most positive or highest level of agreement. Twenty surveys were completed, representing a response rate of 33 %

of its rationale and educational benefit has been surprisingly high (see Fig. 31.1 below). Two other centers have performed more extensive surveys of their residents and have found that while the RRS has an acknowledge benefit of improving patient safety, it has not interfered with resident autonomy and fulfillment of educational needs [34]. A two-phase survey conducted by Stevens and colleagues found that 5 years after implementation of an RRS, residents felt more comfortable obtaining senior help and less concerned over autonomy [35]. Interestingly, interns reported greater confidence in their abilities, suggesting a confidence/competence gap that in some ways reflects the mind-set that led to the development of rapid response systems. Reported levels of cooperation between the primary teams and the MET have been equally encouraging, and in fact, the best relationship between the entities is one where the primary team is engaged in patient care and recognizes the need for additional resources, so calls the RRT. In these cases, the RRT does not necessarily take over the care, but augments ongoing efforts.

Rapid response teams can derive a number of benefits from having a critical care perspective; first and foremost is an understanding of what types of patients and conditions truly benefit from intensive care. This perspective can help inform discussions regarding the advisability of aggressive care and, when appropriate, can facili-tate its initiation in the most efficient manner. Outside of the ER or ICU, a resident is not likely to gain much experience with the rapid evaluation and stabilization of deteriorating patients. Likewise, in contrast to most ICU physicians, many ward attendings are not comfortable with invasive procedures. Therefore, if a patient's condition requires immediate IV access, titration of vasoactive medications, and estimations of fluid status, care is much more likely to be accomplished with an ICU-based team leader. Worldwide, delays of several hours prior to ICU admission are often seen. Patients will likely benefit from a philosophy assuring that intensive care can begin outside of the ICU if needed. Our RRT was developed with the recognition that critically ill patients deserve intensive care regardless of location, so we are configured in personnel and materials to provide invasive pressure monitoring, real-time display of ECG, pulse oximetry, and CO_2 waveforms and the ability to perform point-of-care ultrasonography and blood analysis in any location. Fluids, antibiotics, and vasoactive medications are brought by pharmacists for immediate use. The use of these capabilities serves the additional purpose of engaging the team in rapid analytic and therapeutic decision-making and can provide a robust educational experience for all involved. Residents of all training levels can be involved in a level commensurate with their skills and experience and patient acuity and can certainly learn from seeing more experienced personnel in action.

While much can be said about the different team designs, the important factor is that the literature supports great flexibility in this area. Those departments most concerned about resident education should increase their involvement in the activities and administration of the system to assure that it is shaped according to their needs.

The Value of System Improvement

While the overall intent of an RRS is to provide immediate service to patients in need, its leadership should engage in data collection and periodic examination of system functions including:

- The afferent limb: Calling criteria and education and behaviors related to summoning of help. What are the calling trends? Are certain units calling less? Why? Do nurses feel empowered to call for help when they are simply worried about a patient? Are doctors telling nurses to not call the team? Why?
- Epidemiology: What is the nature of the calls? Are there certain disease processes that are more prevalent in the hospital? Are calling criteria properly aligned with patient needs?
- Monitoring: Are current monitoring practices capable of detecting early deterioration? If not, what modalities may improve detection?
- Education: Do nurses feel like they understand when to call an alert? Do residents feel they are learning during team activations?
- Triage: Do call patterns suggest problems in the patient triage process? How are triage decisions being made?

Needless to say, the RRS is full of opportunities to perform research on the nature and outcome of deteriorating patients. Additionally, the fullest educational yield will be gained by analysis that is directed to not only specific high-yield cases, but also to the general issues of patient safety and care.

Data from cardiac arrests, ICU admissions, quality assurance projects, and disease-specific treatments can be analyzed to understand patient care characteristics and gaps that need to be filled. When possible the RRT should conduct a post-event debriefing—immediately after the event being best. A number of issues typically come up: first, it is important to understand why or why not detection processes functioned as designed and whether there were any other early signs of compromise. In terms of team function, diagnostic impressions, immediate actions, and therapeutic options are always rich areas of discussion. Team leadership, communication, and other dynamics are of high importance as well. The need for teamwork will have a greater presence in emergency care than the care of more routine patients. If an event brings up general care or system issues, review at morning report time or as case conferences can expand the educational yield [36].

Error analysis can provide important insight into whether improvements need to be made in technical training, teamwork, or organizational structure [37, 38]. The overall handling and discussion of errors and "near misses" likely to increase the extent of error reporting if done in a nonjudgmental manner. A system that is nonpunitive and that rewards admission of mistakes creates a healthy climate where there is a greater likelihood of identifying and correcting "latent" sources of future errors [37]. Residents exposed to this "culture of safety" may let this philosophy shape behavior and improve patient care in other settings.

Simulation-based training is a well-accepted modality in nearly all hospital-based residencies. Our analysis of RRT case mix has led to training that captures highly prevalent emergency situations such as sepsis, opiate overdose, mental status change, myocardial ischemia, and mental status change. Internal medicine interns who will continue as categorical residents are put through this course at the conclusion of their first year as an indoctrination to the responsibilities they will soon face as senior residents and team leaders. This curriculum and course (the *SCARED* course—Stanford Course on Active Resuscitation, Evaluation and Decision-making) provides both guidance on how to manage critical events and teams, but also provides direction on the rapid response and provides necessary resources for caring for unstable patients.

The Value of Follow-Up

With fragmentation of health care into clinic, ward, and critical care domains, it is easy to neglect the educational value of following patients through different episodes of care. Many residents may not recognize the difference between those that benefit from intensive care and those for whom ICU admission is an entry point to end of life care. Regardless of rapid response design, insightful follow-up of patients is necessary to truly understand the evolution and natural history of different disease processes. Academic departments have the ability to create expectations regarding patient follow through and incorporate these into their work ethic. Likewise, it is important for residents to convey information regarding a patient's course to nurses and others who cared for the patient; the latter provides important feedback that improves the medical knowledge and judgment of other care providers.

Why Change?

The authors of this textbook have serious doubts concerning the efficacy of the current apprentice mode of residency training to provide the highest quality of care for all patient encounters without the engagement of more senior staff in the management and supervision of care. If it were truly reliable, appropriate feedbacks would be in place and assure that delays in care would be minimized over time and that outcomes would be improved. This clearly is not the case. Instead, the status quo functions under the assumption that each trainee has an unwritten right to work through the management of severe medical problems on his or her own. Unfortunately, management of these illnesses is time sensitive, and the process of unsupervised discovery and learning compromises patient outcome. More and more,

educators are recognizing that having experts on hand to recognize and correct errors facilitates competence and learning to a greater extent than allowing unrecognized errors to play out [39]. A recent report by the US Institute of Medicine calls for increased level of trainee supervision as a necessary measure to improve patient safety [40].

With advancing medical specialization, one frequently sees interdepartmental cooperation at the bedside, where the caregiving team is happy to acquiesce significant portions of a patient's management to the cardiologist, nephrologist, surgeon, or oncologist. Indeed, the latter specialties possess certain types of technology, protocols, and detailed knowledge of pathophysiology that can be pivotal to the optimal management and survival of a patient. In the context of specific organ-based derangements, it is rational to seek this type of support, and most do so willingly without questioning the loss of educational benefit. In fact, most specialty services offer trainee rotations knowing that they carry great educational value that is maximized by interaction with experts in the field. The RRS is an analogous attempt on the part of critical care community to educate others to the presence of critical illness outside of the ICU and to bring the necessary resources to the patient at a time when he or she is likely to benefit [41]. Additionally, there are patients with illnesses that are not likely to respond to intensive care; receiving the input of critical care professionals has allowed many to institute comfort measures with greater confidence.

The Larger Landscape of Medical Education

Many of the changes in health-care delivery associated with medical emergency teams are likely to facilitate the assimilation and assessment of competencies now required in the US Accreditation Council of Graduate Medical Education (ACGME) and the American Board of Medical Specialties. As part of the Outcomes Project, residency review committees of the ACGME have required programs to develop methods for residents to attain and document competency in six different areas: [1]

- Patient care
- Medical knowledge
- Practice-based learning and improvement
- Interpersonal and communication skills
- Professionalism
- System-based practice

Further developments mandated that medical specialty boards identify specific training milestones and that residency programs track competency in these areas at different levels of training. Accordingly, residencies may need to pay more deliberate attention to creating training experiences that can achieve specific competencies. Based on the discussion above, one can envision how resident involvement in rapid response systems can facilitate key areas of resident training, including the development of skills in the management of unstable patients, team leadership, and understanding the connection between team activities and the broader epidemiology of patient deterioration in general.

Summary

Rapid response systems provide a rich opportunity for learning and practicing acute care skills while improving patient care. Senior resident and attending leadership assures that patient care decisions are made in a timely manner and based on higher levels of experience and training while providing adequate mentorship and guidance to lower level trainees. Rapid response systems also provide outstanding opportunities for detailed analysis of patient deterioration and methods that may improve its detection. It is important to note that the RRS is not a panacea. Avoidable cardiac arrests and late calls continue to exist in even the most seasoned efforts [24, 29], so the need to understand and improve systems is a constant need. Interestingly, while systems have ample opportunities for resident education on multiple fronts, the presence of these activities may help strengthen the overall success of a rapid response system.

References

1. Accreditation Council for Graduate Medical Education, Outcome Project. http://www.acgme.org/outcome/. Accessed 2 Oct 2009.
2. Institute of Medicine, Corrigan JM, Kohn LT, Donaldson MS. To err is human—building a safer health system. Washington DC.: National Academy Press; 2000.
3. Cook RI, Render M, Woods DD. Gaps in the continuity of care and progress on patient safety. BMJ. 2000;320(7237):791–4.
4. Petersen LA et al. Does housestaff discontinuity of care increase the risk for preventable adverse events? Ann Intern Med. 1994;121(11):866–72.
5. Buist MD et al. Recognising clinical instability in hospital patients before cardiac arrest or unplanned admission to intensive care. A pilot study in a tertiary-care hospital. Med J Aust. 1999;171(1):22–5.
6. Schein RM et al. Clinical antecedents to in-hospital cardiopulmonary arrest. Chest. 1990;98(6):1388–92.
7. McGloin H, Adam SK, Singer M. Unexpected deaths and referrals to intensive care of patients on general wards. Are some cases potentially avoidable? J R Coll Physicians Lond. 1999;33(3):255–9.
8. Franklin C, Mathew J. Developing strategies to prevent inhospital cardiac arrest: analyzing responses of physicians and nurses in the hours before the event. Crit Care Med. 1994;22(2):244–7.
9. Franklin CM et al. Decreases in mortality on a large urban medical service by facilitating access to critical care. An alternative to rationing. Arch Intern Med. 1988;148(6):1403–5.
10. Sax FL, Charlson ME. Medical patients at high risk for catastrophic deterioration. Crit Care Med. 1987;15(5):510–5.
11. Lighthall GK et al. Use of a fully simulated intensive care unit environment for critical event management training for internal medicine residents. Crit Care Med. 2003;31(10):2437–43.
12. Hillman KM et al. Duration of life-threatening antecedents prior to intensive care admission. Intensive Care Med. 2002;28(11):1629–34.
13. McQuillan P et al. Confidential inquiry into quality of care before admission to intensive care. BMJ. 1998;316(7148):1853–8.
14. Vazquez R et al. Enhanced end-of-life care associated with deploying a rapid response team: a pilot study. J Hosp Med. 2009;4(7):449–52.
15. Hillman K et al. Introduction of the medical emergency team (MET) system: a cluster-randomised controlled trial. Lancet. 2005;365(9477):2091–7.
16. Chan PS et al. Rapid response teams: a systematic review and meta-analysis. Arch Intern Med. 2010;170(1):18–26.
17. Howell MD et al. Sustained effectiveness of a primary-team-based rapid response system. Crit Care Med. 2012;40(9):2562–8.

18. Lighthall GK, Mayette M, Harrison TK. An institutionwide approach to redesigning management of cardiopulmonary resuscitation. Jt Comm J Qual Patient Saf. 2013;39(4):157–66.

19. Sebat F et al. A multidisciplinary community hospital program for early and rapid resuscitation of shock in nontrauma patients. Chest. 2005;127(5):1729–43.

20. Benson L et al. Using an advanced practice nursing model for a rapid response team. Jt Comm J Qual Patient Saf. 2008;34(12):743–7.

21. Devita MA et al. Findings of the first consensus conference on medical emergency teams. Crit Care Med. 2006;34(9):2463–78.

22. Lighthall GK, Markar S, Hsiung R. Abnormal vital signs are associated with an increased risk for critical events in US veteran inpatients. Resuscitation. 2009;80(11):1264–9.

23. Smith GB et al. The ability of the National Early Warning Score (NEWS) to discriminate patients at risk of early cardiac arrest, unanticipated intensive care unit admission, and death. Resuscitation. 2013; 84(4):465–70.

24. Galhotra S et al. Mature rapid response system and potentially avoidable cardiopulmonary arrests in hospital. Qual Saf Health Care. 2007;16(4):260–5.

25. Azzopardi P et al. Attitudes and barriers to a medical emergency team system at a tertiary paediatric hospital. Resuscitation. 2011;82(2):167–74.

26. Trinkle RM, Flabouris A. Documenting rapid response system afferent limb failure and associated patient outcomes. Resuscitation. 2011;82(7):810–4.

27. Boniatti MM et al. Delayed medical emergency team calls and associated outcomes. Crit Care Med. 2014; 42(1):26–30.

28. Calzavacca P et al. Features and outcome of patients receiving multiple medical emergency team reviews. Resuscitation. 2010;81(11):1509–15.

29. Downey AW et al. Characteristics and outcomes of patients receiving a medical emergency team review for acute change in conscious state or arrhythmias. Crit Care Med. 2008;36(2):477–81.

30. Lovett PB et al. Rapid response team activations within 24 hours of admission from the emergency department: an innovative approach for performance improvement. Acad Emerg Med. 2014;21(6):667–72.

31. Bellomo R et al. A prospective before-and-after trial of a medical emergency team. Med J Aust. 2003;179(6):283–7.

32. Bristow PJ et al. Rates of in-hospital arrests, deaths and intensive care admissions: the effect of a medical emergency team. Med J Aust. 2000;173(5):236–40.

33. Goldhill DR, White SA, Sumner A. Physiological values and procedures in the 24 h before ICU admission from the ward. Anaesthesia. 1999;54(6):529–34.

34. Sarani B et al. Resident and RN perceptions of the impact of a medical emergency team on education and patient safety in an academic medical center. Crit Care Med. 2009;37(12):3091–6.

35. Stevens J et al. Long-term culture change related to rapid response system implementation. Med Educ. 2014;48(12):1211–9.

36. Mullan PC, Kessler DO, Cheng A. Educational opportunities with postevent debriefing. JAMA. 2014; 312(22):2333–4.

37. Helmreich RL. On error management: lessons from aviation. BMJ. 2000;320(7237):781–5.

38. Braithwaite RS et al. Use of medical emergency team (MET) responses to detect medical errors. Qual Saf Health Care. 2004;13(4):255–9.

39. Wu AW et al. Do house officers learn from their mistakes? JAMA. 1991;265(16):2089–94.

40. Committee of optimizing graduate medical trainee hours and work schedules to improve patient safety. Resident duty hours, enhancing sleep supervision and safety. Washington D.C.: The National Academies Press; 2008.

41. Hillman K. Critical care without walls. Curr Opin Crit Care. 2002;8(6):594–9.

Optimizing RRSs Through Simulation

32

Melinda Fiedor Hamilton, Elizabeth A. Hunt, and Michael A. DeVita

Introduction

In 2003, a report by the National Registry of Cardiopulmonary Resuscitation (NRCPR) of 207 hospitals within the USA revealed that the majority (86 %) had an organized team to respond to in-hospital cardiac arrests (IHCA), and more recently, a survey of 1000 hospitals from the

M.F. Hamilton, MD, MSc, FAHA (✉)
Department of Critical Care Medicine, University of Pittsburgh Medical Center Director, Pediatric Simulation, Peter M. Winter Institute for Simulation, Education, and Research (WISER), Pittsburgh, PA, USA

Children's Hospital of Pittsburgh Simulation Center, Pittsburgh, PA, USA
e-mail: fiedml@ccm.upmc.edu

E.A. Hunt
Department of Anesthesiology and Critical Care Medicine, The Johns Hopkins University School of Medicine, 600 N. Wolfe Street, Sheikh Zayed Tower, Baltimore, MD 21287, USA

M.A. DeVita, MD, FCCM, FRCP
Department of Surgery, Critical Care, Harlem Hospital Cente, 506 Lenox Avenue, New York, NY 10037, USA

Department of Internal Medicine, Critical Care, Harlem Hospital Center, 506 Lenox Avenue, New York, NY 10037, USA
e-mail: michael.devita@NYCHHC.ORG

American Hospital Association show growth in this practice, with 91 % of respondent hospitals using an organized team to respond to hospital resuscitations [1, 2]. In addition to the existence of these teams, a significant trend in the use of simulation for team training has been reported. The Edelson study cited 62 % of respondent hospitals utilized routine-simulated resuscitation training and 34 % utilized routine cardiac arrest case reviews with debriefing. Mundell et al., via a systematic review and meta-analysis of 182 included studies, report that simulation-based training, in comparison with no intervention, is effective regardless of outcome, level of learner, study design, or specific task trained [3]. Despite the increased number of organized team responses and specialized team training, in-hospital cardiac arrest continues to result in poor patient outcomes. Recent reviews reveal approximately 200,000 adult in-hospital cardiac arrests annually, with an overall survival of only 18–20 % [4]. Emphasis on earlier recognition of patient deterioration, quality of resuscitation, and post-resuscitative care continues, and rapid response systems (RRS) are integral to these continued efforts to improved IHCA outcomes.

Though the majority of hospitals utilize the RRS concept, there is variation in team composition, number of team members, and method of dispatch. The need for training of these teams, however, remains a constant and is quite essential to enhance the quality of care delivered. The principles of team training may be applied across the spectrum of variation and are reviewed in this chapter.

The word "team" typically refers to a group of people that work together on a regular basis, in a coordinated and coherent fashion. Professional athletic teams provide an example of how a classic team functions: team members all have a *common goal* of winning their athletic events; they *practice together* regularly; individuals typically have one *designated role* or position that they play, and in which they become a true expert; team members often develop some type of shorthand to aid in *communication*; and the team typically functions best with a good *team leader* or captain. All of these elements apply to RRS teams.

Unique Aspects of Hospital Crisis Teams

Hospital crisis teams serve a critical purpose: to prevent further deterioration and death in suddenly critically ill patients usually outside critical care areas. To succeed, they must act quickly and correctly. Success improves with effective and efficient function. Delays in action, miscommunication, and errors can increase the likelihood of a fatal outcome for the patient. Such a critical function should be the target of frequent and effective training programs, but, ironically, the training of crisis teams is particularly difficult because of the dynamic nature of the teams. In many ways, crisis teams represent the antithesis of the well-trained athletic team and must overcome major barriers to function effectively.

The Ad Hoc Nature of Crisis Teams

Code teams are usually ad hoc teams—they consist of people who are brought together in a crisis, although they may never have worked together previously. Once the crisis is over, they return to their other patient care activities and may not work together again. It seems impossible to train all of the possible combinations of a code team. A study by Pittman et al. of a cardiac arrest team revealed that 67 % of team leaders had had no communication with the team members prior to the cardiac arrest event, 33 % had "informal" communication prior, and only 7 % had a debriefing session after the cardiac arrest [5]. Unlike the professional athletic team, where the sport is the everyday "job," for crisis teams responding to arresting or deteriorating patients, the crisis is not, and responding to these events is a small fraction of their workload.

The ad hoc nature of crisis teams makes it more difficult to practice communication, organization, group problem-solving, and the integrated functioning skills necessary for teamwork. The difference between a team that practices until they function like a well-oiled machine and the team whose members have literally never met becomes obvious when video recordings of crisis events are reviewed. Crisis team training programs must directly address the fact that the team that assembles for a crisis may not have worked together previously. This poses unique challenges to our need to improve the outcomes for these patients.

Simulation of Crises as Diagnostic Tool

Sullivan and Guyatt published one of the first studies of the use of cardiac arrest simulations in the hospital setting to identify deficiencies in the crisis team response [4]. They concluded: "Mock arrests are an extraordinarily powerful means of revealing suspected and unsuspected inadequacies in resuscitation procedure and equipment, and in motivating physicians and administrators to correct the deficiencies rapidly" [4]. Subsequent work by other teams has similarly revealed that simulation can be a powerful diagnostic tool in revealing inadequacies in a hospital's crisis response [6].

The mock code work by Dongilli et al. provides an example of applying crisis team training principles successfully as a diagnostic tool [7]. Mock codes were performed over several months in an adult hospital that is part of a 22-hospital health institution [6]. The aim was to evaluate the first responders and the elapsed time until appropriate resuscitation maneuvers. Measurements included elapsed time: time to call the operator about the crisis, time to send a voice page to the code team, time to code pagers' tones, and time to first-responder arrival [7]. Analysis of the results revealed that it took up to 4 min for the first responder to arrive at the crisis [7]. In reviewing the hospitals' operator notification procedure, it was discovered that the operators received the call, entered information into the paging system, triggered the belt paging system (which requires 3 min to deliver the page alert), and then paged the code team on the overhead speaker system [7]. This process caused an unnecessary delay in the time to the first responder's arrival to the crisis. The procedure was changed, and the operators were instructed to voice-page the code team immediately after receiving the call and to set off the pagers afterward [7]. After this protocol change, time to arrival of the first responder at the next mock code was improved to 1 min and 46 s and remained around 90 s since [7].

Hunt performed a series of 34 surprise, multidisciplinary mock codes over a 3-year period at three children's hospitals [8]. The mock codes consisted of scenarios of pediatric respiratory distress, respiratory arrest, or cardiopulmonary arrest [8]. Evaluation revealed delays to the assessment of airway, breathing, circulation, administration of oxygen, initiation of chest compressions, and decision to defibrillate, as well as errors in leadership and communication [8]. Hunt concluded that the study identified "targets for educational interventions to improve pediatric cardiopulmonary resuscitation and, ideally, outcomes" [8].

Finally, Prince et al. utilized simulation as part of a multistep restructuring of a hospital code team. Mock codes were performed in the patient care setting, and a number of issues were identified that led to quality and process improvements. These items included, but were not limited to, identification of dysfunctional code activation buttons, delays in lab test results, and the delay of interosseous access (IO) equipment arriving to the crisis scene. Wuality process improvements could then be implemented, including working with biomedical engineering to resolve the dysfunctional activation buttons, implementing the use of ISTAT for codes, and assigning IO equipment delivery to a specific staff person [9].

Simulation of Crises Improves Teamwork and Confidence

In addition to identification of systems issues, medical crisis team simulations can improve teamwork skills and confidence of team members. Frengley et al. found that a simulation-based study day improved teamwork in multidisciplinary critical care unit teams, including improved overall teamwork behavior, leadership, and team coordination and verbalizing situational information. In addition, the majority of post-course evaluation respondents reported increased confidence in managing similar events and emergency events in general [10]. Thomas et al. randomized high-fidelity simulation to practice neonatal resuscitation skills, and the trained participants exhibited more frequent teamwork behaviors and better workload management [11]. Allan et al. developed a specific crisis resource management curriculum for a pediatric cardiac intensive care units and focused on teamwork principles and technical resuscitation skills. Participants perceived improvement in their ability to function as a code member and confidence in a code, and all participants felt the program to be very useful [12]. Similar studies in other disciplines, including nursing, obstetrics, and community hospital settings, show simulation training for crisis events to be useful in improving confidence, comfort, and teamwork [13–15].

Simulation of Crises Improves Patient Outcomes

Most importantly, simulation training for crisis teams has resulted in improvements in actual team performance and patient outcomes. Wayne et al. trained second-year internal medicine residents utilizing a 10-h simulation-based educational intervention, while third-year residents received traditional training, including recent ACLS renewal but no simulation training. After the training period, a 6-month study period was selected, and hospital logs of actual patient cardiac arrest team responses were reviewed. The logs showed simulator-trained residents had significantly higher adherence to AHA standards vs. traditionally trained residents, and, specifically, simulator-trained residents were over seven times more likely to lead an adherent ACLS response than traditionally trained residents. This emphasizes the importance of simulation training; these second-year residents had less clinical experience and less traditional ACLS training (one vs. two provider courses), yet with simulation training, they outperformed more experienced trainees [16]).

In a landmark study published in 2011, Andreatta et al. instituted random mock codes at increasing rates over a 48-month period in a children's hospital at a tertiary care academic medical center. Events were recorded and used for immediate debriefing and feedback. Self-assessment data and hospital records for cardiopulmonary arrest (CPA) rates were examined for the study duration. In 2005, CPA survival rates were 10 %, but after the routine integration of the formal mock code program, the CPA survival rate was increased to approximately 50 %, in increments that correlated with the increasing number of mock code events. This study underlies the importance of simulation training for crisis teams as this all-important education translated to improved patient outcomes [17].

The Process

Crisis team training should focus on organizational skills, not on medical and nursing assessment and treatment skills. Unfortunately, the medical and nursing care knowledge and skills have been the traditional education focus for these teams (i.e., ACLS training). We believe that essential elements in a crisis team training session

include well-written, simulated resuscitation scenarios and skillful debriefing that focuses on organization and team dynamics. General principles to follow for crisis team training scenarios include using lifelike situations, having a specific learning objective or objectives for each scenario (or, more accurately, each debriefing), and incorporating team quality improvement goals. In addition, real-life errors can be replicated to train teams to avoid similar mistakes. Finally, and importantly, scenarios should be tightly focused toward facilitating the learning objective. They can be as short as 1 min if the learning objective is to see how long it takes a person to recognize a crisis, request an RRS response, and have the first responder arrive. On the other hand, if the goal is to focus on diagnosis and triage to an appropriate ICU, the scenario may require as long as 20–30 min. The debriefing should then be directed toward that learning objective. This focus helps the learner understand the points that they should grasp following each simulation session.

In any case, one should not expect to use a simulator and suddenly be able to train teams. Team training requires an organized curriculum and effective teaching directed at achieving specific behaviors. This chapter will address some key elements in developing a crisis team training curriculum.

What to Teach

The first step in developing a curriculum for crisis team training is to create clearly defined educational objectives for the session. Although these objectives will vary slightly at each institution, based on identified deficiencies, the training must openly acknowledge the unique nature of crisis teams and provide a road map to enable the ad hoc group to function well together. The following principles will invariably need to be covered: the team's goals, designated role assignment, communication, and leadership.

Goals of Crisis Response Teams

For crisis teams to function in an organized manner, they must devote time and effort to organization at the beginning of a crisis response. In our opinion, the major reason that crisis team responses tend to be disorganized is that individual members jump into medical and nursing actions prior to organizing the team. Teams are more likely to function well if the individuals have common goals, and they coordinate their efforts. Once organization has occurred, then medical and nursing interventions will proceed more efficiently. This organization step need not delay care if done well.

The first and most important goal of the team is to deliver effective and efficient basic life support throughout the entire episode. This includes assessment of airway, breathing, and circulation and, if necessary, rapid initiation of bag-mask ventilation and chest compressions, rapid defibrillation, and frequent reassessment. If the patient is in a shockable rhythm, the specific goal should be for the first shock to be delivered within 3 min of patient collapse.

The second goal is the effective and efficient delivery of appropriate advanced life support, including diagnosis of the underlying problem and delivery of definitive care. Finally, appropriate triage must occur.

Merely making team members aware of their overall goals and of the time intervals by which a specific resuscitation maneuver should be performed likely will be associated with better performance [18]. In addition to the team goals, each individual member should be aware of the goals for his specific role, as each specific job, if done appropriately, will help meet the overall goals.

Designated Roles: Assignment and Definition

When a crisis occurs in the hospital, the worst-case scenario is to have no plan for dealing with it. This is very unlikely in the twenty-first century. However, it is surprisingly common for a hospital to make a concerted effort to determine who will carry code beepers and how they will be activated, and yet neglect to plan who will perform which resuscitation job, or even what the jobs are. Unfortunately, this often results in important jobs or resuscitation tasks being left undone—for example, a delay of the performance of chest compressions or placement of intravenous/interosseous access.

The key to designing a crisis team response is to determine the specific roles and corresponding responsibilities that are desired and then designate them ahead of time, during training. There are two effective approaches to role assignment. The first is to have very clear roles that need to be assumed; often it does not matter who assumes which role, only that each role is filled by someone with adequate skills for the roles' set of responsibilities. The second approach is to teach each person who carries the code pager what his expected specific role will be when she/he arrives, so she/he knows what he should do. If that role is filled while another remains open, the responders must recognize that circumstance and fill the empty role. Failure to do this may result in failure to perform key tasks and lead to patient harm.

Each institution must also determine how its team will be structured—that is, who will participate in the response. Organizing the team and choosing roles go hand in hand. One must be familiar with available personnel for a crisis team response and choose roles accordingly. For example, one institution may only have four available crisis team responders, while another may have ten. The latter team will be able to expand the number of available roles, i.e., having two crash cart managers instead of one. Once it is clear how many people (and from which disciplines) are available to the team, assignment of the responsibilities for each role is the next step. Explicitly designating roles and responsibilities will remove the ambiguity that contributes to the chaos often seen during a crisis situation.

At the University of Pittsburgh, eight discrete roles were identified that are needed for every crisis team response. Although there were initially six roles, repeated specific errors during training sessions demonstrated the need for clearer and more roles. The team composition was altered, and roles are adjusted and added until the training teams reliably succeeded in meeting the predetermined task completion goals. The educators decided that it is important that all team members be trained to assume any one of several roles that they are capable of performing for several reasons. First, this cross-training improves the team's flexibility: in hospital crisis events, team members arrive in haphazard fashion, yet filling certain roles early (like airway management) is essential for success. Second, learning several roles promotes the understanding of the roles that other team members play. Failure to cross-train may lead to errors of communication, coordination, and role omission. For example, if a responding team has no anesthesiologists, anesthetists, and intensivists or other person with intubation skills arrive, it is common that no one even attempts to manage the airway. Instead, they may wait for the airway expert to arrive. This can happen even though team members often possess sufficient skills to manage the airway until an expert arrives. We acknowledge that some hospitals may not have eight responders available for a team response. In that case, we suggest that responders take on more than one role. For example, one person may take on both the airway manager and airway assistant roles. The use of roles to "bundle" responsibilities can help ease the allocation of tasks to team members. Simulation exercises can help determine the best "bundles" when a team member needs to occupy more than one role in a constrained human resource situation.

At the University of Pittsburgh, all members of the medical emergency team—including residents, fellows, attending physicians, critical care nurses, respiratory therapists, and pharmacists—take part in crisis team training sessions at the WISER simulation center. These full-scale, human simulation training sessions have allowed analysis of team function and were the impetus for changes in team structure.

At the beginning of the team training sessions, MET members who have usually never worked together during a medical crisis are required to complete an online didactic program. Upon arrival at the simulation center, the facilitator reviews key concepts of the didactic and orients the group to the simulator. They then participate in a simulated crisis scenario. We currently have eight scenarios (including a "null" scenario in which the simulated patient is not in a crisis). We have observed that the first attempt by the team is invariably chaotic, and many important resuscitation tasks are either delayed or will not be performed at all. For example, after training over 500 advanced cardiac life support-trained individuals, only one team (usually 16–20 people participate in a crisis team training course) has successfully defibrillated ventricular fibrillation in under 3 min in their first simulator session; by the end of the training program, virtually all teams are successful (see Fig. 32.1 for crisis task performance and Fig. 32.2 for simulated survival during the training sessions).

During the training session, crisis team members familiarize themselves with all goals and the roles that they are individually capable of performing; we ensure this by not allowing any person to play the same role twice during training. After debriefing in which participants determine whether they assumed all the roles of our response, and whether they completed all the tasks associated with each role, they then move on to more simulations. The team participates in four simulations, with debriefings to assess role assignment, task responsibility, and team interaction. Because participants take on different roles in each simulation, they develop an understanding of how the team begins to function more effectively and efficiently when each role is filled and the responsibilities clearly defined. This "roles and goals" approach teaches ad hoc teams to work well together, since no matter who arrives to the crisis response (or the order in which they arrive), they will be able to step into a role and perform the associated responsibilities. One of the key tasks during training is to teach the members important steps in effective management of a crisis team response (Table 32.1).

The University of Pittsburgh has reclassified responsibilities at a crisis response to remove professional "tags" and promote the assumption

Role	Responsibility
1. Airway Manager	Obtain airway equipment, assess and assist ventilation, intubate, check pupils
2. Airway Assistant	Assist airway manager, set up oxygen and suction equipment, suction as needed
3. Bedside Assistant (usually a floor RN)	Check pulse, obtain vital signs, place pulse oximeter, assess patient IVs, push medications
4. Circulation Manager	Check pulse, place defibrillator pads, perform chest compressions
5. Procedure MD	Perform procedures, IVs, chest tubes, capillary blood sugar, arterial blood gas
6. Crash Cart Manager (usually an ICU RN)	Record and prepare drugs, manage and operate defibrillator, deploy equipment: bag valve mask, backboard, defibrillator pads, documentation log
7. Treatment Leader	Assess team responsibilities and data, direct treatment, set priorities, triage
8. Data Manager (usually an ICU RN)	Distribute role tags, record AMPLE, retrieve lab results and chart, record interventions
Optional: Nursing Assistant	Bring capillary blood sugar machine and patient chart to bedside, transport lab samples

Fig. 32.1 Performance improvement of role-related tasks from the first through the third sessions of a human-simulator crisis team training program

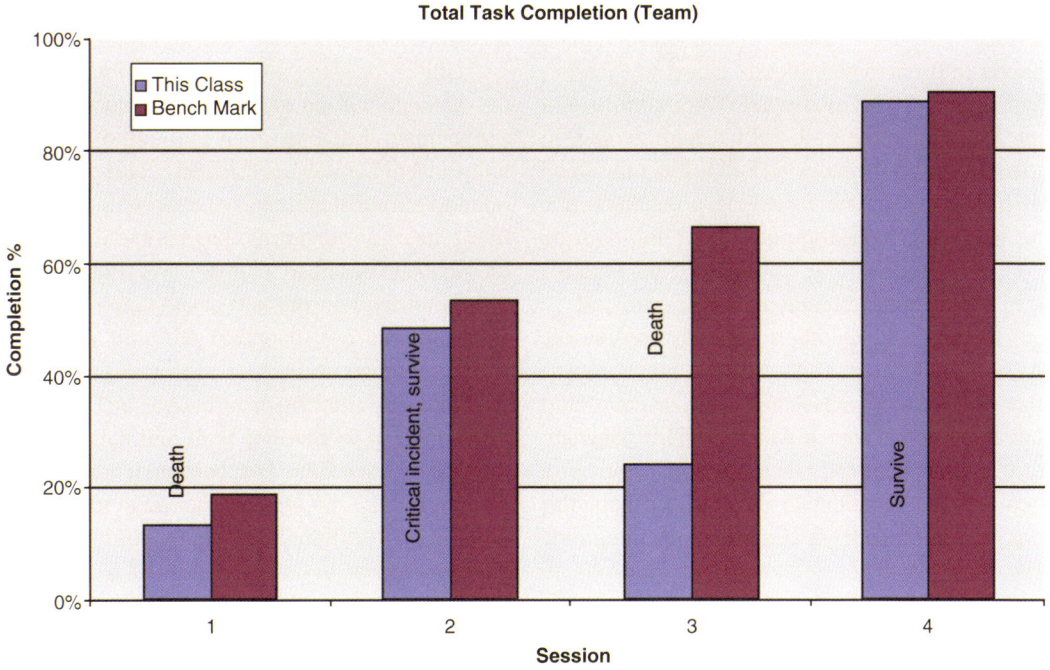

Fig. 32.2 Overall team task completion rate during the first, second, and third scenario sessions of a 3-h training program

of roles, regardless of which professionals arrive [19] (Table 32.2 and Fig. 32.3). Training sessions are multidisciplinary, with nurses, respira-

tory therapists, and physicians all attending a single training session. The group becomes adept at filling roles according to their individual capa-

Table 32.1 Key lessons for crisis team training

Organize the team
Choose roles
Identify and complete responsibilities
Communicate data to relevant person
Analyze data
Diagnose patient
Treat patient

bilities, and they begin to see how individuals can come together for the first time and function as a team. We have also discovered that mapping out positions for each crisis team member is vital; in this way, confusion is kept to a minimum, and each team member can be in the proper position at the bedside to perform his responsibilities [19].

Table 32.2 Roles and goals of crisis team members

Roles	Goals
Airway manager (#1 in Fig. 32.3)	Manages ventilation and oxygenation, intubates if necessary
Airway assistant (#2)	Provides equipment to airway manager, assists with bag-mask ventilation
Bedside assistant (#3)	Provides patient information including AMPLE*, medications delivery
Equipment manager (#4)	Draws up medications, supplies crash cart contents to appropriate team members
Data manager/recorder (#8)	Records vital signs, exam findings, test results, chart
Circulation assistant (#6)	Evaluates pulses, performs chest compressions
Procedure MD (#7)	Performs procedures such as central lines, chest tubes, pulse check
Treatment leader (#5)	Analyzes data, diagnoses, and directs patient treatment

*Allergies, medications, past history, last meal, and event—what happened

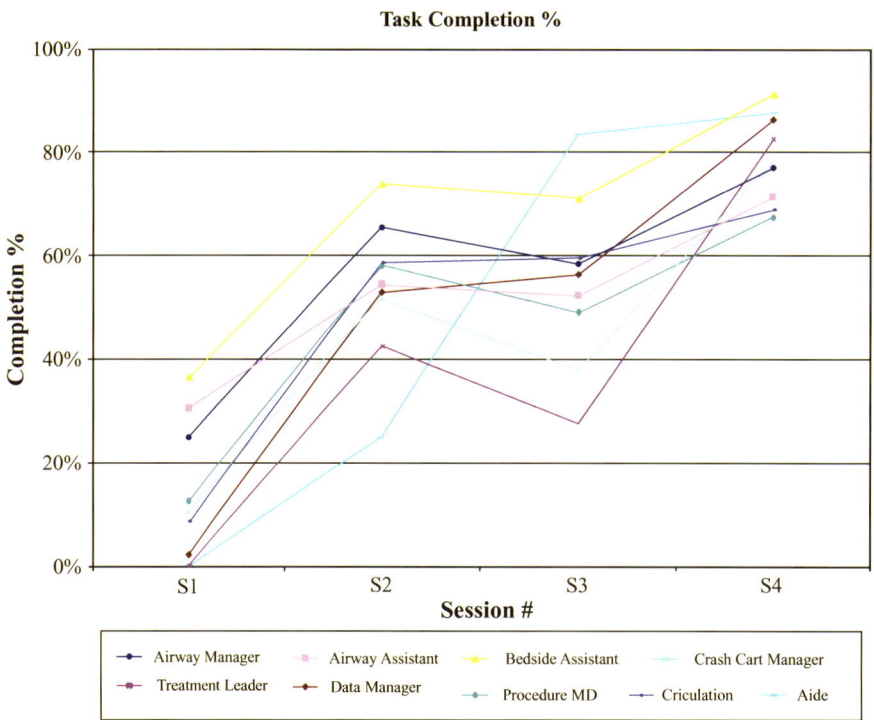

Fig. 32.3 Graphic representation of team roles and goals. Numbers correspond to roles listed in Table 32.2

Full-scale human simulation training has been used to train pediatric crisis response teams as well. At the Johns Hopkins Children's Center, they approach the team structure and function by training individuals on what their jobs will be upon arrival at every crisis they attend. They also avoid the term "Pediatric Code Team" and have explicitly renamed the team the Pediatric Rapid Response Team. The reason is that the team is ideally called for pre-arrest medical crises and prior to any cardiac arrest or "code" occurs. (The medical literature would call for the team being named a medical emergency team rather than a rapid response team because it is physician-led. However, at the Johns Hopkins Children's Center, there is a desire to make it clear that this team is for children, and so the term "pediatric" is used. Further, as the team is for both medical and surgical patients, they avoided the term "medical." Thus the full name is the "Pediatric Rapid Response Team.") The choice of the team's name varies from hospital to hospital, reflecting that hospital's culture, but the performance metrics are similar, and the training goals are similar.

The Johns Hopkins team has ten members, in addition to the floor team, and each member has a specific role. The roles are defined in a hospital protocol, described to individuals during orientation and are practiced during various team training sessions. For example, pediatric residents are trained to understand that during their internship year, any time they respond to a medical crisis their sole job will be to perform compressions if needed. The second-year pediatric residents are trained such that their job will be to defibrillate the patient if needed and otherwise assist with placement of vascular access.

In addition, there are monthly resuscitation training sessions for the residents rotating through the wards. They participate in a series of short mock codes and take turns practicing (1) identifying themselves as the leader, (2) fulfilling the roles they will be expected to perform during actual events, (3) communicating during crises, and (4) performing important resuscitation tasks such as CPR, bag-mask ventilation, defibrillation, and placement of intraosseous needles.

Developing a method to ensure that every important resuscitation task will be completed at every crisis depends on creating (1) clear role definitions, (2) a clear method for determining who will fill each role, and (3) training exercises to allow team members to practice filling the roles and completing the tasks as a cohesive unit.

Communication

Training to ensure effective communication is the next piece to organize. Closed-loop feedback communication is an important method. This term refers to the process whereby a team member will speak to another member and the second member will confirm hearing the message, closing the communication loop. In addition confirmation that the assigned task is completed closes the task performance loop. For example, the team leader says, "Jimmy, can you check for a pulse." Jimmy then states, "I will check the pulse," and completes his job by saying "I still do not feel a pulse." The leader should then confirm receiving this information, "Okay, there is no pulse. Jimmy, please continue CPR." Jimmy confirms, "I am continuing CPR." The closed-loop method of communication serves to lessen chaos and to ensure safe and appropriate management of patient care.

Not only should communication occur in a closed-loop manner, it should be aimed at the specific team member who requires the information, such as the team leader or the crash cart manager; the use of first names is important and effective. The team leader can then analyze data provided by the team members via closed-loop communication, assimilating the information and diagnosing the patient, and then again via closed-loop communication give instruction about appropriate patient treatment.

Simulation of cardiopulmonary arrests and medical crises allows medical emergency team members to practice these communication skills. A particularly effective method is to allow code team members to visualize the effect of communication errors that occurred in the safe environment of the simulation center. For example, during a mock code of a patient in profound septic shock, a pediatric resident orders a 20 cc/kg bolus of normal saline, and when the blood pressure remains low, repeats the order two more times; at the end of the mock code, the resident believes the patient has received 60 cc/kg of normal saline. Upon discussion with the nurses, it becomes clear that they were almost finished preparing the first bolus, but none of the fluid had actually been delivered. They had not even heard the second or third orders and did not realize that the normal saline was a priority, believing that the antibiotics were more important.

Within an RRS team, there are "mini-teams" that have more specific functions, and communication channels must be developed within the group as well as among groups. The three mini-teams are the breathing team, the circulation and patient assessment team, and the diagnosis and treatment team. The breathing team consists of an airway manager and an assistant. They obviously must work closely together and must have one-to-one communication independent of other communication. The circulation team is responsible for determining the presence and quality of circulation and delivering both circulatory assistance and medications. They need to cross-check findings and coordinate tasks that might interfere with each other, like doing chest compressions, placing a central venous catheter, and placing defibrillator pads. Finally the diagnosis and treatment team must assemble all the data, make treatment decisions, and implement them. Recognition of the presence and role of these mini-teams can help improve communication. The goal of the emphasis on organization and communication is to foster a collective consciousness, in which team members coordinate to collect, transmit, and act on data as a group rather than as individuals.

Leadership

Multiple studies demonstrate that poor leadership during cardiopulmonary resuscitation efforts is associated with poor team function [20, 21]. Cooper and Wakelam observed actual cardiopul-

monary arrests and used the Leadership Behavior Description Questionnaire [20]. This study revealed that leaders who participated in tasks in a "hands-on" manner were "less likely to build a structured team, the teams were less dynamic, and the tasks of resuscitation were performed less effectively" [20]. Marsch et al. studied simulated cardiopulmonary resuscitation efforts and observed that "absence of leadership behavior and absence of explicit task distribution were associated with poor team performance" [21].

While good leadership can help ensure good team functioning, a system must be in place to make sure that the team functions well even without an effective leader. For this reason, team members should be taught to assume their roles without needing to be reminded to do it. However, simulation of medical crises and cardiopulmonary arrests will allow the medical emergency team members to practice their leadership skills and actually see the effect of poor leadership. More importantly, training can allow leaders to practice until they can competently head a team.

Debriefing

Debriefing is an essential component of medical emergency team training. Marteau et al. state that there is a "well described tendency to invoke competence after success but not question it after failure" [22]. Their data demonstrated that resuscitation experience without feedback increased confidence, but not competence [22].

The principles of debriefing include timeliness, objectivity, specificity, and balance. Timeliness means that debriefing is most effective for the learner if it occurs immediately after the scenario. This ensures that the experience is fresh in the minds of the trainees, allowing for the greatest learning from feedback and self-assessment.

Debriefing should be objective and specific. It should focus on particulars—not "You did a good job," but rather, "You appropriately applied oxygen to the patient within 30 s." Debriefing can be made very specific using simulation and video recordings. Video review of medical emergency team performance using an objective evaluation instrument allows exact and detailed debriefing.

Finally, debriefing should be balanced. Both successes and errors should be discussed. The key to successful debriefing is to be positive, even if an error is the learning point. The error should be noted, but the focus should be on correct actions. Prior to team training, it should be reinforced that errors will occur during the simulation scenarios just as they occur in the real world. Simulation, however, allows for errors to happen in a safe and educational environment. In the simulated setting, errors can be powerful instructional aids and provide motivation.

What to Measure

RRS team training is important for education, patient safety, and research. For each of these areas, training is most effective if its components can be measured. Measurement can identify deficiencies and demonstrate improvements, if they occur. The key is to measure the correct outcome.

If the aim of RRS team training is education, scenarios should be written with tasks centered on a specific educational goal, such as correct bag-mask ventilation. The measurement will ultimately be a dichotomous value, i.e., "yes" or "no," as to whether the skill was performed effectively. The results help to identify areas on which to focus during debriefing. Institutions may use this technique of successful skill completion to qualify individuals for privileges in a hospital. For example, anesthesiologists may have to successfully demonstrate difficult airway maneuvers in order to receive privileges in their institution.

If the goal of RRS team training is patient safety, measurement could be of patient outcome. However, since many of the outcomes we seek to avoid are rare, it may not be reasonable to look solely at changes in the rates of these outcomes. A second approach can be to observe the adherence to desired procedures or algorithms. As we have seen, Wayne et al. successfully measured adherence to American Heart Association standards, specifically ACLS algorithms [16].

Research using RRS team training can focus on combinations of the above. Measurement of successful tasks completed by a team member, or the entire team, can be compared before and after team training, as well as over time. Studies by Gaba et al. show that both technical and behavioral performance can be assessed via evaluation of videotapes of simulated crisis events [23]. Their results show that cognition and crisis management behaviors vary considerably [23]. This has been seen before and demonstrates the ability of simulation to be used as a "needs assessment tool."

Blum et al. describe the development of an anesthesia crisis resource management course [16]. The course objectives were to understand and improve participant skills in crisis resource management and learn debriefing skills [24]. Course usefulness, debriefing skills, and crisis resource management principles were highly rated by participants [24]. It is interesting to note that course participants were eligible for malpractice premium reductions [24].

More recently, research using RRS team training focuses on improving teamwork, team member confidence, and actual team performance. Most importantly, this research has shown that simulation training for medical emergency teams may actually translate into improved team performance and patient outcomes.

Summary

The past 15 years have shown increases in the number of hospitals with rapid response systems; successful RRS team training may improve the effectiveness and efficiency of these teams and ultimately improve patient outcomes. RRS team training should include clear delineation of the goals of the team, designated role assignments of crisis team members, communication training, and leadership training. The training can be successfully achieved using simulation in combination with well-written scenarios, skillful debriefing, and specific measurements of deficiencies and achievements related to training.

References

1. Peberdy MA, Kaye W, Ornato JP, et al. Cardiopulmonary resuscitation of adults in the hospital: a report of 14, 720 cardiac arrests from the National Registry of Cardiopulmonary Resuscitation. Resuscitation. 2003;58:297–308.

2. Pittman J, Turner B, Gabbott DA. Communication between members of the cardiac arrest team—a postal survey. Resuscitation. 2001;49:175–7.

3. Edelson DP, Yuen TC, Mancini ME, Davis DP, Hunt EA, Miller JA, Abella BS. Hospital cardiac arrest resuscitation practice in the United States: a nationally representative survey. J Hosp Med. 2014;9(6):353–7.

4. Mundell WC, Kennedy CC, Szostek JH, Cook DA. Simulation technology for resuscitation training: a systematic review and meta-analysis. Resuscitation. 2013;84(9):1174–83.

5. Merchant RM, Yang L, Becker LB, Berg RA, Nadkarni V, Nichol G, Carr BG, Mitra N, Bradley SM, Abella BS, Groeneveld PW. American Heart Association get with the guidelines-resuscitation investigators. Incidence of treated cardiac arrest in hospitalized patients in the United States. Crit Care Med. 2011;39(11):2401–6.

6. Sullivan MJ, Guyatt GH. Simulated cardiac arrests for monitoring quality of in-hospital resuscitation. Lancet. 1986;2:618–20.

7. Dongilli T, DeVita M, Schaefer J, Grbach W, Fiedor M. The use of simulation training in a large multi-hospital health system to increase patient safety. Presented at International Meeting for Medical Simulation. Albuquerque, NM; 2004.

8. Hunt EA, Walker AR, Shaffner DH, Miller MR, Pronovost PJ. Simulation of in-hospital pediatric medical emergencies and cardiopulmonary arrests: highlighting the importance of the first 5 minutes. Pediatrics. 2008;121:e34–43.

9. Prince CR, Hines EJ, Chyou PH, Heegeman DJ. Finding the key to a better code: code team restructure to improve performance and outcomes. Clin Med Res. 2014;12(1–2):47–57.

10. Frengley RW, Weller JM, Torrie J, Dzendrowskyj P, Yee B, Paul AM, Shulruf B, Henderson KM. The effect of a simulation-based training intervention on the performance of established critical care unit teams. Crit Care Med. 2011;39(12):2605–11.

11. Thomas EJ, Williams AL, Reichman EF, Lasky RE, Crandell S, Taggart WR. Team training in the neonatal resuscitation program for interns: teamwork and quality of resuscitations. Pediatrics. 2010;125(3):539–46.

12. Allan CK, Thiagarajan RR, Beke D, Imprescia A, Kappus LJ, Garden A, Hayes G, Laussen PC, Bacha E, Weinstock PH. Simulation-based training delivered directly to the pediatric cardiac intensive care unit engenders preparedness, comfort, and decreased anxiety among multidisciplinary resuscitation teams. J Thorac Cardiovasc Surg. 2010;140(3):646–52.

13. Wehbe-Janek H, Lenzmeier CR, Ogden PE, Lambden MP, Sanford P, Herrick J, Song J, Pliego JF, Colbert CY. Nurses' perceptions of simulation-based interprofessional training program for rapid response and code blue events. J Nurs Care Qual. 2012;27(1):43–50.

14. Robertson B, Schumacher L, Gosman G, Kanfer R, Kelley M, DeVita M. Simulation-based crisis team training for multidisciplinary obstetric providers. Simul Healthc. 2009;4(2):77–83.

15. Kegler AL, Dale BD, McCarthy AJ. The use of high-fidelity simulation for rapid response team training: a community hospital's story. J Nurses Staff Dev. 2012;28(2):50–2.

16. Wayne DB, Didwania A, Feinglass J, Fudala MJ, Barsuk JH, McGaghie WC. Simulation-based education improves quality of care during cardiac arrest team responses at an academic teaching hospital: a case-control study. Chest. 2008;133(1):56–61.

17. Andreatta P, Saxton E, Thompson M, Annich G. Simulation-based mock codes significantly correlate with improved pediatric patient cardiopulmonary arrest survival rates. Pediatr Crit Care Med. 2011;12(1):33–8.

18. Kinney KG, Boyd SY, Simpson DE. Guidelines for appropriate in-hospital emergency team time management: the Brooke Army Medical Center approach. Resuscitation. 2004;60:33–8.

19. Fiedor M, DeVita M. Human simulation and crisis team training. In: Dunn WF, editor. Simulators in critical care and beyond. Des Plaines, IL: Society of Critical Care Medicine; 2004. p. 91–5.

20. Cooper S, Wakelam A. Leadership of resuscitation teams: "Lighthouse Leadership.". Resuscitation. 1999;42:27–45.

21. Marsch SCU, Muller C, Marquardt K, Conrad G, Tschan F, Hunziker PR. Human factors affect the quality of cardiopulmonary resuscitation in simulated cardiac arrests. Resuscitation. 2004;60:51–6.

22. Marteau TM, Wynne G, Kaye W, Evans TR. Resuscitation: experience without feedback increases confidence but not skill. BMJ. 1990;300:849–50.

23. Gaba DM, Howard SK, Flanagan B, Smith BE, Fish KJ, Botney R. Assessment of clinical performance during simulated crises using both technical and behavioral ratings. Anesthesiology. 1998;89:8–18.

24. Blum RH, Raemer DB, Carroll JS, Sunder N, Felstein DM, Cooper JB. Crisis resource management training for an anaesthesia faculty: a new approach to continuing education. Med Educ. 2004;38:45–55.

Jack Chen

Following the landmark reports from the Institute of Medicine (IOM) [1, 2] and other studies, numerous intervention programmes have been introduced to improve patient safety [3–7]. However, serious adverse events (SAEs) are still common in acute hospitals, with a conservative estimate of 200,000 in-hospital cardiopulmonary arrests (IHCA) [8] and up to 400,000 potentially preventable deaths each year in the USA [9]. The evaluation of complex system interventions continues to be a challenge. There is little robust evidence about the effectiveness of intervention programmes aimed at system improvement and patient safety [6]. Rigorous evaluation of the systems we use for delivering health care presents a different challenge from the ones used for evaluating simple interventions such as a new drug or new medical technology [10–12].

Characteristics of Complex System Interventions

There is no single and standard way of defining a complex system intervention. The World Health Organization report posits [11] that the current four revolutions that transform health and health systems are (1) life sciences, (2) information and communications technology, (3) social justice and equity and (4) systems thinking to transcend complexity. The authors argued that system-wide and system-level interventions are expected to have profound effects. Such interventions target at and recognise the dynamic architecture and interconnectedness of the health system building blocks (i.e. governance, information, financing, services delivery, human resources, medicines and technologies with people at the centre of such system) [11]. In 2008, the Medical Research Council (MRC) of the UK updated its previous guidance on developing and evaluating complex interventions [12] and posits that despite the fact that there is no sharp boundary between simple and complex interventions, the characteristics that make an intervention complex are (1) the number of interacting components within the experimental and control interventions, (2) number and difficulty of behaviours required by those delivering or receiving the intervention, (3) number of groups or organisation levels targeted by the intervention, (4) number and variability of outcomes and (5) degree of flexibility or tailoring of the intervention permitted.

A complex system intervention in health care often requires changes in the structure, culture and organisational behaviour of an institute, as well as changes in individual practices, all aimed at improving the quality of care [13, 14]. Most of

J. Chen, MBBS, PhD, MBA (Exec) (✉)
Simpson Centre for Health Services Research, South Western Sydney Clinical School, University of New South Wales, Level 1, AGSM Building, Sydney, NSW, Australia
e-mail: jackchen@unsw.edu.au

the quality improvement programmes also share some of these characteristics. Implementing complex system intervention is quite demanding. It may require systematic, multifaceted change strategy including building coalition; academic detailing [15], timely feedback [16], involving opinion leaders [17]; extensive and targeted educational activities; changing organisation structure such as team building; streamlining processes; and providing appropriate staffing.

However, it should be noted that some seemingly simple interventions may also have distinctive system components and interventions delivered are also often, in part, depending on local contexts and settings. For example, there were some system elements necessary to deliver the two different fluids in the SAFE study [17]. The trial involved more than simply delivering a single drug at one point in time. Apart from the fluid type, the fluid regimens were largely determined by the individual hospitals and by individual clinicians within their institutions. Thus the results depended partly on the protocols or systems used for fluid delivery protocols for each patient as well as the two different fluids being compared. The 'Matching Michigan' initiative in England [18] translated the successful Michigan-Keystone program [19] in preventing central line-associated infection into a national initiative but found no significant differences in outcomes between intervention ICU cluster and 'control' ICU cluster and similar pre-ICU treatment effect that cannot be attributed to the campaign that targeted only the participating ICUs. Such results prompted the urge to explore the historical, contextual and local system factors that may interact and modify the intervention effects [18, 20, 21].

Evaluating complex system intervention is sometimes known as health services research, defined as—'a multidisciplinary field of enquiry, both basic and applied, that examines the use, cost, quality, accessibility, delivery, organisation, funding and outcomes of health care services to increase the knowledge and understanding of the structure, processes, and effects of health services for individuals and populations' [22]. An alternative and less formal definition of health

services research states that it provides a framework for exploring the processes and dynamics underlying complex health systems [23]. Thus, this type of research may generate new knowledge about the barriers and enablers to establishing and maintaining best practice within complex systems.

Defining the Theory and Components of Complex System Evaluation

Good system intervention is based on sound theory and explicit causal assumptions of linkage between the intervention, processes, contexts and outcomes that have been described in different disciplines by various frameworks such as theory of change (ToC) [24], logic model for programme evaluation [25], realist evaluation [26], etc. In practice, we must define the underlying theory of the intervention and objectives of the evaluation clearly. Are we satisfied with simply determining clinical outcomes of the intervention, or are we also interested in gaining new knowledge about the processes and their impact within complex systems? Health promotion experts [27, 28] have argued the importance of assessing all three aspects. The conceptual drawback of a focus on only outcome is the lack of any knowledge about why the intervention did or did not produce the expected results. Even if the intervention finally delivers what it promises, we still don't have knowledge of to what degree the intervention could have been improved. Focusing on the final outcomes may also overlook important questions such as how the intervention worked and on what subgroups the intervention worked best.

Evaluation of the Medical Emergency Intervention (MET) is a good example of complex system research [29–36]. The selected clinical outcomes were unplanned admissions to ICU, unexpected deaths and cardiac arrests. However if the implementation of the MET system into a hospital does not produce these expected outcomes, how will we know whether the failure

Fig. 33.1 The critical links leading to successful MET outcomes

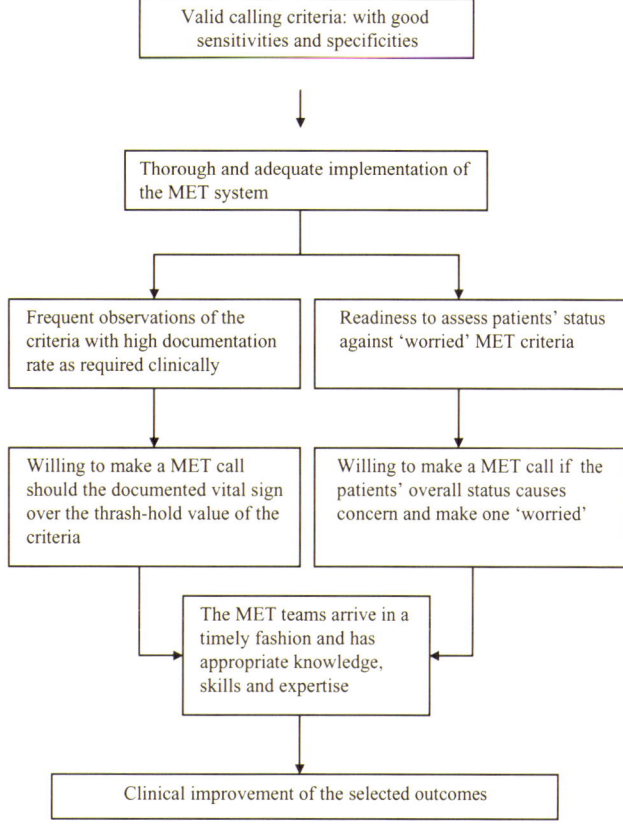

were due to factors such as inadequate implementation [35, 37], suboptimal calling criteria [38], a relative short study period [35], the possible contamination due to the 'rising tide' [35], the lack of critical care skills of the MET team [39] and the tardiness of the MET response [40] or whether the basic concept of early intervention in serious illness just doesn't work. To understand the critical causal theory and processes is perhaps as important as assessing the clinical outcomes (Fig. 33.1).

Other organisational characteristics may also contribute to outcomes. For example, the value placed on building capacity for patient safety may have contributed to the effectiveness of the MET [20, 21]. The nature of the hospital culture may also be an important variable. To complicate matters even more, the implementation of the MET system in itself results in cultural change, such as the need to modify the traditional bal-

ance of power between medical and nursing staff and the need to reconfigure interdisciplinary relationships. All of these factors may impact upon both the processes and outcomes of a complex system intervention such as the MET concept. Therefore we need to consider how many factors other than the simple outcomes can be taken into account when we plan complex system evaluation.

Choosing the Appropriate Research Methodology

We must decide on which paradigms we wish to use for evaluation. For example, do we use quantitative and qualitative methods or perhaps both? If we decide in favour of the latter, what is the sequence, what will the scope be and how might we go about integrating the two methods?

Within an evidence-based approach to medicine (EBM), we tend to classify research evidence based on the design and the features of the evaluation. The single, large randomised controlled trial (preferably double blinded) is the ultimate gold standard. In randomised controlled trials, the emphasis is on the design and the scale of the study. The appropriateness of the rigid EBM approach to patient safety has long been debated [41]. It should be noted that the conventional EBM approach is very different to a research paradigm based on organisational development and organisational learning [42]. The evaluation of the organisational aspects of systems could also adopt the participatory research and action research approach [43, 44]. This paradigm will have less emphasis on the rigour of the design and more emphasis on the development of an iterative and cyclical programme with the potential for supporting a learning culture (such as plan-do-study-act (PDSA) cycle). Researchers who lead and design research exploring organisations and complex systems need to base their thinking within a systems perspective. They need to focus on factors such as the interactions among subsystems and the unexpected benefits or harms of an intervention that may go beyond the original expectations [45, 46].

Randomised controlled trials are useful for comparing a simple intervention such as a new drug or procedure. Experimental and quasi-experimental designs have the highest internal validity for the purposes of complex system evaluations. Complex interventions such as a new system to evaluate early intervention in serious illness usually require complex research methodologies. An intensive care unit is a complex organisation, and patient care can be influenced by many factors such as standards of nursing care and staff morale within the unit. Some of these factors may be as important, or even more important, than a simple intervention such as a new drug. It is often impossible and unethical to adopt a simple RCT design [47] for the evaluation of a system intervention. A system intervention often requires a cluster randomised controlled trial design (cRCT) [48]. However, there can be challenges in using such research methodologies, including:

1. Limited choices in recruiting a control arm: There may be difficulties in finding suitable controls for a cRCT, as the number of units are often relatively small, each with a unique set of characteristics.

2. Contamination (the control group may also adopt the intervention): It is often very difficult to prevent the control units from learning and mimicking the intervention applied to the experimental groups. This is especially true when the intervention has good face validity and is intuitively appealing. In the MERIT study [35], we found that half of the cardiac arrest team calls were not related to a cardiac arrest or death (i.e. they were MET-type calls) during the study period. This may have contributed to the failure to demonstrate a difference. A similar finding also occurred in the ANZ Feeding Guideline Trial [15]. The study found significant changes in the physician feeding behaviour in the interventions groups but not in the hospital discharge mortality rate. However, the data also showed that within patients from control arm ICUs, 37.3 % of them (95 % CI: 28.1–49.6 %) had been fed within 24 h after admitted to the ICU. This was exactly what the evidence-based feeding guideline intended to achieve in the intervention group (60.8 %: 95 % CI: 45.7–80 %). Despite other significant improvement in the process measures, the above two 95CIs were overlapped. This may also in part explain why the study failed to achieve significant improvement in the patient outcome (i.e. hospital discharge mortality).

3. Incomplete implementation of intervention (poor fidelity): For a complex system intervention that targets structural, cultural and behavioural change, not all the units within the experimental group will embrace the changes with the same willingness and commitment. Scepticism, ineptness and a dislike of the unknown may easily derail a great initiative. Furthermore, individuals may also bring their own understanding and value judgement into the recommended changes. The skill sets and the knowledge of individuals may also decide the way that they will bring about the required changes. In the MERIT

study, close to half adverse events in the MET arm which met activating criteria didn't result in a MET call [35]. In the ANZ Feeding Guideline Trial, although the proportion of getting fed within 24 h of admission to an ICU is higher in the intervention group (60.8 % compared to 37.3 % in the control group), it also indicated that close to 40 % of patients within the intervention group weren't treated according to the best available evidence.

4. The need for a large sample size: Due to large variation among units (e.g. ICUs and hospitals) in terms of their size and organisational characteristics, a large number of units are often required in the study in order to achieve generalisability of the study results. These attributes impact significantly on the power of a cluster randomised controlled trial. The greater the variation in these characteristics, the greater the number of the hospitals needed to achieve sufficient statistical power to test the primary and secondary outcomes [49]. Also, the existence of the possible 'contamination' in the control group will effectively dilute the power of a study and confound the results.

5. The limited information to accurately estimate the power of the study: As a result of the relatively high costs of cluster randomised studies, one frequently does not have reliable information on the variations or intra-class correlation coefficients (ICCs) [50, 51] from previous research. The power issue could become even more complicated, as there are often no reported crude ICCs (the ICCs calculation based on the whole sample or the control and the intervention group separately without controlling for other covariates [48]). Even if such information may be available from other studies, the applicability of such ICCs to the current research settings is often questionable. As ICCs reflect certain organisational characteristics, they could be quite different among different health-care systems and settings [52]. Moreover, the information for the conditional ICCs (after adjusting for the key confounding factors such as hospital status, teaching, urban or rural, in the multi-

variate analysis model) is even scarcer. If one mixes all of these hospitals, one may run the risk of comparing 'apples with oranges'. A conditional model (conditional on the key confounding factors) could reduce this problem as a study that is underpowered based on the raw ICCs may have adequate power based on the conditional ICCs.

6. Time frames: Internalisation of system change is a function of time and, thus, may often require a lengthy time frame in order to succeed. For example, it took more than 10 years to demonstrate the effectiveness of trauma systems [53, 54]. This requirement translates into significant costs. For large-scale evaluation projects, such costs may become prohibitive, especially as they are already expensive and cumbersome, compared with the conventional gold standard: a simple randomised controlled trial.

Subsystem Interactions After a Complex System Intervention

When an intervention is applied to a unit or system, there may be unintended or unwanted results stemming from the changes introduced. While the MET system was originally designed to reduce the incidence of cardiac arrest, unexpected deaths as well as unplanned ICU admissions, the introduction of such system may change some aspects of the care in hospitals. For example, several studies explored the relationship between the introduction of a MET system and the issuing of the Not-For-Resuscitation (NFR) Order by the team [55–59]. A study from the MERIT trial showed that the incidence of patients being issued a NFR when attended by a MET team was ten times as high as the rate when attended by a cardiac arrest team [34]. This raises possibility that a MET team may initiate the process of the end-of-life discussion and advanced care planning. Thus, it may act as a de facto palliative care team and could potentially prevent unnecessary resuscitations for some patients. In response to this unintended consequence, a protocol of how MET or rapid response team should respond to end-of-life care issues was developed [60]. Another study from the MERIT data also showed that the introduction of a MET system was associated with significant improvement in the documentation of vital signs at the study period [31].

Cost and Cost-Effectiveness

Implementation of complex system intervention requires leadership and resources. The cost-effectiveness of system interventions should be taken into consideration. It has been widely recognised that well-considered and coordinated interventions are the prerequisite of a successful system change. However, it is also important to know whether the organisation can afford to implement and sustain an intervention such as the MET system. This raises the issue of whether we should incorporate a health economic perspective into evaluation projects. We also need to consider the marginal gain when implementing protracted and extensive system change [61, 62]. For example, the ANZ feeding guideline study applied 18 different implementation strategies in order to achieve a group of recommendations. It may be useful to know what strategy or what combination of these 18 strategies contributed mostly to the observed improvement. Furthermore, are there any strategies redundant, which may be left out without significant reduction of the impact?

Interpreting Study Results of Complex System Interventions

We briefly discussed the possible difficulties in designing and conducting a rigorous study evaluating complex system interventions. There is also the challenge of interpreting the results of an evaluation.

1. The absence of evidence is not evidence of absence: We deliberated on the difficulties in conducting an ideal trial, in having enough power to prove the primary hypothesis, in

avoiding contamination and other confounding factors, in analysing complex relationships and in dealing with multifaceted outcomes. It is more likely than not that a complex system intervention may produce negative results. The word 'negative' is often used incorrectly in these circumstances. In particular, it is incorrect to interpret those inclusive results (such as inadequate powered results) as a negative result [63].

2. Under what types of conditions could the intervention work?

There are often multiple conflicting results from single-centre studies. It may be misleading to propose either positive or negative conclusions on a single-centre trial. Similarly, in complex interventions, it might be more meaningful to discuss results in terms of why and how such interventions may work in certain types of conditions instead of a simple blanket conclusion. For example, using the published data from the MERIT study [32], we might explore the hypothesis that the effectiveness of implementation may be related to the initial incidence of adverse events and that there may be a higher benefit among hospitals that have a higher incidence of the adverse event at baseline. This could mean that for those hospitals which already have successful quality improvement programmes, the net benefit of a MET may be less significant. The MERIT study has shown that the improvement in outcomes after introduction of a MET is largely dependent on the successful implementation of such a system. In other words, as the proportion of emergency team calls (defined as the calls not associated with a cardiac arrest or death) increases, the rate of cardiac arrests and unexpected deaths decreases. This inverse relationship provides support for the notion that early review of acutely ill ward patients by an emergency team is desirable [33].

3. The burden of approval and a Bayesian approach

In view of the evidence-based approach in evaluating complex system intervention, one has to consider the difficulties in assessing the evidence base. The challenge of conducting an adequately powered study in generating level one evidence has not only limited the available studies but has also made meaningful interpretation of results difficult.

Planning and conducting a new trial may take several years, and the availability of the results may take even longer. In the meanwhile, for front-line clinicians, decision-makers and the campaigners for the quality improvement, the decision as whether to implement an intuitively appealing intervention such as intervening early in the case of serious illness remains difficult [41]. In the meantime, researchers and clinicians may turn to other forms of evidence such as those based on the observational studies, process-control techniques and organisational research evidence, qualitative research or expert-based consensus.

Other than a deterministic general view of the right or wrong regarding any particular choice, a Bayesian approach may be employed [64, 65]. This involves summarising the current knowledge based on multiple sources including expert opinions, taking into consideration the individual organisation's own commitment and capacity in instituting the proposed changes, coupled with their own plan-do-study-act (PDSA) model. This type of approach may be a better guide in deciding whether a proposed complex system intervention should be adopted.

Evaluating Complex System Intervention in a Big Data Era

Given the great advance in health information technology, electronic health record and the possibility of real-time multiple source big data, there is an increased possibility that through purposeful building of information infrastructure and linkage of multiple sources of data including large population-based and administrative database, unique opportunities exist to conduct rapid and system-wide evaluation of large-scale system intervention. For example, through the linkage of the admitted patient data collection with the mortality registry in the state of New South Wales,

Australia, it was found that among all 82 public acute hospitals in NSW, the rapid response system uptake increased from 32 % in 2002 to 74 % in 2009. This increase was associated with a 52 % decrease in IHCA rate, a 55 % decrease in IHCA-related mortality rate, a 23 % decrease in hospital mortality rate and a 15 % increase in survival to discharge after an IHCA [29]. Moreover, it was found that reduced IHCA incidence, rather than improved post-cardiac arrest survival, was the main contributor to the reduction in IHCA mortality. Such large data linkage also provided an opportunity for conducting a quasi-experimental study to compare patient outcomes among four large teaching hospitals (one MET hospitals vs three control hospitals) which found similar significant beneficial impact of having a MET on patient outcomes [30]. More recently, there were also growing interests of conducting large-scale, rapid, inexpensive RCT in a big data environment that could be extended to cluster randomised trial to evaluate complex system interventions [66]. These emerging new opportunities hold great promises for researchers and policy-makers to provide timely evaluation of complex system intervention and build a self-learning health system.

Summary

- Evaluating complex system intervention poses unique challenges both to the internal and external validities of the study findings.
- Appropriate designing and conducting a cRCT is demanding. So are the interpretations of the results from such a study. These difficulties may stem from the complexities involving inadequate power of a study, contamination, incomplete implementation of intervention, multiplicity of the results (both planned and unexpected, primary and secondary) and different types of the results (i.e. process, impact and outcomes).
- Unplanned and unexpected results are common after a complex system intervention, and the consequences of such results should also

be explored and understood. Sometimes, the question asked should be 'under what types of conditions such an intervention may work' instead of 'should such an intervention work anywhere, all the time?'

- Embracing a broader evidence base in assessing the results of a complex system intervention and adopting a Bayesian approach in considering whether an intervention be applied to a particular local setting.
- Improvement in health information technology and big data environment may also provide promises in conducting RCT/cRCT, large population-based observational studies and quasi-experimental studies to evaluate complex system interventions.

References

1. Institute of Medicine. Crossing the quality chasm: a new health system for the 21st century. Washington, DC: National Academies Press; 2001.
2. Donaldson MS, Kohn LT, Corrigan J. To err is human building a safer health system. Washington, DC: National Academy Press; 2000.
3. Wong BM, Dyal S, Etchells EE, et al. Application of a trigger tool in near real time to inform quality improvement activities: a prospective study in a general medicine ward. BMJ Qual Saf. 2015;24(4):272–81.
4. McDowell DS, McComb SA. Safety checklist briefings: a systematic review of the literature. AORN J. 2014;99(1):125–37 .e13
5. Wachter RM, Pronovost PJ, Shekelle PG. Strategies to improve patient safety: the evidence base matures. Ann Int Med. 2013;158(5 Part 1):350–2.
6. Shojania KG, Thomas EJ. Trends in adverse events over time: why are we not improving? BMJ Qual Saf. 2013;22(4):273–7.
7. Shekelle PG, Pronovost PJ, Wachter RM, et al. The top patient safety strategies that can be encouraged for adoption now. Ann Int Med. 2013;158(5 Part 2):365–8.
8. Morrison LJ, Neumar RW, Zimmerman JL, et al. Strategies for improving survival after in-hospital cardiac arrest in the United States: 2013 consensus recommendations: a consensus statement from the American Heart Association. Circulation. 2013;127(14):1538–63.
9. James JT. A new, evidence-based estimate of patient harms associated with hospital care. J Patient Saf. 2013;9(3):122–8.
10. Bonell C, Fletcher A, Morton M, et al. Realist randomised controlled trials: a new approach to evaluating complex public health interventions. Soc Sci Med. 2012;75(12):2299–306.
11. de Savigny D, Adam T. Systems thinking for health systems strengthening. WHO; 2009.
12. Craig P, Dieppe P, Macintyre S, et al. Developing and evaluating complex interventions: the new Medical Research Council guidance. BMJ. 2008;337(7676):979–83.
13. Grimshaw J, Eccles M, Tetroe J. Implementing clinical guidelines: current evidence and future implications. J Contin Educ Health Prof. 2004;24(Suppl 1):S31–7.
14. Grimshaw J, Eccles M, Thomas R, et al. Toward evidence-based quality improvement. Evidence (and its limitations) of the effectiveness of guideline dissemination and implementation strategies 1966–1998. J Gen Intern Med. 2006;21(Suppl 2):S14–20.
15. Doig GS, Simpson F, Finfer S, et al. Effect of evidence-based feeding guidelines on mortality of critically Ill adults: a cluster randomised controlled trial. JAMA. 2008;300(23):2731–41.
16. Thomas RE, Croal BL, Ramsay C, et al. Effect of enhanced feedback and brief educational reminder messages on laboratory test requesting in primary care: a cluster randomised trial. Lancet. 2006;367(9527):1990–6.
17. Finfer S, Bellomo R, Boyce N, et al. A comparison of albumin and saline for fluid resuscitation in the intensive care unit. N Engl J Med. 2004;350(22):2247–56.
18. Bion J, Richardson A, Hibbert P, et al. 'Matching Michigan': a 2-year stepped interventional programme to minimise central venous catheter-blood stream infections in intensive care units in England. BMJ Qual Saf. 2013;22(2):110–23.
19. Pronovost P, Needham D, Berenholtz S, et al. An intervention to decrease catheter-related bloodstream infections in the ICU. N Engl J Med. 2006;355(26):2725–32.
20. Bion JF, Dixon-Woods M. Keystone, matching Michigan, and bacteremia zero. Crit Care Med. 2014;42(5):e383–4.
21. Dixon-Woods M, Leslie M, Tarrant C, et al. Explaining Matching Michigan: an ethnographic study of a patient safety program. Implement Sci. 2013;8:70.
22. Field MJ, Tranquada RE, feasley JC Editors : Institute of Medicine. Health service research: workforce and educational issuses. National Academy Press. Washington DC, 1995.
23. Lomas J. Health services research: a domain where disciplines and decision makers meet. In: Sibbald WJ, Bion JF, editors. Evaluating critical care using health services research to improve quality. Berlin: Springer Verlag; 2000. p. 6–19.
24. Taplin DH, Clark H, Collins E, et al. Theory of change technical papers: a series of papers to support development of theories of change based on practice in the field. New York: ActKnowledge; 2013.

25. Millar A, Simeone RS, Carnevale JT. Logic models: a systems tool for performance management. Eval Program Plann. 2001;24:9.
26. Pawson R, Tilley N. Realist evaluation. London: Sage; 1997.
27. Green LW, Kreuter MW. Health program planning: an educational and ecological approach. 4th ed. New York: McGraw-Hill; 2005.
28. Wilson RM, Runciman WB, Gibberd RW, et al. The quality in Australian Health Care study. Med J Aust. 1995;163:458–71.
29. Chen J, Ou L, Hillman KM, et al. Cardiopulmonary arrest and mortality trends, and their association with rapid response system expansion. Med J Aust. 2014;201(3):4.
30. Chen J, Ou L, Hillman K, et al. The impact of implementing a rapid response system: a comparison of cardiopulmonary arrests and mortality among four teaching hospitals in Australia. Resuscitation. 2014;85(9):1275–81.
31. Chen J, Hillman K, Bellomo R, et al. The impact of introducing medical emergency team system on the documentations of vital signs. Resuscitation. 2009;80(1):35–43.
32. Chen J, Flabouris A, Bellomo R, et al. Baseline hospital performance and the impact of medical emergency teams: modelling vs. conventional subgroup analysis. Trials. 2009;10:117.
33. Chen J, Bellomo R, Flabouris A, et al. The relationship between early emergency team calls and serious adverse events. Crit Care Med. 2009;37(1):148–53.
34. Chen J, Flabouris A, Bellomo R, et al. The medical emergency team system and not-for-resuscitation orders: results from the MERIT study. Resuscitation. 2008;79(3):391–7.
35. Hillman K, Chen J, Cretikos M, et al. Introduction of medical emergency team (MET) system—a cluster-randomised controlled trial. Lancet. 2005;365: 2091–7.
36. Hillman K, Chen J, Brown D. A clinical model for Health Services Research—the Medical Emergency Team. J Crit Care. 2003;18(3):195–9.
37. Cretikos MA, Chen J, Hillman KM, et al. The effectiveness of implementation of the medical emergency team (MET) system and factors associated with use during the MERIT study. Crit Care Resusc. 2007;9(2): 206–12.
38. Cretikos M, Chen J, Hillman K, et al. The objective medical emergency team activation criteria: a case-control study. Resuscitation. 2007;73(1):62–72.
39. Flabouris A, Chen J, Hillman K, et al. Timing and interventions of emergency teams during the MERIT study. Resuscitation. 2010;81(1):25–30.
40. Chen J, Bellomo R, Flabouris A, et al. Delayed emergency team calls and associated hospital mortality: a multicenter study. Crit Care Med. 2015. doi:10.1097/CCM.0000000000001192.
41. Leape LL, Berwick DM, Bates DW. What practices will most improve safety? Evidence-based medicine meets patient safety. JAMA. 2002;288(4):501–7.
42. Argyris C. On organizational learning. 2nd ed. Malden, MA: Blackwell Business; 1999.
43. Howard JK, Eckhardt SA. Action research: a guide for library media specialists. Linworth: Worthington, OH; 2005.
44. Johnson AP. A short guide to action research. Boston: Pearson Allyn and Bacon; 2005.
45. Haslett T. Implications of systems thinking for research and practice in management. 07/98 ed. Caulfield East, VIC: Monash University, Faculty of Business and Economics; 1998.
46. Jackson MC. Systems thinking: creative holism for managers. Chichester: Wiley; 2002.
47. Donner A, Klar N. Design and analysis of cluster randomization trials in health research. London: Arnold; 2000.
48. Campbell MK, Elbourne DR, Altman DG, et al. CONSORT statement: extension to cluster randomised trials. BMJ. 2004;328(7441):702–8.
49. Kerry M, Bland JM. Statistical notes: sample size in cluster randomization. BMJ. 1998;316:549.
50. Kerry M, Bland JM. Analysis of a trial randomized in clusters. Br Med J. 1998;316:54.
51. Kish L, Frankel M. Inference from complex samples. J R Stat Soc Series B Stat Methodol. 1974;36:1–37.
52. Campbell MK, Fayers PM, Grimshaw JM. Determinants of the intracluster correlation coefficient in cluster randomized trials: the case of implementation research. Clin Trials. 2005;2(2):99–107.
53. Lecky F, Woodford M, Yates DW. Trends in trauma care in England and Wales 1989–97. Lancet. 2000;355(9217):1771–5.
54. Nathens AB, Jurkovich GJ, Cummings P, et al. The effect of organized systems of trauma care on motor vehicle crash mortality. JAMA. 2000;283(15):1990–4.
55. Calzavacca P, Licari E, Tee A, et al. A prospective study of factors influencing the outcome of patients after a Medical Emergency Team review. Intensive Care Med. 2008;34(11):2112–6.
56. Jones DA, McIntyre T, Baldwin I, et al. The medical emergency team and end-of-life care: a pilot study. Critical Care Resusc. 2007;9(2):151–6.
57. Kenward G, Castle N, Hodgetts T, et al. Evaluation of a Medical Emergency Team one year after implementation. Resuscitation. 2004;61(3):257–63.
58. Parr MJA, Hadfield JH, Flabouris A, et al. The Medical Emergency Team: 12 month analysis of reasons for activation, immediate outcome and not-for-resuscitation orders. Resuscitation. 2001;50:39–44.
59. Young L, Donald M, Parr M, et al. The Medical Emergency Team system: a two hospital comparison. Resuscitation. 2008;77(2):180–8.
60. Higginson IJ, Evans CJ, Grande G, et al. Evaluating complex interventions in end of life care: the MORECare statement on good practice generated by

a synthesis of transparent expert consultations and systematic reviews. BMC Med. 2013;11:111.

61. Drummond MF, McGuire A. Economic evaluation in health care merging theory with practice. Oxford: Oxford University Press; 2001.

62. Folland S, Stano M, Goodman AC. The economics of health and health care. 4th ed. Upper Saddle River, NJ: Pearson Prentice Hall; 2004.

63. Altman DG, Bland JM. Absence of evidence is not evidence of absence. BMJ. 1995;311(7003):485.

64. Hunink MGM, Weinstein MC, Wittenberg E, et al. Decision making in health and medicine: integrating evidence and values. 2nd ed. Cambridge, UK: Cambridge University Press; 2014.

65. Spiegelhalter DJ, Abrams KR, Myles JP. Bayesian approaches to clinical trials and health-care evaluation. New York: Wiley; 2004.

66. Angus DC. Fusing randomized trials with big data: the key to self-learning health care systems? JAMA. 2015;314(8):2.

Rapid Response Systems: Education for Ward Staff Caring for At-Risk and Deteriorating Patients

Gary B. Smith and John R. Welch

Introduction

The education of staff involved in the rapid response system (RRS) constitutes the first 'ring' of the 'chain of prevention' (Fig. 34.1)—a simple approach to the prevention of deterioration in hospital [1]. Sustaining the knowledge, skills and attitudes of medical, nursing and other staff working on general wards is crucial to the functioning of the RRS, as without their involvement, the RRS will be ineffective.

Essential ward staff roles include monitoring, charting and interpretation of patients' vital signs and other clinical variables; identifying 'at-risk' and deteriorating patients; timely administration of simple, first-line treatments; recognising the need for additional, often more experienced, help; and calling the rapid response team (RRT). Ward staff also provide important clinical and resource support to RRT members on their arrival and must assume responsibility for the patient's continuing surveillance and care if the patient remains on the general ward following an RRT visit.

Unlike emergency and critical care department staff, those working on wards are typically generalists and usually work with patients receiving routine, but often complex, care. For any individual staff member, the experience of sudden patient deterioration is relatively uncommon. If deterioration occurs, staff must adjust their working patterns rapidly in order to manage the crisis effectively and prevent life-threatening complications. This is a challenging role and requires staff to be appropriately prepared, especially as wards have fewer resources than specialist areas. Ward staff have usually not enjoyed the same educational opportunities as specialist staff, and numerous reports have identified they do not always possess the knowledge, psychomotor skills and attitudes necessary to recognise or respond to 'at-risk' or deteriorating patients [2–22]. Furthermore, ward staff may have difficulty in identifying their own learning needs [7].

This chapter discusses the crucial contribution of education of ward staff in ensuring safety and improving outcomes of at-risk patients, as well as in staff development.

G.B. Smith, BM, FRCP, FRCA (✉)
Centre of Postgraduate Medical Research & Education (CoPMRE), Faculty of Health and Social Sciences, Bournemouth University, Royal London House, Christchurch Road, Bournemouth, Dorset BH1 3LT, UK
e-mail: gbsresearch@virginmedia.com

J.R. Welch, RN, BSc, MSc
Critical Care Unit (T03), University College Hospital, 235 Euston Road, London NW1 2BU, UK
e-mail: John.Welch@uclh.nhs.uk

M.A. DeVita et al. (eds.), *Textbook of Rapid Response Systems*, DOI 10.1007/978-3-319-39391-9_34

Fig. 34.1 Chain of prevention

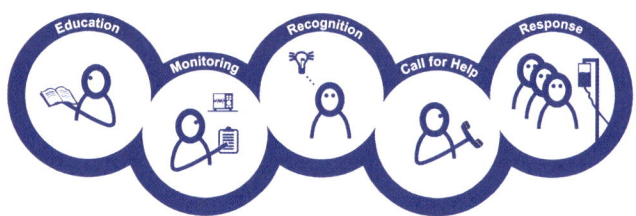

Table 34.1 Examples of level 1 patients (from [23])

Those

• Requiring a minimum of 4-hourly observation

• Requiring continuous oxygen therapy

• Requiring boluses of intravenous fluid

• Epidural analgesia or patient-controlled analgesia in use

• Receiving parenteral nutrition

• Requiring bolus intravenous drugs through a central venous catheter

• With tracheostomy in situ

• With chest drain in situ

• Requiring a minimum of 4-hourly GCS assessment

• Receiving a continuous infusion of insulin

• At risk of aspiration pneumonia

• On established intermittent renal support

• Requiring physiotherapy to treat or prevent respiratory failure

• Requiring more than twice daily peak expiratory flow measurements

GCS: Glasgow Coma Score

The Challenge for Ward Staff

Many medical problems are now managed in community settings, and many low-risk operative procedures are undertaken in day surgery units. Consequently, there has been a trend towards the hospital in-patient population being older and sicker, with patients having multiple comorbidities and undergoing complex medical interventions. Many are admitted as emergencies. All such patients will spend at least some of their hospital stay in a general ward. General ward staff are most likely to care for patients requiring level 1 care (Table 34.1), defined as those '…at risk of their condition deteriorating…' or '…recently relocated from higher levels of care, whose needs can be met on an acute ward with additional advice and support from the Critical

Care team…' [23] (n.b.: the term 'critical care team' would in many circumstances also refer to a RRT). In England in 2001, 12.2% of ward patients required level 1 care (or more); by 2006 this had risen to 21.3% [24, 25].

Evidence for the Need to Improve Education of Ward Staff in Acute Care

Two confidential enquiries have demonstrated deficiencies in ward care for critically ill patients [2, 3]. In the first, 54% of emergency ICU admissions received suboptimal care before their transfer to ICU, and many ICU referrals were delayed [2]. In the second, the initial assessment and/or examination of acute medical patients was deemed unacceptable in 13% of cases, and initial treatment was delayed and/or inappropriate in 26% [3]. Substandard ward care is associated with a higher mortality [2], as is delayed recognition and treatment of patients [26–30], and delayed intensive care unit (ICU) admission [31–33].

In both confidential enquiries, underlying factors leading to substandard care included failures of organisation, lack of supervision, lack of knowledge, failure to appreciate clinical urgency and failure to seek advice. The management of the airway, breathing, circulation, monitoring and oxygen therapy were rated as poor in many cases. Recent publications continue to demonstrate poor clinical monitoring and fail to recognise and/or adequately treat deterioration in hospital [34, 35].

Other studies suggest that medical students are ill-prepared for their initial years as doctors [8–12]. Trainee doctors often possess poor knowledge of aspects of acute care, e.g. pulse oximetry and oxygen therapy [13, 14] and junior doctors frequently make errors when dealing with emergencies [15]. In particular, these relate to incomplete understanding of hospital systems, prioritisation, ethical principles, communication, situation awareness and procedural skills [15]. Rates of error amongst trainees are higher at the beginning of the academic year [36].

Need assessments also suggest significant gaps in nurses' knowledge and competencies [16–20, 22, 37] and teamworking is also reported to be poor [20]. In one recent study, enrolled nurses expressed a lack of understanding of the cause of patient deterioration but indicated a desire to enhance their skills and knowledge through relevant training courses [21]. Specifically, they requested education about '… basic pathophysiology, signs and symptoms of disease process and the relationship between underlying disease processes and changes in the patient's vital signs …'. Experiential learning, including simulated practice, was identified as a favourable learning strategy [21].

Some of these deficiencies may exist because common texts contain insufficient information regarding the assessment and management of critically ill patients [38, 39]. However, newly qualified doctors have also expressed disquiet with the level of acute care training provided at medical school [40, 41]. Common concerns include the transfer of knowledge into practice, acts and omissions, their roles and responsibilities, performing under stress and the medical hierarchy [12]. There is concern that acute care training should have increased emphasis at undergraduate and preregistration level [42–48].

What General Ward Staff Need to Know

The particular competencies required by individual members of the ward team to ensure safe management of at-risk and deteriorating patients will vary but will typically include:

- The rationale for rapid response systems and the role of ward staff in it
- How to measure physiological parameters accurately

- How to observe patients, including patients' vital signs monitoring requirements
- How to record observations accurately
- Normal physiological values and how to interpret observed signs
- How to recognise patient deterioration
- How to use a track and trigger system (e.g. medical emergency team (MET) calling criteria [49], the National Early Warning Score [50])
- An appreciation of clinical urgency
- When and how to perform simple interventions (e.g. airway opening, oxygen therapy, intravenous fluid administration)
- Successful teamworking
- Organisation
- How and when to seek help from other staff
- How to use a systematic approach to delivering information, e.g. RSVP [51], SBAR [52], iSoBar [53]
- The role of ward staff in decisions about cardiopulmonary resuscitation and end-of-life care
- Human factors pertinent to the rapid response system

Detailed guidance by health policy developers regarding the specific acute care competencies required by ward staff has only recently emerged. In 2000, the report of a national review of critical care services by the Department of Health (DH) for England emphasised the need to '…share critical care skills with staff in wards and the community ensuring enhancement of training opportunities and skills practice …'; however, it provided little detail about how this might happen [54]. Specifically, it identified that all ward staff should have competency-based training in high dependency care within 4 years of the report [54], but this ambitious aim has still to be achieved.

In 2005, using a modified Delphi technique, a group of UK healthcare professionals established the Acute Care Undergraduate Teaching (ACUTE) Initiative, which identifies 71 essential and 16 optional competencies for medical graduates. It was proposed that these should form the core competency set for undergraduate training in acute care and resuscitation [44]. This provided a significant challenge, as teaching in acute care is often poorly coordinated, even amongst university medical schools.

In 2007, the National Institute for Health and Care Excellence (NICE) for England and Wales issued guidance on *Acutely ill patients in hospital: recognition of and response to acute illness*, recommending that staff working with acutely ill patients on general wards should be provided with education and training to include competencies in '...monitoring, measurement, interpretation and prompt response to the acutely ill patient appropriate to the level of care they are providing...' [55]. NICE also recommended that staff '...should be assessed to ensure they can demonstrate them...' [56]. Subsequently, the DH in England issued a framework of competencies targeted at hospital staff to complement the NICE guidance on managing acute illness [56].

The DH competencies are based on the principles that patients have needs related to their risk of deterioration and that interventions appropriate to meet those needs must be readily available, as and when required [56]. It identifies six staff roles:

- Nonclinical staff (this group may include the patient's relatives)
- Recorder
- Recogniser
- Primary responder
- Secondary responder
- Tertiary responder (n.b., this grade of response is not provided by ward staff)

A group of expected competencies is assigned to each of these six roles. The competencies are cumulative, and, as the patient severity increases, the competencies also advance in complexity, responsibility and clinical risk. Competencies are not assigned to specific staff groups, professions, grades or levels of seniority but are aggregated on the basis of the role of the staff required to possess them.

Staff designated as 'recorders' will generally measure vital signs, record these and other observations and calculate an early warning score (EWS) or compare the data with the RRT calling criteria in use. 'Recognisers' will monitor the patient's condition, interpret data in the context of the individual patient and adjust the frequency of observations and/or level of monitoring. 'Primary responders' will be capable of interpreting data and starting first-line treatments, e.g. the use of oxygen therapy or intravenous fluid. 'Secondary responders' would be called if the patient fails to improve with first-line treatments and would be capable of formulating a diagnosis, refining and developing the treatment plan and recognising when referral to critical care is needed. 'Tertiary responders' are staff with critical care competencies, e.g. as defined by the Competency Based Training programme in Intensive Care Medicine for Europe [57], or similar initiatives. Therefore, with the exception of tertiary responder roles and some 'secondary responder' functions, the bulk of the DH staff roles are provided by ward staff.

Any member of staff can perform the role of 'recorder', although it is often likely to be done by a nursing assistant. Most commonly, the 'recogniser' or 'primary responder' will be a nurse. However, in some situations, a doctor could undertake this role, and the 'secondary responder' could be a nurse practitioner or consultant nurse provided they have the certified skills, experience and training to respond appropriately. Although clinical staff will perform most interventions, some competencies might be undertaken by nonclinical staff (e.g. porters knowing which gas cylinder to obtain) or even by the patient's visitors (e.g. calling for help [58–60].

The DH competencies are conveniently organised under the following headings: (1) Airway, Breathing, Ventilation and Oxygenation; (2) Circulation; (3) Transport and Mobility; (4) Acute Neurological Care: and (5) Patient-Centred Care, Teamworking and Communication [56]. Table 34.2 provides an example of the roles relating to high-flow and controlled oxygen therapy for 'recorders', 'recognisers', 'primary responders' and 'secondary responders'. Examples of some suggested primary responder competencies to deal with breathing and circulation problems and issues of teamworking and communication are set out in Table 34.3 (from [56]).

Table 34.2 Examples of the roles relating to respiratory rate, oxygen saturation and high-flow and controlled oxygen therapy for 'recorders', 'recognisers', 'primary responders' and 'secondary responders' (modified from [56])

Competency group	Nonclinical staff	'Recorder'	'Recogniser'	'Primary responder'	'Secondary responder'
Respiratory rate	Recognises respiratory arrest and calls 2222	Measures respiratory rate Records result and assigns trigger score for respiratory rate. Has knowledge of what constitutes an abnormal value	Interprets trigger in context of patient and responds in accordance with local escalation protocols. Adjusts frequency of observations in keeping with trigger	Identifies inadequate respiratory effort and institutes clinical management therapies	Evaluates effectiveness of treatment, refines treatment plan if necessary, formulates a diagnosis and recognises when referral to critical care is indicated
High-flow and controlled oxygen therapy	Identifies and collects medical gases if designated.	Identifies and uses masks /nasal cannula/Venturi adapters at appropriate oxygen flow rates. Records oxygen concentration/flow	Follows oxygen prescription. Understands the context when controlled oxygen is required, and applies high-flow oxygen effectively in emergencies	Prescribes oxygen and evaluates effectiveness	Has detailed knowledge of the use of controlled and high-flow oxygen therapy. Evaluates effectiveness of oxygen therapy and revises treatment accordingly
Oxygen saturation		Measures oxygen saturation. Records result and assigns trigger score. Has knowledge of limitations of pulse oximetry, and recognises abnormal result	Interprets measurements in context, and intervenes with basic measures in accordance with local escalation protocols including oxygen and airway support. Adjusts frequency of observations in keeping with trigger	Identifies possible cause of hypoxia, prescribes oxygen therapy and institutes clinical management therapies	Formulates diagnosis, evaluates effectiveness of treatment, refines treatment plan if necessary and recognises when referral to critical care is indicated

In 2004, the Australian Commission on Safety and Quality in Health Care held an open consultation to seek advice about the core skills, knowledge and competencies required by all clinicians for recognising and responding to deterioration, escalating care and providing an initial response until expert help arrives. It also sought comments on processes for assessing competence, mandatory training and the duration, frequency and delivery of training [61]. Overall, there was a lack of consensus in the responses about the minimum standard of training necessary [62]. The competencies that were commonly listed by respondents to the consultation were virtually identical to those already listed at the beginning of this section of the chapter. There was a general

feeling that all clinicians providing direct patient care '…should have at least a minimum standard of training and competency for recognising and responding to clinical deterioration, and that no clinician should be exempt…' [62]. Perhaps surprisingly, there were significantly different views about whether training should be mandated [62].

Some patients referred to RRTs have deteriorated to the point where there is little or no likelihood that they will benefit from aggressive medical intervention and where end-of-life care might be more appropriate [63]. Consequently, it is now recognised that medical students and trainee doctors (and, in our view, nurses) should receive training in competencies relevant to palliative care for patients with serious, life-threatening

Table 34.3 Example competencies for ward staff caring for the acutely ill

Management of breathing

- Identifies inadequate respiratory effort/inadequate ventilation/cause of breathlessness and institutes clinical management therapies
- Has knowledge of which additional diagnostic tests are appropriate (e.g. peak flow, spirometry), institutes them and formulates management plan
- Prescribes nebulisers including appropriate driving gas
- Identifies possible cause of hypoxia, prescribes oxygen therapy and institutes clinical management therapies and evaluates effectiveness
- Undertakes arterial blood gas sampling and measurement and interprets blood gas values
- Has knowledge of indications for continuous positive airway pressure and non-invasive ventilation and identifies risks
- Requests and interprets chest radiograph
- Uses basic airway adjuncts and suction
- Assists with urgent intubation
- Prepares equipment for/assists with chest drain insertion. Manages patient with drain
- Identifies tension pneumothorax as a possible cause of breathlessness. Has knowledge of the management of a tension pneumothorax

Management of circulation

- Identifies abnormal heart rate and institutes clinical management therapies
- Has knowledge of common abnormalities and can interpret ECG in the context of the patient. Responds in accord with local protocols and institutes clinical therapies
- Has knowledge of causes of abnormal blood pressure and which diagnostic investigations are appropriate. Institutes clinical management therapies
- In cases of abnormal fluid balance, identifies when clinical intervention is required and institutes diagnostic investigations and a management plan
- Inserts urinary catheter
- Identifies source of bleeding and clinical impact and initiates definitive management. Commences resuscitation
- Has knowledge of which blood tests are required in both elective and emergency situations. Can request test/s and performs venesection
- Inserts iv cannula in 'difficult' cases
- Identifies need for and initiates fluid challenge for resuscitation and institutes clinical management plan. Prescribes maintenance fluids and drugs
- Has knowledge of indications for and risks of blood products. Prescribes blood products

(continued)

Table 34.3 (continued)

- Identifies low cardiac output and institutes diagnostic investigations and a management plan
- Identifies potential causes of collapse/unresponsiveness relevant to the individual patient
- In-hospital resuscitation
- Understands rationale for the use of emergency drugs and can administer

Teamworking and communication

- Recognises leadership role within team and responsibility to refer to secondary responder. Provides information in a structured format that conveys clinical urgency
- Incorporates within the documentation a management plan and timescale for reassessment. Identifies when referral to the secondary responder will be indicated

illness. Suitable competencies have been defined recently [64].

Challenges in Training Ward Staff in the Immediate Management of Acute Illness

It is a major undertaking to get a critical mass of ward staff trained to detect and manage acute illness, especially if there has been insufficient undergraduate or preregistration education and training. This was highlighted in the report of the multicentre MERIT study where, despite four months of training, ward staff called a MET to only 30% of patients that were subsequently transferred to ICUs, even though these patients met agreed referral criteria [49]. The authors of a separate study concluded that the long-term effectiveness of an educational programme to support the introduction of a MET required periodic and continued training [65].

There are also substantial costs and other challenges involved in developing and sustaining an effective education programme and in releasing both learners and trainers whilst still maintaining clinical services. Organisations should utilise regular reviews of service priorities and patient safety incidents to design suitable educational interventions and should develop a coordinated, cost-effective approach to providing accessible training. This can be achieved only if there is senior leadership and engagement with the whole range of clinical staff [56]. Evaluating the impact of education and training on patient outcomes is crucial.

Baseline knowledge and clinical experience affect learning, but recent changes in the way that staff work and are trained have generally reduced contact time with patients. These points have practical applications in deciding what education is clinically and cost-effective for different staff members. For example, advanced life support skills are better retained if delayed until trainees have 6 months of clinical experience [66, 67]. Organisations should detail the roles and responsibilities of all involved in acute care, clarifying the essential skills pertinent to every member of the ward team and identifying those staff that can be equipped to reliably deliver additional skills. Training can be tailored accordingly, so that individuals focus on what is essential for their particular role, rather than on learning skills they are unlikely to use [68].

Education Essential to the Implementation of a RRS

Since RRTs were introduced, many education programmes for ward staff have focused on the theory behind the RRS and the criteria and process for activating the RRT [69, 70]. Such training is essential to ensure timely referral and a rapid response [71, 72], but rarely provides ward staff with the knowledge of how to prevent deterioration or the actions to take between calling the RRT and its arrival. Common causes of deterioration on general wards lie within the scope of the patient's primary teams' practice [73–75] and studies report that many of the interventions undertaken by RRTs are simple therapies [76–82]. No matter how fast a RRT responds, there will always be an opportunity for ward staff to act before their arrival. Starting some treatments before the RRT arrives may be the most important factor in reducing mortality [65].

Unfortunately, evidence from ward cardiac arrests suggests that ward staff often perform poorly in the moments between patient discovery and arrival of the cardiac arrest team [83, 84].

Current Initiatives in Acute Care Education

Falling hospital cardiac arrest rates have led to calls to reduce the emphasis on widespread advanced life support training and to increase education in the recognition and response to pre-arrest clinical deterioration [68]. Such training should be structured around a systematic approach to assessment and management of *A*irway, *B*reathing, *C*irculation, *D*isability, issues revealed by *E*xposure of the patient (i.e. the ABCDE system) and methods of effective communication and teamworking [68, 85–89]. These principles underpin many of the educational programmes in acute care offered to undergraduate, postgraduate and post-registration staff working outside critical care areas [18, 37, 68, 85–97]. Many such courses utilise educational techniques and technologies derived from long-standing, usually generic, resuscitation courses. On a typical course, learners may be required to read a manual, attend a number of short talks and workshops, view demonstrations of practical techniques and practise some skills, usually using a variety of part trainers or whole patient manikins or standardised patients [98].

The development of specific, short, multi-professional courses teaching a standardised pre-emptive approach to critical illness to general ward staff began in 1999 with the development of the *A*cute *L*ife-threatening *E*vents: *R*ecognition and *T*reatment (ALERT) course in the UK [68, 99]. This one-day course was designed to give ward staff greater confidence and ability in the recognition and management of adult patients who have impending or established critical illness. ALERT focuses on common problems encountered during patient deterioration, e.g. 'the blue and breathless patient' and 'the hypotensive patient'. The course trains staff from different disciplines together, with the purpose of improving communication and multi-professional teamworking. Participants take turns to play all roles including that of the standardised patient. Numerous other similar courses now exist, e.g. COMPASS [88] and AIM [89]. Others [91, 92, 100, 101] have a broader remit, often allocating only a small proportion of course time to teaching about the prevention of critical illness. Not all are multi-professional.

Some acute care courses incorporate e-learning [92, 96] and, more recently, there has been an emphasis on small group interactive teaching and the use of scenarios akin to the real-life practice of learners using immersive human patient simulation [18, 95]. However, simulation-based courses are both labour-intensive and costly, making it difficult to train large numbers of staff. Consequently, hospitals can usually only provide this specialised type of training to individuals once a year at best, despite evidence that knowledge and skills deteriorate over time [102]. The use of e-learning techniques either alone or as part of a blended approach to education is therefore increasing.

Healthcare support workers or assistants (HCSW or HCA) now have a major role in the monitoring and detection of acutely ill patients [103], being responsible for undertaking most routine observations at the bedside. Consequently, educational strategies similar to those used for qualified staff, e.g. short courses [104, 105] and simulation [105], are used for these groups too.

A focused 'little but often, in the clinical area' approach to training may be useful in maintaining some, mainly psychomotor, acute care skills. The use of 'just-in-time' and 'just-in-place' training, in which skills training is provided in situ immediately before its likely usage, is currently being investigated in ICU paediatric airway training [106] and cardiopulmonary resuscitation [107]. Such techniques may find use in acute care.

The Role of the RRT in Educating Ward Staff

RRT members have an important role in educating ward staff, by delivering expert teaching whilst ensuring that the referral of a patient by ward staff is a positive experience. UK RRTs—usually nurse-staffed critical care outreach teams—are expected to 'share' critical care skills with ward staff [54, 108], and this is usually done via a combination of formal and informal teaching [109]. There is great benefit in outreach team members and ward staff undertaking regular, inter-professional reviews of cases together to discuss *what happened*, *what should have happened* and *what has been learned* [110]. Findings of suboptimal care will almost always require an educational response, tailored to addressing skill or knowledge deficits or system failures. Outreach staff often teach on short acute care courses, but can also provide immediate feedback on referrals or work with ward staff to assess and manage more complex 'at-risk' patients. The more reactive nature of the MET system is, perhaps, less well suited to permit such prolonged interactions between ward and RRT staff. Finally, seconding ward staff to work as members of the RRT [111] or enabling members of a patient's primary team to lead a RRT call [112] could provide additional training opportunities for selected staff.

Evidence for Benefit in Acute Care Educational Interventions

It is difficult—if not impossible—to separate the effects of education from other developments aimed at improving processes and patient outcomes in acute care [113]. Perhaps as a result, there is relatively little published research about the direct effects of training ward staff on such indicators.

However, there is evidence that education of ward staff may be a very, perhaps the most, important component of a RRS [65]. In a prospective before-and-after trial of a MET, almost all of the observed reduction in the hospital cardiac arrest rate occurred during the period when ward staff were being educated about and prepared for the introduction of the MET [114]. In another hospital, with an established RRT (ICU Liaison Team), introducing a tool designed to assist in the early identification of unstable ward patients facilitated ICU admission and was associated with a reduced number of ward cardiac arrests [115]. Similarly, in another hospital with an established MET, there was improved use of the RRT and a significant reduction in cardiac arrests following the implementation of specific, objective criteria for MET activation [116, 117]. In one study, staff trained to use an EWS, and SBAR measured respiratory rate twice as frequently and more often alerted a doctor, when presented with the nursing chart of a fictitious patient [118]. However, calculating an EWS and using SBAR remained poor. Communication with a doctor continued to be hampered by the absence of structure and subsequent loss of information [118]. Finally, a Portuguese group has shown a reduction in the long-term effectiveness of a RRS, suggesting that the critical factor was probably '…the staff education, awareness, and responsiveness to physiologic instability of the patients…' [65]. The authors concluded that the effectiveness of a RRS programme '…is dependent not only on the existence of an MET but mainly on the periodic and continued education and training of the entire hospital staff …' [65].

The ALERT course has been shown to improve staff knowledge and attitudes towards managing patient deterioration and improved documentation using an ABCDE assessment structure [119–122]: it has also been used as part of a strategic approach to reducing hospital mortality [123]. A 6-year audit of the UK Resuscitation Council's Immediate Life Support (ILS) course observed a close association between the proportion of healthcare professionals who were ILS trained and the number of emergency alert calls initiated as pre-arrest calls. There was also a significant decrease in cardiac arrests [124]. A prospective, controlled before-and-after introduction of a multi-faceted intervention including an education programme, COMPASS, showed reductions in unplanned admissions to ICU and unexpected hospital deaths [125]. COMPASS was also evaluated as part of a different multi-faceted intervention for paediatric patients, where the combined package led to improved documentation of vital signs and communication and reduced time to medical review [126].

The Acute Illness Management (AIM) was modified for a preregistration nursing programme and delivered within an established module [101]. There was a positive correlation between theoretical learning, high levels of satisfaction amongst participants and a clear perception that the programme enhanced clinical practice and awareness [101]. Another institution has described an in situ simulation-based education programme—The 'First 5 Minutes' programme—to enhance ward staff's response to crises [127]. Specifically, content focuses on the response to cardiac arrest and nurse-initiated defibrillation, but the authors claim that these objectives and activities apply to any patient crisis. Simulation sessions of up to 30 min took place outside the simulation centre in settings similar to a patient room and were offered throughout the day and night. Participants reported increased comfort in managing patients before MET arrival. Staff knowledge was increased; there was improved performance of key tasks before MET arrival and a reduced time to defibrillation [127].

Similar in situ training has been reported during the introduction of a paediatric MET (pMET), using 2-h session integrating the training of the pMET and ward staff [128]. Educational impact was measured by auditing the care of all unplanned paediatric ICU admissions before and after implementing the pMET. Deteriorating patients were recognised earlier by ward staff, more often reviewed by consultants, more often transferred to high dependency and more rapidly escalated to intensive care. Introduction of pMET coincided with significantly reduced hospital mortality. Ward staff responses to deterioration improved even if the pMET was never involved, suggesting that lessons learnt during training had been applied more widely [128].

A comparative study of face-to-face simulation in a ward-like laboratory setting (using a professional actor as a standardised patient) (FIRST2ACT) [129] with a web-based e-simulation programme (FIRST2ACTWeb) showed both to be effective strategies with e-simulation offering greater feasibility. The face-to-face approach was more positively evaluated with respect to the benefits of working in a team and receiving face-to-face debriefing [130]. A small randomised controlled trial (RCT) comparing classroom teaching with a clinical simulation teaching session showed that simulation training was better at improving the performance of ABCDE assessments than classroom teaching [131]. Participants who received simulation teaching were also more likely to be satisfied with their teaching experience [131].

One simulation-based programme—Rescuing A Patient In Deteriorating Situations (RAPIDS) [132]–incorporates detailed debriefing and validated assessment tool (RAPIDS-Tool) [133] to evaluate participants' performance in assessing and managing patient deterioration and in telephone reporting of patient deterioration. An initial evaluation of the RAPIDS course demonstrated significant increases in post-test scores for assessing and managing patient deterioration, and communication, compared to the control group [127]. However, separate data from the same study showed that both groups showed increases in self-confidence scores, but there was no significant correlation between self-confidence and clinical performance and between knowledge and clinical performance [134].

An ambitious 45-h course for undergraduate nurses, utilising didactic lectures, skill labs, medium- and high-fidelity simulations and facilitator-led guided reflection sessions, has been shown to increase participants' knowledge, self-confidence and perceptions of teamwork. The repetitive simulation practice, accompanied by video feedback and reflection, helped participants perfect their performance and develop reasoning skills [135]

The imbalance between the availability of manikin-based simulation and the number of potential staff requiring training has resulted in an increasing use of web-based learning. One study has shown this strategy to be at least as good as manikin-based simulation [136]. The web-based programme—eRAPIDS—uses a range of multimedia tools to provide a narrative about a deteriorating patient. Information about the underlying physiological signs of patient deterioration is presented in an animation showing two nurses in conversation; onscreen text and illustrations are used to explain the tasks

involved in assessing and managing the patient and reporting the findings; and the learner emulates the role of a nurse assessing and managing a deteriorating virtual patient with one or more deteriorating acute medical conditions [137]. Post-performance debriefing is also provided. In a prospective RCT of eRAPIDS, participants reported that the training was relevant to practice and fostered problem-solving. A follow-up study has demonstrated that, post training, nurses had increased knowledge of the physiological changes of deterioration and improved performance in assessing, managing and reporting these signs [138]. Another group used the RAPIDS-Tool to show improved mean assessment and management scores (i.e. the use of ABCDE) after simulation training. However, reporting scores (i.e. use of SBAR) were not significantly different [139].

A two-phase education programme of an e-learning module and simulation scenarios with organised debriefing was evaluated using pre- and post-education knowledge surveys and assessment of time to critical actions in the simulation scenarios [140]. Knowledge scores increase significantly, and there were reductions in both the time to application of the first correct critical intervention and the time to escalate care [140]. A two-centre RCT of clinical simulation versus classroom-based training for undergraduate nurses showed that simulation training led to better systematic assessment and management of the airway, breathing and circulation [141]. The group who received simulation training were significantly more satisfied with their teaching [141]. In a study designed to examine the teamwork skills used by nursing students and RNs to manage deteriorating patients during simulation exercises with patient actors, more experienced staff had a greater ability to work as part of a team. Clinical performance was similar for both groups [142].

Summary

Education of ward staff is essential for an effective rapid response system. Evidence suggests that ward staff can improve patient outcomes by intervening early with simple procedures and by ensuring timely involvement by the RRT when necessary. It is clear that a range of educational methods are required, with flexible and easy access to resources that suit different learning styles and address different sorts of patient need. Skill acquisition must be valued, and be seen to be valued, by both employers and staff, and time and resources are provided for learning and practice. Some theoretical knowledge can be gained by self-instruction, be it using written materials, video or online packages; but motor skills and integration of different components of the required skill set need hands-on practice.

References

1. Smith GB. In-hospital cardiac arrest: is it time for an in-hospital 'chain of prevention'? Resuscitation. 2010;81:1209–11.
2. McQuillan PJ, Pilkington S, Allan A, et al. Confidential inquiry into quality of care before admission to intensive care. BMJ. 1998;316:1853–8.
3. National Confidential Enquiry into Patient Outcomes and Death. An acute problem? London: National Confidential Enquiry into Patient Outcome and Death; 2005.
4. National Patient Safety Agency. Safer care for the acutely ill patient: learning from serious incidents. London: NPSA; 2007.
5. National Patient Safety Agency. Recognising and responding appropriately to early signs of deterioration in hospitalised patients. London: NPSA; 2007.
6. Purling A, King L. A literature review: graduate nurses' preparedness for recognising and responding to the deteriorating patient. J Clin Nurs. 2012;21:3451–65.
7. Cox H, James J, Hunt J. The experiences of trained nurses caring for critically ill patients within a general ward setting. Intensive Crit Care Nurs. 2006;22:283–93.
8. Matheson C, Matheson D. How well prepared are medical students for their first year as doctors? The views of consultants and specialist registrars in two teaching hospitals. Postgrad Med J. 2009;85:582–9.
9. Rolfe IE, Pearson SA, Sanson-Fisher RW, et al. Which common clinical conditions should medical students be able to manage by graduation? A perspective from Australian interns. Med Teach. 2002;24:16–22.
10. Buist M, Jarmolowski E, Burton P, et al. Can interns manage clinical instability in hospital patients? A survey of recent graduates. Focus Health Prof Edu. 2001;13:20–8.

11. Tallentire VR, Smith SE, Skinner J, et al. The preparedness of UK graduates in acute care: a systematic literature review. Postgrad Med J. 2012;88:365–71.
12. Tallentire VR, Smith SE, Skinner J, et al. Understanding the behaviour of newly qualified doctors in acute care contexts. Med Educ. 2011;45:995–1005.
13. Smith GB, Poplett N. Knowledge of aspects of acute care in trainee doctors. Postgrad Med J. 2002;78:335–58.
14. Howell M. Pulse oximetry: an audit of nursing and medical staff understanding. Br J Nurs. 2002;11:191–7.
15. Tallentire VR, Smith SE, Skinner J, et al. Exploring patterns of error in acute care using framework analysis. BMC Med Educ. 2015;15:3.
16. Wood I, Douglas J, Priest H. Education and training for acute care delivery: a needs analysis. Nurs Crit Care. 2004;9:159–66.
17. Derham C. Achieving comprehensive critical care. Nurs Crit Care. 2007;12:124–31.
18. McGaughey J. Acute care teaching in the undergraduate nursing curriculum. Nurs Crit Care. 2009;14:11–6.
19. Cooper S, Kinsman L, Buykx P, et al. Managing the deteriorating patient in a simulated environment: nursing students' knowledge, skill and situation awareness. J Clin Nurs. 2010;19:2309–18.
20. Bogossian F, Cooper S, Beauchamp A, et al. Undergraduate nursing students' performance in recognising and responding to sudden patient deterioration in high psychological fidelity simulated environments: an Australian multi-centre study. Nurse Educ Today. 2014;34:691–6.
21. Chua WL, Mackey S, Ng EKC, et al. Front line nurses' experiences with deteriorating ward patients: a qualitative study. Int Nurs Rev. 2013;60:501–9.
22. Buykx P, Cooper S, Kinsman L, et al. Patient deterioration simulation experiences: impact on teaching and learning. Collegian. 2012;19:125–9.
23. Intensive Care Society. Levels of critical care for adult patients. London: Intensive Care Society; 2009.
24. Chellel A, Fraser J, Fender V, et al. Nursing observations on ward patients at risk of critical illness. Nurs Times. 2002;98:36–9.
25. Smith S, Fraser J, Plowright C, et al. Nursing observations on ward patients—results of a five-year audit. Nurs Times. 2008;104:28–9.
26. Tirkkonen J, Ylä-Mattila J, Olkkola KT, et al. Factors associated with delayed activation of medical emergency team and excess mortality: an Utstein-style analysis. Resuscitation. 2013;84:173–8.
27. Chen J, Bellomo R, Flabouris A, et al. Delayed emergency team calls and associated hospital mortality: a multicenter study. Crit Care Med. 2015;43:2059–65.
28. Quach JL, Downey AW, Haase M, et al. Characteristics and outcomes of patients receiving a medical emergency team review for respiratory distress or hypotension. J Crit Care. 2008;23:325–31.
29. Calzavacca P, Licari E, Tee A, et al. The impact of rapid response system on delayed emergency team

activation patient characteristics and outcomes—a follow-up study. Resuscitation. 2010;81:31–5.

30. Downey AW, Quach JL, Haase M, et al. Characteristics and outcomes of patients receiving a medical emergency team review for acute change in conscious state or arrhythmias. Crit Care Med. 2008;36:477–81.

31. Cardoso LT, Grion CM, Matsuo T, et al. Impact of delayed admission to intensive care units on mortality of critically ill patients: a cohort study. Crit Care. 2011;15:R28.

32. Young MP, Gooder VJ, McBride K, et al. Inpatient transfers to the intensive care unit: delays are associated with increased mortality and morbidity. J Gen Intern Med. 2003;18:77–83.

33. Chalfin DB, Trzeciak S, Likourezos A, et al. Impact of delayed transfer of critically ill patients from the emergency department to the intensive care unit. Crit Care Med. 2007;35:1477–83.

34. Hogan H, Healey F, Neale G, et al. Preventable deaths due to problems in care in English acute hospitals: a retrospective case record review study. BMJ Qual Saf. 2012;21:737–45.

35. Donaldson LJ, Panesar SS, Darzi A. Patient-safety-related hospital deaths in England: thematic analysis of incidents reported to a national database, 2010–2012. PLoS Med. 2014;11(6):e1001667.

36. Haller G, Myles PS, Taffe P, et al. Rate of undesirable events at beginning of academic year: retrospective cohort study. BMJ. 2009;339:b3974.

37. O'Riordan B, Gray K, McArthur-Rouse F. Implementing a critical care course for ward nurses. Nurs Stand. 2003;17:41–4.

38. Cook CJ, Smith GB. Do textbooks of clinical examination contain information regarding the assessment of critically ill patients? Resuscitation. 2004;60:129–36.

39. Powell AGMT, Paterson-Brown S, Drummond GB. Undergraduate medical textbooks do not provide adequate information on intravenous fluid therapy: a systematic survey and suggestions for improvement. BMC Med Educ. 2014;14:35.

40. Cooper N. Medical training did not teach me what I really needed to know. BMJ [Career Focus]. 2003;327:190s.

41. Goldacre MJ, Lambert T, Evans J, et al. Preregistration house officers' views on whether their experience at medical school prepared them well for their jobs: national questionnaire survey. BMJ. 2003;326:1011–2.

42. Harrison GA, Hillman KM, Fulde GW, et al. The need for undergraduate education in critical care. (Results of a questionnaire to year 6 medical undergraduates, University of New South Wales and recommendations on a curriculum in critical care). Anaesth Intensive Care. 1999;27:53–8.

43. Smith CM, Perkins GD, Bullock I, et al. Undergraduate training in the care of the acutely ill patient: a literature review. Intensive Care Med. 2007;33:901–7.

44. Perkins GD, Barrett H, Bullock I, et al. The Acute Care Undergraduate TEaching (ACUTE) initiative: consensus development of core competencies in acute care for undergraduates in the United Kingdom. Intensive Care Med. 2005;31:1627–33.

45. Higginson R, Lewis R, De D, et al. The need for critical care nurse education at preregistration level. Br J Nurs. 2004;13:1326–8.

46. Shen J, Joynt GM, Critchley LA, et al. Survey of current status of intensive care teaching in English-speaking medical schools. Crit Care Med. 2003;31:293–8.

47. Rattray JE, Paul F, Tully V. Partnership working between a higher education institution and NHS Trusts: developing an acute and critical care module. Nurs Crit Care. 2006;11(3):111–7.

48. Whereat SE, McLean AS. Survey of the current status of teaching intensive care medicine in Australia and New Zealand medical schools. Crit Care Med. 2012;40:430–4.

49. Hillman K, Chen J, Cretikos M, et al. Introduction of the medical emergency team (MET) system: a cluster-randomised controlled trial. Lancet. 2005;365:2091–7.

50. Report of a working party. National Early Warning Score (NEWS): standardising the assessment of acute-illness severity in the NHS. London: Royal college of physicians; 2012. ISBN 978-1-86016-471-2.

51. Featherstone P, Chalmers T, Smith GB. RSVP: a system for communication of deterioration in hospital patients. Br J Nurs. 2008;17:860–4.

52. Thomas CM, Bertram E, Johnson D. The SBAR communication technique: teaching nursing students professional communication skills. Nurse Educ. 2009;34:176–80.

53. Porteous JM, Stewart-Wynne EG, Connolly M, et al. iSoBAR—a concept and handover checklist: the National Clinical Handover Initiative. Med J Aust. 2009;190:S152–6.

54. Department of Health. Comprehensive critical care: a review of adult critical care services. London: Department of Health; 2000.

55. National Institute for Health and Clinical Excellence. NICE clinical guideline 50 acutely ill patients in hospital: recognition of and response to acute illness in adults in hospital. London: National Institute for Health and Clinical Excellence; 2007.

56. Department of Health. Competencies for recognising and responding to acutely ill patients in hospital. London: Department of Health, National Health Service; 2009.

57. Competency Based Training programme in Intensive Care Medicine for Europe and Other World Regions. Available online at: http://www.cobatrice.org/en/index.asp. Accessed 25 Nov 2015.

58. Ray EM, Smith R, Massie S, et al. Family alert: implementing direct family activation of a pediatric rapid response team. Jt Comm J Qual Patient Saf. 2009;35:575–80.

59. Odell M, Gerber K, Gager M. Call 4 Concern: patient and relative activated critical care outreach. Br J Nurs. 2010;19:1390–5.

60. Vorwerk J, King L. Consumer participation in early detection of the deteriorating patient and call activation to rapid response systems: a literature review. J Clin Nurs. doi: 10.1111/jocn.12977. Accessed 25 Nov 2015.

61. Australian Commission on Safety and Quality in Health Care. National safety and quality health service standards: training and competencies for recognising and responding to clinical deterioration in acute care. Consultation paper. Sydney: Australian Commission on Safety and Quality in Health Care; 2014.

62. Australian Commission on Safety and Quality in Health Care. National safety and quality health service standards: training and competencies for recognising and responding to clinical deterioration in acute care. Consultation report and options for action. Sydney: Australian Commission on Safety and Quality in Health Care; 2014.

63. Tan LH, Delaney A. Medical emergency teams and end of life care: a systematic review. Crit Care Resusc. 2014;16:62–8.

64. Schaefer KG, Chittenden EH, Sullivan AM, et al. Raising the bar for the care of seriously ill patients: results of a national survey to define essential palliative care competencies for medical students and residents. Acad Med. 2014;89:1024–31.

65. Campello G, Granja C, Carvalho F, et al. Immediate and long-term impact of medical emergency teams on cardiac arrest prevalence and mortality: a plea for periodic basic life-support training programs. Crit Care Med. 2009;37:3054–61.

66. Jensen ML, Lippert F, Hesselfeldt R, et al. The significance of clinical experience on learning outcome from resuscitation training-a randomised controlled study. Resuscitation. 2009;80:238–43.

67. de Ruijter PA, Biersteker HA, Biert J, et al. Retention of first aid and basic life support skills in undergraduate medical students. Med Educ Online. 2014;19:24841.

68. Smith GB, Welch J, DeVita MA, et al. Education for cardiac arrest—treatment or prevention? Resuscitation. 2015;92:59–62.

69. Jones D, Baldwin I, McIntyre T, et al. Nurses' attitudes to a medical emergency team service in a teaching hospital. Qual Saf Health Care. 2006;15:427–32.

70. Johnson AL. Creative education for rapid response teams. J Contin Educ Nurs. 2009;40:38–42.

71. Cretikos MA, Chen J, Hillman KM, et al. The effectiveness of implementation of the medical emergency team (MET) system and factors associated with use during the MERIT study. Crit Care Resusc. 2007;9:205–12.

72. Jones D, Bates S, Warrillow S, et al. Effect of an education programme on the utilization of a medical emergency team in a teaching hospital. Intern Med J. 2006;36:231–6.

73. Prado R, Albert RK, Mehler PS, et al. Rapid response: a quality improvement conundrum. J Hosp Med. 2009;4:255–7.

74. Kollef MH, Chen Y, Heard K, et al. A randomized trial of real-time automated clinical deterioration alerts sent to a rapid response team. J Hosp Med. 2014;9:424–9.

75. Tobin AE, Santamaria JD. Medical emergency teams are associated with reduced mortality across a major metropolitan health network after two years service: a retrospective study using government administrative data. Crit Care. 2012;16:R210.

76. Pirret AM. The role and effectiveness of a nurse practitioner led critical care outreach service. Intensive Crit Care Nurs. 2008;24:375–82.

77. Ball C, Kirkby M, Williams S. Effect of the critical care outreach team on patient survival to discharge from hospital and readmission to critical care: non-randomised population based study. BMJ. 2003;327:1014–6.

78. Dacey MJ, Mirza ER, Wilcox V, et al. The effect of a rapid response team on major clinical outcome measures in a community hospital. Crit Care Med. 2007;35:2076–82.

79. Story DA, Shelton AC, Poustie SJ, et al. The effect of critical care outreach on postoperative serious adverse events. Anaesthesia. 2004;59:762–6.

80. Story DA, Shelton AC, Poustie SJ, et al. Effect of an anaesthesia department led critical care outreach and acute pain service on postoperative serious adverse events. Anaesthesia. 2006;61:24–8.

81. Kenward G, Castle N, Hodgetts T, et al. Evaluation of a medical emergency team one year after implementation. Resuscitation. 2004;61:257–63.

82. Flabouris A, Chen J, Hillman K, et al. Timing and interventions of emergency teams during the MERIT study. Resuscitation. 2010;81:25–30.

83. Hunziker S, Tschan F, Semmer NK, et al. Hands-on time during cardiopulmonary resuscitation is affected by the process of teambuilding: a prospective randomised simulator-based trial. BMC Emerg Med. 2009;9:3.

84. Einav S, Shleifer A, Kark JD, et al. Performance of department staff in the window between discovery of collapse to cardiac arrest team arrival. Resuscitation. 2006;69:213–20.

85. Frost PJ, Wise MP. Early management of acutely ill ward patients. How junior doctors can develop a systematic approach to managing patients with acute illness in hospital. BMJ. 2012;345:e5677.

86. Smith GB, Osgood VM, Crane S. ALERT™—a multiprofessional training course in the care of the acutely ill adult patient. Resuscitation. 2002;52:281–6.

87. Resuscitation Council UK Immediate Life Support Course Manual 4th edition. London: Resuscitation Council UK; January 2016.

88. http://www.health.act.gov.au/professionals/compass. Accessed 25 Nov 2015.

89. http://gmccsi.org.uk/aim-courses. Accessed 25 Nov 2015.
90. Ellison S, Sullivan C, Quaintance J, et al. Critical care recognition, management and communication skills during an emergency medicine clerkship. Med Teach. 2008;30:e228–38.
91. Cave J, Wallace D, Baillie G, et al. DR WHO: a workshop for house officer preparation. Postgrad Med J. 2007;83:4–7.
92. Gruber P, Gomersall C, Joynt G, et al. Teaching acute care: a course for undergraduates. Resuscitation. 2007;74:142–9.
93. MacDowall J. The assessment and treatment of the acutely ill patient—the role of the patient simulator as a teaching tool in the undergraduate programme. Med Teach. 2006;28:326–9.
94. Shah IM, Walters MR, McKillop JH. Acute medicine teaching in an undergraduate medical curriculum: a blended learning approach. Emerg Med J. 2008;25:354–7.
95. Fuhrmann L, Østergaard D, Lippert A, et al. A multi-professional full-scale simulation course in the recognition and management of deteriorating hospital patients. Resuscitation. 2009;80:669–73.
96. Collins TJ, Price AM, Angrave PD. Pre-registration education: making a difference to critical care? Nurs Crit Care. 2006;11:52–7.
97. Liaw SY, Scherpbier A, Klainin-Yobas P, et al. A review of educational strategies to improve nurses' roles in recognizing and responding to deteriorating patients. Int Nurs Rev. 2011;58:296–303.
98. Leung JY, Critchley LA, Yung AL, Kumta SM. Introduction of virtual patients onto a final year anesthesia course: Hong Kong experience. Adv Med Educ Pract. 2011;2:71–83.
99. http://www.alert-course.com. Accessed 25 Nov 2015.
100. Soar J, Perkins GD, Harris S, et al. The immediate life support course. Resuscitation. 2003;57:21–6.
101. Steen CD, Costello J. Teaching pre-registration student nurses to assess acutely ill patients: an evaluation of an acute illness management programme. Nurse Educ Pract. 2008;8:343–51.
102. Hamilton R. Nurses' knowledge and skill retention following cardiopulmonary resuscitation training: a review of the literature. J Adv Nurs. 2005;51:288–97.
103. James J, Butler-Williams C, Hunt J, et al. Vital signs for vital people: an exploratory study into the role of the healthcare assistant in recognising, recording and responding to the acutely ill patient in the general ward setting. J Nurs Manag. 2010;18:548–55.
104. Watson D, Carberry M. Training HCAs to recognise patient deterioration. Training HCAs to recognise patient deterioration. Nurs Times. 2014;110:73–84.
105. Bedside Emergency Assessement for Hospital Support Workers (BEACH). http://www.alert-course.com/?page_id=226. Accessed 25 Nov 2015.
106. Nishisaki A, Colborn S, Watson C, et al. Just-in-time simulation training improves ICU physician trainee airway resuscitation participation without compromising procedural success or safety. Circulation. 2008;118:S1453.
107. Niles D, Sutton RM, Donoghue A, et al. "Rolling Refreshers": a novel approach to maintain CPR psychomotor skill competence. Resuscitation. 2009;80:909–12.
108. Department of Health and NHS Modernisation Agency. The National Outreach Report. London: Department of Health; 2003.
109. McDonnell A, Esmonde L, Morgan R, et al. The provision of critical care outreach services in England: findings from a national survey. J Crit Care. 2007;22:212–8.
110. Cronin G, Andrews S. After action reviews: a new model for learning. Emerg Nurse. 2009;17:32–5.
111. Plowright C, O'Riordan B, Scott G. The perception of ward-based nurses seconded into an outreach service. Nurs Crit Care. 2005;10:143–9.
112. Sarani B, Sonnas S, Bergey MR, et al. Resident and nurse perceptions of the impact of a medical emergency team on education and patient safety in an academic medical center. Crit Care Med. 2009;37:3091–6.
113. Hutchings A, Durand MA, Grieve R, et al. Evaluation of modernisation of adult critical care services in England: time series and cost effectiveness analysis. BMJ. 2009;339:1130.
114. Bellomo R, Goldsmith D, Uchino S, et al. A prospective before-and-after trial of a medical emergency team. Med J Aust. 2003;179:283–7.
115. Green AL, Williams A. An evaluation of an early warning clinical marker referral tool. Intensive Crit Care Nurs. 2006;22:274–82.
116. DeVita MA, Braithwaite RS, Mahidhara R, Stuart S, Foraida M, Simmons RL, Members of the Medical Emergency Response Improvement Team (MERIT). Use of medical emergency team responses to reduce hospital cardiopulmonary arrests. Qual Saf Health Care. 2004;13:251–4.
117. Foraida MI, DeVita MA, Braithwaite RS, et al. Improving the utilization of medical crisis teams (Condition C) at an urban tertiary care hospital. J Crit Care. 2003;18:87–94.
118. Ludikhuize J, Borgert M, Binnekade J, et al. Standardized measurement of the modified early warning score results in enhanced implementation of a rapid response system: a quasi-experimental study. Resuscitation. 2014;85:676–82.
119. Hutchinson S, Robson WP. Confidence levels of PRHOs in caring for acutely ill patients. Postgrad Med J. 2002;78:697.
120. Viner J. Implementing improvements in care of critically ill, ward-based patients. Prof Nurse. 2002;18:91–3.
121. Smith GB, Poplett N. Impact of attending a one-day course (ALERT™) on trainee doctors' knowledge of acute care. Resuscitation. 2004;61:117–22.
122. Featherstone P, Smith GB, Linnell M, et al. Impact of a one-day inter-professional course (ALERT™) on attitudes and confidence in managing critically ill adult patients. Resuscitation. 2005;65:329–36.

123. Wright J, Dugdale B, Hammond I, et al. Learning from death: a hospital mortality reduction programme. J R Soc Med. 2006;99:303–8.

124. Spearpoint KG, Gruber PC, Brett SJ. Impact of the immediate life support course on the incidence and outcome of in-hospital cardiac arrest calls: an observational study over 6 years. Resuscitation. 2009;80:638–43.

125. Mitchell IA, McKay H, Van Leuvan C, et al. A prospective controlled trial of the effect of a multifaceted intervention on early recognition and intervention in deteriorating hospital patients. Resuscitation. 2010;81:658–66.

126. McKay H, Mitchell IA, Sinn K, et al. Effect of a multifaceted intervention on documentation of vital signs and staff communication regarding deteriorating paediatric patients. J Paediatr Child Health. 2013;49:48–56.

127. Tasota FJ, Clontz A, Shatzer M. What's the 4-1-1 on "the first five"? Nursing. 2010;40:55–7.

128. Theilen U, Leonard P, Jones P, et al. Regular in situ simulation training of paediatric medical emergency team improves hospital response to deteriorating patients. Resuscitation. 2013;84:218–22.

129. Buykx P, Kinsman L, Cooper S, et al. FIRST2ACT: educating nurses to identify patient deterioration. A theory-based model for best practice simulation education. Nurse Educ Today. 2011;31:687–93.

130. Cooper S, Cant R, Bogossian F, et al. Patient deterioration education: evaluation of face-to-face simulation and e-simulation approaches. Clin Simul Nurs. 2015;11:97–105.

131. Merriman CD, Stayt LC, Ricketts B. Comparing the effectiveness of clinical simulation versus didactic methods to teach undergraduate adult nursing students to recognize and assess the deteriorating patient. Clin Simul Nurs. 2014;10:e119–27.

132. Liaw SY, Rethans JJ, Scherpbier A, et al. Rescuing A Patient In Deteriorating Situations (RAPIDS): a simulation-based educational program on recognizing, responding and reporting of physiological signs of deterioration. Resuscitation. 2011;82:1224–30.

133. Liaw SY, Scherpbier A, Klainin-Yoba P, et al. Rescuing A Patient In Deteriorating Situations (RAPIDS): an evaluation tool for assessing simulation performance on clinical deterioration. Resuscitation. 2011;82:1434–9.

134. Liaw SY, Scherpbier A, Rethans J-J, et al. Assessment for simulation learning outcomes: a comparison of knowledge and self-reported confidence with observed clinical performance. Nurse Educ Today. 2012;32:e35–9.

135. Hart PL, Brannan JD, Long JM, et al. Effectiveness of a structured curriculum focused on recognition and response to acute patient deterioration in an undergraduate BSN program. Nurse Educ Pract. 2014;14:30–6.

136. Liaw SY, Chan SW, Chen FG, et al. Comparison of virtual patient simulation with mannequin-based simulation for improving clinical performances in assessing and managing clinical deterioration: a randomized controlled trial. J Med Internet Res. 2014;16:e214.

137. Liaw SY, Wong LF, Chan SW, et al. Designing and evaluating an interactive multimedia web-based simulation for developing nurses' competencies in acute nursing care: randomized controlled trial. J Med Internet Res. 2015;12:e5.

138. Liaw SY, Wong LF, Ang SB, et al. Strengthening the afferent limb of rapid response systems: an educational intervention using web-based learning for early recognition and responding to deteriorating patients. BMJ Qual Saf. 2016;25:448–456. doi: 10.1136/bmjqs-2015-004073. Accessed 25 Nov 2015.

139. Bell-Gordon C, Gigliotti E, Mitchell K. An evidence-based practice project for recognition of clinical deterioration: utilization of simulation-based education. J Nurs Educ Pract. 2014;4:69–76.

140. Ozekcin LR, Tuite P, Willner K, et al. Simulation education: early identification of patient physiologic deterioration by acute care nurses. Clin Nurse Spec. 2015;29:166–73.

141. Stayt LC, Merriman C, Ricketts B, et al. Recognizing and managing a deteriorating patient: a randomized controlled trial investigating the effectiveness of clinical simulation in improving clinical performance in undergraduate nursing students. J Adv Nurs. 2015;71:2563–74.

142. Endacott R, Bogossian FE, Cooper SJ, et al. Leadership and teamwork in medical emergencies: performance of nursing students and registered nurses in simulated patient scenarios. J Clin Nurs. 2015;24:90–100.

Gabriella Jaderling and David Konrad

Introduction

Rapid response systems have evolved as an organized approach to improve patient safety by addressing unmet needs of deteriorating patients on general wards [1]. Being based on education and increased awareness, these systems induce a complex change across the whole hospital that can be more difficult to quantify than a novel drug or a single intervention. How then do we best measure the effects of what we do and what tools do we have to assess our outcomes? Should we measure the process or the outcomes, or both? And what are the best outcomes to measure?

Measuring safety and evaluating complex interventions is challenging as they are dependent on a number of interlinked processes such as educational efforts, resources, team-building, administrative support and the context in which they are implemented. Process measures such as staff satisfaction, impact of education or effects on end of life care are just as important to investigate as the traditional outcomes of cardiac arrest rate and mortality. Thus, multiple studies with different methodologies, both quantitative and qualitative will be necessary [2]. Well-designed and -performed observational studies from different types of hospitals and different parts of the world will be valuable and should be regarded as such [3]. It is hardly ethical to perform a randomized controlled trial at the individual level to evaluate the effect of an intervention that is based on providing highly qualified care when an acute life threatening condition is identified, nor does it lend itself to blinding.

We need to assess all aspects of introducing a fundamental system change: has the process itself been successful? Are the calling criteria adequate? Are they being used? Are they being responded to in a timely fashion? These questions might be best assessed using qualitative studies and will be fundamental when trying to evaluate if the intervention has any effect on outcome. If we can not ascertain that the process has been successful we can not say whether the intervention is effective.

Rapid response systems have in the recent years become widely adopted and evaluated but there has been conflicting evidence of their effect [4–7]. Several single center studies have shown positive results [8–13] but it is not always easy to draw any conclusions as different outcomes have been used, inclusion criteria vary and cultural and structural differences among hospitals may play an important role in the implementation and maintenance of the RRS [14, 15]. Do we measure the same things? The use of historical controls in

G. Jaderling, MD, PhD (✉) • D. Konrad, MD, PhD
Perioperative Medicine and Intensive Care,
Karolinska University Hospital,
171 76 Stockholm, Sweden
e-mail: gabriella.jaderling@karolinska.se

© Springer International Publishing Switzerland 2017

M.A. DeVita et al. (eds.), *Textbook of Rapid Response Systems*, DOI 10.1007/978-3-319-39391-9_35

before–after studies is an important limitation as changes in case mix and seasonal variation must be taken into account. Generalization of single center studies is problematic and the restraints must be understood. The commitment and enthusiasm of a local investigator may be key to the success of implementation in one setting which may not be reproducible elsewhere [3]. The study population may differ greatly as well as the local resources, such as staffing of academic vs non-teaching hospitals. With these limitations in mind, there is no need to dismiss these studies [16]. Commonly viewed, observational studies do not hold the same scientific worth as large RCT's and may not lend themselves to generalization as easily although they do give important input as to whether implementation was successful and relevant goals for outcome have been reached. This provides important feedback to the system in question and may also point to possible areas of improvement as well as being able to inspire and promote further research.

Standardization of the RRS Process

Initiating RRS

When setting up an RRS in a hospital a considerable amount of time must be put into preparations before the launch and a thorough literature review should include methods of organizational change. Based on a hypothesis (early identification and intervention of the at-risk patient in the general ward improves outcome) the problem is identified. In our institution this was done by performing a prevalence study to calculate how many patients fulfilling the criteria we would find at a given time [17]. This also allowed us to validate the criteria chosen by restricting and extending them within the study.

The introduction of a complex intervention is largely dependent upon good support among all involved: clinicians, nursing staff, and management. It is helpful if a network is formed for continuous evaluation and feedback processes since a multidisciplinary approach is necessary in the implementation as well as in the evaluation and the research [18].

If a reliable baseline of the relevant outcomes is not available a pilot study should be performed in order to assess these. This will also aid in determining possible barriers to implementing the protocol and offer insight into how to overcome them. Surveys of the opinions of clinicians and nursing staff can provide useful information for the present implementation and also outline practice variability and differences in attitudes among different centers [19].

Trial design is a crucial step and should involve epidemiological and statistical expertise from the start. As with any other clinical research, the trial is to be designed to answer a clearly defined question.

Data Collection

A great deal of information can be gathered from each call and later sorted and compiled for different purposes. Quantitative information based on the events surrounding the call is well suited to integrate into a database. Standardization of the collection and reporting of RRS data is important for consistency and will facilitate comparisons across institutions. One example of reporting forms can be found in a publication from Australia [20] and guidelines for uniform reporting have further been proposed by an international consensus group in the Utstein style, with a comprehensive set of recommended core and supplemental data elements [21]. Unless automated data collection is a reality, data may need to be gathered from different sources, such as a RRS paper form, patient's electronic charts and hospital records. There is always the risk of data not being collected consistently considering that many calls are made during off-hours and not seldom under pressed circumstances. To ensure capture of all calls, our experience has been that the form needs to be as short as possible and easy to complete. An example of the form used to record RRS calls by clinicians responding to calls at Karolinska is presented in Fig. 35.1. A protocol should then exist to fuse these bits of information reliably and accurately into a usable database. It should be limited to a few trained staff to collect and record data in order to ease standardization.

Ward: **Patient ID:**

Date: **Date of birth:**

RRT call time: **Gender:**

RRT arrival time:

RRT return time:

Reason for calling:

☐ Respiratory rate < 8   ☐ Heart rate < 40   ☐ Reduced consciousness

☐ Respiratory rate > 30   ☐ Heart rate > 130   ☐ Intuition

☐ SpO2 < 90   ☐ Systolic BP < 90   ☐ None fulfilled

Vital parameters:

   - **At time of call:**

Respiratory rate: SpO2: O_2 l/min: Heart rate: Blood pressure: GCS: Temp:

   - **At RRT assessment:**

Respiratory rate: SpO2: O_2 l/min: Heart rate: Blood pressure: GCS: Temp:

Treatments and disposition:

☐ IV volume   ☐ CPAP/BiPAP   ☐ X-ray/US/CT   ☐ Consultant

☐ O2   ☐ Inhalations   ☐ IV access   ☐ ECG

☐ Bloodgas/labs   ☐ Medication:

☐ Other treatments:

☐ Remain in ward   ☐ Transfer to ICU   ☐ Transfer to HDU   ☐ Other:

Limitation of medical treatment: (date of documentation:)

☐ No limitation   ☐ Should be discussed

☐ Do Not Resuscitate   ☐ Do Not Intubate   ☐ Not for ICU

Fig. 35.1 Case report form used at Karolinska, to be filled out by the team leader at each RRT call

This database can then be used in itself to describe the RRS process for internal evaluation and analysis of events or fused with further information such as a hospital database for outcome assessment of mortality and cardiac arrest. The minimum data necessary for process and outcome evaluation includes information on the setting, patient demographics, events and outcome (Table 35.1). A standardized and reliable documentation for limitations of medical treatment such as do not resuscitate orders is paramount but can be a challenging issue that should be dealt with on a hospital wide basis. This may differ greatly between hospitals and even between different clinics within the same hospital and is possibly the most difficult factor to control for.

A channel for qualitative information gathering can be through regular meetings with contact persons in each ward and by setting up an easily accessible way to reach the RRS team, for instance through an e-mail address on the hospital's intranet. Further useful information to assess is changes in attitudes, decision-making and acceptance of the system. Questionnaires and in-depth interviews with staff can be of use to explore satisfaction with the system as well as to identify areas for improvement [22, 23].

Table 35.1 RRS database case form—minimum set

Hospital information
Bed allocation
Outcome statistics—annually
Response team information
Composition
Structure
Coverage
Activation criteria
Patient information
ID number
Age
Gender
Location/type of ward
Type of admission (acute/elective)
Admitted—date
Discharged—date
Previous RRS call
Previous ICU care
RRS call information
Call date
Call time
Response time
Time spent on ward
Call reason (criteria activated)
RRS outcome
Clinical findings
Interventions
Transfer to/left on ward
Patient outcome
Discharge diagnosis (ICD-10)
Operated—date
Limitations of medical treatment—date
Mortality—date

Evaluation

The success of the system is dependent upon all parts of it being functional and thus all different parts need to be evaluated. Demographic data on the hospital as well as the set-up of the team needs to be reported in order to describe the context in which the system is working [21].

The afferent limb of any RRS is defined as the function that detects and identifies a medical emergency and consequently triggers an adequate response [18]. It needs to be evaluated on a regular basis to see whether it is functioning properly. Have the educational efforts been adequate? Is the awareness widespread? Are the calling criteria being used enough? This is hard to measure accurately without considerable effort and we may see more of automated and continuous monitoring in the future [24, 25]. Delays in triggering need to be recognized as they have an impact on the result [26, 27] and the underlying causes might best be assessed with qualitative studies.

The efferent limb is the crisis response component and can be of different constitutions, nurse-led or physician-led [18] but share the property of responding to a trigger and bringing critical care experience to the acutely ill patient. Response times should be measured and reported as well as the competency of the team and the equipment immediately available. Cooperation and communication skills connecting the two limbs should be given consideration and perhaps assessed using video analysis of the system at work [2] or other forms of team training [28, 29].

The time frame may be of importance and reflect a direct dose–response relationship [30, 31]. The effects of implementing system changes are not instantaneous. In comparison one can look at the introduction of organized trauma systems which have taken at least 10 years before a reduction in mortality could be shown [32]. Any new system introduction needs time to mature and set properly [33].

Outcome

To set up standardized tools of assessment we first need to decide what outcomes are of importance and the next step must be to have an adequate baseline of what we want to measure. In a recent consensus study, complete agreement was not achieved among the expert panel as to what the best endpoints for validating a risk stratification tool within a track-and-trigger system would be [34]. Clinical outcomes generally considered to be the best possible choices, and also commonly used, are unexpected deaths, cardiac arrests and unplanned ICU admission. In one pilot study an audit tool of patient-centered outcomes for evaluating and benchmarking RRS performances has further been suggested [35]. Mortality can be easily assessed but the time to follow-up should be taken into account. How long of a follow-up is adequate? ICU mortality or even hospital mortality may not be the most useful measures of the success of a treatment as they are influenced by local admission and discharge policies. Cardiac arrests are also commonly used due to their dichotomous nature but the form of registration needs to be considered. Are there reliable accounts of the number of cardiac arrests in the hospital? Cardiac arrests occurring in high-surveillance areas such as ICUs, operating rooms and emergency departments should not be included as these patient populations are not the focus of RRSs. Again, limitations to escalate care must clearly be stated as this could influence a change in the number of unexpected deaths/cardiac arrests. It is becoming apparent that part of the RRS activities include discussions of care at the end of life and whether patients would benefit from cardiopulmonary resuscitation or not [36–38]. A limitation of medical treatment can be present before the call or decided during the call, in which case it is recorded with ease. However, a discussion initiated during the call could actually trigger a decision being made at any point thereafter. It can also be reconsidered and changed several times during a patient's stay depending on the clinical conditions.

Conclusion

The process of implementing and upholding a functioning RRS is clearly a multidimensional web of events and to make an assessment of it the process needs to be defined down to its separate elements and viewed accordingly. Three phases can be discerned: pre-implementation, implementation, and evaluation.

Proper preparation is fundamental for successful implementation. It must be decided which type of RRS is suitable for a particular institution and valid calling criteria chosen. Education and information for the entire hospital includes distributing written materials as well as repeated sessions with staff where questions and concerns can be addressed directly. Baseline information needs to be collected in order to be able to later assess effects of the intervention.

The implementation is performed and data collection standardized, for which there are comprehensive recommendations to aid in the setting up of useful information gathering [21]. A good database format from the start is key for future research. Standardization will provide us with a common nomenclature and enable easier comparisons between different centers over the world.

Evaluation and reevaluation is important for understanding the process and for being able to amend it if necessary. Questionnaires can be used to assess staff satisfaction. Feedback from clinicians and nursing staff is reviewed and answered as soon as possible. Continuous education is important considering staff turnover. The educational part of the RRS is probably the most crucial part of success and as such needs to be a never-ending process.

References

1. Hillman K, Parr M, Flabouris A, Bishop G, Stewart A. Redefining in-hospital resuscitation: the concept of the medical emergency team. Resuscitation. 2001;48: 105–10.
2. Hillman K, Chen J, May E. Complex intensive care unit interventions. Crit Care Med. 2009;37:S102–6.
3. Bagshaw SM, Bellomo R. The need to reform our assessment of evidence from clinical trials: a commentary. Philos Ethics Humanit Med. 2008;3:23.
4. Hillman K, Chen J, Cretikos M, Bellomo R, Brown D, Doig G, Finfer S, Flabouris A. Introduction of the medical emergency team (MET) system: a cluster-randomised controlled trial. Lancet. 2005;365: 2091–7.
5. Chan PS, Jain R, Nallmothu BK, Berg RA, Sasson C. Rapid response teams: a systematic review and meta-analysis. Arch Intern Med. 2010;170:18–26.
6. Cretikos MA, Chen J, Hillman KM, Bellomo R, Finfer SR, Flabouris A. The effectiveness of implementation of the medical emergency team (MET) system and factors associated with use during the MERIT study. Crit Care Resusc. 2007;9:206–12.
7. Chen J, Bellomo R, Flabouris A, Hillman K, Finfer S. The relationship between early emergency team calls and serious adverse events. Crit Care Med. 2009;37:148–53.
8. Buist MD, Moore GE, Bernard SA, Waxman BP, Anderson JN, Nguyen TV. Effects of a medical emergency team on reduction of incidence of and mortality from unexpected cardiac arrests in hospital: preliminary study. BMJ. 2002;324:387–90.
9. Bellomo R, Goldsmith D, Uchino S, Buckmaster J, Hart GK, Opdam H, Silvester W, Doolan L, Gutteridge G. A prospective before-and-after trial of a medical emergency team. Med J Aust. 2003;179:283–7.
10. Bellomo R, Goldsmith D, Uchino S, Buckmaster J, Hart G, Opdam H, Silvester W, Doolan L, Gutteridge G. Prospective controlled trial of effect of medical emergency team on postoperative morbidity and mortality rates. Crit Care Med. 2004;32:916–21.
11. Priestley G, Watson W, Rashidian A, Mozley C, Russell D, Wilson J, Cope J, Hart D, Kay D, Cowley K, Pateraki J. Introducing critical care outreach: a ward-randomised trial of phased introduction in a general hospital. Intensive Care Med. 2004;30:1398–404.
12. DeVita MA, Braithwaite RS, Mahidhara R, Stuart S, Foraida M, Simmons RL. Use of medical emergency team responses to reduce hospital cardiopulmonary arrests. Qual Saf Health Care. 2004;13:251–4.
13. Konrad D, Jäderling G, Bell M, Granath F, Ekbom A, Martling C. Reducing in-hospital cardiac arrests and hospital mortality by introducing a medical emergency team. Intensive Care Med. 2010;36:100–6.
14. Winters BD, Pham JC, Hunt EA, Guallar E, Berenholtz S, Pronovost PJ. Rapid response systems: a systematic review. Crit Care Med. 2007;35:1238–43.
15. Winters BD, Weaver SJ, Pfoh ER, Yang T, Pham JC, Dy SM. Rapid-response systems as a patient safety strategy: a systematic review. Ann Intern Med. 2013;158:417–25.
16. Bellomo R, Bagshaw SM. Evidence-based medicine: classifying the evidence from clinical trials—the need to consider other dimensions. Crit Care. 2006;10:232.
17. Bell MB, Konrad D, Granath F, Ekbom A, Martling CR. Prevalence and sensitivity of MET-criteria in a Scandinavian University Hospital. Resuscitation. 2006;70:66–73.
18. Devita MA, Bellomo R, Hillman K, Kellum J, Rotondi A, Teres D, Auerbach A, Chen WJ, Duncan K, Kenward G, Bell M, Buist M, Chen J, Bion J, Kirby A, Lighthall G, Ovreveit J, Braithwaite RS, Gosbee J, Milbrandt E, Peberdy M, Savitz L, Young L, Harvey M, Galhotra S. Findings of the first consensus conference on medical emergency teams. Crit Care Med. 2006;34:2463–78.
19. Delaney A, Angus DC, Bellomo R, Cameron P, Cooper DJ, Finfer S, Harrison DA, Huang DT, Myburgh JA, Peake SL, Reade MC, Webb SA, Yealy DM. Bench-to-bedside review: the evaluation of complex interventions in critical care. Crit Care. 2008;12:210.
20. Cretikos M, Parr M, Hillman K, Bishop G, Brown D, Daffurn K, Dinh H, Francis N, Heath T, Hill G, Murphy J, Sanchez D, Santiano N, Young L. Guidelines for the uniform reporting of data for medical emergency teams. Resuscitation. 2006;68:11–25.
21. Peberdy MA, Cretikos M, Abella BS, De Vita M, Goldhill D, Kloeck W, Kronick SL, Morrison LJ, Nadkarni VM, Nichol G, Nolan JP, Parr M, Tibballs J, van der Jagt EW, Young L. Recommended guidelines for monitoring, reporting, and conducting research on medical emergency team, outreach, and rapid response systems: an Utstein-style scientific statement: a scientific statement from the international liaison committee on resuscitation (American Heart Association, Australian Resuscitation Council, European Resuscitation Council, Heart and Stroke Foundation of Canada, InterAmerican Heart Foundation, Resuscitation Council of Southern Africa, and the New Zealand Resuscitation Council); the American Heart Association emergency cardiovascular care committee; the council on cardiopulmonary, perioperative, and critical care; and the interdisciplinary working group on quality of care and outcomes research. Circulation. 2007;116:2481–500.
22. Jones D, Baldwin I, McIntyre T, Story D, Mercer I, Miglic A, Goldsmith D, Bellomo R. Nurses' attitudes to a medical emergency team service in a teaching hospital. Qual Saf Health Care. 2006;15:427–32.
23. Bagshaw SM, Mondor EE, Scouten C, Montgomery C, Slater-Maclean L, Jones DA, Bellomo R, Gibney RT. A survey of nurses' beliefs about the medical emergency team system in a Canadian Tertiary Hospital. Am J Crit Care. 2009;19(1):74–83.
24. Hravnak M, Edwards L, Clontz A, Valenta C, Devita MA, Pinsky MR. Defining the incidence of cardiorespiratory instability in patients in step-down units using an electronic integrated monitoring system. Arch Intern Med. 2008;168:1300–8.

25. Bellomo R, Ackerman M, Bailey M, Beale R, Clancy G, Danesh V, Hvarfner A, Jimenez E, Konrad D, Lecardo M, Pattee KS, Ritchie J, Sherman K, Tangkau P. A controlled trial of electronic automated advisory vital signs monitoring in general hospital wards*. Crit Care Med. 2012;40:2349–61.

26. Calzavacca P, Licari E, Tee A, Egi M, Downey A, Quach J, Haase-Fielitz A, Haase M, Bellomo R. The impact of rapid response system on delayed emergency team activation patient characteristics and outcomes-a follow-up study. Resuscitation. 2009;81(1):31–5.

27. Quach JL, Downey AW, Haase M, Haase-Fielitz A, Jones D, Bellomo R. Characteristics and outcomes of patients receiving a medical emergency team review for respiratory distress or hypotension. J Crit Care. 2008;23:325–31.

28. DeVita MA, Schaefer J, Lutz J, Wang H, Dongilli T. Improving medical emergency team (MET) performance using a novel curriculum and a computerized human patient simulator. Qual Saf Health Care. 2005;14:326–31.

29. Wallin CJ, Meurling L, Hedman L, Hedegard J, Fellander-Tsai L. Target-focused medical emergency team training using a human patient simulator: effects on behaviour and attitude. Med Educ. 2007;41:173–80.

30. Jones D, Bellomo R, Bates S, Warrillow S, Goldsmith D, Hart G, Opdam H, Gutteridge G. Long term effect of a medical emergency team on cardiac arrests in a teaching hospital. Crit Care. 2005;9:R808–15.

31. Jones D, Bellomo R, DeVita MA. Effectiveness of the medical emergency team: the importance of dose. Crit Care. 2009;13:313.

32. Nathens AB, Jurkovich GJ, Cummings P, Rivara FP, Maier RV. The effect of organized systems of trauma care on motor vehicle crash mortality. JAMA. 2000;283:1990–4.

33. Jones D, Bates S, Warrillow S, Goldsmith D, Kattula A, Way M, Gutteridge G, Buckmaster J, Bellomo R. Effect of an education programme on the utilization of a medical emergency team in a teaching hospital. Intern Med J. 2006;36:231–6.

34. Pedersen NE, Oestergaard D, Lippert A. End points for validating early warning scores in the context of rapid response systems: a Delphi consensus study. Acta Anaesthesiol Scand. 2015;60(5):616–22.

35. Morris A, Owen HM, Jones K, Hartin J, Welch J, Subbe CP. Objective patient-related outcomes of rapid-response systems—a pilot study to demonstrate feasibility in two hospitals. Crit Care Resusc. 2013;15:33–9.

36. Chen J, Flabouris A, Bellomo R, Hillman K, Finfer S. The medical emergency team system and not-for-resuscitation orders: results from the MERIT study. Resuscitation. 2008;79:391–7.

37. Jones DA, Bagshaw SM, Barrett J, Bellomo R, Bhatia G, Bucknall TK, Casamento AJ, Duke GJ, Gibney N, Hart GK, Hillman KM, Jaderling G, Parmar A, Parr MJ. The role of the medical emergency team in end-of-life care: a multicenter, prospective, observational study*. Crit Care Med. 2012;40:98–103.

38. Jaderling G, Bell M, Martling CR, Ekbom A, Konrad D. Limitations of medical treatment among patients attended by the rapid response team. Acta Anaesthesiol Scand. 2013;57:1268–74.

The Impact of Rapid Response Systems on Not-For-Resuscitation (NFR) Orders

Arthas Flabouris and Jack Chen

Background

Rapid response teams (RRT) evolved as a system based approach for the recognition of, and response to, the acutely ill hospital inpatient. They evolved following revelations that hospital inpatients who suffer adverse events such as a cardiac arrest or unanticipated admission to an intensive care unit (ICU) had documented physiological abnormalities prior to these events [1–10], had an inadequate or no escalation response to these physiological abnormalities [4] when a timely escalation of care may have been beneficial [11].

Formal hospital policies relating to orders of not-for-resuscitation (NFR) were first published in the mid-1970s [12, 13]. Interestingly, these policies were preceded by a period of less formal application of the withholding of cardiopulmonary resuscitation from patients by staff who would deem it to be of no benefit to certain patients [14]. Such decision making was occurring in isolation to the patient and their wishes.

At that same time, a strong ethical framework was evolving that was promoting aspects of patient autonomy. Unilateral decision making was being less supported in favour of decisions that involved a multidisciplinary input, the wishes and values of the patient or, in the absence of a competent patient, their surrogate. Guidelines for the process of generating formal NFR orders were developed so as to increase competent patient participation in the decision making process. Formal NFR orders increased patient participation in such decision making and so reduced the likelihood of terminally ill patients receiving inappropriate resuscitation measures, improved quality of life at the terminal stages and bereavement adjustment [15–17].

Not for resuscitation orders set out the patient's, or their surrogates', expressed wishes of what should be done in the event of a cardiac or respiratory arrest. They are not meant to affect other aspects of care [18]. However there is variability and uncertainty in the way clinicians interpret NFR orders, what they understood them to mean in respect to appropriateness of a wide variety of other treatment options [19, 20], as well as to how well they document their indication, discussions associated with them as well as the level of medical seniority involved [21].

A. Flabouris (✉)
Intensive Care Unit, Royal Adelaide Hospital and
Faculty of Health Sciences, School of Medicine,
University of Adelaide, North Tce, Adelaide, South
Australia 5001, Australia
e-mail: Arthas.Flabouris@health.sa.gov.au

J. Chen
Simpson Centre for Health Services Research, South
Western Sydney Clinical School, University of New
South Wales, Level 1, AGSM Building, Sydney, New
South Wales, Australia
e-mail: jackchen@unsw.edu.au

Not-For-Resuscitation Decision Making

The current hospital inpatient population is older and more likely to have chronic disease and significant comorbidities. Whereas in the past death was relatively sudden, being in a younger group and usually from serious infection, trauma or obstetric related, nowadays death is associated with gradual deterioration of a chronic illness. This course may be predictable for certain conditions and demonstrate typical physiological disturbances as death approaches [22]. It may also be precipitated by acute deterioration associated by acquiring an acute and unrelated illness (e.g., sepsis and septic shock due to a respiratory infection in a patient with severe congestive cardiac failure).

Among Australian acute hospital inpatient deaths, 90% have a preceded NFR order [23, 24] and this rate differs significantly from that of other countries. In comparison, 79% of hospital deaths in the USA [25] and approximately 50–60% among a group of European countries, which varied from 73% in Switzerland to 16% in Italy [26].

Studies that have revealed highly variable patterns of NFR decision making, have also explored factors behind this variability. Factors such as patient's age [27, 28], gender [29], diagnosis [30, 31], physician specialty [32, 33] and the investment they feel they may have had in the patient's care [34, 35], physician's confidence in discussing [36] and explaining [37] resuscitation orders with patients and their surrogates, hospital characteristics [38], and family personal or religious reasons [34, 35] have all been shown to contribute to this variability. The prescription of NFR orders often occurs in conflict to patients prior expressed wishes [32], and to documented patient advanced directives [39].

Similarly, as the majority of day-to-day care of the patient is undertaken and supported, often distant to senior consultant physicians, by junior medical staff and nursing staff who are often under-resourced, poorly trained for and disempowered to make significant decisions, such as initiating discussions relating to patient treatment choices [40].

Even when a commitment to initiate end of life discussions has been made by the patient's admitting team there are other impediments to timely NFR orders such as insufficient time to have such discussions, acute or unexpected patient deterioration, actively treating the patient for a reversible condition and not knowing the patient well enough [34, 35, 41].

In contrast, critical care physicians have been shown to contribute more positively towards the process of end of life decision making. This may be because such decisions are occurring more commonly within the ICU environment [42], and such patients are more likely to die with an NFR order, have a shorter ICU length of stay and fewer interventions [43].

Rapid Response Teams and Not-For-Resuscitation Orders

These circumstances described above are not dissimilar to the antecedents for rapid response teams. For example the latter evolved from a failure of a hospital wide systematic approach to potentially preventable cardiac arrests and unanticipated ICU admissions. The factors that contributed to such failures included increasing medical specialization, ageing patient population with more comorbidities and the reliance on junior medical staff who are often ill equipped and trained in the recognition and management of an acutely ill patient [44, 45].

A program based upon identifying hospital inpatents for whom advanced care planning could be initiated, training of staff to recognize, respond to, and facilitate end of life discussions, documentation, and supportive clinical care has been developed with the expressed intention of improving patient end of life treatment option documentation, reducing risk of unnecessary aggressive medical care, and increasing the likelihood of attaining the patients expressed wishes for end of life care [46].

As intended RRT are called to attend acutely ill patients, based upon criteria that reflect acute physiological disturbance and thus expose the patient to increased risk of harm or even death.

Fig. 36.1 Proportion of each event for which an NFR order was documented, at the time of that event by the MET or the cardiac arrest team

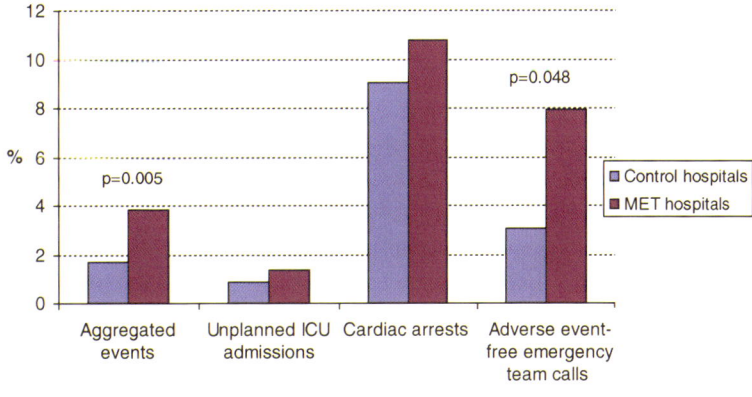

It is not improbable that some of these patients may in fact be dying, as expected, but as yet have been failed to be recognized as dying and failed to have a management plan that excludes aggressive life support measures. As RRT typically consist of critical care based staff, who are potentially better positioned to identify and manage dying patients and to withhold futile resuscitation measures, it is theoretically plausible that RRT may influence NFR ordering. In fact, observational studies have shown that an NFR order is issued at the time of an RRT call for between 4 and 25% of all calls [47–49]. Initiation of NFR orders has been recorded by many studies to occur more commonly than critical care type interventions such as endotracheal intubation, basic and advanced life support, and vasopressor/inotropic support [50].

Furthermore, the MERIT study [23] showed the rate of NFR orders issued at the time of an event was almost threefold higher within MET hospitals compared with that of the non-MET hospitals. A subsequent analysis of the MERIT study data relating to NFR orders, identified that among MET hospitals there was a significant increase in the proportion and rate of NFR orders issued for all the events combined, when compared to control hospitals. This difference was due predominately to a significantly higher number of NFR orders issued during RRT attendance not related to either a cardiac arrest or death or unplanned ICU admission. Among MET hospitals, 8% of RRT were associated with issuing an NFR order, compared to 3% of calls in the control hospitals (Fig. 36.1). In terms of overall NFR orders, MET related NFR orders are a relatively small proportion (Table 36.1).

In reality, this figure may be an underestimation, as it is possible that emergency team attendance may have prompted a subsequent consideration of an NFR order being issued post an emergency team attendance. A future exploration of such processes would be important and would require consideration of the many logistic and educational factors that appear to influence the activities and impact of RRT [51, 52].

Rapid Response Teams and Patients with PreExisting Not-For-Resuscitation Orders

The allocation of NFR orders, did not preclude a patient from having an emergency team attendance, particularly so for hospitals allocated a MET, which were three times more likely to attend to patients with a prior NFR order, than a typical cardiac arrest team. RRT calls to patients with preexisting NFR orders is a more common occurrence than calls at which NFR orders are issued by the RRT. Such patients can make up to 20–35% of all RRT calls [53–55]. It is not uncommon for patients with preexisting NFR orders to be the subject of an RRT within the 24 h prior to their death, and often out of hours or have had a prior RRT call (Table 36.2) [56, 57].

Table 36.1 Number of events per 1000 admissions during which an NFR order was issued (aggregate and by each of our event types)

Outcome	Control hospitals		MET hospitals		Weighted mean	
	Mean(SD)	Range	Mean(SD)	Range	difference (95%CI)[a]	P
Aggregated events	0.31 (0.26)	0.00–0.80	0.69 (0.51)	0.15–1.94	0.52 (0.14–0.90)	0.009**
Deaths	0.16 (0.11)	0.00–0.34	0.18 (0.11)	0.00–0.37	0.00 (−0.09–0.10)	0.969
Unplanned ICU admissions	0.06 (0.13)	0.00–0.40	0.07 (0.12)	0.00–0.37	0.02 (−0.06–0.09)	0.621
Cardiac arrests	0.16 (0.11)	0.00–0.37	0.15 (0.14)	0.00–0.46	0.01 (−0.10–0.11)	0.892
Adverse event-free emergency team calls	0.04 (0.09)	0.00–0.27	0.40 (0.42)	0.00–1.32	0.49 (0.20–0.78)	0.002**

[a]The P values were derived using the weighted t-test to compare the rates between 11 control hospitals and 12 MET hospitals;
**$P < 0.01$;

This would suggest that although there may be a proportion of patients with an NFR order for whom an RRT is either called in error or, for whom other critical care interventions are also not appropriate, but are not stipulated to be so within the existing framework for NFR orders. There are also such patients for whom it is deemed appropriate that they receive critical care type supports, other than cardiopulmonary resuscitation. This is not uncommon as not all patients with an NFR are near their end of life or die during their hospital admission. Typically, approximately 30% are discharged home [58, 59]. In a review of patients with a prior NFR order, these patients had a higher respiratory rate, lower SaO2 and were just as likely to receive a critical care type intervention (Table 36.2) [57]. They were however less likely to be admitted to an ICU and more likely to be left on the ward at the time of an RRT call. They were also more likely to be documented not for further RRT calls in comparison to patients without a prior NFR order [57].

These findings suggest that patients with existing NFR orders encounter acute physiological disturbances that require some form of intervention. This may not necessarily be an RRT attendance, but in the absence of an alternative type response, the RRT becomes the default response. In particular, there is a perception by clinicians that NFR orders lead to less care than they believe should occur. This belief may lead to doctors being less willing to fill out NFR orders, even in circumstances where they do not think CPR would be appropriate, for fear of diminishing the overall level of care that the patient receives [60].

Table 36.2 Comparison of patients with, and those without a preexisting NFR order at the time of a MET attendance

	Preexisting NFR (N=198)	No preexisting NFR (N=1060)	P Value
Age (years, median, IQ)	81 (72, 87)	70 (53, 81)	<0.01
Gender (% males)	56.4%	54.3%	0.55
Cardiac arrest call	9 (4.5%)	134 (12.6%)	<0.01
Time of MET (hrs, median, IQ)	11:00 (7:23, 16:42)	12:50 (7:55, 18:20)	0.06
Scene time (mins, median, IQ)	17 (6, 33)	20 (10, 35)	0.02
Pulse on arrival (median, IQ)	99 (79, 125)	99 (78, 124)	0.96
Respiratory rate on arrival (median, IQ)	24 (18, 30)	20 (16, 26)	<0.01
SBP on arrival (mmHg) (median, IQ)	117 (91, 145)	120 (90, 148)	0.53
SaO2 on arrival (median, IQ)	93 (85, 97)	97 (93, 99)	<0.01
Arrival GCS = 15	41 (24.3%)	479 (51.7%)	<0.01

Rapid Response Teams and Orders Other than Not-For-Resuscitation

With the demise of the conventional cardiac arrest team and in this new era of an RRT, evidence is emerging that there may be a need for specific orders in hospitals with RRT relating to the appropriateness or not of the attendance of RRT, and if so, the desirable level of RRT intervention, e.g., a "not for RRT" order or a "modified RRT" order.

In one observational study, RRTs, in comparison to admitting teams, were less likely to document a NFR (64.6% vs 98.6% of all orders, $p < 0.01$) or an NFICU (37.5% vs 82.0% of all orders, $p < 0.01$) order, but more likely to document a NF RRT (64.6% vs 44.0% of all orders, $p = 0.04$) or a modified RRT (8.3% vs 0% of all orders, $p = 0.04$) order [21]. Such a process would require either modification to existing NFR discussions and documentation processes or development of a separate parallel process. These are important considerations as RRT are becoming increasingly prevalent and active and information related to RRT becomes more public as it spreads beyond medical media and to the broader media.

In light of this high variability of NFR orders and the many factors identified as contributing to this variability, it would be expected that the introduction of an RRT would have a differential impact upon each environment into which it is introduced. It also highlights the importance of the need for generic and uniform international guidelines for the issuing of not just, NFR orders, but also those associated with RRT activity such as not for RRT or modified RRT orders. In particular as calls to patients with existing NFR orders who are close to their time of death are not uncommon [50, 56], and for whom an emergency response team, equipped with the critical care resources and skills to prevent unexpected adverse events has commonly become, in the absence of an alternative, the default response to such patients.

Rapid Response Teams and Palliative Type Care

In essence, RRT appear to not only identify and respond promptly to acutely ill patients with the purpose of preventing progression to more serious event (e.g., cardiac arrest, ICU admission), but also identify and respond to patients with RRT calling criteria that may be dying, with the purpose of preventing progression to another type of serious event (e.g., inappropriate resuscitation during the end stage of life). With the former patient, acute resuscitation measures are indicated and associated with improved patient outcomes, while with the latter, patient specific

palliative care services and/or management are indicated. Wether earlier identification of patients for whom palliative type of end of life care is indicated by RRT results in better outcome (e.g., improved quality of life) for such patients has not been explored. Theoretically that may be a possibility as RRT attendance may result in avoidance of unnecessary aggressive life support measures and earlier palliative care referral, factors that have been associated with improved quality of life [17, 61].

The question of wether the RRT should respond to patients with preexisting NFR orders is an increasingly important one as future RRT activity is likely to continue to escalate as RRT uptake continues to grow [62] and new measures are introduced to assist in identifying the deteriorating patient [63]. It also raises the issue of RRT training, as currently RRT members are trained to deliver basic and advanced life support, but less likely to be given the skills to manage end of life decision making and care. Table 36.3 outlines the potential advantages, disadvantages, and potential alternatives in response to this question.

Among the participating hospitals within the MERIT study, there was a wide extent of variability in the issuing of NFR orders. Factors such as teaching hospital status, location (urban vs. metropolitan), hospital size (number of beds), and MET allocation could only account for <50% of the variance in such orders [23]. This would suggest that it is important that each hospital examine how best their RRT can serve to identify and respond to patients with end of life needs, and possible alternative responses.

Summary Points

- There are similarities between the health system factors that contribute to variability and weaknesses in the application of NFR orders to hospital inpatients and those that form the basis of the evolution of RRT.
- There is theoretical plausibility for RRT to influence the issuing of NFR orders, supported by evidence from a large cluster randomized trial that following the introduction of a MET, and in comparison to conventional cardiac

Table 36.3 Patients with pre-existing NFR orders: Pros and Cons of Rapid Response Team attendance and possible alternatives

Pros of RRT attendance for patients with preexisting NFR orders	Cons of RRT attendance for patients with preexisting NFR orders	Possible alternatives
Timely response	Adds to escalating RRT workload and potentially diverts RRT from other deteriorating patients Creates a negative attitude towards RRT activity Fatigue and stress among RRT members Exposes RRT and ward staff to potential conflict and negative perceptions of each other RRT members not trained for palliative care medicine	"Acute" palliative care teams Identifying positives of RRT response or defining an expected scope of RRT practice for such patients RRT and ward staff debrief and counselling. Support by senior clinicians
Improved administration of palliative care during episodes of acute physiological disruption Support ward nursing and junior medical staff with end of life care decisions	Patient less likely to participate in treatment choices associated with reduced suffering because of acute deterioration	Early palliative care referral with predetermined management plans in the event of acute deterioration Training of ward nursing and junior medical staff to have the skills and confidence to deal with end of life care decisions Greater senior medical support with end of life care decisions
Patient not subjected to discomfort of critical care type therapies (including basic and advance life support) that are not likely to benefit them or ICU admission	Patient are subjected to the discomfort of critical care type therapies (including basic and advance life support) that are not likely to benefit them as the patient and their wishes may be unknown to the RRT	Early palliative care referral with predetermined management plans in the event of acute deterioration Training of RRT in end of life care
Precipitates discussions in respect to orders broader than that of NFR, e.g., "not for RRT" and avoids risk of subsequent RRT attendance and intervention	RRT unfamiliar to the patient and family, usually after hours and during an acute period of reduced patient interaction are negotiating "not for RRT, modified RRT" and other limitations beyond that of existing NFR order	Educate admitting teams to consider expanding, where appropriate, end of life care discussions to include aspects of "not for RRT, modified RRT"

arrest teams, more NFR orders were issued at the time of a MET call.

- RRT activity may be associated with other hospital system changes that could potentially further influence the issuing of NFR orders as well as the type of orders (not for RRT, modified RRT, etc.) being issued.
- Observational studies have revealed that up to 24% of all RRT calls involve the issuing of NFR orders.
- Observational studies have also revealed that up to 35% of all RRT calls involve patients with preexisting NFR orders, often within 24 h of their time of death.
- There is the potential of patient benefit for a closer association between critical care based RRT and palliative care services.

- The future role of RRT in end of life decisions and care would need to be continually evaluated as RRT activity continues to increase and hospital wide strategies to better identify and manage patients at their end of life evolve.

References

1. Schein RMH, Hazday N, Pena M, et al. Clinical antecedents to in hospital cardiopulmonary arrest. Chest. 1990;98:1388–92.
2. Franklin C, Mathew J. Developing strategies to prevent in hospital cardiac arrest: analysing responses of physicians and nurses in the hours before the event. Crit Care Med. 1994;22:246–7.
3. Smith A, Wood J. Can some in-hospital cardio-respiratory arrest be prevented? Resuscitation. 1998; 37:133–7.

4. McQuillan P, Pilkington S, Alan A, et al. Confidential inquiry into quality of care before admission to intensive care. BMJ. 1998;316:1853–8.

5. Goldhill DR, White SA, Sumner A. Physiological values and procedures in the 24 h before ICU admission from the ward. Anaesthesia. 1999;54:529–34.

6. McGloin H, Adam SK, Singer M. Unexpected deaths and referrals to intensive care units of patients on general wards. Are some cases potentially avoidable? J R Coll Physicians Lond. 1999;33:255–9.

7. Hillman KM, Bristow PJ, Chey T, et al. Antecedents to hospital deaths. Intern Med J. 2001;31:343–8.

8. Hillman KM, Bristow PJ, Chey T, et al. Duration of life-threatening antecedents prior to intensive care admission. Intensive Care Med. 2002;28:1629–34.

9. Hodgetts TJ, Kenward G, Vlackonikolis I, et al. Incidence, location and reasons for avoidable in-hospital cardiac arrest in a district general hospital. Resuscitation. 2002;54:115–23.

10. Kause J, Smith G, Prytherch D, Parr M, Flabouris A, Hillman K, and for the Intensive Care Society (UK) & Australian and New Zealand Intensive Care Society Clinical Trials Group ACADEMIA Study investigators. A comparison of Antecedents to Cardiac Arrests, Deaths and EMergency Intensive care Admissions in Australia and New Zealand, and the United Kingdom—the ACADEMIA study. Resuscitation. 2004;62:275–82

11. Rivers E, Nguyen B, Havstad S, et al for the Early Goal-Directed Therapy Collaborative Group. Early goal-directed therapy. N Engl J Med. 2001;345(19):1368–77

12. Clinical Care Committee of the Massachusetts General Hospital. Optimum care for hopelessly ill patients: A report of the Clinical Care Committee of the Massachusetts General Hospital. N Engl J Med. 1976;295:362–4.

13. Rabkin MT, Gillerman G, Rice NR. Orders not to resuscitate. N Engl J Med. 1976;295:364–6.

14. Burns JP, Edwards J, Johnson J, Cassem NH. Do-not-resuscitate order after 25 years. Crit Care Med. 2003;31:1543–50.

15. Fukaura A, Tazawa H, Nakajima H, et al. Do not resuscitate orders at a teaching hospital in Japan. N Engl J Med. 1995;333:805–8.

16. Stern SG, Orlowski JP. DNR or CPR—the choice is ours. Crit Care Med. 1992;20:1263–72.

17. Wright AA, Baohui Z, Ray A, et al. Associations between end-of-life discussions, patient mental health, medical care near death, and caregiver bereavement adjustment. JAMA. 2008;300(14):1665–73.

18. Decisions relating to cardiopulmonary resuscitation. A joint statement from the British Medical Association, the Resuscitation Council (UK) and the Royal College of Nursing 2007.

19. Uhlmann RF, Cassel CK, McDonald WJ. Some treatment withholding implications of no code orders in an academic hospital. Crit Care Med. 1984;12:879–81.

20. LaPuma J, Silverstein MD, Stocking CB, Roland D, Siegler M. Life sustaining treatment. A prospective study of patients with DNR orders in a teaching hospital. Arch Intern Med. 1988;148:2193–8.

21. Sundararajan K, Flabouris A, Keeshan A, Cramey T. Documentation of limitation of medical therapy at the time of a Rapid Response Team call. Aust Health Rev. 2014;38:218–22.

22. Murray SA, Kendall M, Boyd K, Sheikh A. Illness trajectories and palliative care. BMJ. 2005;330:1007–11.

23. The MERIT Study Investigators. Introduction of medical emergency team (MET) system—a cluster-randomised controlled trial. Lancet. 2005;365:2091–7.

24. Jones DA, McIntyre T, Baldwin I, Mercer I, Kattula A, Bellomo R. The medical emergency team and end-of-life care: a pilot study. Crit Care Resusc. 2007;9:151–6.

25. The Support Principal Investigators. A controlled trial to improve care for seriously ill hospitalized patients. JAMA. 1995;274:1591–8.

26. van Delden JJ, Lofmark R, Deliens L, et al. Do-not-resuscitate decisions in six European countries. Crit Care Med. 2006;34:1686–90.

27. Bedell SE, Pelle D, Maher PL, et al. Do-not-resuscitate orders for critically ill patients in the hospital. How are they used and what is their impact? JAMA. 1986;256:233–7.

28. Youngner SJ, Lewandowski W, McClish DK, et al. 'Do not resuscitate' orders: incidence and implications in a medical-intensive care unit. JAMA. 1985;253:54–7.

29. Stolman CJ, Gregory JJ, Dunn D, et al. Evaluation of the do not resuscitate orders at a community hospital. Arch Intern Med. 1989;149:1851–6.

30. Schwartz DA, Reilly P. The choice not to be resuscitated. J Am Geriatr Soc. 1986;34:807–11.

31. Wachter RM, Luce JM, Hearst N, et al. Decisions about resuscitation: inequities among patients with different diseases but similar prognoses. Ann Intern Med. 1989;111:525–32.

32. Hofmann JC, Wenger NS, Davis RB, et al. Patient preferences for communication with physicians about end-of-life decisions. SUPPORT investigators. Study to understand prognoses and preference for outcomes and risks of treatment. Ann Intern Med. 1997;127:1–12.

33. Murphy BF. What has happened to clinical leadership in futile care discussions? Med J Aust. 2008;188:418–9.

34. Kuiper MA. Dying: domain of critical care medicine? Crit Care Med. 2012;40:316–7.

35. Bouley G. The rapid response team nurse's role in end of life discussions during critical situations. Dimens Crit Care Nurs. 2011;30:321–5.

36. Sulmasy DP, Sood JR, Ury WA. Physicians' confidence in discussing do not resuscitate orders with patients and surrogates. J Med Ethics. 2008;34:96–101.

37. Lynn J, Teno JM, Phillips RS, et al. Perceptions by family members of the dying experience of older and seriously ill patients. SUPPORT Investigators. Study to understand prognoses and preferences for outcomes and risks of treatments. Ann Intern Med. 1997;126:97–106.

38. Sidhu NS, Dunkley ME, Egan MJ. "Not-for-resuscitation" orders in Australian public hospitals: policies, standardised order forms and patient information leaflets. Med J Aust. 2007;186:72–5.

39. Morrell ED, Brown BP, Qi R, Drabiak K, Helft PR. The do-not-resuscitate order: associations with advance directives, physician specialty and documentation of discussion 15 years after Patient Self-Determination Act. J Med Ethics. 2008;34:642–7.

40. Tulsky JA, Chesney MA, Lo B. See one, do one, teach one? House staff experience discussing do-not-resuscitate orders. Arch Intern Med. 1996;156:1285–9.

41. Micallef S, Skrifvars MB, Parr MJ. Level of agreement on resuscitation decisions among hospital specialists and barriers to documenting do not attempt resuscitation (DNAR) orders in ward patients. Resuscitation. 2011;82:815–8.

42. Prendergast TJ, Luce JM. Increasing incidence of withholding and withdrawal of life support from the critically ill. Am J Respir Crit Care Med. 1997;155:15–20.

43. Kollef MH, Ward S. The influence of access to a private attending physician on the withdrawal of life-sustaining therapies in the intensive care unit. Crit Care Med. 1999;27:2125–32.

44. Hillman K, Flabouris A, Parr M. A hospital-wide system for managing the seriously ill: a model of applied health systems research. In: Sibbald WJ, Bion JF, editors. Update in intensive care and emergency medicine, Vol 35-Evaluating critical care, using health services research to improve outcome. Berlin: Springer; 2000.

45. Lam S, Flabouris A. Medical trainees and public safety. In: DeVita MA, Hillman K, Bellomo R, editors. Medical emergency teams, implementation and outcome measurement. 2006, ISBN: 0-387-27920-2

46. Austin Health, Respecting Patient Choices. http://www.respectingpatientchoices.org.au/. Accessed Dec 2008.

47. Parr MJ, Hadfield JH, Flabouris A, Bishop G, Hillman K. The Medical Emergency Team: 12 month analysis of reasons for activation, immediate outcome and not-for-resuscitation orders. Resuscitation. 2001;50(1):39–44.

48. Kenward G, Castle N, Hodgetts T, et al. Evaluation of a medical emergency team one year after implementation. Resuscitation. 2004;61(3):257–63.

49. Buist MD, Moore GE, Bernard SA, Waxman BP, Anderson JN, Nguyen TV. Effects of a medical emergency team on reduction of incidence of and mortality from unexpected cardiac arrests in hospital: preliminary study. BMJ. 2002;324:387–90.

50. Tan LH, Delaney A. Medical emergency teams and end-of-life care: a systematic review. Crit Care Resusc. 2014;16:62–8.

51. Cretikos MA, Chen J, Hillman KM, Bellomo R, Finfer SR, Flabouris A. The effectiveness of implementation of the medical emergency team (MET) system and factors associated with use during the MERIT study. Crit Care Resusc. 2007;9(2):206–12.

52. Buist M, Bellomo R. The medical emergency team or the medical education team. Crit Care Resusc. 2004;6:88–91.

53. Jaderling G, Calzavacca P, Bell M, et al. The deteriorating ward patient: a Swedish—Australian comparison. Intensive Care Med. 2011;37:1000–5.

54. Calzavacca P, Licari E, Tee A, et al. Features and outcome of patients receiving multiple medical emergency team reviews. Resuscitation. 2010;81:1509–15.

55. Casamento AJ, Dunlop C, Jones DA, Duke G. Improving the documentation of medical emergency team reviews. Crit Care Resusc. 2008;10:24–9.

56. Jones DA, Bagshaw SM, Barrett J, et al. The role of the medical emergency team in end-of-life care: a multicenter, prospective, observational study. Crit Care Med. 2012;40:98–103.

57. Coventry C, Flabouris A, Sundararajan K, Cramey T. Rapid response team calls to patients with a pre-existing not for resuscitation order. Resuscitation. 2013;84:1035–9.

58. Downar J, Rodin D, Barua R, Lejnieks B, Gudimella R, McCredie V, Hayes C, Steel A. Rapid response teams, do not resuscitate orders, and potential opportunities to improve end-of-life care: a multicentre retrospective study. J Crit Care. 2013;28:498–503.

59. Chen J, Flabouris A, Bellomo R, Hillman K, Finfer S, The MERIT Study Investigators. The medical emergency team system and not-for-resuscitation orders: results from the MERIT Study. Resuscitation. 2008;79:391–7.

60. Fritza Z, Fulda J, Haydocka S, Palmer C. Interpretation and intent: a study of the (mis)understanding of DNAR orders in a teaching hospital. Resuscitation. 2010;81:1138–41.

61. Temel JS, Greer JA, Muzikansky A, et al. Early palliative care for patients with metastatic non-small-cell lung cancer. N Engl J Med. 2010;363(8):733–42.

62. Chen J, Ou L, Hillman KM, Flabouris A, Bellomo R, Hollis SJ, Assareh H. Cardiopulmonary arrest and mortality trends, and their association with rapid response system expansion. Med J Aust. 2014;201:167–70.

63. Kansal A, Havill K. The effects of introduction of new observation charts and calling criteria on call characteristics and outcome of hospitalised patients. Crit Care Resusc. 2012;14:38–43.

ERRATUM to: Dying Safely

Magnolia Cardona-Morrell and Ken Hillman

Erratum to:
Chapter 27 in: M.A. DeVita et al. (eds.), Textbook of Rapid Response Systems,
DOI 10.1007/978-3-319-39391-9_27

Chapters 27 was originally published with an incorrect figure. The chapter has been updated with the correct figure.

The updated original online version for this chapter can be found at
http://dx.doi.org/10.1007/978-3-319-39391-9_27

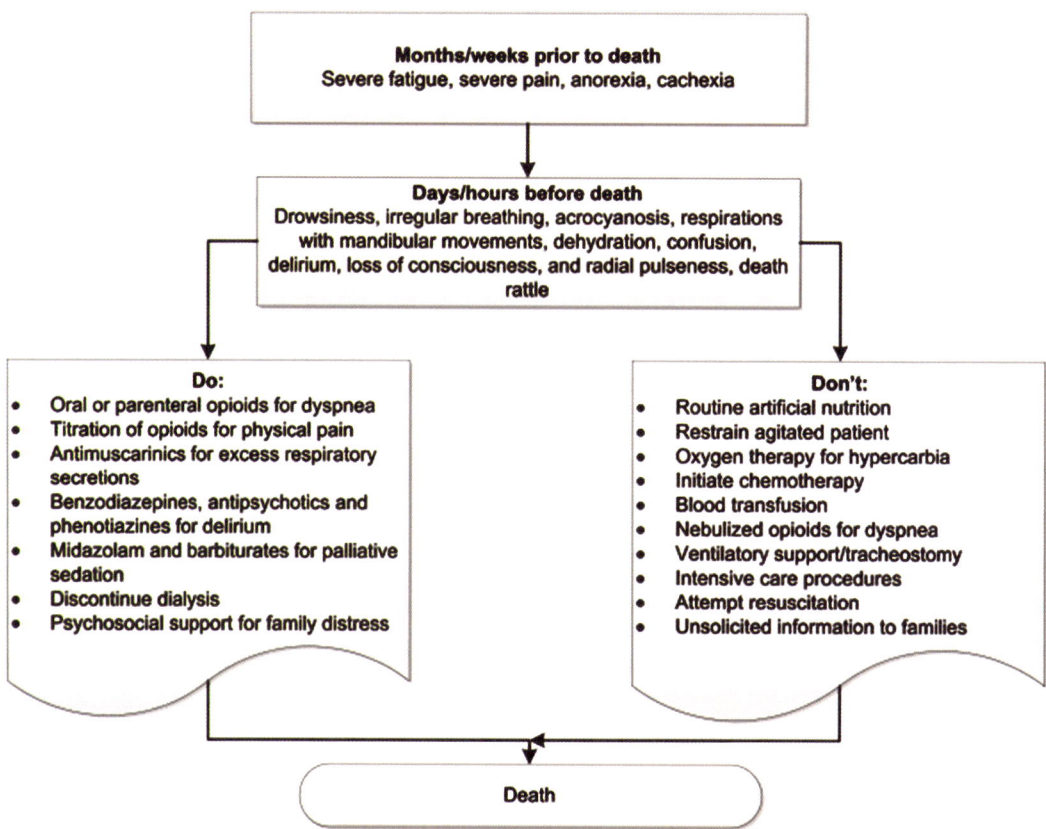

Fig. 27.1 To treat or not to treat: Journey from signs and symptoms to safe death

Index

25954898R00230

Printed in Great Britain
by Amazon